Textbook on

Medicolegal Issues

Related to Various Medical Specialties

Textbook on
Medicolegal Issues
Related to Various Medical Specialties

THIRD EDITION

Editors

Satish Tiwari
MD(Pediatrics) LLB FIAP
Professor
Department of Pediatrics
Medical College, Amravati
Maharashtra, India
Founder President
Indian Medico-Legal and Ethics Association

Mahesh Baldwa
MBBS DCH MD LLB LLM FIAP PhD(Law) MBA MA(Psy)
Founder President
Medicolegal Chapter/Group of Central Indian Academy of Pediatrics
Senior Medicolegal Advisor and Senior Consultant Pediatrician
Baldwa Hospital, Mumbai, Maharashtra, India
External Faculty Maharashtra National Law University

Mukul Tiwari
MD DCH FIAP
Consultant Pediatrician
Apex Hospital
Gwalior, Madhya Pradesh, India
Chairperson, Medicolegal Group of IAP 2015–2017
President, IMLEA 2020–2022

Alka Kuthe
MBBS DGO LLM(Criminology) and PG Diploma in Human Rights Education
Consultant Gynecologist and Medicolegal Counselor
Department of Obstetrics and Gynecology
Kuthe Accident Hospital and Maternity Nursing Home
Amravati, Maharashtra, India
Chairperson FOGSI MTP Committee 2025–2027
Chairman IMA Maharashtra Medicolegal Cell 2023, 2024
Chairman AMOGS Medicolegal Cell 2018–2020

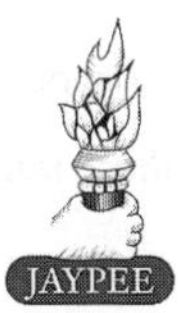

JAYPEE BROTHERS MEDICAL PUBLISHERS
The Health Sciences Publisher
New Delhi | London

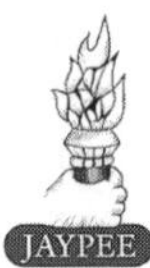

Jaypee Brothers Medical Publishers (P) Ltd

Headquarters
EMCA House, 23/23-B
Ansari Road, Daryaganj
New Delhi 110 002, India
Landline: +91-11-23272143, +91-11-23272703
+91-11-23282021, +91-11-23245672
e-mail: jaypee@jaypeebrothers.com

Corporate Office
4838/24, Ansari Road, Daryaganj
New Delhi 110 002, India
Phone: +91-11-43574357
Fax: +91-11-43574314
e-mail: jaypee@jaypeebrothers.com

Overseas Office
JP Medical Ltd.
83, Victoria Street, London
SW1H 0HW (UK)
Phone: +44-20 3170 8910
e-mail: info@jpmedpub.com

EU GPSR Authorised Representative
Logos Europe, 9 rue Nicolas Poussin
17000, La Rochelle, France
Phone: +33 (0) 6 67 93 73 78
e-mail: contact@logoseurope.eu

Website: www.jaypeebrothers.com
Website: www.jaypeedigital.com

Inquiries for bulk sales may be solicited at: jaypee@jaypeebrothers.com

Textbook on Medicolegal Issues / Satish Tiwari, Mahesh Baldwa, Mukul Tiwari, Alka Kuthe

First Edition: 2012

Third Edition: **2026**

ISBN: 978-93-5696-777-9

Printed at: Samrat Offset Pvt. Ltd.

Disclaimer

In last few years, The CPA 2019 has replaced the CPA 1986, NMC has replaced MCI, BNS/BNSS have replaced IPC/CrPC, etc. Care has been taken by the authors/contributors/editors to update the chapters as per the latest changes in the various sections. If, in some chapters the recent updates have been missed inadvertently; readers are requested to refer to the specific provisions/sections in the new laws or Acts.

Contributors

Aarti Avinash Kinikar MBBS MD DCH DNB MRCP-UK PGDHHM
Professor and Head
Department of Pediatrics
Byramjee Jeejeebhoy Government Medical College
Pune, Maharashtra, India

Abhyuday Tiwari MBBS MD(Dermatology)
Consultant Dermatologist
Department of Dermatology, Apex Hospital
Gwalior, Madhya Pradesh, India

Alka Kuthe MBBS DGO LLM(Criminology) and PG Diploma in Human Rights Education
Consultant Gynecologist and Medicolegal Counselor
Department of Obstetrics and Gynecology
Kuthe Accident Hospital and Maternity Nursing Home
Amravati, Maharashtra, India
Chairperson FOGSI MTP Committee 2025–2027
Chairman IMA Maharashtra Medicolegal Cell 2023, 2024
Chairman AMOGS Medicolegal Cell 2018–2020

Alok Gupta MBBS MD(Pediatric Medicine)
Chief of Pediatrics, Counselor and Environmentalist
Department of Pediatrics
Mansarovar Polyclinic
Jaipur, Rajasthan, India

Amitabh Shanker Saxena MBBS(AFMC) MD(Psychiatry) Dip NB(Psychiatry) PGDMLE(NLSIU) MSc(Defence and Strategic Studies) LLB
Senior Medical Officer
Department of Master Control Center
Air Force, Army College of Medical Sciences
New Delhi, India

Amit Padvi MBBS MD Fellowship in Pediatric Anesthesiology
Formerly Worked as Assistant Professor
Department of Anesthesia
Faculty Member, Department of Pediatric Anesthesia
Seth GS Medical College and KEM Hospital
Mumbai, Maharashtra, India

Amrita Mishra BAMS MS *Prasuti Tantra Stree Rog*(Obstetric and Gynecology) PhD MBA Clinical Research and Healthcare FAIMER Fellow
Associate Professor
Department of *Prasuti Tantra Stree Rog*
RA Podar Medical College (Ayurved)
Worli, Mumbai, Maharashtra, India

Anjan Bhattacharya MBBS DCH(London) MRCP(London) FRCPCH(UK)
Senior Consultant Developmental Pediatrician and Head
Child Development Center
Apollo Multispeciality Hosptal, Kolkata
Royal College Examiner for MRCP Child Health and DCH (UK) Examinations
Director, Post Graduate Diploma in Early Intervention for Neurodevelopmental Disorders (CCPTR; MAKAUT, WB)
WB University of Technology
Kolkata, West Bengal, India

Anurag Verma MBBS MD(Medicine) LLB PGDMLS LLM
Consultant Physician
Medicolegal Consultant
MIC Pvt Ltd, Apex Insurance Ltd
Vice President (North Zone) IMLEA
Member of Medicos Legal Action Group
Associate Professor
HD College of Law
Kashipur, Uttarakhand, India

Anurag Yadav MBBS DNB(Radiodiagnosis)
Co-Chairperson and Professor of Radiology
Department of Imaging
Sir Ganga Ram Hospital
New Delhi, India

Arun Gupta MBBS MD(Pediatrics)
President, Delhi Medical Council
Vice President Legal Committee, IMA
Fortis Hospital
New Delhi, India

Arun Manglik MBBS MD(Pediatrics) DNB(Pediatrics)
Pediatrician, Department of Pediatrics
Ankur Clinics, ILS Hospitals
Kolkata, West Bengal, India

Ashish Jain MBBS DCH PGCC CCIML LLB
Senior Consultant Pediatrician and
Medicolegal Advisor
Department of Pediatrics
Tulip Chest and Child Care Clinic
Gurugram, Haryana, India

Ashok Banga MBBS MD(Pediatrics)
Consultant Pediatrician
Director, Chirayu Hospital
Gwalior, Madhya Pradesh, India

Astha Khushwah MBBS DNB(Radiodiagnosis)
Resident, Department of Imaging
Sir Ganga Ram Hospital
New Delhi, India

Atul Bhargava PhD Management (Healthcare) MBA
Healthcare Service Management PGDMLS PGDCLP
PGDHHM PGDFSQM Masters in Clinical Psychology
BCBR AI and ML Certified DRDO(Pune)
Expert Committee Member
MBA Hospital Management
and Academic Counselor for PGDHHM,
PGDFSQM (IGNOU)
CICP, Auditor CSSD, Endosafe, I Comply CAHO
Auditor AORN, Consultant (MNC), IMLEA
ISQUA Fellowship
Infection Control Academy of India Professional
Member
IFCAI Professional Member

Avinash Bansal MBBS MD(Pediatrics) PGD-AP
PGDMLE DHA
Head
Department of Neonatology, Pediatrics and
Adolescent Medicine
BVP Hospital and Research Center
Kota, Rajasthan, India

Bhupendra Kumar Gupta MBBS MD(Pediatrics)
DM(Neonatology)
Consultant Neonatologist and Pediatrician
Department of Pediatric and Neonatology
Apollo Sage Hospital
Bhopal, Madhya Pradesh, India

Brij Bhushan Sahni MBBS MD(Pediatrics) FIAP
Ex-Chief Consultant Pediatrics and
Chief Medical Officer
Department of Pediatrics
Tata Main Hospital, Dhanbad
Presently Consultant Pediatrician
Dhanbad, Jharkhand, India

Chandrika Rao MBBS DCH MD(Pediatrics)
Postgraduate Diploma in Medical Law and Ethics
Professor
Department of Pediatrics
Convener Medical Education
Ramaiah Medical College and Hospitals
Bengaluru, Karnataka, India

Charu Mittal MBBS MD DNB(Obstetrics and
Gynecology)
Private Practitioner
Department of Obstetrics and Gynecology
Nidaan Hospital
Gwalior, Madhya Pradesh, India
Ex-Assistant Professor
Department of Obstetrics and Gynecology
Medical College
Baroda, Gujarat, India

CM Chhajer MBBS MD(Pediatrics)
Associate Professor
Department of Pediatrics
Geetanjali Medical College
Udaipur, Rajasthan, India

Deepshikha MBBS MD DNB(Pediatrics)
Specialist
Assistant Professor
Department of Pediatrics
Tata Main Hospital and Manipal Tata Medical College
Jamshedpur, Jharkhand, India

Deepshikha Sahu MBBS MS DNB MNAMS
Consultant and Owner of Matrika Gynec and Surgicare Center
Jabalpur, Madhya Pradesh, India
Consultant
Aditya Superspeciality Hospital and Trauma Center
Jabalpur, Madhya Pradesh, India

Devaraj V Raichur MBBS MD(Pediatrics) MBA(Hospital Administration) MA(History) LLB
Professor and Head
Department of Pediatrics
JGMM Medical College
Hubballi, Karnataka, India

Dilip Walke MBBS MD
Consultant Gynecologist
Department of Obstetrics and Gynecology
Jupiter Hospital Baner and Medipoint Hospital, Aundh
Pune, Maharashtra, India

Divyangee V Mundhe MBBS DNB(General Surgery) Fellowship in Minimal Access Surgery
Consultant
Department of General and Laparoscopic Surgery
Mundhe Patil Surgical Hospital
Parbhani, Maharashtra, India

Dnyanesh DK MBBS MD(Pediatrics) LLB
Professor and Head
Department of Pediatrics
JN Medical College
KLE Academy of Higher Education and Research Centre
Belagavi, Karnataka, India
Consultant Pediatrician
KLE'S PK Hospital
Belagavi, Karnataka, India

Gautam Biswas MBBS MD(Forensic Medicine)
Professor and Head
Department of Forensic Medicine and Toxicology
DMC and Hospital
Ludhiana, Punjab, India

Geeta Bansal MBBS MD(Pediatrics) PGD-AP MSCCFT
Director
Department of Pediatrics and Adolescents
Nishtha Shishu and Kishore Swasthya Kendra
Kota, Rajasthan, India

Girish Kumthekar MBBS MD(Obstetrics and Gynecology) LLB(Specialization) Dip Reproductive Medicine(Germany)
Consultant Obstetrician, Gynecologist, Infertility Specialist and Med-Legal Consultant
Past Associate Professor
Dr VM Government Medical College
Solapur, Maharashtra, India
Ashwini Sahakari Rugnalaya, Navjeevan Fertility and IVF Center
Solapur, Maharashtra, India

Gita Guin MBBS MS LLB FICOG
Professor
Department of Obstetrics and Gynecology
Government NSCB Medical College
Jabalpur, Madhya Pradesh, India

Gouri Gore MBBS(Mumbai) MS(Obstetrics and Gynecology) Mumbai
Consultant Gynecologist
Department of Obstetrics and Gynecology
Surya Hospital, Chembur and Zen Multispecialty Hospital
Chembur, Mumbai, India

Ira Shah MBBS MD(Pediatrics) DNB FCPS DCH(Gold Medalist) DPID(UK)
Professor and Head
Department of Pediatrics Infectious Diseases and Pediatric GI, Hepatology
BJ Wadia Hospital for Children and Nowrosjee Wadia Maternity Hospital
Mumbai, Maharashtra, India
Nodal Officer, Pediatric DR-TB (State)
Center of Excellence and Pediatric HIV/ART Center, BJ Wadia Hospital for Children and Nowrosjee Wadia Maternity Hospital
Mumbai, Maharashtra, India

Ishita Banerjee MBBS MD(Pediatrics) LLB PGDMLE
Consultant
Department of Pediatric Cardiology
Heartline Cardiac Care Center
Prayagraj, Uttar Pradesh, India

Jayesh Nareshchandra Panot MBBS DNB(Pediatrics)
Associate Professor and Deputy Medical Superintendent
Department of Pediatrics
Rajiv Gandhi Medical College and Chhatrapati Shivaji Maharaj Hospital
Thane, Maharashtra, India

JK Gupta MBBS DCH FIAP LLB LLM
Consultant Pediatrician
Yashi Child Care
Kanpur, Uttar Pradesh, India
National Chairperson Medicolegal Chapter of Indian Academy of Pediatrics 2022–2025

Jyoti Bindal MBBS MS(Obstetrics and Gynecology) LLB PG Diploma in Hospital Management
Vice Chancellor
Sri Aurobindo University
Indore, Madhya Pradesh, India

Kanya Mukhopadhyay MBBS MD DNB DM(Neonatology)
Professor of Neonatology
Department of Pediatrics
PGIMER
Chandigarh, India

Kishan Singh Rawat MBBS MD(Radiology)
Senior Consultant
Department of Radiology
Sir Ganga Ram Hospital
New Delhi, India

Kritika Tiwari MBBS DNB(Pediatrics)
Consultant, Department of Pediatrics
Matushree Gomati Hospital
Mumbai, Maharashtra, India

Kumar Diwakar MBBS MD(Pediatrics) Fellowship Neonatal-Perinatal Medicine University of Calgary
Consultant Neonatologist
Department of Neonatology
Lancashire Women and Newborn Centre
Burnley General Hospital
Burnley, Lancashire, England, United Kingdom

Mahesh Baldwa MBBS DCH MD LLB LLM FIAP PhD(Law) MBA MA (Psy)
Founder President
Medicolegal Chapter/Group of Central Indian Academy of Pediatrics
Senior Medicolegal Advisor and Senior Consultant Pediatrician
Baldwa Hospital, Mumbai, India
External Faculty, Maharashtra National Law University

Manisha Bhandari LLB
Legal Practitioner, Department of Law and Judiciary, Supreme Court and High Court
New Delhi, India

Milind Shah MBBS MD DGO DFP FICOG FIAOG
Professor and Head
Department of Obstetrics and Gynecology, Gandhi Natha Rangaji Homoeopathic Medical College
Solapur, Maharashtra, India
Honorable Secretary General, (FAOPS) Federation of Asia Oceania Perinatal Societies
President, ISPAT (Indian Society of Prenatal Diagnosis and Fetal Therapy)

Mukul Tiwari MD DCH FIAP
Consultant Pediatrician, Apex Hospital
Gwalior, Madhya Pradesh, India
Chairperson, Medicolegal Group of IAP 2015–2017
President, IMLEA 2020–2022

(Col) Murli Janardan Sabath MBBS MD(Hospital Administration) PGDMLE
Senior Advisor and Faculty Hospital Administration
Veteran Armed Forces Medical Services
New Delhi, India

Namita Padvi MBBS MD DNB(Fellowship in Pediatric Anesthesiology) Emirates Hospital Dubai
Former Assistant Professor
Department of Anesthesia
Topiwala National Medical College and
BYL Nair Charitable Hospital
Mumbai, Maharashtra, India

NB Mathur MBBS MD FNNF
Professor and Head
Department of Pediatrics
Faculty of Medical Sciences, University of Delhi
New Delhi, India
Former Director Professor and Head
Department of Neonatology
Maulana Azad Medical College
New Delhi, India
Past President, National Neonatology Forum
New Delhi, India

Neeraj Nagpal MBBS MD FIMSA FISG FIAMS
Managing Trustee, Medicos Legal Action Group
Director, Hope Gastrointestinal Diagnostic Clinic
Mohali, Punjab, India

Neetu Jain MBBS DNB(Medicine) FCCP(USA) EDRM(Europe) FICCM
Senior Consultant
Department of Pulmonary, Critical Care and Sleep Medicine
PSRI Hospital, New Delhi, India
and
Tulip Chest and Child Care Clinic
Gurugram, Haryana, India

NL Sridhar MBBS MD(Pediatrics) LLB
Professor, Department of Pediatrics
Apollo Institute of Medical Sciences and Research
Jubilee Hills, Hyderabad, Telangana, India

Padmakumar K MBBS MD DNB MNAMS PGDMLE FIAMLE
Professor and Head
Department of Forensic Medicine
Jubilee Mission Medical College and Research Institute
Thrissur, Kerala, India

Pallavi Nigam Sethi MBBS MD(Dermatology and STD) PGDCD PGDCC
Consultant Dermatologist
Department of Dermatology and Cosmetology
Heritage Hospital
Sosyo Circle
Surat, Gujarat, India

Piyali Bhattacharya MBBS DCH MD(Pediatrics) FIAP FRCP(London)
Consultant Pediatrician
Department of General Hospital
SGPGIMS (Sanjay Gandhi Postgraduate Institute of Medical Sciences)
Lucknow, Uttar Pradesh, India

Pramod Kumar Nigam MBBS MD(Dermatology and STD) MBA PG Diploma in Human Law(NALSAR) FIAD FAMS FRCP(Glasgow)
Former Director cum Professor and Dean
Department of Dermatology
STD and Leprosy
Administration, Government Medical College,
Mahasamund, Chhattisgarh, India
and
Pt JNM Medical College
Raipur, Chhattisgarh, India

Prasant Kumar Saboth MBBS MD(Pediatrics)
Professor
Department of Pediatrics
IMS and SUM Medical College and Hospital
Bhubaneswar, Odisha, India

Preeti Srivastava MBBS(Gold Medalist) DNB(Pediatrics) Fellowship Pediatric Neurology (KK Children's Hospital, Singapore) ASEPA-ASNA EEG Certified (Singapore)
Senior Consultant and Unit Head
Tata Main Hospital
Jamshedpur, Jharkhand, India
Assistant Professor
Manipal Tata Medical College
MAHE
Jamshedpur, Jharkhand, India

Priyamvada Bhasin MBBS MS(Ophthalmology)
Medical Director
Department of Ophthalmology
Ratan Jyoti Netralaya, Ophthalmic Institute and Research Centre
Gwalior, Madhya Pradesh, India

Pukhraj Bafna MBBS MD DCH FIAP PhD
Head, Department of Medicine
CDCRI
Rajnandgaon, Chhattisgarh, India

Purendra Bhasin MBBS MS(Ophthalmology)
Director
Department of Ophthalmology
Ratan Jyoti Netralaya, Ophthalmic Institute and Research Center
Gwalior, Madhya Pradesh, India

Rahul Madhav Dawre MBBS MD(Pediatrics)
Associate Professor
Department of Pediatrics
Byramjee Jeejeebhoy Government Medical College
Pune, Maharashtra, India

Rajendra Borkar MBBS MD(Pediatrics)
Consultant
Department of Pediatrics
Jawaharlal Nehru Medical College
Sawangi (Meghe)
Wardha, Maharashtra, India

Rajinder Gulati MBBS MD(Pediatrics) FIAP
Consultant Pediatrician
National Health Mission Punjab
UCHC cum Mother Child Hospital
Ludhiana, Punjab, India

Rajneesh Kumar Sharma BSc BHMS MD(Homeopathy) DI(Homeopathy) London hMD(UK) PhD
Homeo Cure and Research Institute
Vaibhav Homeopathic Pharma, Sparsh Multispecialty Hospital
(NABH Accredited)
Kashipur, Uttarakhand, India

Ravisankar TN MBBS PGDMLE MBA
Senior Family Physician
Department of Family Medicine
Sudar Hospitals
Chennai, Tamil Nadu, India

Rishi Bhatia MBBS MS(Surgery) LLB PGDMLE PGDMLS
General and Laparoscopic Surgeon
Medicolegal Advisor UP Nursing Home Association and UP IMA
Meerut, Uttar Pradesh, India
Past President Indian Medico-Legal Ethics Association

Rohini Deshpande MBBS MD(Obstetrics and Gynecology) FRCOG(London) FMAS Dip(Endoscopy) Clermont-Ferrand France
Past Secretary
Indian Medico-Legal and Ethics Association
Department of Obstetrics and Gynecology
Ramkrishna Hospital
Solapur, Maharashtra, India

Ruchita Shukla MBA(HR)
Assistant Professor
Department of Management Studies
Rukmini Devi Institute of Advance Studies
New Delhi, India
Director, Human Medico-Legal Consultants Pvt Ltd
Amravati, Maharashtra, India

Rupali Patil Jain MBBS DORL DPAA LLB PGDMLS PGDHHM
Consultant ENT Surgeon Arihant Hospital, Warud
Amravati, Maharashtra, India
Medicolegal Consultant SSH Legal Firm,
Mumbai, Maharashtra, India
Faculty, Allergy Course by Dr Anand Sumandeep University, Vadodara, Gujarat, India

Samarjit Singh Ghuman MBBS MD(Radiodiagnosis)
Vice-Chairman
Department of Imaging
Sir Ganga Ram Hospital
New Delhi, India

Sandeep Jhajra Dayanand MBBS MD FNNF DM(Neonatology)
Consultant and Unit Incharge
Department of Pediatrics
Tata Main Hospital
Jamshedpur, Jharkhand, India
Associate Professor, Manipal Tata Medical College
Jamshedpur, Jharkhand, India

Sandhya Satish Khadse MBBS MD(Pediatrics)
Professor and Dean
Department of Pediatrics
MGM Medical College, Nerul
Navi Mumbai, Maharashtra, India

Satish Tiwari MBBS MD(Pediatrics) LL.B FIAP
Professor
Department of Pediatrics
Medical College, Amravati
Maharashtra, India
Founder President
Indian Medico-Legal and Ethics Association

Satish V Agrawal MBBS MD(Mumbai) DCH DNB(Pediatrics)
Consultant
Department of Pediatrics
Agrawal Children Hospital
Amravati, Maharashtra, India
Founder President
Indian Medico-Legal and Ethics Association
Maharashtra State Branch, India

Seema Sud MBBS DNB(Radiodiagnosis)
Chairperson
Department of Imaging
Sir Ganga Ram Hospital
New Delhi, India

(Late) Shantanu Abhyankar MBBS MD(Obstetrics and Gynecology) FICOG
Ex-Medical Director
Modern Clinic, Wai (Satara)
Maharashtra, India

Sheikh Minhaj Ahmed MBBS MD DNB MNAMS FIAP
Consultant Pediatric Intensivist
Lilavati Hospital and Research Center
Mumbai, Maharashtra, India

Shivakumar F Kumbar MBBS DA LLB(Specialization) LLM MBA(Hospital Management) MA(Journalism) PGMLS PGMLE CDM(IIAM) CCEPC Bio-Ethics(UNESCO) FIAMS IASMPMM(Sexual Medicne)
Senior Specialist
Department of Anesthesiology, District Hospital
Dharwad, Karnataka, India
Anesthesiologist, Medicolegal Consultant, Accredited Mediator, Member of Mediation Cell – District Consumer Commission, Medical Journalist

Shivali Vaid BDS MDS
Professor and Head
Department of Oral and Maxillofacial Pathology and Microbiology, Maharana Pratap College of Dentistry and Research Centre
Gwalior, Madhya Pradesh, India

Suchismita Mallick MBBS DNB(Anesthesiology) Fellowship in Pain Management(Aesculap Academy) PGDPML(National University of Juridical Science)
Professor and Head
Department of Anesthesiology
Sarat Chandra Chattopadhyay Govt Medical College Hospital
Howrah, West Bengal, India

Sudhir Mishra MBBS MD(Pediatrics) FIAP
Consultant Pediatrician
Ex-Head, Department of Pediatrics
Tata Main Hospital and Manipal Tata Medical College
Jamshedpur, Jharkhand, India

Sumanta Ghosh Maulik MBBS MD(Anesthesiology) DPM PGDMLE MBA(Healthcare Management)
Professor and Head
Department of Anesthesiology
Burdwan Medical College
Burdwan, West Bengal, India

Sushila Baldwa MBBS MD DGO
Consulting Obstetrician and Gynecologist
Baldwa Hospital and Apollo Clinic
Nakoda Foundation
Mumbai, Maharashtra, India
Formerly Faculty at BJ Medical College and Sassoon General Hospital
Pune, Maharashtra, India

Sushil Kumar MBBS MD(Pediatrics)
Specialist, Assistant Professor
Department of Pediatrics
Tata Main Hospital and Manipal Tata Medical College
Jamshedpur, Jharkhand, India

Tapas Sarangi MBBS MD(Pediatrics)
Head Consultant
Department of Pediatrics
Tata Main Hospital
Noamundi, Jharkhand, India

Tarvinder Bir Singh Buxi MBBS MD(Radiology)
Advisor
Department of Imaging
Sir Ganga Ram Hospital
New Delhi, India

Tulsi Prasad MBBS MD(Pediatrics)
Consultant Pediatrician
Department of Pediatrics
Rani Children Hospital
Ranchi, Jharkhand, India

Varsha Baldwa MBBS MD FRCP(Australia)
Consultant, TissuPath
Melbourne, Australia
Formerly Consultant, PD Hinduja Hospital
Mumbai, Maharashtra, India
Formerly Consultant, GS Medical College and KEM Hospital
Mumbai, Maharashtra, India
GMC Surat, Gujarat, India
GMC Kota, Rajasthan, India

Vijay Kuthe MBBS D Ortho
Consultant, Department of Orthopedics
Kuthe Accident Hospital; and Maternity Nursing Home Amravati, Maharashtra, India
Founder Member, Amravati Orthopedic Association
President, Amravati Orthopedic Association 2007–2008

VP Singh MBBS MD(Forensic Medicine) LLB PGDMLE
CC in Healthcare Quality Management
Professor
Department of Forensic Medicine
Dayanand Medical College and Hospital
Ludhiana, Punjab, India

Zahabiya Nalwalla MBBS MD(Pediatrics)
Fellowship in Pediatric Infectious Diseases Fellowship in Pediatric Gastroenterology
Clinical Associate
Department of Pediatric Infectious Diseases
Nowrosjee Wadia Maternity Hospital
Mumbai, Maharashtra, India

Preface to the Third Edition

यदा यदा हि धर्मस्य ग्लानिर्भवति भारत ।
अभ्युत्थानमधर्मस्य तदात्मानं सृजाम्यहम् ।।

("Whenever there is decay of righteousness, O Bharata, and there is exaltation of unrighteousness, then I myself come forth; for the protection of the good, for the destruction of evil-doers, for the sake of firmly establishing righteousness, I am born from age to age").

From: Bhagavad Gita, An Ancient Hindu Epic

The third edition of *"The Textbook of Medicolegal Issues Related to Different Specialties"* is before you. As a groundbreaking work in its field, it is a source of great satisfaction that the first two editions were widely successful and well received by the medical community. While many medicolegal issues are shared across specialties, each branch also faces unique challenges. This edition strives to provide a comprehensive resource, addressing a wide range of topics tailored to the needs of various specialties.

The practice of medicine is as old as the mankind itself. It might have begun when one caveman gave herbs to another caveman for some ailment. The medicolegal aspect of it must have begun when the herb caused worsening of symptoms and the second caveman accused the first caveman of giving him a bad herb.

Although previously considered more of an art, the technical and scientific discoveries in the medical field over the late-19th and 20th centuries gradually made it a science and in the second half of the 20th century it has been accorded the status of a profession. Earlier, medical professionals were put on a higher pedestal compared to other professionals as they dealt with human life, which is more precious than worldly possessions. In the later half of the 20th century, there has been an unprecedented explosion in science and technology which have influenced the concepts of medical practice. Some strong factors have emerged which changed this relationship of faith and trust; doubts and hostility seeped into it. This change is reflecting in an ever-increasing number of medicolegal cases. Erosion in the relationship began in the later half of the 20th century and has increased gradually since then. Consumer law, which was enacted in 1986 and repealed and re-enacted in 2019, gave another severe blow to the relationship. Consumerism, autonomy and e-knowledge, by-products of social progress, are other factors which have been pivotal in changing the relationship. The model of the doctor–patient relationship has changed. Doctor is no more the demi-god! The new model is *doctor–patient partnership*.

However, ironically, medicine is a service which will always require ethics and human touch and cannot be governed by pure and cold science alone. A patient who considers his doctor as merely a service provider and walks into his clinic with preconceived notions of his illness and treatment options derived from websites which may not be accurate at all times is at risk of entering into an unhealthy and combative relationship. Nonetheless, writing is clear on the wall. Medical practice is changing and doctors have to adapt to changes sooner than later. This book is intended to provide the reader with much desired knowledge and wisdom to face different medicolegal situations, keep abreast of relevant laws as applicable to practicing doctors, and prevent, solve, and understand the day-to-day legal problems.

As per ancient Sanskrit saying "विजयते ते सत्त्वं I" (Your strength will win), it means you can be successful in any battle provided it is for a valid reason and you are strong by your inner strength as well. Medical science being uncertain, we need to make ourselves strong by all means, by skill, by knowledge—both medicolegal and specialty related. Knowledge and skill increase confidence, courage, and competence.

It is a well-known fact that ignorance breeds and feeds uncertainty. Uncertainty breeds and feeds unfounded fears. Unfounded fears may never become true or actually happen in one's life but make life stressful and unlivable. In the light of knowledge, let us drive away these unfounded legal fears, of allegations and litigations. Let medicine and law join forces to provide fearless, improved care and ensure peace of mind for all.

The chapters from previous editions have been thoroughly updated and revised to include recent case laws. Additionally, 10 new chapters have been introduced, covering topics that were not included in earlier editions. The editors extend heartfelt gratitude to the authors who, despite our pressing demands, have graciously shared their expertise and made invaluable contributions to this endeavor.

Satish Tiwari
Mahesh Baldwa
Mukul Tiwari
Alka Kuthe

Preface to the First Edition

Hani-Labh, Jivan-Maran, Jas-Apjas Bidhi Hath
(Loss-Profit, Life-Death, Fame-Defame is in the hands of destiny)

— ***Tulsidas's Ramcharitmanas***

No person on this earth is immortal. It is important to understand that doctors can never predict the future of any patient as the dynamic human body does not obey the linear laws of deterministic predictability. A very sick patient may stand long hours of surgery and recover completely while relatively healthy patient may succumb to minor stress or allergic reactions.

The term "Medicolegal" incorporates the basics of two professions, i.e. Medicine and Law. Although doctors encounter the law at every turn during the practice of their profession, they frequently have insufficient knowledge of it. A doctor confronts it when, as the treating doctor, he is summoned to a court of law in a personal injury lawsuit; he meets it when he is called as an expert in connection with a claim against a colleague and when he is faced in his office or clinic by unforeseen situations, like sudden unexpected death, patient-generated violence, etc. It will be better to accept the change and brace ourselves with the knowledge to cope with the change.

With passing time, the standards of medical care are rising as also the patients' expectations. This race may convert medical practice into a battleground between the doctors and patients. In India, medical law is yet to crystallize. Nothing can be said with absolute certainty on many issues as the final word is yet to come. The legal system wants medical practitioners to follow standard practices; setting standards is, however, a difficult task. Medicine is a vast and ever-changing field. It is also equally important to take into account the needs of the individual patient, available infrastructure, resources and the regional limitations. Therefore, a lot of information, documentation and know-how is needed. In the last few years, the medicolegal scenario has changed further.

Every relationship is a dynamic process and doctor–patient relationship is no different. It has gone a sea-change since its beginning thousands of years back. It will be a futile exercise to look back and remember the good old days when the doctor was all powerful, a Semi-God. With the change in medicosocial dynamics, cases against doctors are witnessing a phenomenal rise, constant upgradation of the practicing doctor vis-á-vis the fast-changing laws of the country. Medical professionals fumble when they confront a court case against them with allegations of negligence or deficiency in medical service. It will be quite useful for today's doctors to be well-equipped with medicolegal knowledge if they want to practice their profession safely, without the hassle of too many cases slapped on them. Doctors in the West have been quicker to respond to the need for such knowledge. There is ample literature generated from the West, which analyzes the issues of legal aspects of medical practice and doctor-patient relationship thoroughly. There is scanty literature on this subject in India where the volume of patients is many times more than that of most of the Western countries. We should have our literature, studies and observations suited to our milieu. With the phenomenal increase in the patient volumes in India, the need for indigenous literature is going to be even greater in the future.

Each branch of medicine has its own medicolegal issues. There are different books on medicolegal issues pertaining to different branches of medicine, but no single book which comprehensively deals with medicolegal issues in most of the vulnerable branches together is available. This book was envisioned with the same objective in mind. The editors sincerely hope that this book will serve to fill the void effectively. The book looks beyond the problems and moves on to solutions. The editors hope that doctors from different specialities will find in this book constructive suggestions and solutions towards many of the issues which plague them.

An endeavor has been made to include the information related to almost all the branches in allopathic medical science and to create a perfect blend of clinical practice and various laws applicable to its varied aspects. It covers major issues which a doctor is likely to face during his/her professional career with case laws and important Supreme Court judgments in simple language, so that a doctor can easily understand its legal implication and apply it. A section on *the Acts* and certain important tips in the form of algorithms for *Safe Practice* while managing the patient, have been added, which would help the doctors to follow uniform standards, which, in turn, will help in better patient care.

Lastly, we welcome feedback and suggestions from the esteemed readers that will make the book more useful.

Human mind is like a parachute, it works best when it is open

Satish Tiwari
Mahesh Baldwa
Mukul Tiwari
Alka Kuthe

Contents

PLATE 1

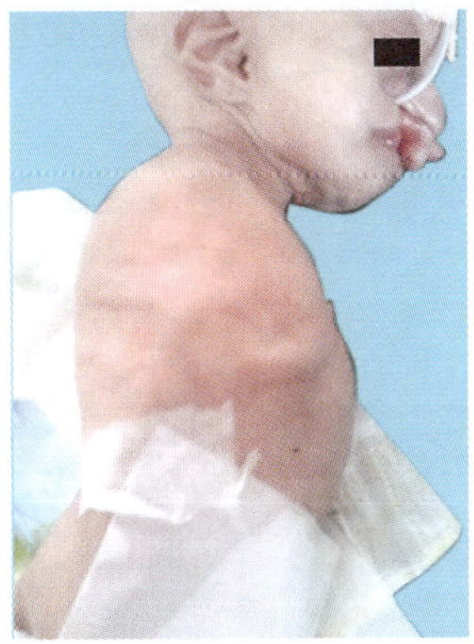

Fig. 29.1.1: Newborn with cleft lip and palate and amelia. ***(Chapter 29)***

Courtesy: Dr Rajendra S Kulhari, SPMC, Bikaner.

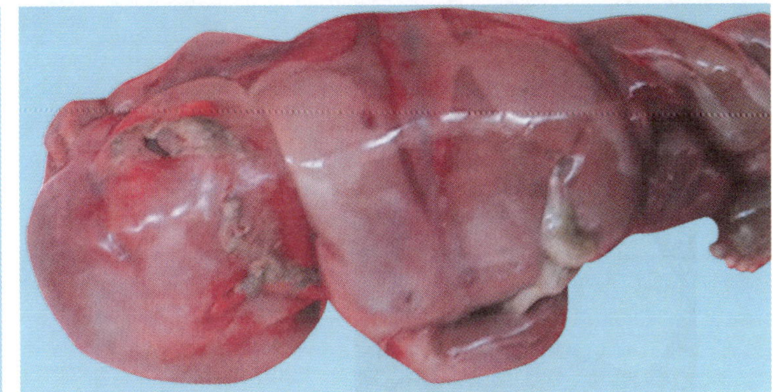

Fig. 29.1.2: Nonimmune hydrops fetal is showing generalized edema. ***(Chapter 29)***

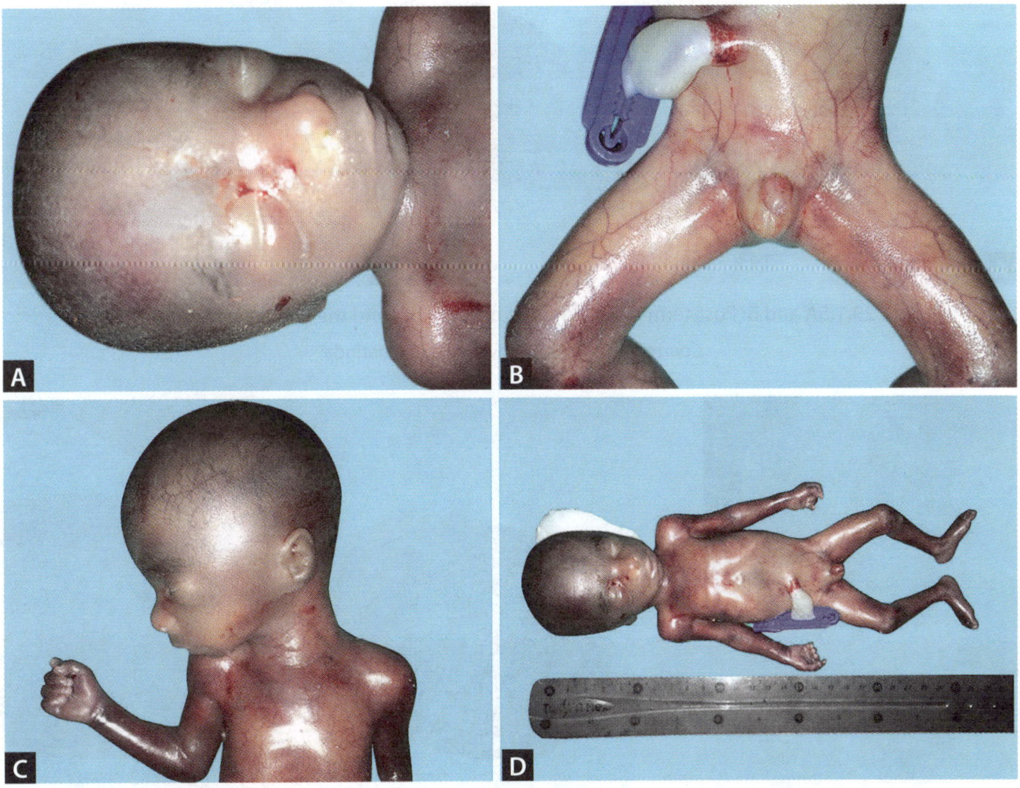

Figs. 29.1.3A to D: Fetus of 21–22 weeks' gestation (weight 365 g). ***(Chapter 29)***

PLATE 2

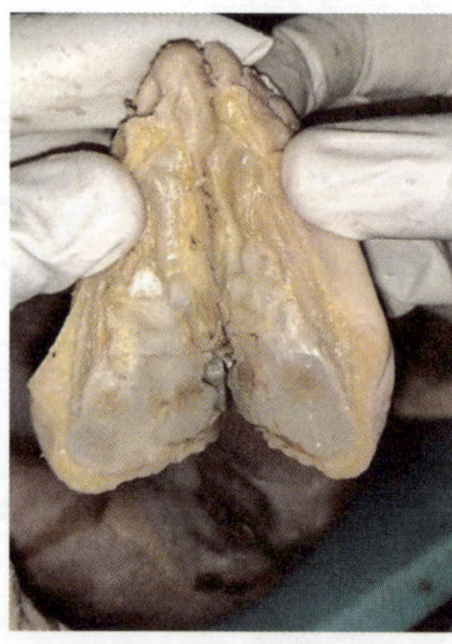

Fig. 29.1.4: Ossification centers of calcaneum (5th month) and talus (7th month). ***(Chapter 29)***

Courtesy: Dr Murugesa Bharathi, IGMC and RI, Puducherry.

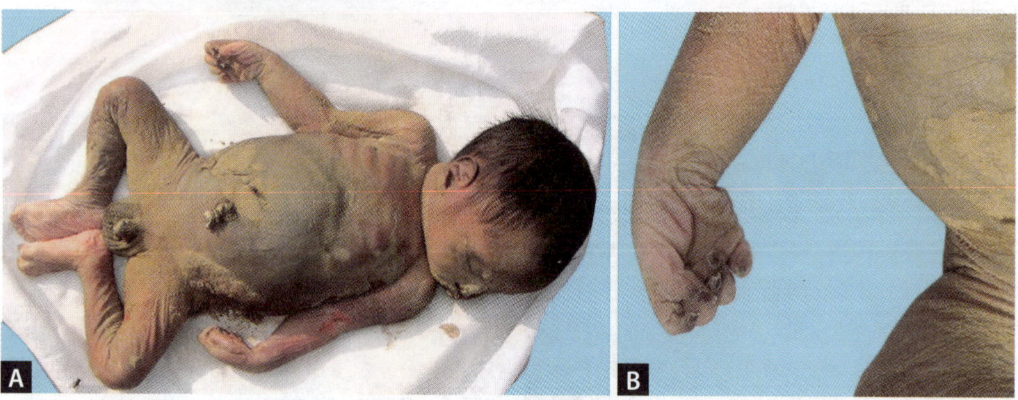

Figs. 29.1.5A and B: Post-term baby. Note the nails are beyond the fingertips. ***(Chapter 29)***

Courtesy: Dr Parmod Goyal, AIMSR, Bhatinda.

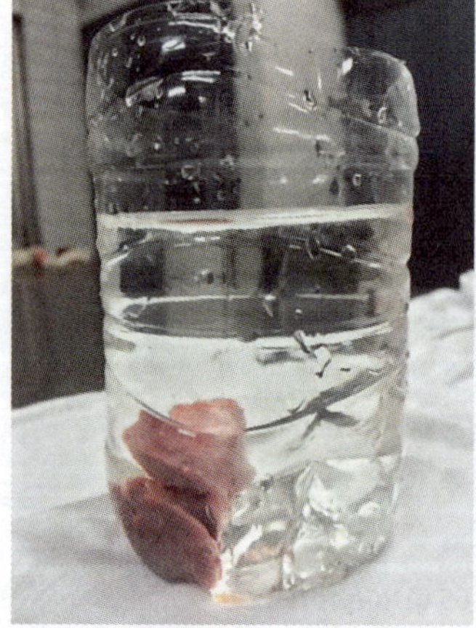

Fig. 29.1.6: Hydrostatic test showing sinking fetal lungs (negative test). ***(Chapter 29)***

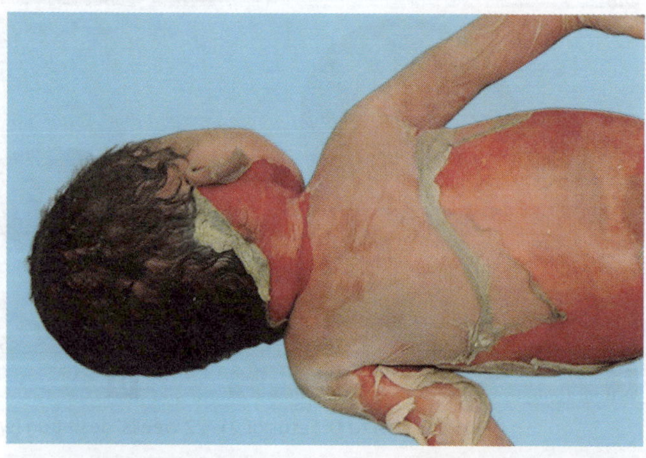

Fig. 29.1.7: Deadborn fetus showing skin maceration. ***(Chapter 29)***

Courtesy: Dr Joseph Prahlow, Kalamazoo, MI, US.

PLATE 3

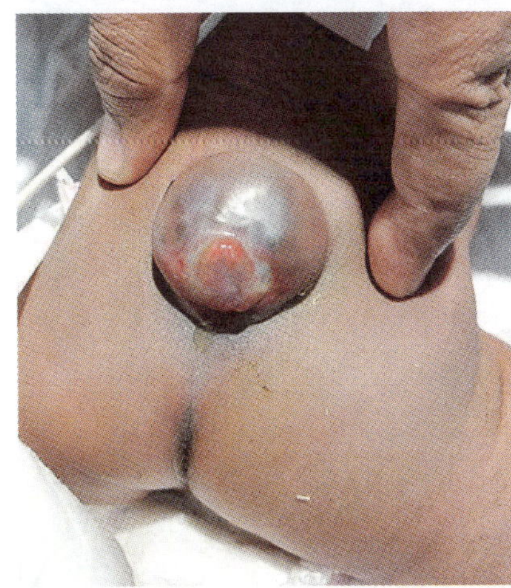

Fig. 29.1.8: Meningomyelocele. ***(Chapter 29)***

Courtesy: Dr Narinder S Bhatti, Jalandhar.

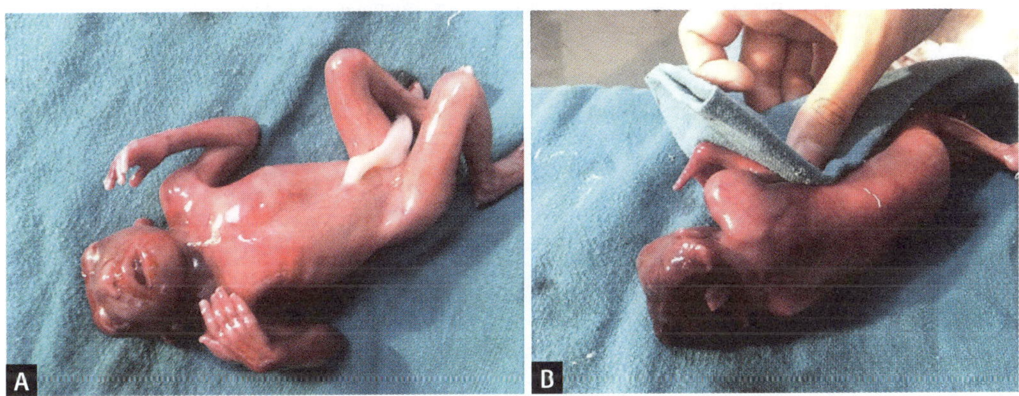

Figs. 29.1.9A and B: Anencephaly at 18 weeks' gestation. ***(Chapter 29)***

Courtesy: Dr Meenakshi, Jalandhar.

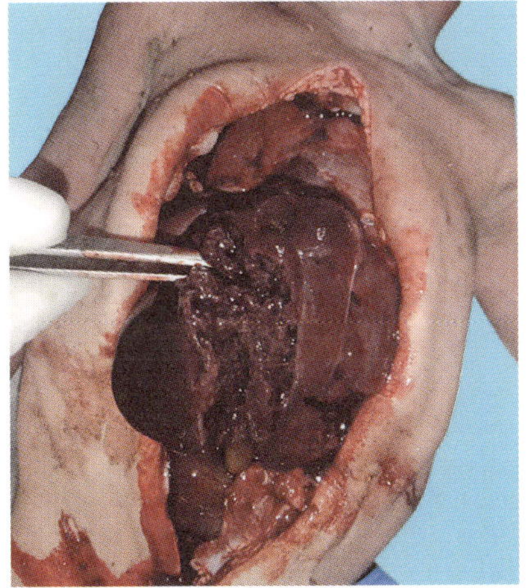

Fig. 29.1.10: Laceration of liver with hemoperitoneum. ***(Chapter 29)***

Courtesy: Dr Shalender K Saharan, SPMC, Bikaner.

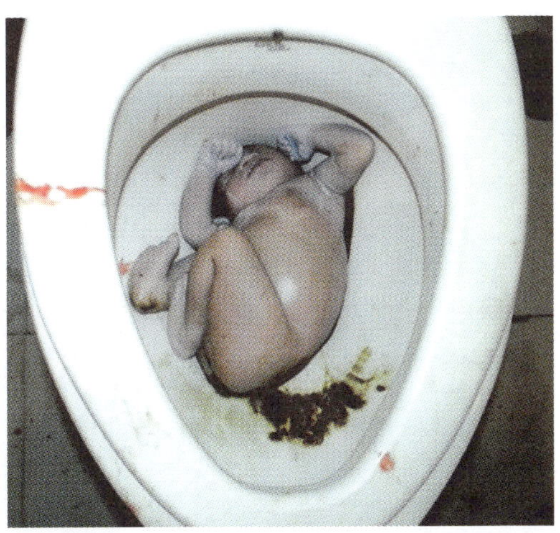

Fig. 29.1.11: Precipitate labor. ***(Chapter 29)***

Courtesy: Dr Viswakanth B, KIMS and H, Mangaluru.

PLATE 4

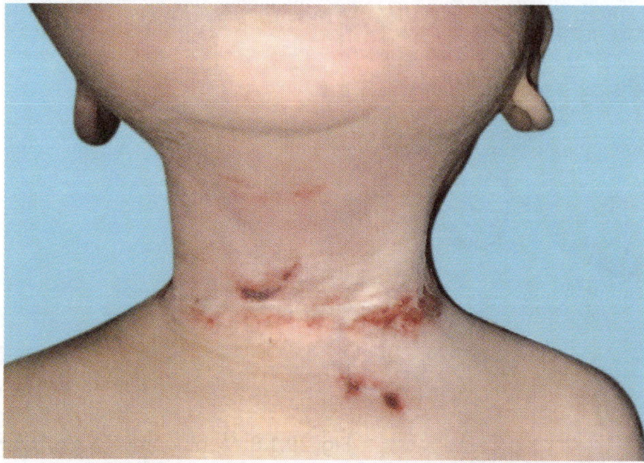

Fig. 29.1.12: Ligature strangulation. ***(Chapter 29)***

Courtesy: Dr Sandeep Haridas, Swami Ramanand Teerth Rural GMCH, Maharashtra.

SECTION

1

Basics

Section Editor: Arun Manglik

Section Outline

CHAPTER 1

Introduction

Rishi Bhatia

Human culture is built upon the foundation of values that form the basis of an ethical society—honesty, integrity, respect, pursuit of excellence, civic duty, accountability, and loyalty. When we scan the history of human civilization, it becomes evident that the evolution of ethical concepts has preoccupied philosophers, ethicists, sociologists, theologians, professionals, and indeed all of the society. Since the dawn of the civilization, by trial and error, it has become established that a society and more so it is medical profession, a public-oriented and noble profession, that can survive and thrive only by observance and practice of certain rules of conduct guided by ethical, moral, legal, and social values of the land. The prime object of the medical profession is to render service to humanity with full respect for the dignity of a human being. A doctor's role is to cure when possible and to relieve pain and suffering always. Sometimes, he may fail in the role while trying his best.

The science and practice of medicine have continued to change with the times and advancement of knowledge, but the fundamental principles of professional behavior have remained unchanged. Even in the presence of conflict between traditional age old ethos and customs and changing values and orientations, the code of conduct, rules, and obligations coined together as "medical ethics" still uphold, foster, and guarantee the mode of conduct and behavior of the members of medical profession as to the obligation of the doctor to the (1) patient, (2) fellow doctors, (3) state through the health professionals, and (4) the society. It differs from "law" or "legislation" as ethics are governed and guided by moral sense and conscience and not by any statute or an act of legislation. Ethical code, though not legislation, is equally forceful as it has the approval of the profession at large. Ethics and laws share the social purpose of encouraging right conduct. Laws achieve this purpose through the sovereign power of government, while ethics do so with the help of the profession itself. In all actions, conscience has the last say—it guides the doctor to do what is good and not to do what is bad.

The beginnings of recorded medical practice in India date back to the advent of Aryan invaders. Originating in Central Asia, they settled in the northern Indian plains around 1500 BC. They brought with them, in Sanskrit, the beginnings of the Vedas. The three principal Vedas were *Rig, Sam*, and *Yajur*. A later addition—the Atharvaveda—was the principle source for information on medicine during the early Vedic period. Much useful information is also found in the Ayurvedic classics—*Charaka Samhita, Sushruta Samhita*, and *Bhela Samhita* (around 600 BC). *Charaka Samhita* (600 BC) had outlined the code of conduct for the "would be physicians" of India. *Sushruta Samhita* (300 BC), equally ancient, outlines conduct of surgeons and surgical procedures in those days. "*Bhagvat*" is another ancient Hindu scripture that tells "show goodwill and sympathy to the sick and show feeling of satisfaction on his recovery, in spite of someone having ill will towards you"—the above mentioned attitude will fulfill the ethical requirements for the doctor.

The Hippocratic Oath of the Greek Physician written in 460 BC was intended to be affirmed by each doctor on entry to medical profession which states, "Premium non nocere" which means "First, do no harm"—although almost 25 centuries old, its basic principles are equally valid today. The World Medical Association, established in 1914, made a modern restatement of Hippocratic Oath known as "Declaration of Geneva" and "International Code of Medical Ethics" (1947, 1968, 1983, and 2000) mainly based upon the Hippocratic Oath. The declaration was also adopted by the Medical Council of India (MCI). In India, different systems of medicine prevail and different system have different "Code of Ethics," but the guiding principle is the same. In order to deserve the patient's respect and confidence, the medical man has to conduct himself in a disciplined and dignified manner, as embodied in the code of ethics. As per the Medical Council Amendment, Act No. 24 of 1964, the Council has prescribed standards of professional conduct and etiquette, the Indian Medical Council Regulations 2002, a code of ethics for the medical practitioners.

In the past, doctors were considered "demigods." The family physician or general practitioner (GP) was part of the family, who knew not only the physical but also the mental health of every family member. Not only were the health problems discussed with him but also matrimonial issues, not to speak of feuds between mothers and daughters-in-law. In the good old days that have passed, it was rare for doctors to be sued. The era has changed now; it is now easy to form a public opinion against the medical profession. People in general are becoming more and more "medicophobic." There is an increasing distrust between the doctors and the patients. Medicolegal problems have increased exponentially in every discipline of medical science.

The Consumer Protection Act (CPA), which was enacted in 1986, was dormant till the 90s. With the sudden outpouring of superspecializations, the CPA too became a popular weapon and the relationship between the patient and the doctor shifted to become that of a consumer and a supplier of services as decided by the Supreme Court of India in "Indian Medical Association vs. VP Shantha and others" (decided on November 13, 1995). So the practice of medicine, which had started as an art and subsequently became a science, has finally got the status of "business." Today, medical care services are commodities in a heavily commercialized society. The CPA has done harm to the doctors but not much good to the patients either. The new CPA 2019 has changed territorial and pecuniary jurisdiction to facilitate patients and also online complaint has increased chances of more litigations. As going for a redressal system in the consumer forum is cheap and easy, the number of litigations is on the rise, some on genuine grounds but mostly for financial gains. The doctor-patient relationship has deteriorated drastically in the last two decades. This trend is disturbing to doctors, who want to practice honestly, ethically, and without the fear of lawsuits and violence from patients. Fear of lawsuits and violence from patients and relatives have made doctors defensive, which in turn has resulted in even more deterioration in doctor-patient relationship and the vicious cycle goes on. Doctors have become somewhat overcautious in their approach toward their patients with the result that at times, the patients are being overinvestigated and overtreated. It is, therefore, not surprising that there have been more lawsuits and escalation in insurance premiums. The pressure of high-cost medical service is putting a burden on healthcare budgets and is adversely affecting the healthcare system.

New education policy has initiated teaching in medical colleges in Hindi as well as in regional languages. As a new-course curriculum, Foundation Course has been added in undergraduate syllabus for development of attitude, communication and other skills, and orientation and ethical issues. But our medical students are not taught about CPA and other acts related to medical profession. There are no study sessions where case scenarios in skillful communications and difficult situations are played and solutions discussed. Unethical practice is getting entry into medical profession. Private medical colleges necessitate huge capital investments by their students. On graduation, there arise a need to recover these investments and generate profit on them as soon as the doctor starts practice. Under these circumstances, it is not surprising that students emerging from medical colleges are ill-equipped to ponder the nature and consequences of their own actions toward patients and their families.

Recently, consumerism and judicial activism have evoked remarkable judgments in the National Consumer Disputes Redressal Commission and Supreme Court of India. Every doctor and hospital has the duty to give emergency life-support treatment to every patient coming with life-threatening conditions without waiting for consent or medicolegal formalities. It has been well settled by the Supreme Court in the famous case "Parmanand Katara vs. Union of India and Others" (AIR 1989 SC 2039). In another case, "Paschim Bangla Kheth Mazdoor Samiti and Others vs. State of West Bengal and another" (AIR 1996 SC 2426), the Supreme Court held that hospital cannot refuse such patients on grounds of "no vacant bed" and/or "no neurosurgeon facility available." National Commission in "Pravat Kumar Mukherji vs. Ruby General Hospital and Ors" 2005 CTJ 605 (CPNC) has ruled that no admission can be refused for non payment of fee when the patient is critically ill. Landmark judgment of the Supreme Court ("Jacob Mathew vs. State of Punjab" criminal appeal No. 144–145 of 2004) has given relief to medical profession in cases of death of patients during treatment. For such cases of criminal negligence u/s 304-A IPC or 106-A BNS against doctors, expert opinion is to be taken before proceeding against doctors. Further, a constitution bench of five judges in Lalita Kumari vs. Government of UP and ors (WP Criminal No. 68 of 2008) judgment dated November 12, 2013, holds that preliminary inquiry is to be conducted time bound, not exceeding 7 days before registration of first information report (FIR) in medical negligence cases [para 111, (vi)c].

Now IPC has been replaced by BNS since July 2024. BNS has discriminated Allopathic doctor (MBBS registered under NMC/SMC) from doctors of other Pathies. BNS 106(1) states: "Whoever causes death of any person by doing any rash or negligent act not amounting to culpable homicide, shall be punished with imprisonment of either description for a term which may extend to 5 years, and shall also be liable to fine; and if such act is done by a registered medical practitioner while performing medical procedure, he shall be punished with imprisonment of either description for a term which may extend to 2 years and shall also be liable to fine. Explanation: For the purpose of this sub-section, "registered medical practitioner" means a medical practitioner who possesses any medical qualification recognized under the National Medical Commission Act 2019 and whose name has been entered in the National Medical Register or a State Medical Register under that Act.

In spite of changing scenario of medical profession, the government (Central and States) has not done remarkable duty for providing safe and standard medical services. The Supreme Court had directed in "Jacob Mathew vs. State of Punjab" case that "Statutory Rules or Executive Instructions incorporating certain guidelines need to be framed and issued by the Government of India and/or the State Governments in consultation with the Medical Council of India," but so far MCI has not been consulted and no such permanent rules or guidelines have been framed. The government has given guidelines temporarily issued by the Supreme Court in this case. The Supreme Court in this case has observed "The investigating officer and the private complainant can not always be supposed to have knowledge of medical science so as to determine whether the act of the accused medical professional amounts to rash or negligent act." In a judgment ("Martin F D'Souza vs. Mohd Ishfaq" decided on February 2, 2009), the Supreme Court observed, "The Court and Consumers are not experts in Medical Science and must not substitute their own views over that of specialists." Therefore, the Supreme Court directed that before issuing notice to the doctor or hospital, the Consumer Forum or Civil Court should refer the matter to a competent doctor or committee of doctors. Despite such guidelines and orders by the Supreme Court in different cases, FIRs are being lodged against doctors for medical negligence without expert opinion and without investigations. So the government must amend the CPA and Indian Penal Code (IPC)/*Bharatiya Nyaya Sanhita* (BNS) to safeguard medical professionals and to consider taking expert opinion in every case against medical profession before the case is admitted in any court or registered in police station. As submitted by the Directorate General of Health Services (DGHS) and observed by the Supreme Court in "Parmanand Katara vs. Union of India and Ors" (AIR 1989 SC 2039) case, "Article 21 of the constitution casts the obligation on the State to preserve life." Therefore, it should be the duty of State (Government) to reimburse the expenses for treatment of life-saving conditions of patients brought in emergency to the private hospital if patient is unable to pay because one cannot refuse life-saving treatment of critically ill patient as directed by the National Commission in "Pravat Kumar Mukherji vs. Ruby General Hospital" 2005 CTJ 605 (CPNC). But the government has not given any serious thought about the problem of expenses done on such patients when the duty of the State to preserve life is being carried out by private hospitals and doctors. Government should float health insurance policy for private hospitals and doctors to reimburse expenses on treatment of life-threatening emergencies in hospitals. The Medical Termination of Pregnancy (MTP) Act needs amendment to check termination of pregnancy by oral drugs (e.g., misoprostol and mifepristone) taken directly from chemists by patients without prescription of authorized and qualified medical practitioner because by this method, unlawful termination of pregnancy has become easier.

The MTP Act amendment on March 25, 2021, facilitated termination of pregnancy up to 20 weeks by one registered medical practitioner (RMP) and up to 24 weeks by two RMPs with certain preconditions. It permitted the MTP during widowhood or for divorcee. It did not permit MTP for unmarried women. On World Safe Abortion Day, the Supreme Court of India on September 29, 2022, quoting the violation of right to equality before law under Article 14 of the constitution, adjudicated that every women married or unmarried or single has the right to abortion between 20 and 24 weeks, thus extending the limitation of Rule 3B of MTP Rules 2003 (as amended in 2021). The court has broadened woman's right to abortion, seeing the women as the ultimate decision maker, thus giving abortion as a constitutionally protected "reproductive right."

The Medical Termination of Pregnancy (MTP) Act needs amendment to check termination of pregnancy by oral drugs (e.g., Misoprostol and Mifepristone) taken directly from chemists by patients without prescription of authorized and qualified medical practitioner because by this method, unlawful termination of pregnancy has become easier. Termination of pregnancy by medical method with drugs like Misoprostol and Mifepristone without prescription of qualified doctor and over the counter sale of such drugs should be included as punishable crime in the Act like termination of pregnancy by unqualified doctor written in the Act.

With the advent of the Clinical Establishment Act 2010 to regulate clinics and hospitals, the National Medical Commission Act 2019 to regulate medical education, the Indian Council of Medical Research (ICMR) Consensus Guidelines on "Do Not Attempt Resuscitation 2020," Telemedicine Practice Guidelines 2020, Assisted Reproductive Technology (Regulation) Act 2021 to regulate in vitro fertilization (IVF) centers, sperm banks, etc., and Surrogacy (Regulation) Act 2021 to regulate surrogacy have been implemented.

The current ethicolegal issues under debate are Central Act on medical professionals protection against violence, capping of compensation against medical negligence, patient confidentiality in digitalization of medical records, doctors' advertisement and social media, and sponsorship of pharma companies for updating knowledge of doctors. To control and regulate all these, much more is to be done by the government after consulting the medical experts in the field. The future of medicolegal issues is under struggle to thrive for better and safe medical services.

CHAPTER

Ethical Issues in Medical Practice

Pukhraj Bafna

INTRODUCTION

Medical ethics for all practical purposes may be defined as a code of conduct accepted voluntarily by medical practitioners within the profession. In order to understand medical laws and ethics, it is helpful to understand the differences between medical law and ethics. A law is defined as a rule of conduct or action prescribed or formally recognized as binding or enforced by a controlling authority such as local state and federal governments. Ethic is considered a standard of behavior and a concept of right and wrong beyond what the legal consideration is in any given situation. Moral values serve as a basis for ethical conduct. Legally, medical ethics are not enforceable by law but are defended by the state medical council.

The four pillars of medical ethics—(i) beneficence, (ii) nonmaleficence, (iii) autonomy, and (iv) equity, may be enough for an individual medical practitioner faced with an ethical conundrum, but they are hardly sufficient to inform the choices of civil society. The practice of medicine according to ethical principles requires that decisions regarding treatment, preventive or interventional strategies or quality of life of patients in relation to life support treatment, should be based on evidence as far as possible.

Ethics is primarily concerned with four rational approaches:

1. *Deontology*: Which involves a search for well-founded rooms that can serve as the basis for making moral decisions.
2. *Consequentialism*: As the basis for ethical decision-making, on an analysis of the likely consequences or outcomes of different choices and actions.
3. *Principlism*: Uses ethical principles as the basis for making moral decisions.
4. *Virtual ethics*.

It is important that, physicians know and exemplify the core values of medicine especially compassion, competence, and autonomy. These values, along with respect for fundamental human rights, serve as the foundation of medical ethics. Besides its adherence to these three core values, medical ethics differs from the general ethics applicable to everyone by being professed in an oath.

From its beginning in the remote past, the practice of medicine was permeated by a code of ethical conduct which has evolved through the centuries. Oaths and Codes vary from one country to another and even within countries, but they have many common features including promises that, physicians will consider the interests of their patients above their own, will not discriminate against patients on the basis of race, religion or other human rights grounds, will protect the confidentiality of patient information, and will provide emergency care to anyone in need.

HISTORY OF MEDICAL ETHICS

Charak Samhita

In India, an ethical dimension of medical practice was first practiced by Charak, 2000 years ago. The student had to take an elaborate oath in a sacred ceremony. The oath covered every aspect of physician's code including his personal, academic, professional, and social conduct. It is a classic in the history of medical ethics. Great emphasis was placed on the training of physicians which took place in gurukuls or in universities such as Takshashila. In short, the Charak Oath was:

"Not for the self,
Not for the fulfilment of any worldly
Material desire or gain,
But solely for the good of suffering
Humanity,
I will treat my patient and excel all".

Ethics was not discussed as a separate subject in the manner of protocol for medical debate in the ancient texts. They were dissolved in the concepts and procedures which were invisible. The physician had to so conduct himself that the patient would look upon him as his father and mother.

Hippocrates (460–377 BC) a Greek physician, is considered the father of Western medicine. He set down a code of ethical conduct for physicians known as HIPPOCRATIC OATH, the oldest code of medical ethics. In the past, medical ethics were concerned mainly with physician-patient relationship, inter-physician relationship, referral of patients, and health care decisions. Hippocratic Oath, even after 25 centuries, is still a beacon light to guide us in our pursuit of an ethical practice. Though, Hippocrates is traditionally considered the author of this oath but, its authorship is actually unknown.

THE HIPPOCRATIC OATH

I swear by Apollo the physician, by Aesculapius, Hygeia and Panacea, and I take to witness all the Gods, all the Goddesses, to keep according to my ability and my judgment, the following Oath:

"To consider dear to me as my parents him who taught me this art; to live in common with him and if necessary, to share my goods with him to look upon his children as my own brothers, to teach them this art if they so desire without fee or written promise to impart to my sons and the sons of the master who taught me and the disciples who have enrolled themselves and have agreed to the rules of the profession, but to these alone, the percepts and the instruction. I will prescribe regimen for the good of my patients according to my ability and my judgment and never do harm to anyone. To please no one will I prescribe a deadly drug, nor give advice which may cause his death. Nor will I give a woman a pessary to procure abortion. But I will preserve the purity of my life and my art. I will not cut for stone, even for patients in whom the disease is manifest; I will leave this operation to be performed by practitioners (specialists in this art). In every house where I come I will enter only for the good of my patients, keeping myself far from all intentional ill-doing and all seduction, and especially from the pleasures of love with women or with men. Be they free or slaves. All that may come to my knowledge in the exercise of my profession or outside of any profession or in daily commerce with men, which ought not to be spread abroad. I will keep secret and will never reveal. If I keep this oath faithfully, may I enjoy my life and practice my art, respected by all men and in all times; but if I swerve from it or violate it, may the reverse be my lot".

THE ROLE OF THE WORLD MEDICAL ASSOCIATION

As the only international organization that seeks to represent all physicians, regardless of nationality or specialty, the World Medical Association (WMA) has undertaken the role of establishing general standards in medical ethics that are applicable worldwide. From its beginning in 1947, it has worked to prevent any recurrence of the unethical conduct exhibited by physicians in Nazi Germany and elsewhere. During the Second World War, gross violation of medical ethics was reported. The WMA's first task was to update the Hippocratic Oath for 20th century use; the result was the Declaration of Geneva, adopted at the WMA's second general assembly in 1948. It has been revised several times since, most recently in 1994. The second task was the development of an international code of medical ethics, which was adopted at the third general assembly in 1949 and revised in 1968 and 1983. This code is currently undergoing further revision. The next task was to develop ethical guidelines for research on human subjects. This took much longer than the first two documents; it was not until 1964 that the guidelines were adopted as the Declaration of Helsinki. This document has undergone periodic revision, most recently in 2000.

DECLARATION OF GENEVA

(As amended at Sydney, 1968)

- At time of being admitted as a member of the medical profession.
- I will solemnly pledge myself to consecrate my life to the service of humanity.
- I will give to my teachers the respect and gratitude which is their due.
- I will practice my profession with conscience and dignity.
- The health of my patient will be my first consideration.
- I will respect the secrets which are confided in me, even after the patient has died.
- I will maintain by all the means in my power, the honor and the noble traditions of the medical profession.
- My colleagues will be my brothers.
- I will not permit considerations of religion, nationality, race, party politics or social standing to intervene between my duty and my patient.
- I will maintain the utmost respect for human life from the time of conception even under threat; I will not use my medical knowledge contrary to the laws of humanity.
- I make these promises solemnly, freely and upon my honor.

INTERNATIONAL CODE OF MEDICAL ETHICS

Duties of Doctors in General

A doctor must always maintain the highest standards of professional conduct. A doctor must practice his profession uninfluenced by motives of profit. The following practices are deemed unethical:

- Any self-advertisement except such as is expressly authorized by the national code of medical ethics.
- Collaboration in any form of medical service in which the doctor does not have professional independence.
- Receiving any money in connection with services rendered to a patient other than a proper professional fee, even with the knowledge of the patient.
- Any act or advice which could weaken physical or mental resistance of a human being may be used only in his interest.
- A doctor is advised to use great caution in divulging discoveries or new techniques of treatment.
- A doctor should certify or testify, only to that, which he has personally verified.

Duties of Doctors to the Sick

- A doctor must always bear in mind the obligation of preserving human life.
- A doctor owes to his patient complete loyalty and all the resources of his science.
- Whenever an examination or treatment is beyond his capacity, he should summon another doctor who has the necessary ability.
- A doctor shall preserve absolute secrecy on all he knows about his patients because of the confidence entrusted in him.
- A doctor must give emergency care as a humanitarian duty unless he is assured that others are willing and able to give such care.

Duties of Doctors to Each Other

- A doctor ought to behave to his colleague as he would have them behave to him.
- A doctor must not entice patients from his colleagues.
- A doctor must observe the principles of "The Declaration of Geneva" approved by the World Medical Association.

DECLARATION OF HELSINKI

(Revised 1975)
Recommendations guiding medical doctors in biomedical research involving human subjects.

Introduction

It is the mission of the medical doctor to safeguard the health of the people. His or her knowledge and conscience are dedicated to the fulfilment of this mission.

The Declaration of Geneva of the World Medical Association binds the doctor with the words: The health of my patient will be my first consideration, and the International Code of Medical Ethics declares that, "Any act or advice which could weaken physical or mental resistance of a human being may be used only in his interest."

The purpose of biomedical research involving human subjects must be to improve diagnostic, therapeutic and prophylactic procedures and the understanding of the etiology and pathogenesis of the disease.

In current medical practice, most diagnostic, therapeutic or prophylactic procedures involve hazards. This applies a fortiori to biomedical research.

Medical progress is based on research which ultimately must rest in part on experimentation involving human subjects. In the field of biomedical research, a fundamental distinction must be recognized between medical research in which the aim is essentially diagnostic or therapeutic for a patient and medical research, the essential object of which is purely scientific and without direct diagnostic or therapeutic value to the person subjected to the research.

Special caution must be exercised in the conduct of research which may affect the environment, and the welfare of animals used for research must be respected.

Because it is essential that the results of laboratory experiments be applied to human beings to further scientific knowledge and to help suffering humanity, the World Medical Association has prepared the following recommendations as a guide to every doctor in biomedical research involving human subjects. They should be kept under review in the future. It must be stressed that the standards, as drafted, are only a guide to the physicians all over the world. Doctors are not relieved from criminal, civil, and ethical responsibilities under the laws of their own countries.

The NMC Shapath or Oath

The National Medical Commission (NMC) proposes replacing the age-old Hippocratic Oath with a modified "*Maharshi Charak Shapath*" for Indian medical graduates, emphasizing service to humanity and ethical conduct. Charaka, is a prominent figure in Ayurveda and considered as the father of Indian medical science. The NMC's Undergraduate Medical Education Board (UGMEB) proposed this change, citing the importance of upholding ethical standards and the principles. This is a set of instructions by a teacher to prospective students and includes respect for the autonomy and dignity of patients and also:

- Dedication to the service of humanity.
- Respect for human life and patient autonomy.
- Maintaining confidentiality and practicing with conscience and dignity.
- Upholding the honor and traditions of the medical profession.

Professional Secrecy

In medical ethics, secrecy is an important component. The informations received by physician have to be kept confidential and not to be divulged without the written consent of the patient. The doctor may fall into litigation if he fails to keep the medical secrecy.

Confidentiality of Medical Records

During the treatment of the patient whatever medical records have been originated, all have to be kept confidential. With the written permission of the patient only they can be made public.

They can be produced if court of law desires. On suspicion of negligence, police has the power to seize the medical records. The medical records can be used for academic benefit by keeping the identity of the patient secret.

Privileged Communication

The physician has to keep all the information confidential which has been acquired during the treatment of the patient, but to perform his legal duty and responsibility towards society; the disclosure of information called privileged communication may be required. It is in two ways:

1. *Absolute privilege*: Means any statement made in the court of law or parliament or state assembly.
2. *Qualified privilege*: Notification or births, deaths, reporting of a color-blind bus driver to manager of the bus depot, notifiable disease to municipal authorities is not a breach of secrecy or crime. The statement must not be malicious and must be made in good faith to a person who has right to receive it. Only relevant information is to be provided to the concerned authorities and not the whole case file of the patient.

Ethics of Relations with Fellow Colleagues

A few principles have been laid down to be observed while dealing with fellow colleagues:

- Hold your fellow colleagues as your brothers.
- Do not criticize your colleagues in the presence of patients.
- In the difference of opinion, talk to the colleague directly rather than through the patient.
- Do not entice the patient from your colleague.
- Send the patient back to your colleague after a consultation if he has been referred to you.
- Do not involve in fee splitting with your colleagues.
- Possibly an assistant should not open practice in the same area where his senior is practicing.

ETHICAL CHALLENGES IN HEALTH CARE

Ethical climate of the time and the current ethical dilemmas override geographical boundaries and are experienced in various forms around the world. Although, significant international consensus exists on some basic ethical issues such as the duty to seek informed consent, to protect the confidentiality of identifiable health data and to respect the rights of participants in clinical trials, new technologies continuously challenge that consensus. They require us to think, how widely accepted ethical principles can be applied to newly arising dilemmas. Health care technologies hold both a promise and a threat but, medical ethics is about balancing the harms and benefits of any intervention.

Today in India, the state and state-run institutions are no longer the focal point of health care development and provision. In fact, corporations and private providers, who are primarily unregulated, increasingly control the development of health care technology and its use. These developments give rise to ethical questions such as those related to appropriateness and equitable distribution of technologies, the need for setting priorities in research, the role of governments and/or independent agencies in regulating research and the use of health care technologies, and the control of intellectual properties.

Ethical Issues in Clinical Practice

Medical technologies dominate present day clinical practice. However, advances in technological know-how have not necessarily been accompanied by the systemic changes in public policy that are required to make these benefits accessible and affordable. In a largely market based health care system, there is a heavy burden on the poor to pay for services, this creates a dichotomy between those who have the means to pay and therefore, have access to technology based care and those who cannot afford to pay and do not have access. This dichotomy is particularly apparent in treatment of chronic diseases, including cases in which organ transplantation may be necessary. Another challenge that has emerged is linked to the fact that hi-tech treatment oriented solutions are given more attention, leading to the neglect of simpler prevention focussed responses.

Particular ethical issues have arisen in the use of technological means to prolong life. Families have gone to court demanding the right to withdraw life support and allow their loved ones to die a "natural" death. These documented cases represent just the tip of the iceberg.

Similarly, in the field of artificial reproduction and reproductive health, the possibility of using technological means to predict or even influence the characteristics of fetus has created a whole range of ethical debates. Debates on ethics of assisted reproductive technologies have brought to the fore the intersections between gender, society, national policy and regulation, and ethical practice.

Other ethical issues related to the use of technology in health care are in the arena of professional education, one example is the training of paraprofessional health workers to conduct medical abortions. A key challenge is the expansion of access to the benefits of health care technologies at the same time as ensuring their safe and scientific use. There are virtually no institutional mechanisms to monitor the use of technology by the broad array of health workers (registered and unregistered) practicing in countries like India.

Ethical Issues in Research

Research on health care technologies has been a hotly debated subject in bioethics, particularly in fields such as vaccine and drug development, genomics, artificial reproduction, and stem cell research. The burgeoning number of law suits in the western world is evidence of the contentiousness of these issues.

Other issues that are relevant in the discussions of the ethics of the research on health care technologies include the participation (or exclusion) of vulnerable as well as the quality of informed consent. There is often a very fine line between treatment/care and research because both are undertaken in the same setting by the same professional. Thus, the condition of consent, including the motivations for participation in research must be critically examined.

Setting priorities in research on health care technologies also pose several ethical dilemmas. Not only there is a need for attention to the ethical dimensions of medical research that is being undertaken, but the ethical implications of neglected areas of research also need to be considered. Developing affordable technologies and scaling up available affordable technologies have also not received adequate attention.

Ethical Issues in Public Health and Policy

Any technology, when used on a wide scale, has important consequences for the society. This is particularly evident in the case of food and agricultural technology. Large numbers of people, all over the world, still suffer from malnutrition. Developing nations have limited political clout when it comes to issues such as gene modification, intellectual property rights, biodiversity, conservation, and the erosion of traditional farming practices. Despite nearly a decade of discussions on labeling, marketing restrictions and banning genetically modified foods, many constituencies continue to view current regulations as extremely weak. Further, some argue that developing nations have become laboratories for research on food technologies, agriculture, and biotechnology. Others contend that these developments will make significant contributions to end world hunger, poverty, and malnutrition.

Another example of the profound impact of technology on human society is in the development and deployment of vaccines. Ensuring appropriate coverage, a necessary condition for the effective use of vaccines, brings into focus the state's roles and responsibilities in health care delivery. Firstly, the state has to enlist community support and participation, and, secondly, it has to make resources available to ensure coverage. Both these aspects raise several ethical dilemmas related to individual freedom, the use of state power as well as the welfare function of the state. Questions remain about the future availability of these vaccines and their costs.

While technology has vastly expanded the range of healthcare options, it has led to a massive increase in the cost of health care. Prohibitive costs have meant that health care has become out of reach for a significant proportion of the population, and this has led to indebtedness and further exacerbation of poverty. Paradoxically, the growth of medical technology has leveled international barriers. Medical tourism has become a popular policy option for developing countries that have a large trained professional workforce and access to technology. While it is conjectured that the revenues from medical tourism will benefit the local population, there is little documented evidence to support this contention. On the contrary, the development of hi-tech infrastructure necessary to promote medical tourism has led to human, financial and material resources being diverted away from institutions accessible and available to the local population. The superimposition of a highly modernized health care system on societies where primary care remains a pressing need is fraught with ethical dilemmas.

Ethical issues also emerge at the intersections of policies on trade and health. For example, intellectual property rights, compulsory licensing, and international trade agreements have had important implications for drug pricing and access in developing countries. The balancing of economic and health concerns merits close attention.

PRESENT DAY ETHICS: REGULATORY VACUUM

We are constantly witnessing new developments—medical tourism, corporate medicine, holistic medicine, and a host of others—whose regulatory and ethical dimensions are far from clear. The existing bodies such as the MCI, State Medical Councils, etc., were set up for different purposes long ago and have neither the competence nor the moral authority to uphold ethical standards in the practice of medicine. Unfortunately, our professional associations have failed to develop effective elaborate mechanisms to ensure the ethical conduct of members as the BMA and AMA have done to their credit in UK and USA.

Today, the medical profession is completely unprepared and untrained to look at the rising tide of clinical trials scientifically and get involved without violating the ethical code of the profession. The ultimate victim of unethical practices in medicine will be the people who may be unaware of their rights, unable to give informed consent and too poor to seek remedies.

The need for a body to uphold ethics in the practice of medicine has never been more acute than at present. It is not only most desirable but essential that a council for medical ethics is set up in India by an act of parliament to serve as an ethical watchdog of the medical profession for the benefit of public. The council should be empowered to deliberate on all complaints of unethical conduct of medical doctors and institutions and warn, admonish, censure, and order punishments; and its decisions should not be questionable in a court of law. Unless we take a bold step now, we shall be guilty of building a grand medical mansion on ethical sands, which would fall when the rains come and winds blow.

KEY LEARNING POINTS

- Ethical issues are very important in the present era of commercialization of medical services.
- Hippocratic Oath is considered as the oldest code of medical ethics.
- Maintain professional secrecy and confidentiality.
- Follow the ethical principles in research.
- A doctor must practice his profession uninfluenced by motives of profit.

BIBLIOGRAPHY

1. Ann Sommerville, Keynote address. The second national bioethics conference 2007, Moral and ethical imperatives of health care technologies: scientific, legal and socio-economic perspectives: Ind J Med Ethics. 2006;3:35-7.
2. Beauchamp TL, Childress JF. Principles of biomedical ethics, 3rd ed. New York and Oxford: Oxford University press; 1989.
3. Beecher HK. Ethics and clinical research New Engl J Med. 1966;274:1354-60.
4. Gillon R. Medical ethics: Four principles plus attention to scope. BMJ. 1994:309;184.
5. Indian Council of Medical Research Ethical guidelines for biomedical research on human subjects. New Delhi: ICMR: 2000. [online] Available from http://icmr.nic.in/ethical.pdf.
6. Kasturiaratchi N, Le R, Seeberg J, (Eds.), Health ethics in six SEAR countries. Health ethics in South-East Asia, Volume 1. WHO Regional office for South-East Asia. [online] Available from http:// www.who.int/ethics/regions/en/searo_ethics.pdf.
7. Medical Council of India. Indian Medical Council professional conduct Etiquette and Ethics Regulations, 2002. Gazette of India dated 06.04.02 part III section 4. [online] Available from http://www.medclik.com/his/mci.asp.
8. Sharma RK. Legal Aspects of Patient Care. 2003 medical ethics.
9. Singh S. Ethics in research: A box of tissues. Psychiatr Bull. 2007;31(3):81-2.
10. Valiathan MS, AS Paintal Memorial Oration. Indian J Chest Dis Allied Sci. 2006;48:7-11.
11. World Medical Association Declaration of Helsinki. Ethical Principles for Medical Research Involving Human Subjects. Adopted by the 18th World Medical Assembly. June 1964, amended in 1975, 1983, 1989, 1996 and 2000 with notes of clarification added in 2002 and 2004. [Cited 2007 Mar 12]. [online] Available from http://www.wma.net/e/policy/b3.htm.

2.1 Ethical Issues in Medical Research

NB Mathur

INTRODUCTION

Ethics are the set of rules that govern our expectations of our own behavior. Research institutions and their researchers must follow ethical guidelines in conducting publishing and governing research activities. Ethics in clinical research aim to implement the acceptable conditions for exposure of some individuals to acceptable risks for the benefit of society. Research on human subjects involves ethical, legal, and administrative concerns. The objectives of research ethics include (1) to guard/protect human participants, their dignity, rights and welfare; (2) to make sure that research is directed in a manner that assists welfares of persons, groups and/or civilization as a whole, and (3) to inspect research schemes for ethical reliability on controlling risk, protection of privacy of participants and ensure informed consent. Institutional ethics committees (EC) are responsible for overseeing that the rights of the subjects of research are protected and their dignity and welfare is ensured.

REGULATORY FRAMEWORK

To address these challenges, India has established a robust regulatory framework for research ethics. The primary regulatory body for research ethics in India is the Indian Council of Medical Research (ICMR). The ICMR has developed the National Ethical Guidelines for Biomedical and Health Research Involving Human Participants, which outlines the ethical principles that should be followed in research involving human participants.

In addition to the ICMR, other regulatory bodies in India that oversee research ethics have developed their own ethical guidelines for research. These include the Department of Science and Technology (DST), the Department of Biotechnology (DBT), and the Central Drugs Standard Control Organization (CDSCO). These cover a wide range of topics including animal research, stem cell research, and genetic research.

INDIAN COUNCIL OF MEDICAL RESEARCH GUIDELINES

These guidelines have included the four fundamental principles of ethics viz. autonomy, non-maleficence, beneficence, and justice. The guidelines include chapters on general principles of research ethics, ethical issues, responsible conduct of research, ethical review process including constitution of institutional EC, informed consent process, vulnerability and vulnerable population, clinical trials of drugs and other interventions, public health research, social and behavioral sciences research for health, human genetics testing, biological materials, biobanking and datasets, and research during emergencies and disasters.

General Principles of Ethics in Research

- *Principle of essentiality:* The research should be for the advancement of knowledge that benefits patients and all others in healthcare as also the ecological wellbeing of the planet.
- *Principles of voluntariness, informed consent, and community agreement:* The participants should be well-informed of the objective and nature of research, their role, any benefits and harms, consequences and all the risks involved. It should be ensured that the information to participants avoids technical jargon and is in the language they understand. They should have the right to choose to voluntarily participate or not in the research. Before asking for written consent, the prospective participant must be explained about the research and any queries should be answered. The written Informed Consent Document (ICD) has two parts—(1) Participant information sheet (PIS) providing information on known facts about research which has relevance to participation. (2) Informed Consent Form—an acknowledgement by the study subject that the PIS has been understood and the person is willing to be enrolled. For children between 7 and 12 years, verbal assent is required and for 12–18 years old, written assent signed by the child is required. Essential elements of ICD are given in **Box 2.1.1**.
- *Principle of nonexploitation:* Research participants should be compensated or remunerated for their involvement. Research protocol should state provision of compensation through insurance or any other means such as free treatment covering all risks. The population which is vulnerable or dependent must be protected from any harm or possibility of abuse.
- *Principle of privacy and confidentiality:* Research data should not disclose identity of the participant and should ensure privacy, autonomy, and dignity of participants.
- *Principle of precaution and risk minimization:* All precautions should be taken to prevent research participant from any harm and risk should be minimized **(Table 2.1.1)**. Beneficence and nonmaleficence are principles of maximizing the likely benefits and minimizing the likely harms to the participants of research. Harms to the participant could be physical, mental trauma or embarrassment, social disadvantage, breach of privacy and loss of confidential data.

Box 2.1.1: Essential elements of informed consent document (ICD).

- Statement mentioning that it is research
- Purpose and method of research
- Duration of participation, frequency of contact, number of participants, type of data collected, and methods
- Expected benefits to participants or community as outcome of research
- Any risks, discomfort, or inconvenience from participation
- Extent of confidentiality of records
- Any payment for participation in research
- In case of injury related to research, the treatment will be free or compensation will be provided
- Freedom to withdraw from research at any time
- How to contact members of research team for questions related to research and chairperson or member secretary for ethical issues

Table 2.1.1: Categorization of risk in research.	
Less than minimal risk	• Research on databases available in public domain, meta-analysis • Probability of anticipated harm or discomfort is nil
Minimal risk	• Research related to clinical history and examination, investigations such as X-ray, examining body fluids such as urine and saliva noninvasively or sampling hair • Probability of anticipated harm or discomfort is as in routine life in general population or as in performing routine tests where serious harm or adverse effect is unlikely
Minor increase over minimal risk or low risk	• Routine research on children and adolescents and persons not capable of giving consent • New diagnostic technique on pregnant and lactating women. Denying or postponing the required proven care to the controls. Minimally invasive procedures causing brief pain such as drawing blood for testing • Personal identifiable data causing social risk, psychological harm, and discomfort • Probability of anticipated harm or discomfort is little more than minimal
More than minimal risk or high risk	• Research involving interventional study using drugs, devices, or invasive procedures (lumbar puncture, biopsy, endoscopic procedure, IV sedation for diagnostic procedure) • Probability of anticipated harm or discomfort is more than minimal

- *Principle of professional competence:* Researchers should be qualified in the field of research. There should be no bias in study design, analysis and interpretation of data, and publication of research. The researcher should be open to sharing results and accepting constructive feedback.
- *Principle of accountability and transparency:* The research should be transparent and conducted honestly. There should be honesty with the study subjects, methods used, and results presented. All agreements and promises with stakeholders must be honestly abided and no false promises made. The research data should be available for 5 years for scrutiny.
- *Principle of the maximization of public interest and of distributive justice:* The research should be used for benefit of all humans irrespective of social class.
- *Principle of institutional arrangements:* Institutional arrangements required for the research should be made transparent. Institutional EC **(Table 2.1.2)** should be constituted in every institution conducting research. The institutional EC should have 7–15 members and quorum is constituted by five members, including at least one is from outside the institution. The EC needs to register itself with the Ministry of Health and Family Welfare, Department of Health Research as per the Drugs and Clinical Trial Rules 2019, chapter IV, Rule 122DD and the amendment of the Drugs and Cosmetic Rules through GSR 72(E) in 2013. The registration, if provisional, is valid for 2 years and if final for 5 years. The EC members include medical, scientific, nonmedical, and nonscientific persons. They are responsible for protecting the rights and safety of research subjects in clinical trials. The EC should grant approval to the protocol after reviewing and satisfying itself about the investigators, resources available in the institution, appropriateness of study design, adequacy of information for consent, and protection of confidentiality of subjects. The EC is responsible for analyzing and reporting

Table 2.1.2: Composition of Ethics Committee (EC) and qualification of members conforming with the national guidelines.

• Chairperson • Vice Chairman (Optional) • Nonaffiliated to institution	• Should have earlier served in an EC • May be from any field
Member Secretary from the same institution. Having an additional secretary is optional	• Well-versed with ethical issues and research • Should be communicative and willing to put in extra time
Basic medical scientists from same or other institutions	For drug trials a pharmacologist is preferable
Clinicians from same or other institutions	Reputed, trained, and qualified experts
Legal experts from same or other institutions	Recognized degree in law preferably with some training in medicolegal field
Social scientist, philosopher, or theologian from same or other institutions	Degree, expertise, or training in any of the following fields: Social, religious, behavioral, or philosophical. Should preferably be working with a health-related nongovernment organization familiar with local moral and cultural issues
Lay persons not pursuing career in medical or health science in the previous 5 years and from other institution	Should be from the local community or a community representative, literate, familiar with local language, moral and cultural issues. Should preferably be pursuing some community welfare activity

serious adverse events. The records of EC can be inspected by the Central Drugs Standard Control Organization and any queries raised need to be answered by EC.

- *Principle of public domain:* The results of research should be made public. The trial should be made public before start of recruitment via clinical trial registry systems such as www.ctri.in. Responsible publication of research involves responsibly publishing to promote and uptake research or knowledge.
- *Principle of compliance:* The ethical principles should be complied with by all those associated with the research.

ADVANTAGES OF RESEARCH ETHICS

The basic objectives of research are promoted by research ethics. Mutual trust and respect among researchers and participants are crucial as research requires cooperative working in an accountable manner without jeopardizing the rights and welfare of participants. Ethics in research are the foundation of positive public opinion and public support for clinical research. Ethical research enhances reliability of clinical researchers among public.

CHALLENGES

One of the significant challenges facing ethics in clinical research in India is the lack of awareness about research ethics, ethical guidelines, and principles that govern research. The researcher may not have the necessary training to conduct research ethically. This can lead to unethical practices, such as exploiting research participants or failing to obtain informed consent. In some cases, researchers may hold a position of authority or influence over research participants, which can make it difficult for participants to refuse to participate in the research or to report any ethical violations. This hampers a fair and unbiased research process. Another issue is the functioning of institutional ethics committees, which may not be optimal.

EDUCATION AND TRAINING IN RESEARCH ETHICS

An important step in research ethics is the promotion of research ethics education and training. Universities, medical colleges and research institutions in India should offer courses and workshops on research ethics, which provide researchers with the necessary knowledge and skills to conduct research ethically. The ICMR offers online course on Ethics Review of Health Research which is technically supported by the World Health Organization (https://nie.gov.in).

CONCLUSION

In conclusion, ethics in research in India require ongoing attention and improvement. There are challenges to ethical research practices, such as the lack of awareness among researchers, suboptimally functioning EC and power imbalances between researcher and participant. However, the regulatory framework and the registration of EC by research institutions are encouraging. By continuing to promote education and training in research ethics, establishing EC in all institutions undertaking research, emphasizing on well-prepared project initiation documentation (PID) and involving research participants in the research process, ethics in medical research can be further improved.

KEY LEARNING POINTS

- Indian Council for Medical Research (ICMR) has published the National Ethical Guidelines for Biomedical and Health Research Involving Human Participants.
- These guidelines have included 12 general principles of ethics in medical research elaborating the four fundamental principles of ethics viz. autonomy, nonmaleficence, beneficence, and justice.
- The research participants should be well-informed of the objective and nature of research, their role, any benefits and harms, consequences and risks involved, and written consent obtained by the researcher using the written Informed Consent Document.
- Institutional ethics committees are responsible for ensuring that the research protects the rights, and welfare of the human subjects.
- There is a need to promote Research Ethics Education and the ICMR offers online course on Ethics Review of Health Research (https://nie.gov.in).

BIBLIOGRAPHY

1. Central Drugs Standard Control Organisation. (2019). Guidelines for Ethics Committee. [online] Available from https://cdsco.gov.in/opencms/resources/UploadCDSCOWeb/2018/UploadPublic_NoticesFiles/Guidelines%20for%20Ethics%20Committee%20CDSCO.pdf [Last accessed May, 2024].
2. Department of Science and Technology, Government of India. (2017). Guidelines for Research Ethics. [online] Available from https://dst.gov.in/sites/default/files/Guidelines_for_Research_Ethics_2017.pdf [Last accessed May, 2024].
3. Indian Council of Medical Research. (2017). National Ethical Guidelines for Biomedical and Health Research Involving Human Participants. [online] Available from https://www.icmr.gov.in/neglected_diseases/NT/ICMR_National_Ethical_Guidelines_2017.pdf [Last accessed May, 2024].
4. New Delhi Indian Council of Medical Research and Department of Biotechnology. (2017). National Guidelines For Stem Cell Research. [online] Available from https://dbtindia.gov.in/sites/default/files/National_Guidelines_StemCellResearch-2017.pdf [Last accessed May, 2024].

3

CHAPTER

Rights/Duties of Patients and Doctors

Prasant Kumar Saboth, Murli Janardan Sabath

INTRODUCTION

There is an international consensus growing toward ensuring entitlement of a patient to certain amount of protection from physicians, healthcare providers, and the State. Various countries and societies have already initiated codification of these in form of Charter of Patient's Rights. Rights can be described as those legal, social, or ethical principles of entitlement which forms the fundamental freedom one is allowed of. As per Merriam Webster's dictionary, "*Rights are something to which one has a just claim*, in other words, *a privilege to which one is justly entitled*; something that one may properly claim as due".

The United Nations General Assembly held in Paris on 10 December 1948, recognized that the foundation of freedom, justice, and peace in the world largely depends upon the inherent dignity and equal and inalienable rights of all members of human family. The Universal Declaration of Human Rights (UDHR) proclaimed by the UN General Assembly is considered as a milestone document in the history of human rights which is applicable as a common standard of achievement for all people and all nations.

THE INDIAN PERSPECTIVE

Inspired by international charters and guided by national level provisions, the National Human Rights Commission (NHRC) has recommended Charter of Patient's Rights, the draft of which was shared by the Ministry of Health and Family Welfare (MoHFW) with government of all States and Union Territories (UTs) for review. This document primarily acts as a guide for the Union as well as State Governments to formulate concrete operational mechanisms to protect patient's rights and to make these rights functional and enforceable by law.

The Charter of Patient's Rights has been drafted with an aim to educate citizens and generate widespread awareness among public about the kind of treatment they deserve as patients and human beings, in healthcare settings and what they should expect from the government and their healthcare providers. Citizens can play a vital role in elevating the standards of healthcare if they have adequate awareness of their rights and if they know their responsibilities since they also have an obligation to respect the privileges of the healthcare providers.

Health being a state subject, it is for the respective State/UT government to develop effective operational mechanism to adopt, implement, and monitor the Charter of Patients' Rights along with allocation of budget for promotion of Patients' Rights Charter and setting up grievance redressal mechanism for patients. NHRC advisory also recommends that respective State/UT government to prominently display the Charter of Patients' Rights in both, public and private healthcare facilities as well as on their respective websites.

The National Council for Clinical Establishments which has been setup in the MoHFW under the Clinical Establishments Act, 2010 in the year 2021, has further updated the aforesaid Charter of Patients' Rights and shared the same with the States and UTs for implementation, where the Clinical Establishments Act is applicable.

National Health Authority (NHA) is mandated to implement the *Ayushman Bharat Pradhan Mantri-Jan Arogya Yojana* (AB PM-JAY) which empanels a pan-India network of >25,000 hospitals for providing healthcare services to the scheme's beneficiaries. NHA has shared the Charter of Patients' Rights recommended by NHRC and issued a communication to various State Health Agencies (SHA) to ensure observance of Patients' Rights Charter across all empaneled hospitals and to display it at prominent areas in the hospital premises.

CHARTER OF PATIENTS' RIGHTS

The National Council for Clinical Establishments has approved the following rights of patient and his/her representative:

Right to Information

- The doctor and the healthcare establishment should ensure that every patient is provided adequate and relevant information such as nature and cause of illness, provisional as well as confirmed diagnosis, investigations proposed and decision for clinical management and its possible complications.
- The treating physician has a duty to ensure that this information is communicated to the patient in a simplified manner in an easy language known to them and at their level of understanding.
- The patients and their caretakers also have a right to know the identity and professional status of care providers in the hospital, hence the hospital authorities have a responsibility to provide such details routinely for information of the public.
- Every patient and his/her designated caretaker have the right to access factual information regarding the expected cost of treatment and on completion of treatment, to receive an itemized bill with details of expenses along with receipt of payments made.
- Every clinical establishment shall display details of services and rates to be charged at a conspicuous place, both in local as well as in English language.

Right to Records and Reports

- A patient or his caregiver is entitled to access his/her medical records and investigation reports while being hospitalized and the hospital should provide the same within 72 hours when required.

- The medical records and reports will be made available to the patient at the time of discharge. Copies of the same may also be made available, wherever applicable, after paying appropriate fees for photocopying.
- In cases of death, the hospital authorities have a responsibility to provide the authorized relative of the patient with death certificate and case summary along with copies of investigations.

Right to Emergency Medical Care

All hospitals both in the government and in the private sector are duty bound to provide basic emergency medical care to an injured person without demanding or waiting for any payment/advance. Supreme Court in its judgment on Parmanand Katara versus Union of India (1989) case has made it clear that basic emergency care should be provided to such patients irrespective of their paying capacity.

Right to Informed Consent

- Prior to any potentially hazardous test, invasive procedure or complex treatment which carries certain risks, it is the duty of the treating doctor to provide all relevant information to the patient and his/her caregiver regarding the main risks that are involved in the procedure.
- Unless the patient/caregiver is convinced and an informed consent has been obtained in writing in the manner explained under Drugs and Cosmetic Act Rules 2016, the treating doctor may not proceed with the procedure or treatment.
- It is the duty of the hospital management to ensure that a proper policy is in place to provide consent forms for patients in an obligatory manner and all doctors are instructed to seek informed consent of the patients and allow their participation in the decision-making process.

Right to Confidentiality, Personal Dignity, and Privacy

- The hospital management has a duty to ensure that all data concerning the patients should be kept under secured safe custody and insulated from data theft and leakage.
- Healthcare providers must maintain strict confidentiality about any health-related information of their patients, unless essential in specific circumstances in the interest of public health considerations or if required in court of law.
- Patients have the right to their privacy, the healthcare establishment should ensure that its staff upholds the human dignity of every patient in all situations.
- During physical examination of a female patient by a male practitioner, presence of another female person or attendant should be ensured at all times.

Right to Second Opinion

- Every patient has the right to seek a second opinion or consultation from any clinician of his/her choice.

- The healthcare establishment should respect the patient's right and provide all necessary medical records and information required for seeking such opinion without any extra cost or delay.

Right to Non-discrimination

- Every patient has the right to receive treatment without any discrimination based on his or her illnesses or conditions, including human immunodeficiency virus (HIV) status or other health condition, religion, caste, ethnicity, gender, age, sexual orientation, linguistic, or geographical/social origins.
- The hospital management has a duty to ensure that all doctors and other staff are adequately oriented to avoid any form of discriminatory behavior or treatment with any person under the hospital's care.

Right to Safety and Quality of Care

- Patients have the right to a safe and secure environment within the hospital premises.
- Every patient has a right to receive appropriate healthcare as per currently accepted standards, norms, and standard guidelines in a professional manner in complete consonance with the principles of medical ethics.
- Patients and their caretakers have a right to seek redressal in case of perceived medical negligence or damage caused due to deliberate deficiency in service delivery.

Right to Choose Alternative Treatment Options, if Available

- Patients and their caretakers, after considering all aspects of their clinical situation, may choose between alternative treatment options, if these are available.
- A patient may take the option of refusing care after considering all available options, however, with responsibility for any consequences arising out of such a decision.
- Patient cannot be forced to buy medicines from hospital pharmacy or undergo tests in laboratory designated by hospital.

Right to Patient Education

- Patients have the right to be educated about facts relevant to his/her medical condition and healthy lifestyle practices, their rights and responsibilities, entitlements in term of appropriate health insurance schemes and how to seek redressal of their grievances.
- The hospital management and treating physician have a duty to provide such education according to standard procedure and communicate in simple and easy language the patients understand.

Right to Protection and Compensation for Patients Involved in Clinical Trials, Biomedical, and Health Research

- Every person/patient who is approached to participate in a clinical trial has a right to due protection in this context.

- All clinical trials must be conducted in compliance with the protocols and Good Clinical Practice Guidelines issued by Central Drugs Standard Control Organization, Directorate General of Health Services, Government of India as well as all applicable statutory provisions of Amended Drugs and Cosmetics Act, 1940 and Rules, 1945.
- Participation of patients in clinical trials must always be voluntary based on informed consent, given after provision of all relevant information.

Right to Grievance Redressal

- Every patient and their caregivers have the right to give feedback, make comments, or lodge complaints about the healthcare they are receiving or had received from a doctor or hospital.
- In case they feel aggrieved due to infringement of any of their rights mentioned in this charter, they may lodge a written complaint with the concerned official designated for the purpose by the healthcare establishment.
- They can further complain with an official mechanism constituted by the government such as Patients' Rights Tribunal Forum or Clinical Establishments Regulatory Authority as the case may be.
- The patient has right to a fair and prompt hearing of his/her concern and may appeal to a higher authority in the healthcare provider organization and also insist on the outcome of the complaint in writing.

RESPONSIBILITIES OF PATIENT

While promoting their rights, patients, and caretakers should follow their responsibilities toward the hospital and healthcare providers so that doctors and hospital staff can perform their work satisfactorily.

- *Honest disclosure of information:* Patients should disclose all health-related information to their doctor, without concealing any relevant information, so that correct diagnosis and treatment can be facilitated.
- *Treatment compliance:* Patients should not only cooperate with the doctor during examination, diagnostic tests, and treatment, but should also follow doctor's advice and instructions.
- *Cooperation with hospital and hospital staff:* Patients should follow the appointment time, cooperate with hospital staff and fellow patients, avoid creating disturbance to other patients, and maintain cleanliness in the hospital.
- *Payment of fees or other charges on time*: Patients should pay their dues in time as and when asked for by the hospital or the treating doctor as the case may be.
- *Refrain from violence against doctor and hospital staff:* Patients should respect the dignity of the doctor and other hospital staff as human beings and as professionals. Whatever the grievance may be, patient/caregivers should not resort to violence in any form and damage or destroy any property of the hospital or the service provider.

  The rights and responsibilities of patients are given in **Table 3.1**.

Table 3.1: Rights and responsibilities of patients.

Rights of patients	*Responsibilities of patients*
• *Right to information*: ○ Adequate relevant information about the nature, cause of illness, proposed investigations and care, expected results of treatment, possible complications, and expected costs ○ Information on the rates charged for each type of service provided and facilities available ○ Every clinical establishment shall display details of services and rates to be charged at a conspicuous place, both in local as well as in English language • *Right to clinical records and itemized bill*: Access a copy of the case papers, patient records, investigation reports and detailed bill (itemized) • *Right to informed consent*: Doctor has to obtain informed consent of the patient prior to specific tests/treatment (e.g. surgery, chemotherapy, etc.) • *Right to second opinion*: Patient has right to seek second opinion from an appropriate clinician of his/her choice, with records and information being provided by the treating hospital • *Right to confidentiality, human dignity, and privacy during treatment*: To have ensured presence of a female person, during physical examination of a female patient by a male practitioner • Right to nondiscrimination about treatment and behavior on the basis of human immunodeficiency virus (HIV) status • Right to choose alternative treatment if options are available • Right to proper referral and transfer • Release of dead body of a patient cannot be denied for any reason by the hospitals • *Right to choose source for obtaining medicines or tests*: Patient cannot be forced to buy medicines from hospital pharmacy or undergo tests in laboratory designated by hospital • Right to protection and compensation for patients involved in clinical trials, biomedical, and health research • Right to patient education • *Right to be heard and seek redressal*: Every hospital shall establish a grievance redressal mechanism to address grievances of the patients in a time bound manner	• To provide all health-related information • To cooperate with doctors during examination, treatment • To follow all instructions • To pay hospitals fees as agreed on time • To respect dignity of doctors and other hospital staff • Never resort to violence

PROFESSIONAL CODE OF CONDUCT

The Ethics and Medical Registration Board of the National Medical Commission has made certain regulations emphasizing professional conduct of Registered Medical Practitioners which has been published under the Gazette Notification named *"National Medical Commission Registered Medical Practitioner (Professional Conduct) Regulations, 2023*. As per these regulations it shall be deemed that each registered medical practitioner at the time of application has read and agreed to abide by the regulations made by NMC.

The erstwhile Medical Council of India in 2002 also adopted similar regulations for professional conduct & etiquette of Medical practitioners.

As per the NMC regulations, a physician shall not aid or abet or commit any unethical acts as given below:

- *Self Advertising*: A medical professional must not directly or indirectly engage in self advertising for financial gains.
- Running an open shop (dispensing of drugs and appliances by physicians) is unethical.
- Rebates and commission in any form or kind such accepting gifts, gratuity, commission, etc., are strictly unethical and prohibited for all medical professionals.
- Physicians should avoid unethical practices such as practice of secret remedies, euthanasia, violation of human rights, etc.
- In relation to pharmaceutical companies, medical professions are prohibited from accepting any gift, travel facilities, hospitality, or monetary gains.
- *Adultery or improper conduct:* Abuse of professional position by committing adultery or improper conduct with a patient or by maintaining an improper association with a patient will render a physician liable for disciplinary action as provided under the relevant sections of the National Medical Commission Act or the concerned State Medical Commission rules.
- A medical practitioner shall not endorse any drug or product of the industry publicly. Any study conducted on the efficacy or otherwise of such products shall be presented to and/ or through appropriate scientific bodies or published in appropriate scientific journals in a proper way.
- A registered medical practitioner should not get involved in sex determination or illegal abortion.
- A physician should not issue medical certificates without any substantial reasons and evidence.

DUTIES OF DOCTORS

A registered medical practitioner with qualification as approved by the National Medical Commission has to make declaration to follow the Code of Medical Ethics in his professional activities. The various chapters under these regulations elaborate the wide ambit of duties a physician owes in general, toward his patients, toward his colleagues in profession, etc., along with legal and disciplinary implications.

The duties of medical professionals are given in **Table 3.2**.

Table 3.2: Duties of medical professionals.

Duties in general	*Duties toward patients*	*Duties toward other doctors and paramedical staff*	*Duties toward public*
• Every self employed RMP shall display his/her unique registration ID assigned by EMRB in the prescription or other receipts issued to the patients. The seal/stamp shall be clearly placed below the RMP's signature • Maintaining good medical practice • Membership in Medical Society and participation in Continuing Medical Education Program organized by professional bodies for at least 30 hours every 05 years • *Maintenance of medical records:* Every physician shall maintain the medical records pertaining to his/her indoor patients for a period of 3 years. If requested by patients or their authorized attendants or legal authorities, the documents should be issued within 72 hours • Every RMP shall prescribe using generic names of drugs written legibly and in judicious dosage • Consultation fees, if charged shall be made known to patient before examination or treatment. Does not apply to those in Govt service	• Obligations to the sick. No physician shall arbitrarily refuse treatment to a patient • A physician should maintain patience, delicacy, and professional secrecy • The patient must not be neglected. Once having undertaken a case, the physician should not neglect the patient, nor should he withdraw from the case without giving adequate notice to the patient and his family • The boundaries of doctor–patient relationship should be respected and especially sexual boundary violations must be avoided	• Unnecessary consultations should be avoided except in doubtful and difficult conditions • While referring a patient to a specialist, the attending physician should provide a case summary of the patient to the specialist, who should then communicate his opinion in writing to the attending physician • *Fees and other charges:* A physician shall clearly display his fees and other charges on the board of his chamber and/or the hospitals he is visiting. However, no patient to be refused treatment in emergency due to inability to pay • All physicians should be ready to render gratuitous service to all physicians and their immediate family, dependents in time of need	• Physicians, as good citizens, are responsible for dissemination of appropriate scientific advice on public health issues in public interest without self promotion • They should cooperate with the authorities in administration of sanitary/public health laws and regulations • A physician should notify the concerned public health authorities of every case of communicable disease under his care, in accordance with the laws/rules and regulations • When an epidemic occurs, a physician should not abandon his duty for fear of contracting the disease himself

SUMMARY

Hospitals and medical professionals have a responsibility toward patients and their caretakers to render the requisite care with due compassion and sincerity while making every effort to respect their personal dignity, privacy, and all other rights. Patients while promoting their rights too owe a moral obligation to follow the laid down principles of the hospital environment and allow doctors and healthcare providers to perform their role without any obstruction and in a satisfactory manner. There is a need for government and healthcare organization to build an environment to educate the patients and their care givers regarding these rights and responsibilities.

KEY LEARNING POINTS

- Rights and responsibilities of patients have to be defined and every healthcare worker should be aware of them.
- Hospitals should make adequate efforts to educate patients about their rights and to make them aware of their responsibilities too.
- Confidentiality, personal dignity, and privacy of patients should be respected. Presence of a female attendant or another female should be ensured if a female patient is examined by a male medical professional.
- Informed consent of patients or their family members should be obtained prior to each procedure or intervention, where risks are involved.

BIBLIOGRAPHY

1. Universal Declaration of Human Rights (UDHR). United Nations General Assembly; 1948.
2. Health Care as a Human Right. National Human Rights Commission, India; 2015.
3. Ministry of Health and Family Welfare. (2022). Charter of patients' rights. [online] Available from https://pib.gov.in/PressReleaseIframePage.aspx?PRID=1797699 [Last accessed May, 2024].
4. Clinical Establishment Act; 2010.
5. National Medical Commission Registered Medical Practitioner (Professional Conduct) Regulations, 2023- reg. (https://www.nmc.org.in/rules-regulations/national-medical-commission-registered-medical-practitioner-professional-conduct-regulations-2023-reg/).
6. Patients Charter by National Accreditation Board for Hospitals (NABH). [online] Available from https://nabh.co/Images/pdf/Patient_Charter-DMAI_NABH.pdf [Last accessed on Nov, 2024].
7. The Consumer Protection Act; 1986.
8. Drugs and Cosmetic Act 1940, Rules 2016.
9. Protocols and Good Clinical Practice Guidelines. Central Drugs Standard Control Organisation, Directorate General of Health Services, Govt. of India. [online] Available from https://cdsco.gov.in/opencms/resources/UploadCDSCOWeb/2018/UploadImmunization/Clinical.pdf [Last accessed on Nov, 2024].
10. Indian Council of Medical Research. National Ethical Guidelines for Biomedical and Health Research Involving Human Participants. New Delhi; 2017.

CHAPTER 4

Legal Hurdles in Medical Practice

Suchismita Mallick

INTRODUCTION

"Ignorantia juris non excusat"—as the Latin dictum follows, ignorance of law is not excused and liability of person is not escaped if he is unaware of the law. Therefore, it is of paramount importance to be aware of not only medicine but the laws relating to one's medical practice as well.

Under the ambit of the Article 21 of the golden triangle of the Indian constitution which embodies the right to life and as per the World Health Organization (WHO) declaration of health being a fundamental right, right to life and health is an integral part of human life and therefore protected by the law. Under the Indian constitution, health is primarily a state subject. There are ethical practice guidelines laid down by regulatory bodies, for example, the National Medical Commission (NMC) at the individual level. The various legislations such as the Clinical Establishment Act (CEA), the Drugs and Cosmetic Act (DCA), and Pre-Conception and Pre-Natal Diagnostic Techniques (PCPNDT) Act, the Indian Council of Medical Research (ICMR) rules relating to research and judicial pronouncements, especially concerning fundamental rights, all add up to the legal side of clinical practice. The legal angle has gained more importance with deterioration of the doctor-patient relationship, evolving from a paternalistic relationship to a consumer-based model in current times of commercialization of medical practice and corporatization of healthcare facilities. The fiduciary nature of the relationship and the implicit trust between the physician and the patient has been eyed skeptically. With increased patient awareness, civil and criminal laws and special acts to regulate the medical profession have created several legal hurdles for a clinician.

CODE OF ETHICS REGULATIONS

The NMC follows the Professional Conduct, Etiquette and Ethics Regulations, 2002, implements it for all physicians. It describes in detail the duties of a physician to their patients in its eight chapters. It includes duties relating to consultation of patients, to the fellow colleagues, to the public, unethical acts, and misconduct.

Duties of the clinician include maintaining good character, following the principles of good medical practice, confidentiality, prescribing drugs, recordkeeping for 3 years, and to abide by the law of the land. The medical records may either be computerized or noncomputerized system. Clinicians have a legal and professional obligation to complete the certificate or medicolegal report truthfully.

Ethical guidelines for biomedical research on human participants, 2006—the principles of voluntariness, informed consent, confidentiality, transparency, risk minimization, and compensation need to be maintained in medical research.

Unethical acts are illegal advertising, patenting, or copyrighting medical applications and dealing with pharmaceutical companies for monetary benefits or favors where conflicting interests are present. Active euthanasia/mercy killing is prohibited in our country. However, passive euthanasia, whereby withholding treatment will lead to demise of the patient and the concept of an advance will, whereby the patient can direct the court to withhold life support in his critical state, is gaining acceptance after the landmark Aruna Shanbaug case and Common Cause Case. A medical board of three medical experts, a waiting period of 15 days, and a division bench of two judges is the process through which these cases have to be decided.

The acts of misconduct makes the doctor liable for disciplinary actions from the medical commission such as deregistration or suspension. It includes violation of regulations and laws, for example, PCPNDT, failure to maintain confidentiality, discrimination against patients, not maintaining records or not taking informed consent for procedures, conviction by the court of law, and failure to follow ICMR guidelines in clinical drug trials.

Informed consent is also extremely important in the eyes of the law—what is consented to is not actionable (volenti non fit injuria) is a principle of tort law and liability of a doctor is much diminished in its presence. The word "informed consent" was first used by Justice Cardozo in 1957 in a medical malpractice suit of Salgo vs. Leland Stanford Jr University Board of Trustees. The informed consent has two categorical parts, the information and the consent. It can also be described in five parts: Competence, disclosure, understanding, voluntariness, and consent. The judgement of the Supreme Court in Indian Medical Association vs. VP Shantha and others brought the medical profession under the Consumer Protection Act (CPA) of 1986 and absence of an informed consent was a medical service deficiency under section 2 and therefore a vital part of a legal defense. The form must show the diagnosis, nature, and extent of the procedure, written in simple comprehensible language, preferably in vernacular and legible handwriting. It has to be obtained well in advance except for emergency procedures and not on the day of operation. It should ideally be signed by the patient if he is a competent adult. In case of being illiterate, thumb impression can be taken and witnessed and attested by a third party with no conflict of interest. The consent also needs to be signed by the physician as this is an agreement which is bilateral in nature between the concerned parties and needs to be signed by both the patient and the physician. The other essentials of a consent include documentation of date and time, patient information—name, age, and registration number, doctor information—name and registration number, witness information—name and signature of witness, type of surgery, anesthesia, blood transfusions, risks, need for perioperative critical care and ventilator, whether the patient will be photographed and information relating to the case will be used for academic purpose or publication or for teaching purposes for medical courses, the method of disposal of tissues or body parts, risks and benefits and alternate procedures, and consequences of refusal to treatment, all need to be mentioned. It also should document that all of the above facts were explained to the patient in a comprehensible and simple way. An incomplete consent form, and blanket consent or no consent in case of repeat procedure or change of procedure are all potential sources of litigation for a clinician and results in a weak case in the court of law.

In spite of this elaborate code of ethics and guidelines, the unethical acts, especially concerning the pharmaceutical industry and various other deviations from the abovementioned guidelines, even more so with rampant practice of unlicensed medicine, continue due to lack of adequate monitoring and reporting. In 2023, the NMC introduced the professional conduct regulation which tried to handle this with rules concerning generic drug prescriptions and stringencies concerning the sponsorship of medical conferences by pharmaceutical companies, but it has been put on hold. In rural or peripheral setups, the standard guideline of maintaining the doctor-patient ratio, where a general practitioner can see maximum of 40 patients in 200 minutes and a specialist, 20 patients in 200 minutes is recommended for proper functioning of a medical facility. However, the ratio is disturbed and the huge patient load and the multitude of tasks that a doctor faces inevitably lead to deviation from guidelines and negligence issues.

IMPORTANT LEGISLATIONS

It is troublesome for a physician to set up a clinic with such varied rules and regulations and corruption is prevalent in these sectors where the very purpose of the acts are overlooked. Few of the Acts relevant to medical practice—the PCPNDT Act, Pharmacy Act, DCA, Narcotic Drugs and Psychotropic Substance (NDPS) Act, Mental Health Act, Transplantation of Human Organs and Tissues Act (THOTA), Epidemic Disease Act, and National AIDS Control Organization (NACO) guidelines.

Drugs and Cosmetics Act (DCA): The shortcomings of this act remain over-the-counter drug selling in India, corruption in giving license for setting up of pharmacy, inadequate pharmacovigilance, improper storage and handling of drugs and vaccines, and lack of reporting of adverse events to drugs. Medical device regulation is usually under DCA. Handful of devices are regulated and most devices are not regulated for safety standards. Medical technology is mostly imported and follows its own safety standard guidelines and therefore the physician is at risk using them.

Insurance Regulatory and Development Authority (IRDA)—majority of insurance providers are funded by third-party agencies and there is lack of uniformity in the insurance provided and lack of transparency on their part and they enjoy the autonomy in setting up their own rules and regulations. The government sector health insurance is limited in the amount of compensation and not adequate to compensate for private setups.

Separate electrical license, fire safety license, building license, permit from Atomic Energy Regulatory Board (AERB) for X-ray, etc., trade license, pollution license from Pollution Board, and compliance with Biomedical Waste Management Rules 2016 under Environmental Protection Act, all are essential.

Medical Termination of Pregnancy (MTP) Act: This act advises on the scenarios of timing of abortion within 12 weeks and beyond 12 weeks up to 20 weeks. The subsection to this describes situations when a medical practitioner can terminate the pregnancy in good faith, for example, life risk of the woman or risk of grave physical or mental injury or in case of an abnormal baby. Grave injury can be rape or failure of contraception or mental anguish suffered by the pregnant woman on account of it. Mental illness and mental retardation and teenage pregnancy are few interesting situations where there is a scope of violation of bodily autonomy of women. The Suchitra Srivastava case was an example of this instance. The Supreme Court stayed the high court order of termination of pregnancy of a mentally retarded person and upheld the right to bodily autonomy of the woman and reproductive rights and personal liberty under Article 21 of the constitution. In the Niketa Mehta case, the question of the right to abortion came face to face with disability rights. The lady in case was 26 weeks pregnant and appealed for an abortion as a cardiac defect was diagnosed prenatally in the fetus. But the court dismissed the petition and denied abortion in this case stating that the court cannot overstep the legislature and refused to expand the scope of section 5 of the MTP Act. Thus, the right to bodily autonomy was not maintained in this case. This was in turn challenged by the human rights law network which filed a petition against the 1971 act. The court accepted the petition and the decision remains pending.

Clinical Establishment Act

The CEA is applicable for all clinical establishments including government, private sector, single doctor chamber or clinic, and to all recognized systems of medicine including Homeopathy, Ayurveda, Unani, or Siddha, thereby putting modern medicine and alternate systems at par with each other. Only exception is the armed force clinical facilities. It is a special legislation whereby the central government under Article 252 can enact a law on a state subject. This act needs to be ratified by the states for applicability. So far, 11 states have ratified this act. The other states have enacted their own clinical establishment acts and tailored the original act according to the needs of the state. It is a three-tiered system with councils existing at the central, state, and district levels. It provides guidelines for clinical establishments for minimum standards of staff, service, and other facilities. Electronic recordkeeping, emergency medical care, display of rates charged, compliance of standard guidelines all need to be maintained. Registration under this act is mandatory. Provisional registration is provided without any inspection and minimum license fees being ₹12,500 for a 15-bedded clinic. Permanent registration is given for a period of 5 years and it is nontransferrable. There is a time for public objection within 30 days. The registration can also be cancelled after a show cause notice if violations of rules occur. A clinic not registered under this act is punishable with a penalty extending up to ₹5 lakhs and even a person serving in an unregistered facility is punishable with a penalty. Its stringent guidelines for maintaining minimum standards and on the other hand, legalizing alternate forms of medicine at par with modern evidence-based medicine is somewhat self-contradictory. It has its own protocols and guidelines with particular importance to infectious diseases and any deviation in practice can be treated as negligence by the regulatory commission. It is also supposed to cap the price or rates for different procedures and bring some uniformity and regulations. In private sectors, the profit on drugs and consumables range from around 100 to 1,700% and this makes up about 40–50% of a patient's bill. The CEA has the responsibility to regulate the charges and rates and advises fair price shop for any facility with more than 100 beds. Although the efforts continue, the price capping has not been successful and is subject to extensive litigations.

LEGAL COMPLAINT MECHANISM

A patient may seek legal redressal in multiple ways simultaneously also. Legal action sought might be under the tort law or breach of contract in a civil suit for which monetary compensation is claimed or lodge a complaint under the Indian Penal Code (IPC) sections in a criminal lawsuit. They can also complain to the medical council and also institute a complaint under the CPA.

Civil Lawsuit

A patient or a family member can institute a civil case for breach of duty to care and consequent damage or negligence and its liability under the tort law. The complaint has to be filed according to the territorial and pecuniary jurisdiction of courts as described in the code of civil procedures. A civil suit can also be filed on the basis of violation of the Indian Contract Act. There is an implicit or written explicit contract between a doctor and a patient and therefore, both are liable if violation of contract occurs, for example, in case of negligence of doctors or nonpayment by patients. Damages under the tort law is calculated on the basis of general damages.

Criminal Law Cases

Actions against criminal offences are initiated by the state and results in punitive actions. It is only applicable in medical practice for gross negligence or rash acts and comes under IPC sections, for example, 304, 336–338, and 340–342 (wrongful confinement of patient). These offences are all cognizable offences, i.e., a doctor can be arrested without warrant. BNS sections equivalent of IPC are: IPC 340 (BNS 340), IPC 342 (BNS 339), IPC 304 (BNS 105), IPC 336, 338 (BNS 125,125B) Section 50 of the same code also states that the offence must be informed and he can arrange for a lawyer and seek anticipatory bail under section 437 of Code of Criminal Procedure 1973. The Supreme Court has also laid down rules concerning the criminal prosecution of a physician, wherein the police officer investigating the case has to take a medical opinion of an expert from the government sector and the case considered from the Bolam principle and cannot arrest a doctor in a routine manner.

MEDICAL NEGLIGENCE

Negligence is an *act of commission* or *omission* which a prudent man of average skill would not undertake. The burden of proof is usually on the plaintiff in a negligence suit. The concept of negligence according to Indian jurisprudence, it is described in the Law of Torts. It is the breach of legal duty to take due care that a reasonable man with average standard of care would do or commit something that a prudent person would not commit, resulting in a consequential damage. Negligence can be described in three ways, namely a state of mind with the intention or *mens rea,* a careless conduct and the breach of duty to take care that is imposed by either common or statute law. Criminal negligence requires a gross deviation from standard practice and a rash and reckless behavior with total disregard for the consequences. The degree of care is usually proportional to the risk undertaken. Professional people have a higher accountability to maintain their standards with the reasonable degree of care according to the level of skill. As long as they follow an accepted practice, they are not considered negligent. As Lord Denning MR said that in case of a professional man, an error of judgment is not negligence. Indian courts also concur on that opinion and stated that wrong diagnosis is not negligence and the difference of opinion among specialists cannot be the ground to prove negligence of a professional. The standard for reasonable competence remains in the ability to meet average practice standards as was said in the Bolam case (1957) WLR, which is accepted both in the developed countries and in India. *Res ipsa loquitur* is a situation of gross negligence where things speak for themselves and hence, there is no need to prove. Hospital's liability with respect to medical negligence can be direct or vicarious liability. Direct liability refers to the deficiency of the hospital in providing proper environment or qualified staff for treatment. Vicarious liability means the liability of an employer for the negligent act of its employees. "Good faith" is an act done or believed with due care in the best interest of the patient with a reasonable skill and care exercised for the discharge of duty. IPC Section 88–92 involve acts causing harm but done with consent of the patient and with good faith and are crucial to defense in the court of law.

CONSUMER PROTECTION ACT

The CPA was enacted to protect the interest of the consumer and it is a quasi-judicial body functioning at district Forum, State Commission, National Commission, and finally at the Supreme Court. It has equivalent powers to that of a civil court and a person can present his/her own case and complainant can be the aggrieved or any beneficiary or voluntary organization. The landmark case of IMA vs. VP Shantha brought the medical profession under the purview of this act in 1986. Medical profession is considered a "service" as in Section 2(1)(o) of the CPA. The complaint is lodged as a deficiency of service and medical and nonmedical negligence are included under it. A party can file a complaint with nominal fees and speedy remedy is the goal of the CPA in contrary to the civil courts. All hospitals and private and government-paying sections are all included under the CPA except government and charitable hospitals which function free of charge or when a doctor is rendering the service free of charge or as a personal service. A payment of a token amount for registration does not bring them under the purview of the CPA. Filing of a suit is barred by a time limitation of 2 years from the time of the incident, but in special cases, it can be extended. Any notice from the consumer court needs to be answered in a 30-day time period with to the point, clear answers backed up with an affidavit from experts or colleagues supporting the physicians point with relevant references. It is important to intimate the professional indemnity provider and insurance companies as well.

CONCLUSION

With the increase in number of litigations, the concept of defensive medicine arises. Maintaining the code of ethics, proper communication, empathy, and documentation and taking proper, informed consent, following the standard guidelines of practice or adhering to the Bolam principle, maintaining due diligence and exercising adequate skill necessary for the risk undertaken and protocolization of medicine can all lead to better outcome. Few defenses against medical cases include adherence to Bolam principle or standard of care, therapeutic misadventure, which was done in good faith, contributory negligence, doctrine of *res judicata*, suit barred by limitation, and expert opinion. However, the society and the legal systems need to take into account the innumerable difficulties faced by a clinician in the daily practice and need to realize the austere environments and limited resources available to them at times and not subject the physicians to unnecessary litigation and create an atmosphere of mistrust between the doctor–patient relationship and defensive medicine.

KEY LEARNING POINTS

- Ignorance of law is no excuse.
- Follow the various laws of the land to avoid litigations.
- Ethical practice is beneficial in long-run.
- Follow the accepted norms or standard operating protocols.

BIBLIOGRAPHY

1. Civil law, criminal law, judicial precedents.
2. Clinical Establishment Act.
3. Code of Ethics Regulations, 2002 & 2023.
4. Consumer Protection Act 2019.
5. Medical negligence.

5

CHAPTER

Communication Skills

Sandhya Satish Khadse

INTRODUCTION

"Disseminate the practice of health care relationship and communication that integrates best medical practice with patients' and clinician's values, needs, and choices".

"Communication is a transactional process in which messages are filtered through the perceptions, emotions, and experiences of those involved". From womb to tomb we communicate. We learn to express ourselves through appearance, style of speech, body language, and a lot more. An important part of personality is the way an individual communicates. Medical field does not remain immune to these phenomena. In fact, communication is the glue that cements the physician-patient relationship.

These are quite simply, the skills that allow human beings to communicate with each other in an effective way. For pediatricians communication skills consist of:

- The ability to talk with relatives, listening to them must be a two way process and it is an essential part of communication.
- The ability to communicate sufficiently well with patients and relatives so as to understand their concerns, problems and beliefs and to elicit relevant information.
- The ability to explain patient's illness and its treatment. The explanation should be clear, complete and in language that relatives can easily understand. The treatment option should be explained clearly and completely, so that they can make informed decisions about treatment.
- The ability to convince relatives to follow the treatment plan. This is especially important when embarking on prolonged, expensive, difficult or culturally unacceptable treatment for a patient.
- The ability to establish a relationship with the relatives and patient, based on mutual respect and trust.
- Some skills, like being able to put all classes of relatives at their ease, being able to generate confidence and being comfortable holding conversations on nonmedical subjects with relatives and patients.

IMPORTANCE OF COMMUNICATION SKILLS

There are several advantages to possessing good communication skills **(Box 5.1)**. In general, a doctor with these skills is more likely to have happy, satisfied patients, than an equally technically competent doctor who does not bother about communication.

Box 5.1: Advantages of good communication.

- Patient satisfaction, leading to regular visits and referrals
- Feeling of empowerment and control
- Adherence to treatment plan
- Loyalty even if treatment is not immediately effective
- Less chance of complaints and legal actions in the event of a mistake

Even if a physician's diagnosis and treatment are accurate, thoroughly rationale and successful, poor communication leaves relatives unhappy and resentful. On the other hand, answering all questions without hesitations enhances patient's and relative's belief in doctor's expertise. This is especially so with chronic or incurable disease, which are associated with anxiety, stress and uncertainty for the whole family. A doctor who offers supports, empathy and clear and complete explanations at every step can help alleviate this to a significant extent. Good communication also enhances adherence to long-term therapy. On the other hand, lack of communication can lead to treatment discontinuation and therapeutic failure. This can extend to depression and despair, all to anger and complaints.

Most complaints in health care systems both public and private arise from poor communication. Very few people can judge the quality of doctor's examination, diagnosis, or prescription. Obviously, relatively few complaints originate in poor performance in these areas. Relatives are annoyed by the doctor's refusal to spend time with them, refusal to hear complaints, give clear explanations, a casual or callous approach to patient's problem, and lack of courtesy and care, are followed by poor treatment outcomes, complaints, quarrels, and legal actions are likely. On the other hand, good communication can play a significant part in avoiding complaints and malpractice claims.

BARRIERS TO GOOD COMMUNICATION

Traditionally, we have not paid much attention to communicating well. Even today few of us appreciate the importance of communication skills, hardly any make a concerted effort to learn and apply such skills. This is perhaps the single biggest barrier to good communication. Unless we accept the contribution of good communication to patient outcomes and relative's satisfaction, poor communication is likely to remain the norm in the medical field.

Even doctors, who realize the importance of good communication, are not always successful in implementing it. Many of us do not know what patients want from us **(Box 5.2)**.

Some Other Barriers to Good Communication

Lack of Time

Most doctors see a large number of patients every working day. This is true of both government and private hospitals. History taking, physical examination, and prescription writing are of course, essential parts of clinical encounter. When time is short, it is communication with relatives that is sacrificed. We can overcome this partially, by deputing some explanations to paramedical staff.

Box 5.2: What patients want?

- Clarity and directness
- Listening and attention
- Honesty and empathy
- More and better information about their illness, treatment plan, and expected outcome
- More openness about the hazards and side effects of treatment
- More information about the relief of symptoms and other concerns
- Advice on what they can do to help themselves
- Information on other treatments available
- A supportive, nonjudgemental, empathizing doctor
- Plan that is easy to follow
- Demonstrations, videos, and audiovisual help

Arrogance

Arrogance is deeply ingrained into doctors. We expect our patients and their relatives to follow our commands unquestioningly. We do not understand the need for explanations and often give none.

Shyness

Relatives may be very shy and not ask the question they have in their minds. On the other hand, the doctor may be shy and either ignore questions or give minimal and incomplete answers. Shyness on either side stands in the way of adequate information being imparted.

Language and Jargon

In any major city of India, there is likely to be large population of people from other states and linguistic groups. Communication with them needs special efforts.

Most such people will bring an interpreter with them while coming to us. It is necessary to give interpreter the information in small chunks and have him translate it for the relatives as you go along. This is especially important with the prescription; explain one drug at a time and have it translated.

A major problem occurs when the relatives speak English. As soon as we meet English-speaking relatives, we start speaking in technical hypermedical language. This leaves the relatives confused and uninformed. While talking in English, it is essential to make an effort to talk in language that a nonmedical person can understand.

Deafness

Deafness is the major cause of poor communication and a special concern when our relatives are accompanied by their relatives. When we suspect a hearing impairment, we must speak loudly, slowly and distinctly. Other useful measures are voice amplification if a device is available, a quiet room to improve signal to voice ratio; use written communication; and asking the family, at the end of consultation, if they have understood everything and if they have any question.

An important measure is to have relatives repeat the prescriptions instruction, to ascertain they have been understood. This ensures that the patient will receive the medication as it has been prescribed.

Phones

Earlier, a telephone would buzz discretely on a receptionist's desk, and a consultation would be uninterrupted. Today, there is a phone in everyone's pocket and hands and calls can interrupt and hinder communication terribly.

Information Needs

When faced with a chronic/permanent condition most patients or relatives want to know:
- What treatment can achieve best for their patients, relief of symptoms and prolongation of life, shortening of course of the disease?
- Expected progress of patients during treatment.
- What to expect by way of improvement, side-effects, fresh problems, etc.?
- Chances of complete cure.
- Treatment options.

The last point is especially important. Complementary and alternative medicine is a growing business and their remedies are often advertised and promoted aggressively. It is necessary to explain treatment goal, explain how our treatment works and convey them the unscientific basis and unreliability of advertised "magic remedies".

STRATEGIES FOR IMPROVING COMMUNICATION

Check What the Relatives Know

With intelligent and knowledgeable relatives, the discussion can begin at a higher level. However, assessing the relative's knowledge is important, because some of their knowledge or understanding may be faulty. Many relatives get their knowledge from magazines, lay books, and websites. Most of these sources have no system of review or control of the information published.

Assess What the Relatives Want to Know

Some relatives want to know every little fact and details about their patient's condition. Others simply want a prescription and an assurance that all will be well. It is important to assess the relative's desires and communicate accordingly.

Assess the Understanding

The patients may not fully understand what is being told to them. They are upset about the individual being sick. They have poor comprehension skills they have language problems; there could be many reasons. If the patients indicate that they do not fully understand what is being told to them, stopping the explanations for that session might be appropriate and take it up next time. Understanding can be improved by giving time to absorb and by repetition.

At the end of consultation, patients can be asked to repeat some information, to ensure it has been understood.

Listening Skills

Most of us hardly allow the patients or relatives to speak. As soon as they start their description of the problem we start asking questions and attempt to keep the consultation focused. However, this often leads to incomplete description of the problem. Listening well is an important part of communication. This requires the provision of adequate time with patient's willingness to listen to their relatives concern. A quiet room, lack of interruptions, provision of chairs for the sitting at an appropriate distance, good eye contacts are helpful to enhance listening and learning from the patients or relatives.

Build Confidence

The relative's confidence must be bolstered. We need to accept what the relatives say without judging it. A little specific praise for the relative's efforts so far helps significantly in building confidence and helping relatives to cope. Some suggestions for future care improve their confidence that they will be able to manage the situation. Giving false hope is wrong, but we can give information in positive manner.

Truth

Patients like to know the truth, but the bald truth can be harsh and shocking. Patients deserve to know the truth, but its delivery should be tempered with common sense and empathy.

If the facts are particularly unpleasant, they can be delivered in small parts spread out over two or more visits. However, if patients express a desire to know everything, it must be told to them. Withholding information leads to distress.

Simplicity and Clarity

Not all relatives have good educational and intelligence level. Explaining things in simple, clear and direct language is very important. Clarity and directness are particularly important with patients of low comprehension abilities. Many people do not comprehend words like 'growth or tumor', 'cancer' sound shocking, but may be necessary to drive home.

Be Tolerant

Patients react in various ways and we should be prepared. Blame, anger, and a sudden outpouring of grief; all these are common reactions. We should be ready to deal with these emotions with understanding and support.

Empathy

Relatives of sick patients are going through difficult experience. They appreciate the fact that doctors understand their situational difficulties. While sympathy has overtones of pity and is likely to be resented, empathy is simply an understanding of relative's plight.

Table 5.1: Factors effecting communication skills.

DO's	*DONT's*
• Greet the patient and relatives with name • Smile • Sit down while talking • Try to talk in a patients language • Direct the conversation to relevant direction • At the end of consultation, ask if relatives have any questions • Engage the relatives in a dialogue • Give time for relatives to absorb and understand content of your explanation and then to ask questions • Use videos and demonstrations • Give true facts and honest experiences	• Look at your watch frequently • Appear to be in hurry • Use too many medical terms • Talk with your hand on the door handle or foot outside the door • Interrupt all the time • Start examination and then write out a prescription before the main problem has been identified • Give long lectures as explanations • Ignore concern mentioned by relatives • Say that the relatives would not understand about the illness and it is very complicated to understand • Get irritated with cross questioning or scientific references quoted by the relatives

Online training in communication skills is feasible, desirable, and associated with increased confidence in key skills.

Behaviors linked to positive patient outcomes are verbal ones like empathy, patient centred questioning, friendliness, courtesy, explanations, humour, summarization, and clarification and nonverbal ones like head nodding, forward lean, uncrossed arms, arm symmetry, and less mutual gaze.

Apart from these broad principles, many small factors affect communication positively or negatively **(Table 5.1)**.

WHO IS AT FAULT?

Let us be introspective by asking certain questions:

- Do we wish the patient when he/she enters the clinic room?
- How many times do we listen?
- How much time do we allow the patients/family members to talk?
- How often do we make a deliberate effort to elicit patients' ideas and concerns, emotions, and problem which have impact on their health? How often do we thank them? And lastly,
- How many of us are aware/knowledgeable about science of communication?

At some point during the course of a terminal illness, a meeting between health care professionals and the patient/family is necessary to review the disease course and develop end-of-life goals of care. Learning the process step of a Family Conference is an important skill for physicians, nurses, and others who are in a position to help patients and families.

Family Conference Process Steps

- *Why*: Clarify conference goals in your own mind. What do you hope to accomplish?
- *Where*: A room with comfort, privacy and circular seating.

- *Who*: Relatives legal decision-maker/health care, power of attorney; family members, social support; key health care professionals.
- Introduction and relationship building—introduce self and others; review meeting goals; clarify if specific decisions need to be made. Establish ground rules: each person will have a chance to ask questions and express views; no interruptions; identify legal decision maker, and describe importance of supportive decision making. If you are new to the patient/family, spend time seeking to know the "person"—ask about hobbies, family, etc.
- Determine what the patient/family already knows.
- Review medical status—review current status, prognosis and treatment options. Ask each family member in turn if they have any questions about current status, plan, and prognosis. Respond to emotional reactions.

Family discussion with a nondecisional patient—ask each family member what do you think should be done? Ask if the family would like you to leave room to let family discuss alone.

Wrap-up

Summarise consensus, disagreements, decisions and plan. Caution against unexpected outcomes. Identify family spokesperson for ongoing communication.

Document in the chart—who was present, what decisions were made, follow-up plan.

Delivering Bad News

Create an appropriate physical setting—a quiet, comfortable, room, turn off beeper, check personal appearance, have participant's including you, sitting down. Determine who should present? Ask the patients whom they want to participate-clarify relationships to the patients. Decide if you want others present (e.g., nurse, consultant, and social worker) and obtain patient/family permission.

Think through your goals for the meeting as well as possible goals of the patient. Make sure you know basic information about the patient's disease, prognosis, and treatment options.

Special circumstances—when relatives/family members do not speak the language of discussion. Obtain a skilled medical interpreter.

Percepting self-reflection—residents will invariably have strong emotions when they have to give bad news. In these situations, residents should not spontaneously discuss their own emotional reaction with a perceptor; therefore, they should be introducing this topic. "This is a really hard case, how are you doing?"

Physicians often have strong emotional reactions when a patient encounters bad news. Normalise the experience for the resident; "It is normal to have strong feelings."

Information for Relatives and Families about Ventilator Withdrawal

The physician's counselling of families is a critical aspect of care for the dying patient who is to be removed from the ventilator. Ideally the family will be involved in the decision to withdraw the ventilator. Before the withdrawal, the following issues should be discussed:

- **Potential outcome of ventilator withdrawal:** Assuming all other life sustaining treatments have been stopped, including artificial hydration and nutrition, there are several potential outcomes—rapid death within minutes (typically patients with sepsis on maximal blood pressure support) death within hours to days, or stable cardiopulmonary function leading to a different set of care plans, including potential hospital discharge. If the later possibility is realistic, future management plans should be discussed prior to ventilator removal, since some families may desire to resume certain treatments, notably artificial hydration/ nutrition.

- **The procedure of ventilator withdrawal:** Never make assumptions about what the family understands; describe the procedure in clear, simple terms, and answer any questions. Families should be told before-hand the steps of withdrawal and whether or not it is planned/desired to remove the endotracheal tube. In addition, they should be counseled about the use of oxygen and medication for symptom control. Assure them that the patients comfort is of primary concern. Explain that breathlessness may occur, but that can be managed. Confirm that you will have medication available to manage any discomfort. Ensure they know that the patient will likely need to be kept asleep to control their symptoms.

  If asked, explain that they can show love and support through touch, wiping of the patient's forehead, holding a hand and talking to him or her.

Support the Decision

Even though a family is able to make a definite, decision for ventilator withdrawal, such a decision is always emotionally charged. Families will constantly second-guess themselves, especially if the death appears to linger following ventilator withdrawal. Physician support, guidance and leadership are crucial, as the family will be looking to the physician to ensure them that they are "doing the right thing". Furthermore, support needs to continue following death during the bereavement period.

Role of Consent

Under section 13 of the Indian Contract Act 1872, "consent" is defined and states that two or more persons are said to consent when they agree to the same thing in the same sense. In the case of a minor, relatives of the minor, being the natural guardian, or a guardian appointed by a court, shall be the person competent to contract for and on behalf of the minor.

INFORMED CONSENT

Informed consent is a part of a physician's duty to disclosure; however, this duty has an exception. In the event, the physician is of a considered opinion that, the patient is in a highly disturbed condition or so anxious that the information given would not be processed rationally or that it would only cause significant psychological harm then the doctor may choose not to inform the patient about the treatment or procedure.

The other exception is where the patient prefers not to be informed. These exceptions are known as "Therapeutic Privilege".

In case informed consent is obtained then in case of medical mishap the doctor has a better defence and courts generally have taken a view that where the patient underwent the surgery with full knowledge of attendant risk, the doctor cannot be held liable.

Good communication is an art that can be acquired, developed and improved by experience however; it can also be taught and assessed by means of structured programs. Formal training is not easily available to doctors in job or practice. We can improve our communication skills with some personal efforts. This will lead to better patient/relative satisfaction and perhaps better clinical outcomes. Our patients and their families value compassion, explanation and reassurance as much as diagnosis, treatment and care. Times have changed so have our patients and their relatives. In today's scenario, patients are health care consumers and doctors are providers. Hence, a good communication skill is an essential component of overall care and these simple skills allow human being to communicate with each other in an effective way.

"The patient will never care how much you know, until they know how much you care"— **Terry Canale in his American Academy of Orthopaedic Surgeons Vice Presidential Address.**

KEY LEARNING POINTS

- Communication skills are important to improve doctor–patient relationship.
- Please remove barriers while communicating with patients/relatives.
- Improving communication is the best option to diminish the chances of allegations of negligence.
- Delivering the "Bad news" is an art.
- Communication skill can help in decision making in critical cases.

BIBLIOGRAPHY

1. Ambuel B, Weissman D. Fast fact and concept. #016; Conducting a Family conference. 2nd edition August, 2005.
2. Bhushan SJ. Medical Negligence and Compensation. Bharat Law Publications, Jaipur, 2nd edition, 1999. pp. 11-14.
3. Canale T. The Oschner Journal. 2010;10(1):38-43.
4. Charles VG, David EW. Fast Fact and Concept #85 Ventilator Withdrawal Protocol [part1].
5. Faulkner A. Breaking Bad news—a flow diagram. Palliative Medicine. 1994;8:45-51.
6. Hawken SJ. Good communication skills: Benefits for doctors and patients. NZFP. 2005;3293):185.
7. Iverson VK. Pocket protocols–notifying survivors about sudden unexpected death. Galen Press Inc, Tucson, Arizona,1999.
8. Kemper KJ, Foy JM, Larry Wissow, et al. Enhancing communication skills for pediatric visits through on-line training using video demonstrations. BMC Medical Education. 2008;8:8.
9. Lee W. Communication Skills and Doctor Patient Relationship. Hong Kong Medical Diary. Vol. 2 No. 3, March 2006.
10. Mehta PN. Communication skills talking to parents. Indian Pediatrics. 2008;45(4):301-4.
11. Palmer RN. A Physician's Guide to Clinical Forensic Medicine. Humana Press, New Jersey, 2000. pp. 17-23.
12. Patankar CV, Bhalerao UD. Communication, We Need to Learn. For Being Doctors. Knowledge update program Vol 4. Maharashtra University of Health Sciences, Nashik.
13. Ptacek JT, Eberhardt TL. Breaking Bad news: A review of the literature. JAMA. 1996;157:323.
14. Rubenfeld GD, Crawford SW. Principles and practice of withdrawing life sustaining treatment in the ICU in managing death in the intensive care unit. In: Curtis JR, Rubenfeld GD (Eds). Oxford University Press, 2001. pp. 127-147.
15. Singhal SK. The Doctor and Law. MESH Publishing House, Mumbai. 1st edition, 1999. pp. 166-9.
16. Weissman D. Fast Facts and Concepts#11 delivering bad news part 2-talking to patients and precepting trainees. June 2000. End of Life Physician Education Resource Centre. www.eperc.mcw.edu. [Last accessed April, 2014].
17. Weissman DE. Decision making at a time of crisis near the end of life. JAMA. 2004;292:1738-43.

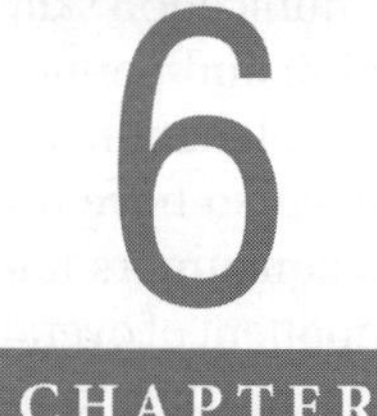

6

CHAPTER

Doctor–Patient Relationship

Mukul Tiwari, Abhyuday Tiwari

INTRODUCTION

"I wouldn't demand a lot of my doctor's time. I just wish he [or she] would brood on my situation for perhaps five minutes, that he would give me his whole mind just once, be bonded with me for a brief space, survey my soul as well as my flesh... Without some such recognition, I am nothing but my illness"

—Anatole Broyard (Essayist)

Doctor–patient relationship (DPR) is as old as the origins of human race. It started when one caveman gave herbs to another caveman for some malady. It is often said that the practice of medicine started as an art, then evolved as a science and has now become a trade. But the truth is that practice of medicine is a combination of all three. It is not for a doctor to treat this as art alone, science alone, or profession alone if he wants to make his practice successful and gratifying.

The doctor–patient relationship is central to the practice of medicine and is essential for the delivery of high-quality health care in the diagnosis and treatment of disease. Patients must have confidence in the competence and trustworthiness of their doctor. They must feel they can confide in him as they would in their parents and siblings. Establishment of good rapport with a patient is the most important. Some medical specialties, such as psychiatry and family medicine need a good doctor–patient relationship more than others, such as pathology or radiology. The doctor–patient relationship forms one of the foundations of contemporary medical ethics. Most medical schools and universities in the developed countries teach medical students from the beginning, even before they set foot in hospitals, to maintain a professional rapport with patients, uphold patients' dignity, and respect their privacy but unfortunately, developing countries are slow to catch up this trend.

The archetype "good old doctor with his walk-in clinic" is vanishing. With the advancement in technology, humanistic aspect of the medicine which used to be its hallmark and its crowning glory, is taking a back seat. It is quite reasonable of the society to expect its doctors to be noble and selfless beings but alas! of late many strong factors have come into play, which interfere with doctors' efforts to uphold that image.

Doctor–patient relationship is deteriorating globally and situation is appalling in developed world of Europe or USA where litigation is routine. The conditions in India are also worsening. If we say that society is at fault for this or that a huge global conspiracy is being plotted against the doctors then we would be behaving like an ostrich who buries his head in the sand to avoid the reality. The writing is clear on the wall and we had better read it; the societal factors are changing and we have to change the way we practice. I hope most of the doctors have read the book "Who Moved My Cheese?" by famous author Dr Spencer Johnson, It tells the readers how to adapt to changes in life.

No situation can be totally hopeless; there is a saying *"When we say that a person or a situation is hopeless we close the door in the face of the God"*. It is my belief and conviction that doctor–patient relationship which is undergoing severest strain in today's times can be surely improved. Despite all the constraints it is possible even today to practice competent and caring medicine while combining use of science and technology. We should always remember that despite changing pattern of health care, medicine will always be conducted on a human-to-human basis.

WHAT IS A FIDUCIARY RELATIONSHIP?

The word, Fiduciary derives from the Latin word for "confidence" or "trust". This bond of "trust" between the doctor and patient is essential to begin the process of healing. It is the foundation for physician–patient relationship. The patient–doctor relationship surpasses ethnic, sociocultural and economic considerations. It is based on the premise that the doctor will put the needs of the patient first. For a sound DPR doctors should not only understand biomedical aspects of treatment as well as psychological, social, and cultural dimension of health and illness.

TRADITIONAL CONCEPT OF DOCTOR–PATIENT RELATIONSHIP

Parson's Theory

Talcott Parsons, a social scientist in 1951, theorized the concept of doctor–patient relationship. Parsons believed that amount of illness is controlled through socially prescribed roles for doctor and patients, which facilitate interaction and ensure that both parties work together to return people to a state of health and normal role performance as quickly as possible. His description of roles of doctor and patient is presented as an "ideal type" model.

Parsons viewed the role of the doctor as complementary to the role of patient. Just as the patient is expected to cooperate fully with the doctor, doctors are expected to apply their specialist knowledge and skills for the benefit of the patient, and to act for the welfare of the patient and community rather than in their own self-interest. Doctors are also expected to be objective and emotionally detached, and to be guided by the rules of professional practice. Conformity with these general expectations is an essential requirement for carrying out the tasks of diagnosis and treatment, especially when this involves the need to know intimate details about the patient that are not usually shared between strangers or the conduct of an intimate physical examination **(Table 6.1)**.

Parsons also viewed doctors as enjoying considerable autonomy in executing their professional skills and occupying a position of authority in relation to the patient.

Hippocratic Oath

Hippocratic Oath was the first treatise on doctor–patient relationship. It sets two sets of duties:

- *Duties to the patient*: "Benefit" the sick and keep them from harm.
- *Prohibitions*: Abortion and poisoning.
- Duties to other doctors.

Table 6.1: Parsons analysis of the roles of patients and doctors.	
Patient: Sick role	***Doctor: Professional role***
• Exempted from responsibility for sickness; seen as being unable to get better without professional help • Can legitimately withdraw from normal activities and social responsibilities, e.g., paid work, family duties, housework • Must seek competent treatment from professional health expert • Under a social obligation to get better as quickly as possible	• Must be objective and remain detached, not impose own values • Must not act in self interest (e.g., money and career) but in patient's interests; obey professional code of practice • Must apply a high degree of knowledge and skill to treat the patient • Given right to examine patient intimately, prescribe treatment and wide autonomy in medical practice

Drawbacks:

- It is doctor-centered.
- It is silent about patient's rights.

American Medical Association Codes Prior to 1960

It was largely built on the Hippocratic Oath and was, like Hippocratic Oath, also silent about patient rights.

Paternalism

Both the Hippocratic Oath and the American Medical Association Codes prior to 1960 are paternalistic. In paternalism the principles of beneficence and nonmaleficence take priority over principle of autonomy. Paternalism has following characteristics:

View about Doctor

- The doctor is a quasi-parent
- He is benevolent
- He always knows best
- The control he exercises over the patient is in the best interest of the patient
- He is skilled and wise. He is an authority not only in medicine but also in morality.

View about Patient

- The patient is a quasi-child
- He is dependent
- He is incapable of understanding complex medical information
- He is incapable of making a wise choice concerning his health
- It is in his best interest to be left out of the decision-making process.

Paternalism is fast losing ground. Much of US medical ethics of the past forty years consists of a critique of paternalism and defense of patient rights. The principle of autonomy comes before the principle of beneficence.

Critique of Paternalism

- Doctor's duty of beneficence may conflict with the principle of respect for patient autonomy.
- Patient and physician may disagree on the relative value of health in comparison with other values such as religion.
- Doctors are not infallible.
- Some issues dealing with health care are not strictly medical and doctors are not necessarily more qualified than the patient to make decisions about them.

Respect for Patient Autonomy

- Noninterference with patient's choices
- Treating patient as an end in himself
- Patient is an adult; capable of making his own choices. Has self-determination.

Alternative Models of Doctor–Patient Relationships

The paternalistic model of doctor-patient relationship is obviously inadequate; patients ought to be treated in a way which respects their individuality and their capacity to choose. What kind of relationship ought the doctor and the patient to have? Some more models have been proposed by different authors.

Robert Veatch's Model

In an influential article "Models for Ethical Medicine in a Revolutionary Age" Robert Veatch distinguished four models of doctor-patient relationship:

1. Engineering Model

- The patient makes all the important decisions
- The doctor is a "hired gun." His job is to provide factual information and carry out the patient's wishes.

2. Priestly Model

- The doctor makes all the important decisions; he is the patient's guardian
- The doctor always knows what is best for the patient both in medical and in moral matters
- The doctor always does what is best for the patient
- Patient accepts the authority of the doctor passively.

3. Collegial Model

- Doctor and patient are colleagues; they share the same goals
- They participate equally in solving problems
- Relationship is built on trust.

4. Contractual Model

- Doctor and patient enter into an agreement to pursue mutually acceptable goals using mutually acceptable means

- Patient makes decisions that are important and reserves the right to withdraw from the contract if his values and those of the doctor conflict
- Doctor provides technical expertise and skills but reserves the right to withdraw from the contract if his values and those of the patient conflict.

Assessment of Veatch's Models

Engineering model

Strengths:
- Respects patient's autonomy
- Emphasizes doctor's knowledge and expertise.

Weaknesses:
- Doctor may be asked to perform actions with which he does not agree
- Gives the patient too much power.

Priestly model

Strengths:
- Emphasizes doctor's knowledge and expertise.

Weaknesses:
- Ignores the autonomy of the patient
- Makes the doctor an expert in morality.

Collegial model

Strengths:
- Emphasizes the importance of shared decision-making
- Emphasizes the importance of trust.

Weaknesses:
- Patient's trust may be abused
- Doctor's knowledge outweighs that of the patient.

Contractual model

Strengths:
- The values and rights of the doctor and those of the patient are equally important
- Emphasizes the importance of shared decision-making.

Weaknesses:
- Does not encourage a trusting relationship between the doctor and the patient; it is too legalistic
- It is too individualistic.

Stewart and Roter Model

Stewart and Roter Model has Four Patterns (Table 6.2)

1. **Paternalistic:** The paternalistic approach is typified by a doctor centered style. It relies on closed questions designed to elicit yes or no answers. The doctor will tend to use a disease centered model and be focused on reaching a diagnosis, rather than the patient's unique experience of illness.

Table 6.2: Doctor and patient involvement in Stuart and Roter model.

	Patient control		***Doctor control***	
	High	***Low***	***High***	***Low***
Paternalistic		X	X	
Consumeristic	X			X
Default		X		X
Mutuality	X		X	

Table 6.3: Doctor–patient relationship in Szaz and Hollender model.

Model	***Physician's role***	***Patient's role***	***Application***	***Prototype***
Activity-passivity	Autocrotic warm/detached dominant needs strong figure	Passive	Critical care acute patient, coma anesthesia, trauma delirium	Parent-infant
Guidance-cooperation	Warm/detached makes plans advises informative	Cooperates may be given choices	Above and acute infections chronic care minor illness	Parent-child (adolescent)
Mutual participation	Usually warm discusses plan interactive helps patient help self interpretive	Uses expert advise, active role in own care interactive	Most chronic illnesses psychoanalysis	Adult-adult

2. **Consumeristic:** Here the patient knows exactly what they want and forces the doctor into a patient centered approach.
3. **Default:** This is where the patient centered style fails. The doctor is trying to relinquish control but the patient is unwilling to accept it. The result is an impasse.
4. **Mutuality:** The doctor uses open questions to encourage the patient to talk about his complaint. This approach relies on taking time to listen and trying to understand the patients point of view.

Szaz and Hollender Model

Szasz and Hollender delineated 3 basic models of the doctor-patient relationship. These are tabulated in **Table 6.3**.

ADVANTAGES OF A SOUND DPR

- Improves treatment outcome
- Improves compliance with medical treatment
- Improves clinician satisfaction
- Improves patient satisfaction
- Reduces medical malpractice risk

BASIC PRINCIPLES OF A SOUND DPR

A sound DPR is based on following principles of medical ethics:

- **Principle of autonomy:** Respect the patient's right to self determination. An informal consent involves disclosure and discussion of the nature of the problem to be treated; the proposed treatment; its risks and likelihood of success; alternative treatments and their risks and likelihood of success; and the risks and likely outcome of no treatment at all.

- **Principle of beneficence:** Prevent harm. Always work for good of the patient.
- **Principle of nonmalificence:** First do no harm (primum non-nocere).
- **Fiduciary trust:** Always act in the patient's interests.
- **Principle of justice:** Give each patient his or her right or due.
- **Veracity:** Tell the truth and be honest with your patients.
- **Confidentiality:** Do not disclose private information obtained during clinical contact with the patient, unless the patient expressly permits you to do so.

FACTORS BEHIND DETERIORATING DOCTOR–PATIENT RELATIONSHIP

- **Commercialization of medical education:** Medical education has become quite expensive and more so in private medical colleges. The graduates who come out after spending a heavy sum are less likely to view and treat this profession as missionary.
- **Poor communication skills:** Communication skills are very important buffers against lawsuits and violence. Whenever communication fails problems begin. Most physicians have been trained in a biomedical model and have little or no training from a biopsychosocial perspective. They often don't consider that how they communicate with patients is at least as important as what they communicate. Doctors who don't take the time to help patients understand their medical problem and its treatment fare badly with their patients. Doctors often blame patients when communication breaks down. But researchers have found that many doctors have shaky interviewing skills. For example, many doctors do more talking than listening. A new study published this year journal of the American Medical Association (JAMA) found that 72% of the doctors interrupted the patient's narrative.
- **Increased specialization and lack of primary care doctors:** This problem is more in metro cities. Specialists and super-specialists can't spare much time and "personal touch" is lacking. Old practice of friendly family doctor was good and should be revived. A family doctor can also facilitate better understanding between patients and specialists.
- **Commercialization of society:** The society has become consumerist. Money culture is prevailing over noble values such as sacrifice and honor. A doctor has to earn money to maintain a decent living and to meet the expenses and expectations of his family as well. Still, doctors have to remember that once they have chosen this noble profession of their own free will they should uphold its nobleness.
- **Turbulent society:** Because of increasing conflicts and tensions in the society, people are edgy and ready to fight at the smallest pretext. Violence is everywhere in the society. This tendency extends to people's relations with all service providers including doctors.
- **Role of media:** Increased reports in media about medical errors, the power of the drug industry and the flaws in health care administration is increasing public distrust of doctors. Also, increased reports about violence and lawsuits against doctors, which encourage others to follow suit.
- Giving negative feedback to patients about "rival" colleagues is a popular pastime for many doctors. This is also responsible for a decline in the feeling of respect for doctors.
- Unethical and greedy attitude of some doctors (their number is small) tarnishes the reputation of entire community and nurtures distrust against doctors in general. In some places there is also tendency to give and expect money for referral of patients.

- **Lack of holistic attitude:** Doctors should not only be well equipped with the biomedical aspects of patient care but also understand the psychological, social, and cultural dimension of health and illness. Doctors often ignore theses aspects. A study of 21 doctors at an urban, university-based clinic found that when patients dropped emotional clues or talked openly about emotions and problems, the doctor seldom acknowledged their feelings. Instead the conversation was directed back to technical talk.
- **Rise of managed care:** In USA rise of managed care hospitals is fast spoiling DPR. Doctors are forced to advise less than needed admissions, investigations and delay or restrict hospitalizations.
- **The IT revolution and the "informed patient":** Before the IT revolution knowledge of medicine was doctor's domain; the patient's role was only to listen and comply. The Internet has opened up the floodgates of information. There are thousands of sites ready to offer information and not just basic information but to latest developments and different treatment options. The "informed" patient thus enters doctor's office with a load of information all of which may not be fitting to his case.

THE e-PATIENT REVOLUTION

Internet search for health related information is increasing exponentially and had increased from 54 million in 1998 to 110 million (US figures) in 2002 and has been increasing since. Searching for health related information is a very popular pastime (80%), next only to emailing (93%) and product research before a buy (83%). The typical e-patient belongs to the younger age group, is better educated, comes from higher income group and women search more for a health topic than males. The search is for specific medical condition (63%), medical treatment or procedure (47%), diet and nutrition (44%), exercise and fitness (36%).

Why Doctors Don't Love e-Patient?

In medical fraternity there has been lot of resistance to e-revolution and informed patients, the reason quoted are as follows:

- Medical information on the net is not always reliable
- The belief that human touch will be lost
- The perception that informed patients are problem patients.

The Positive Side of e-Revolution

Although some doctors are skeptical of e-revolution eventually it may turn out to be beneficial for both. Physicians, Gerber and Eiser have suggested that the e-revolution offers opportunities to improve the DPR by sharing the knowledge. Patients still trust the doctor offered information more than that offered by the net. The Physician can now assume the role of consultant helping his patient sort the information on the net to decide informed and intelligent treatment options.

There is fair evidence to support this view—A study by McKay et al. found that patients who participated in an online diabetes education and support group lowered their blood glucose levels more than controls did. A Harris online poll found that patients who use the

Internet to look for health information are more likely to ask more specific and informed questions of their doctors and to comply with prescribed treatment plans.

Doctors have found that it may take less time to explain complex medical information to Internet users than to nonusers.

WHAT ARE THE RESPONSIBILITIES OF THE PATIENTS?

- A patient is responsible for providing to the health care provider, to the best of his or her knowledge, accurate and complete information about present complaints, past illnesses, hospitalizations, medications, and other matters relating to his or her health
- A patient is responsible for reporting unexpected changes in his or her condition to the health care provider
- A patient is responsible for reporting to the health care provider whether he or she comprehends a contemplated course of action and what is expected of him or her
- A patient is responsible for following the treatment plan recommended by the health care provider
- A patient is responsible for keeping appointments and, when he or she is unable to do so for any reason, for notifying the health care provider or health care facility
- A patient is responsible for his or her actions if he or she refuses treatment or does not follow the health care provider's instructions
- A patient is responsible for assuring that the financial obligations of his or her health care are fulfilled in a timely manner
- A patient is responsible for following health care facility rules and regulations affecting patient care and conduct.

HOW TO IMPROVE THE RELATIONSHIP?

- Doctors should try to adapt to the model of doctor-patient partnership. In this concept doctor and patient become partners working together through dialogue and counseling to achieve maximum benefit for the patient and peace and happiness for the doctor.
- Honesty pays. Maintain transparency and honesty; patients always appreciate these qualities and they are good buffers against hostile behavior from patients and lawsuits.
- *Communication skills are important*: Maintain, at all times, dialogue with patients/relatives. Answer and satisfy their queries in clear, understandable language with lots of eye contact. Do not look confused shaky or to be hiding facts. Check posture and body language. Give them a reasonable time. A fascinating study of time perception found that when doctors sat down during an office visit, the patients always thought the visit was longer than when the doctors remained standing, even though the length of both visits was exactly the same. Other simple gestures, such as leaning forward, have been found to help the patients relax, as well as improve satisfaction and recall.
- Keep them informed about patient's condition, prognosis, and a rough estimate of expenditure, without exaggeration or understatement.
- *Give them back*: Doctors should strive to improve their services as an ongoing process. It should not look as if the doctor is only milking the patients and giving nothing in return. A part of the earned money should be ploughed back into better facilities for patients.

- Avoid unnecessary admissions and investigations. Doctors can make more use of clinical sense. Whenever some tests/admissions are necessary reasons of their necessity can be discussed with the patients.
- *Show genuine concern*: Develop true empathy for your patients; falseness shows through one's skin. Doctors' attitude should not look mechanical/haughty but humane enough. Today's patients will not accept the humiliating status of a "dysfunctional biological body".
- *Humor helps*: A well meaning humor immediately earns the goodwill of the patients and relatives. Use more humor in your workplace. Did you see "Patch Adams"? If not see it now.
- *Know your limits*: Never attempt efforts to treat an illness which is beyond your level of expertise. In such cases always ask for a second opinion or refer to a center where the level of expertise is enough to deal effectively with illness.
- *Keep qualified and competent staff*: Incompetent staff may land you in a soup at any time. Suppose you are running an ICU with no qualified duty doctor to replace you at night. In such a situation you should be ready to keep awake the whole night. If you would prefer to sleep you should never keep serious patients who require supervision from qualified doctors and not from paramedical staff.
- *Proper documentation*: Always maintain proper documentation of cases. Never try to manipulate the records.
- *Staff behavior*: Junior doctors and paramedical staff should be trained to be humble and not give unqualified comments and answers to questions asked by patients and relatives. Their unqualified answers often lead to confusions between doctors and patients.
- Develop a system to communicate test results to patients. No news is good news, patients often assume, but according to a survey published in Archives of Internal Medicine, one in three doctors do not always inform patients of abnormal test results, especially if the results are mildly abnormal.
- *Respect patient's narrative*: Rely on patients as experts in the experience of their own illness. Traditionally, doctors have viewed the patient as "an unreliable narrator" and to chart patient observations in subjective language that implies certain skepticism, such as "the patient believes" or "the patient denies." Rotter and Hall recommend that patient's unique knowledge about his illness is just as important to treatment outcome as the doctor's scientific knowledge. They conclude, "The medical visit is truly a meeting between experts."

WHAT ARE DIFFICULT PATIENTS?

In one survey doctors rated 15% of their patients as "difficult". While one doctor's difficult patient may be another doctor's favorite, there are some common characteristics of "pain in the neck" patients. These patients are those that do not trust or agree with the doctor, present too many problems for one visit, do not follow instructions, are demanding or controlling and they may be consistently rude and irritable. They may present as overly helpless or melodramatic. Patients may use the doctor as a scapegoat for their anger. All difficult patients are less likely to receive as good medical care as patients who convey more positive attitudes. Doctors are profoundly influenced by the demeanor, comments, and attitudes of their patients. The difficult patients are more likely to be single and often have a history of unexplained physical symptoms, depression, panic states, obsessive-compulsive disorders, or physical abuse, according to a study of rheumatology patients at the University of Washington Medical Center.

WHAT CAN PATIENTS DO TO IMPROVE THE RELATIONSHIP?

The entire burden of improving the DPR should not lie on the doctors alone; patients can take a step forward to do their bit. Here are a few tips:

- *Learn how to tell your story*: Tell your problems in a coherent manner instead of weaving a spider web and confusing the doctor. Many patients tend to start with interpretation, "I think I have bronchitis" rather than plain facts, "I've been coughing for two weeks." Use concrete examples to explain how illness affects your daily life. For example, "I'm getting worse" is less helpful than "We've been buying milk in quarts because I can't lift gallons anymore." Everyday details also help the doctor understand how the medical data translates into real life
- Study your doctor's individual style. What are his/her likes and dislikes, strengths and weaknesses? Optimistic or pessimistic? Intense or mellow? Organized or absent-minded? Cautious or a risk-taker? The more you understand how your doctor thinks, the more likely you'll know which approaches will work and which won't
- Learn about your illness so you can ask the right questions and help make decisions. Patients who take an active role in their care do better and earn more respect from the doctor. Donald AB Lindberg, MD, Director, National Library of Medicine, says "An informed patient is always the best, even though that puts more pressure on us to keep up to date"
- Accept realistic treatment goals. Many chronic diseases can be managed, but not cured. "In this age of hype, patients have come to expect the impossible, doctors frequently grope in the dark, not because they are delinquent in learning, but because the science does not reach there" says Lown, a renowned DPR analyst
- Should make wise & informed decision about choosing his doctor or the hospital. Having done this, full trust and faith should be reposed in the doctor
- Should provide full information about the illness, allergies, past illnesses, preferences for the kind of medication (syrup/tablets/capsules), family history and all the relevant social and family background
- Should not hesitate to ask as much information as he wants and clarify the instructions without any hesitation
- Report immediately in case of any adverse drug reactions or other adverse happenings
- Should understand beforehand the risk involved in a procedure or operation
- Should ask the doctor for any alternative or choice available. This is his right
- Should know that medical science is a biological science and lots of decisions are made on the basis of experience and personal judgments. Even though the science has advanced many things cannot be still fully explained or predicted
- Avoid shopping around with multiple doctors and alternative systems
- Avoid believing in hearsay and rumors
- Carefully read the consent for any procedure, try to understand its implications and ask for clarifications, if required
- Should differentiate between a complication or mishap and negligence and not blame the doctor for everything that goes wrong.

RIGHTS OF DOCTORS

Doctors don't just have duties; they also have some rights:

- A doctor has a right to turn away a patient before starting treatment but he should provide minimal basic care especially in an emergency situation
- He has a right to select the drugs from wide range of options available, allowed by drug licensing authority of his country
- A doctor can also select the investigations and method of treatment depending upon various factors
- He/she should obtain a written refusal in case the patient does not want to do as advised
- If the doctor, for some reasons can't continue to look after the patient, he/she can delegate the rights/powers to look after the patient to properly trained colleagues, usually with the willingness of patient. However, a better alternative for the practitioners is to start group practice so that one of the regular consultants is always available
- A doctor can decide regarding visits, fees to be charged and maintenance of the patient's record including its secrecy in certain specific situations.

TOMORROW'S DOCTOR

Tomorrow's successful doctors will be the ones who will fulfill the following criteria:

- Will know fully about and understand the rights of patients
- Will be able to communicate effectively with individuals and groups
- Will accept the moral and ethical responsibilities involved in providing care to individual patients and communities
- Will respect patients regardless of their lifestyle, culture, beliefs, race, color, gender, sexuality, disability, age, social or economic status
- Will respect right of patients to be fully involved in care decisions, including the right to refuse treatment or take part in teaching/research
- Will recognise their obligation to understand and deal with patients' healthcare needs by consulting them (and their relatives or carers).

WHAT CAN BE THE ROLE OF MEDICAL ASSOCIATION?

These bodies can play a major role in improving doctor-patient relationship. With the help of media they can arrange seminars inviting doctors and public where both can interact and public can discuss their grievances and doubts with the doctors. This will establish an atmosphere of cordiality and transparency which will improve trust and faith of the patients for doctors. They can establish their own grievances redress cells where complaints of patients can be looked into and if the concerned doctors have really erred then some sort of out of court settlement can be arranged. They can arrange TV shows, talk shows and write newspaper articles to discuss various issues which confuse public hence, leading to mistrust and anger. American Academy of Pediatrics (AAP) regularly informs parents about various medical issues through its website. IMA can adopt a similar approach. These efforts will go a long way in improving doctor patient relationship.

KEY LEARNING POINTS

- DPR is deteriorating very rapidly throughout the world.
- The traditional fiduciary relationship has become consumer and service provider.
- A sound DPR improves patient's satisfaction.
- The e-patient or Google doctors may create more problems.
- Doctors as well as patients/relatives should work for improving DPR.
- Society and policy makers also have major responsibility toward strengthening a healthy DPR.

BIBLIOGRAPHY

1. Beauchamp TL, Childress JF. Principles of Biomedical Ethics, 4th edition. Oxford: Oxford University Press,1994.
2. E-patient-9 Humphrey Taylor The Harris Poll® #21, May 1, 2002. http://www.harrisinteractive.com/news/allnewsbydate.asp?
3. Gerber BS, Eiser AR. The patient-physician relationship in the internet age: future prospects and the research agenda. J Med Internet Res. 2001;3:e15.
4. Harris Interactive. The increasing impact of e-Health on consumer behavior. Health Care News. 2001;1:1.
5. Key communication skills and how to acquire them. Peter Maguire, director, Carolyn Pitceathly. BMJ. 2002;325:697-700.
6. McKay HG, King D, Eakin EG, et al. The diabetes network Internet-based physical activity intervention: a randomized pilot study. Diabetes Care. 2001;24:1328-34.
7. Parsons T (1951). The Social System, Glencoe, Free Press.
8. "Responsibilities of patient"—www.acash.org/newsletter1.
9. "Rights of patient"—www.cgsiindia.org/knowyourright.
10. Simon RI, Shuman DW. The doctor patient relationship. Focus, Fall. 2007;5:423-31.
11. Steinmetz D, Tabenkin H. The 'difficult patient' as perceived by family physicians. Fam Pract. 2001;18: 495-500.
12. Szasz T, Hollender M. A contribution to the philosophy of medicine. Arch Int Med. 1956;97:585-92.
13. Tiwari S. Legal aspects in medical practice. Indian Pediatrics. 2000;37:961-6.
14. "Tomorrow's doctors"—www.gmc-uk.org/education/undergraduate.
15. Veatch RM. The foundations of bioethics. Bioethics. 1999;13:206-17.
16. www.nvcc.edu/home/aaoudjit/descript.htm.
17. www.ucel.ac.uk/shield/docs/notes_doctor_patient.pdf.

SECTION

2

Medical Negligence

Section Editor: Murli Janardan Sabath

Section Outline

CHAPTER 7

Record Maintenance

JK Gupta

"Nothing is more devastating to an innocent physician's defense against the allegations of medical malpractice than an inaccurate, illegible or skimpy medical record."

—Brad Cohn
Chairman, MIEC Board of Governors,
California, USA.

INTRODUCTION

Medical records form an essential part of medical care of a patient for present and future and are vital not only for patient but also for medical personnel providing care. As a written collection of information about a patient's healthcare, they are used in the management and planning of healthcare facilities and services, for medical research, and for the production of healthcare statistics. This will be the only way for the doctor to prove that the treatment was carried out properly. Moreover, it will also be of immense help in the scientific evaluation and review of patient management issues. Medical recording needs the concerted effort of a number of people involved in patient care. The doctor is the prime person who has to oversee this process and is primarily responsible for history, physical examination, treatment plans, operative records, consent forms, medications used, referral papers, discharge records, and medical certificates. There should be proper recording of nursing care, laboratory data, reports of diagnostic evaluations, pharmacy records, and billing processes.

HISTORY OF RECORDKEEPING

The Atharvaveda gives the earliest documentation of medical records in India. An astrologer, horrendous quack doctor Forman recorded over 10,000 consultations between 1596 and 1603. In the late 1590s, Forman taught Napier his methods. Napier's record survives in full, from 1598 to his death in 1634. These contain roughly 40,000 consultations. In 1880s, physicians at Mayo Clinic, Minnesota, kept the patient records in personal leather-bound ledger. This was replaced in 1907 with patient-based records which is still used today. In 1928, the Association for Record Librarians of North America was founded by the American College of Surgeons. They recognized the necessity of the comprehensive, long-term medical records on individual patients. In the

United Kingdom (UK), the first major attempt to standardize medical record came in 1965 with publication of the Tunbridge report. Initially, the records were kept for physician's own epidemiological interest. Slowly, as art and science of medical and surgical services got complex and institutionalization approach developed, the records became means of communication to other team members also. Public hospital and medical colleges started to have medical records department for research and statistical purpose. Today, maintenance of records is mandatory from ethical and legal point of view. Good medical records are best defense against litigation.

WHAT IS A MEDICAL RECORD?

The medical record is a legal document providing a chronicle of patient's medical history and care. The medical record is an important compilation of facts about a patient's life and health. It includes documented data on past and present illnesses and treatment written by the healthcare professionals and planned for future. The medical record "must contain sufficient data to identify the patient, support the diagnosis or reason for attendance at the healthcare facility, justify the treatment, and accurately document the results of that treatment." The main purpose of the medical record is to record the facts about the patient's health history with emphasis on the events affecting the patient during the current admission or attendance at the healthcare facility, and for the continuing care of the patient when they require healthcare in the future. For good patient care, the patient should have one medical record with all admissions filed in that and kept in the one place. The physical medical record is the property of the hospital and the information in the medical record is the property of the patient and cannot be released without the consent of the patient.

CRITERIA FOR AN IDEAL MEDICAL RECORD

Always remember the five "C's—*c*lean, *c*omplete, *c*hronological, *c*omprehensive, and *c*orrect." Records should be without manipulation and overwriting or tempering. If any changes have to be made, then it should be struck with single line and rewritten alongside with initials. Vital information needs to be highlighted such as allergies and drug sensitivities, high-risk medical conditions, human immunodeficiency virus (HIV) status, history of violent tendencies, and known abuser of healthcare services.

WHY MEDICAL RECORD IS IMPORTANT?

Medical recordkeeping is important for two main reasons:

1. *Medical reason*: Medical recordkeeping is important to evaluate existing patient management strategies and to develop institute- and doctor-based disease statistics. For chronic disorders and old cases, records are of immense helping tools for treating clinicians. Multispecialty treatment concept cannot work out without proper medical recordkeeping.
2. *Legal reason*: Medical recordkeeping is not only an obligation on doctors and clinical establishments as per present Medical Council of India (MCI) Rulings and Clinical Establishment and other Acts but is also a defense in modern era of litigations.

"Poor records mean poor defense, no record means no defense." If any legal problem arises, then properly maintained records are of utmost importance. They are the most important proof of what treatment was actually administered to the patient.

TYPES OF MEDICAL RECORD

Hospital Record Directly Related to Patient Management

- *Outpatient department (OPD) record*: Copy of prescription, OPD case register, and vaccination card copy
- *Inpatient record*: Complete indoor case sheets bed head ticket (BHT), including registration details, patient self-declaration proforma, doctor order sheet, nursing notes, patient photo ID, written consents, referral letter copies, discharge card copy, investigation reports copy, follow-up details record, death certificate copy, medicolegal cases (MLC) papers, operation theater (OT) notes papers, procedure performed details, payment receipts, and provisional and final bills raised and settled
- Copy of certificates issued and certificate register
- Medicolegal record

Hospital Record Not Directly related to Patient Management but Necessary

Other administrative records and documents required under different laws:
- Records under Pre-Conception and Pre-Natal Diagnostic Techniques (PCPNDT) Act
- Medical Termination of Pregnancy (MTP) Act
- Bio-Waste and Environment Protection Act
- Other records not related to patient
- Accounts and related record
- Service record of staff, leave, absence, and qualification
- Gratuity, Employee Provident Fund Act, and other labor laws
- Hospital housekeeping and maintenance record, lift and electric equipment maintenance, intensive care unit (ICU)/neonatal ICU (NICU) sterilization roster
- OT instruments and equipment list, autoclave schedule observed
- Asepsis maintenance protocol observed throughout the hospital

ESSENTIAL DETAILS OF THE MEDICAL RECORD

- *Patient particulars*: Personal data of patient, detailed postal address, e-mail, contact numbers, photo ID, and Aadhaar Card
- "Personal declaration proforma" filled in writing of patient or attendant giving above details with essential past and personal history, socioeconomic status, and annual income
- Chief complaint, history of present illness and medical, family , developmental, and dietic history
- Detailed physical examinations, vitals charting, and nursing notes

- Diagnosis provisional and final, differential diagnosis
- Investigation, charting, and reports
- Serious consent, consent for procedure, and daily prognosis explanation consent sheet
- Referral letter and reference notes
- Treatment done and planned
- Telephonic consultation from senior doctors should also be noted down by junior doctors and nursing staff with date and time of noting and endorsement afterward
- Copy of discharge card, death summary, high-risk screening notes, and follow-up plan

RISKS AND WARNINGS

Risks and warnings need to be highlighted before start of treatment. History of allergies or drug sensitivity and high-risk medical condition should be highlighted with red pen. History of violent tendency, HIV, hepatitis B, hepatitis C virus-(HCV)-positive status, and known abuser of healthcare services should also be highlighted.

DOCUMENTATION OF NEONATAL RESUSCITATION IN MEDICAL RECORD

Time of arrival at resuscitation, perinatal risk factors, procedure performed before arrival of doctor, vital signs and Apgar score, details of resuscitation procedure performed, outcome of resuscitation, need of hospitalization, and referral to be documented with noting of time. Examination of congenital anomalies and injury sustained if any. In case stillborn with congenital anomalies, samples must be sent for karyotyping and genetic evaluation. Stopping of resuscitation in case of nonsurvival must be followed with standard norms with proper explanation to attendants. Last menstrual period (LMP), estimate date of delivery (EDD), gestational age, mother's blood group and thyroid status, antenatal history, and ultrasonography (USG) fetal well-being finding must be documented.

MEDICOLEGAL IMPORTANCE OF DISCHARGE CARD OR TRANSFER NOTES

Outpatient department papers, discharge card, referral letter, and death certificate are the most important record because these are directly issued to patient party during the course of treatment and there is no chance of making correction of mistakes. Receiving signed copies of these should be preserved with indoor records. Most of the times, these are the documents with which litigation is filed. Discharge card and transfer notes are the summary documents which reflect the treatment received. The discharge card and transfer notes should mirror the case notes of the patient records with a brief summary. Discharge card must mention condition of the patient at the time of admission and at the time of discharge, treatment given in hospital and course of the stay of the patient, operation notes, complete diagnosis, treatment suggested at the time of discharge, investigation, follow-up schedule, prognosis, danger sign and care at home explained, undertaking of patient/attendant on discharge card itself about understanding of the treatment prescribed, follow-up schedule, danger sign, prognosis, home care, and high-risk screening.

MEDICAL CERTIFICATE

Always remember that medical certificate should be issued on letterhead of doctor or hospital and a copy of the same must be preserved. It must contain date, time, identification mark, mobile number, and signature attested and it must be issued for legitimate purpose only on utmost need. As per clause 1.3.3 of Indian Medical Council Act Regulation 2002, register of medical certificates must be maintained by every physician.

ALWAYS AVOID

Always avoid overwriting, scratching, or scoring. In case corrections have to be made, then strike the whole sentence and corrected notes should be written freshly with signature to avoid suspicion of tempering. Do not alter notes retrospectively.

Correction of the personal identification data of patient such as name, age, and father/husband name should only be done after getting notarized affidavit from patient.

Always avoid rendering the papers whether OPD or indoor incomplete. All the columns of BHT should be properly filled and page should be numbered and all the investigations, nursing notes, referral notes, copy of discharge card, death certificate, and bills should be properly annexed. Avoid leaving any paper loose.

COMMON PROBLEM OF OUTPATIENT DEPARTMENT RECORD RETENTION

Customary patient retains OPD records. All the OPD prescriptions, investigations, and imaging are handed over to patient and attendants in original. Doctors are left with no documentation regarding OPD records. The patient is expected to preserve papers and bring it to clinic and hospital for follow-up consultation. Doctors are at mercy of patient party for OPD record. OPD records may actually be lost or may be hidden by patient at the time of litigation which may prove disastrous to the defense of doctors. Preservation of OPD records is a very cumbersome exercise for any doctor as it is voluminous. Time restrain is also an issue which aids to reluctance in OPD recordkeeping.

Electronic Recordkeeping in Outpatient Department

Ideal answer may be preparing record in two copies and one may be preserved by patient and another by doctor. But it is very difficult in practice. So the best way would be to preserve record in electronic format which is also admissible by courts under section 65B of Indian Evidence Act. Now as per clause 1.3.4 of Indian Medical Council Regulation 2002, efforts shall be made to computerize medical records for quick retrieval. As per rule 13(d), National Medical Commission Ethics and Medical Regression Board (NMC EMRB) notifications published on August 2nd, 2023, "Efforts shall be made to computerize patient's medical records for quick retrieval and security. Within 3 years from the date of publication of these regulations, the RMP shall ensure fully digitized records." So time has come for every doctor and hospital to go for electronic recordkeeping.

Training of Doctors and Staff Regarding Medical Recordkeeping

There should be orientation programs for all doctors and nursing staff for proper notes making and recordkeeping.

Medical Record Department

Large hospitals and all public hospitals have medical record department for managing medical records. The medical record department staffs under the leadership of the medical record officer (MRO) or medical record clerk incharge is responsible for the maintenance of medical records and medical record services. The hospital administration must provide security and sufficient storage space for medical records and an adequate working area for medical record staff. The medical record department staff must safeguard medical records from tampering, loss, and unauthorized use. They are responsible for seeing that the patient's right to privacy and the confidentiality of the information stored within the medical record are maintained at all times.

HOW LONG TO PRESERVE AND MAINTAIN RECORDS?

Registered medical practitioner (RMP) is not obliged to preserve OPD medical record; only indoor records have to be preserved for 3 years by him/her.

As per clause 1.3.1 of Indian Medical Council Act Regulation 2002, "Every physician shall maintain the medical records pertaining to his/her indoor patients for a period of 3 years from the date of commencement of the treatment." The NMC EMRB notification dated August 2nd, 2023, also reiterates the same—"Every self-employed RMP shall maintain medical records of patients (inpatients) for 3 years from the date of the last contact with the patient for treatment, in a standard proforma laid down by the NMC."

Recordkeeping in telemedicine consultation by RMP.

In teleconsultation also, recordkeeping has been made mandatory. Telemedicine guideline has been regarded as annexure 5 of MCI regulation 2002 and is binding on every doctor. Section 3.7.2.1 of the guidelines mentions that it is incumbent on RMP to maintain logs or record of telemedicine interaction (e.g., phone logs, email records, chat/text record, video interaction logs, etc.). Section 3.7.2.2 mentions that patient records, reports, documents, images, diagnostics, data, etc. (digital or nondigital) utilized in the telemedicine consultation should be retained by the RMP. Guideline 11 Telemedicine Guidelines of NMC ERB Notification 2023 in Duties and Responsibilities of RMPs reiterate the same "It is incumbent on RMPs to meticulously maintain the following records/documents for three years from the date of the last consult with the patient."

Retention period for government hospitals.

As per the Directorate General of Health Services (DGHS) vide letter No. 10-3/68-MH dated 31-8-68 (published in "Hospital Manual" in 2002), medical records should be maintained as follows: Inpatient medical records—10 years, outpatient records—5 years, medicolegal registers—10 years.

As per office memorandum of DGHS, No. A-12034/3/2014-MH-II/MH-I dated October 28th, 2014, medical record of indoor patients may be stored in digitized form for at least 10 years or as per availability. For future, all medical records of indoor patient should be digitized on regular and continuous basis and kept indefinitely for future reference, since it contains valuable data which may be required for research and policy planning purpose. Hospital may store medical records in hard copy form inpatient medical records for 3 years, OPD records for 3 years, and medicolegal register and case sheets for 10 years or till the disposal of ongoing case related to these records.

Retention of medical records as per National Accreditation Board for Hospitals & Healthcare Providers/National Accreditation Board for Testing and Calibration Laboratories (NABH/NABL).
Retention period for NABH/NABL is 7 years for inpatient case sheets and 5 years for outpatient case sheets. All other records, summaries (admission, discharge, or death), laboratory reports, preanalytical reports, etc., are required to be retained for a minimum of 5 years.

RETENTION PERIOD OF MEDICAL RECORDS AS PER VARIOUS ACTS

- *Clinical Establishment Act*: As per Uttar Pradesh Clinical Establishment Rule 30-1, retention period for indoor medical record is 3 years as per MCI regulation 1.3.1 and 1.3.2.
- *PCPNDT Act 1994*: Section 29 of the PCPNDT Act 1994 requires proper maintenance of records for a period of 2 years or until disposal of proceeding.
- *MTP Act 1971 Regulation 2003*: As per Rule 5 of MTP Act 1971 Regulation 2003, Form III or Admission register for termination of pregnancies should be kept for 5 years.
- *Retention of Record as per Income Tax Act 1961*: As per section 44AA and Rule 6F, professionals like doctors are obliged to maintain daily case register Form 3C, inventory, cash book, general ledger, carbon copies of bills issued, and original bills received for a period of 6 years from the end of relevant assessment year.

Section 271A mentions that if professional failed to maintain said documents mentioned earlier, assessing officer may impose penalty up to ₹25,000.

LIMITATION PERIOD VERSUS RECORD RETENTION PERIOD

Limitation period is often confused with record retention period while both are different entities with different legal meanings. Record retention period is that period for which record has to be preserved as per statutory duty while limitation period is that period during which person has right to file litigation.

There are two types of statute:

1. *Statutes in which specific limitation period is prescribed are governed by their own limitation provision*:
   a. In Consumer Protection Act (CPA) 2019, section 69 clearly mentioned limitation period for filing complaint which is 2 years and delay may be condoned by forum if forum is convinced by the complainant that there is sufficient cause for delay in filing litigation. Similar was provisioned in CPA 1986 section 24A.
   b. In Criminal Procedure Core (CrPC) 1973 also, specific limitation period is prescribed under section 468 for filing criminal complaint.

2. *Statutes in which no specific limitation period is prescribed are governed by Limitation Act 1961*, for example, Civil Procedure Core.

Section 29-2 of the Limitation Act 1961, specifically says that where any special or local law prescribes for any suit, appeal, or application, a period of limitation different from the period prescribed by the schedule prescribed in the Limitation Act, then specific limitation period provisioned in that statute will prevail.

Retention Period of Indoor Medical Record for Child Patient by Pediatrician

It has been a great confusion that record preservation period for child is 21 years. But it is totally a myth. Section 6(1) of the Limitation Act 1961 which is "disability section" says, "Where a person entitled to institute a suit or make an application for the execution of a decree is, at the time from which the prescribed period is to be reckoned, a minor or insane, or an idiot, he may institute the suit or make the application within the same period after the disability has ceased, as would otherwise have been allowed from the time specified therefore in the third column of the schedule." So a minor may institute the suit after his disability period which is age of majority 18 years is over. This limitation clause is applicable only to those statutes in which specific limitation clause is not provisioned.

As per information received in Right to Information (RTI) reply from MCI [MCI-211(2)](RTI)/2019-Ethics/17871 dated 02-01-2020, retention period for indoor medical record of child patient for pediatrician is same 3 years as mentioned in MCI regulation 2002 clause 1.3.1.

Record Maintenance for Consumer Cases

In the CPA, nowhere record maintenance has been mentioned. In Limitation Clause of CPA, i.e., section 69 CPA 2019 or section 24A section 1986, 2-year limitation period from the cause of action is mentioned and delay may be condoned if forum is satisfied by the complainant that there was justified sufficient cause in filing litigation. Since the Limitation Act is not applicable in CPA as it has its own limitation clause, preserving medical record till age of majority plus 2 years is not applicable in Consumer Cases. So maintaining medical record as per various abovementioned acts is recommended. Still it is wiser that medical record should be preserved for longer period in view of increasing number of consumer litigations.

24×7 CCTV Audio–Video Recordings or Mobile Call and Voice Recording as Record

Closed-circuit television (CCTV) cameras are fitted in clinic and hospital by doctors mostly for safety purpose. But at times, these may be needed as proof of treatment given or negligence committed. In privacy and criminal issues, such type of recording may be needed. Display sign board of under CCTV surveillance must be placed. In era of internet and smart phones, call recording may be done by either party and many times it is admissible in court. So be cautious in telephonic interaction with attendants and anybody. Recording of consultation may be done where both parties agree. Audio-video consent has definitive added value in consent taking procedure and if done after consent of patient party and if preserved properly, it may be good defensive tool in litigation. Many clinics and hospitals are now equipped with counseling room with inbuilt audio-visual recording facility. Do not resuscitate (DNR) consent and organ transplantation consent must be audio-video recorded.

Issuing of Medical Record

As per clause 1.3.2 of MCI regulation 2002, if any request is made for medical records either by the patients/authorized attendant or legal authorities involved, the same should be duly acknowledged and documents shall be issued within the period of 72 hours by authorized person. As per Regulation 13-B of NMC ERB regulation 2023, medical record should be issued within 5 days of making request and as per regulation 13-C, in case of medical emergencies, efforts should be made to make the medical records available at the earliest. As soon as request of medical record is made, authority of record seeker must be checked and it must be issued to the patient or kin after verifying their relation and identity by ID proof, otherwise it may give rise to confidentiality issues. Medical record may have to be issued to third-party administrator (TPA) Company or Police or may have to be submitted in court of law, but whenever issued, it must be issued to authorized person with proper receiving.

Issued record must be complete, pages must be numbered, all columns must be filled, consultant notes and nursing notes must be complete, signatures must contain names of signee, and cutting over writing must be avoided as it will amount to tempering. As soon as request is made to issue medical record, consultants and concern nursing staff must be communicated immediately to fill up the vacant column and to complete the record by all means. So it is advisable that every record must be completed at the time of stay of the patient as a healthy habit as one may not get time again to fill up shortcoming if any. Remember, in criminal case, medical record would be forfeited by police official in no time. So contemporaneous charting is must for all. In Raghunath Raheja vs. The Maharashtra Medical Council and Ors, Bombay High Court held that doctors cannot hide behind confidentiality when the patient party demands medical records.

Medical Record and Right to Information Act 2005

Right to Information Act, under section 2(f) of the RTI Act, provided access to records held by private bodies through regulatory public authority as ordained by any law in force. Section 2(f) says, “information” means any material in any form, including records, documents, memos, e-mails, opinions, advices, press releases, circulars, orders, logbooks, contracts, reports, papers, samples, models, and data material held in any electronic form and information relating to any private body, which can be accessed by a public authority under any other law for the time being in force. With this definition, the right of the citizen is expanded beyond public bodies and extended to private bodies, also provided there is any legal access. As per Clinical Establishment Act, clinics and hospitals are obliged to preserve medical records for 3 years and these needs to furnish district health authorities on demand. So this provides legal access to health record through district health authorities under the RTI Act 2005.

Chief Information Commission held in NP Bhatia vs. IHBAS that the patient's right to obtain his medical record is not only protected under the RTI Act but also under the regulation of Indian Medical Council, which is based on world medical ethics, and also as a "consumer" under the CPA 1986. In case Shri Prabhat Kumar vs. Directorate of Health Services GNCTD, Delhi in File No. CIC/SA/A/2014/000004, the appellant claimed that the death summary of his father prepared by the team of Doctor led by Dr Vivek Nangia of Fortis Hospital is insufficient, unsatisfactory, ambiguous, vague and does not have complete facts and sought complete Death Summary Report and disclosure of the real facts and circumstances leading to death of his father under the RTI Act Central Information Commission (CIC) directed Fortis Hospital to furnish certified copies of entire medical record including a note explaining the cause of death of the father of the appellant, certified copies of documents based on which the causes were ascertained. Rejecting the claim by Fortis Hospital, CIC has held that malpractice by private hospitals amounting to medical terrorism. The CIC called that the government, MCI, and other regulatory authorities have to see that license to practice medicine will not become license to kill and extort and come to the rescue of the helpless patient. On tendency to ask information under RTI in sub judice case, CIC in RK Morarka vs. Central Bank of India Appeal No 908/ICPB/2007/F.No.PBA/07/211 on September 17th, 2007, has held that, "This commission has consistently taken a view that if information sought relates to a pending proceeding before a competent court/tribunal, then the said information should be obtained only through court/tribunal and not under the provision of RTI Act." In case of nonavailability of record after prescribed retention period, CIC has held in TV Varghese vs. BSNL (Appeal No. 251/ICPB/2006, dated 2.1.2007) case that "When the records are not available due to the expiry of the period of preservation according to the departmental rules for destruction of old records, there is no question of providing such information even if the disclosure of such information is not prohibited under section 8(1)(j) of the RTI Act."

Protection of Records

Medical record should be protected from insects, fire, water, and theft. Insecticide spray must be used in record room and naphthalene balls may be used along with. Keep fire extinguisher available in record room. Records should be protected from dampness, water, and floods. To avoid theft, windows and ventilators should be properly covered with frame. If record is lost, then FIR must be lodged.

How to Destroy Records?

Give a public notice in one English and one Vernacular newspaper with a time limit of usually 1 month from date of publication in which anyone wants the relevant paper can come and take the copy of the medical record needed.

After 1 month, destroy record for everyone except where litigation is going on or prelitigation process of notice is going on.

Evidentiary Value of Medical Record

Whenever there is an issue of medical negligence or otherwise, Indian Legal System relies on documentary evidences which has to be filed in the form of medical record. Medical records are medicolegal documents and treating doctor can be cross-examined pertaining to such records. These are the most important evidence when compensation for damage or prosecution or acquittal has to be decided by court. Medical records are primary evidence under section 62 of Indian Evidence Act. It is usually agreed that documentation of facts during treatment is genuine and unbiased. Erasing of entries is not permitted and questionable in court. Medical record can be summoned in court in original form in course of proceeding. Electronic records are also admissible under section 65B of Indian Evidence Act. Under section 91 CrPC, it is required to handover medical record to the police, but one should keep a copy of receiving of handed over medical record.

IMPORTANT CASE LAWS RELATED TO RECORD MAINTENANCE

No negligence in failure to supply the medical records unless there is legal duty to issue it—in *Poona Medical Foundation vs. Marutturao Tikare case,* the National Commission has held that there can be no question of negligence by the reason of failure to supply the medical records unless there is legal duty on the hospital to give the records.

Patient not admitted as indoor patient, hospital not required to maintain the medical record—in *Sh Mahesh Prasad Aggarwal & Ors. vs. M/S. Kamayani Patients Care India Original petition no. 39 OF 2003 NCDRC on 3 January, 2013,* the important question was whether the deceased was indoor patient in the opposite party—hospital. Opposite party—hospital has proved that deceased was not admitted in the opposite party—hospital as indoor patient rather treated as outdoor patient. In these circumstances, Notification dated 11.3.2000 issued by the MCI is not applicable to the present case and opposite party—hospital was not required to maintain the medical record of deceased.

Patient has right to claim medical records pertaining and hospitals are under obligation to maintain them and provide them. In *Kanaiyalal Ramanlal Trivedi vs. Dr Satynarayan Vishwakarma,* it was held by honorable court that without confusion, patient has right to claim medical records pertaining to his treatment and the hospitals are under obligation to maintain them and provide them to the patient on request. The hospital and doctor were guilty of deficiency in service as case records were not produced before the court to refute the allegation of lack of standard care.

Duty to produce medical record in the court, adverse inference could be drawn for not producing the records. In *Dr Shyam Kumar vs. Rameshbhai Harmanbhai Kachiya,* it was held by honorable commission that it is the duty of the person in possession of the medical records to produce it in the court and adverse inference could be drawn for not producing the records. Not producing medical records to the patient prevents the complainant from seeking an expert opinion.

Destroying the case sheet is an attempt to suppress certain facts. In *SA Quereshi vs. Padode Memorial Hospital and Research Centre,* it was held by court that the plea of destroying the case sheet as per the general practice of the hospitals appeared to the court as an attempt to suppress certain facts that are likely to be revealed from the case sheet. The opposite party was found negligent as he should have retained the case records until the disposal of the complaint.

Issues of tampering of medical records needs to be examined in civil court, in *Harenbalal Das vs. Dr Ajay,* it was held by court that issues of tampering of medical records need detailed examination in a civil court rather that in Consumer Court.

Not maintaining confidentiality of patient information can be an issue of medical negligence. In *Dr Tokugha Yeptomi vs. Apollo Hospital Enterprises Ltd and Anr*, it was held by the Supreme Court that not maintaining confidentiality of patient information can be an issue of medical negligence. The HIV status of a patient was known to others without the consent of the patient.

Records show no pain, so not performing X-ray justified—Dr S Ali vs. Dr Lahari—in an accidental injury, doctor did not perform X-ray of shoulder as patient never complained pain. Patient alleged negligence and alleged no record was given. District forum dismissed the case as complainant did not specify which fact was overlooked by doctor.

Bill suggested that treatment was given—PP Ismail vs. KK Radha—in this case, patient with accidental fracture of leg operated in hospital had drill bits left during operation. Later on, left out drill bits were removed by another surgeon. Hospital contended that surgeon was not attached to the hospital. But surgeon charges in bill suggested that surgeon was attached. So hospital held vicariously liable.

Record destroyed—S Qureshi vs. Padode Memorial Hospital and Research Centre—in this case, arthroscopy that was performed for knee ailment later on developed deformity. Doctor failed to explain cause as record was destroyed. Court held that doctor is liable and observed that an educated person would not destroy record when case is pending.

Allegation of not informing negated by informed consent—C Anjani Kumar vs. Madras Medical Mission—it was alleged that possibility of vocal cord palsy was not informed, but this allegation was negated as there was informed consent which showed that it was properly explained.

Incomplete record spell deficiency in service—*Dr Paramjit Singh Grewal vs. Charanjit Singh Chawla* NC 2006—in this case, the National Commission observed that doctor recorded X-ray as OK even though separated chip of humerus was not rightly placed. While performing the operation, the doctor did not maintain proper written record of treatment given and rationale of treatment. Court held deficiency in service. The doctor in his admission stated that he had informed the complainant for the replacement of shoulder when he could not get relief even after open reduction. "I orally informed but not mentioned in the discharge card." Court held not maintaining proper record amounts to deficiency in service.

Records not produced in court—in *Kanhaiyalal Raman Lal Trivedi vs. Dr Satya Narayan Vishwakarma*, the hospital and doctor were guilty of deficiency of service as case records were not produced before the court to refute the allegations of lack of standard care.

Alleged tampering/manipulation of record—in *Meenakshi Mission Hospital and Research Centre vs. Samuraj and Anrs*, the National Commission held that hospital was guilty of negligence as name of anesthetic was not mentioned in operation notes, though anesthesia was given by two anesthetics. There were two progress cards about the same patient on two separate papers.

MEDICOLEGAL CASES

Medicolegal cases are the cases where attending doctor after taking history and clinical examination of the patient thinks that some investigation by law-enforcing agencies is essential so as to fix the responsibility regarding the case in accordance with the law of land. Injuries due to accidents and assault, suspected or evident cases of suicides or homicides (even attempted cases), confirmed or suspected cases of poisoning and burns, cases of injuries with likelihood of death, sexual offences, suspected or evident criminal abortion, all patients brought to the hospital in suspicious circumstances/improper history (e.g., found dead on road), unconscious patients where cause of unconsciousness is not clear, child abuse, domestic violence, person under police custody or judicial custody, patients dying suddenly on operation table or after parenteral administration of a drug or medication, case of drunkenness brought dead, and natural disaster are some examples of MLC. The police should be informed under section 39 of Criminal Procedure Code, the attending MO is legally bound to inform the police about the arrival of a MLC. Any failure to report the occurrence of a MLC may invite prosecution under sections 176 and/or 202 of Indian Penal Code (IPC).

CONFIDENTIALITY OF MEDICAL RECORDS

Medical records can be used as a personal or impersonal document. Personal document—this information is confidential and should not be released without the consent of the patient except in some specific situations. Impersonal document—the record loses its identity as a personal document and patient permission is not required. These records could be used for research purposes. Confidentiality is an important component of the rights of the patient. The hospital is legally bound to maintain the confidentiality of the personal medical records. The patient can claim negligence against the hospital or the doctor for a breach of confidentiality. However, there are certain situations where it is legal for the authorities to give patient information. They are as follows: (1) During referral, (2) when demanded by the court or by the police on a written requisition, (3) when demanded by insurance companies as provided by the Insurance Act when the patient has relinquished his rights on taking the insurance, and (4) when required for specific provisions of workmen's compensation cases, consumer protection cases, or for income tax authorities. The maintenance of confidentiality is an important issue in the era of electronic data storage. There should be checks in place so that only those who are authorized can access the patient data.

ELECTRONIC HEALTH RECORD STANDARDS FOR INDIA 2016

In September 2013, the Ministry of Health and Family Welfare notified the Electronic Health Record (EHR) Standards for India. Ministry of Health and Family Welfare e-Health Section vide its Notification Q-11011/3/2015 e-Gov dated 30.12.2016 issued EHR standard guidelines which say that preservation of medical records assume significant importance in view of the fact that an EHR of a person is an aggregation of all electronic medical records of the person from the very first entry to the most recent one. Hence, all records must compulsorily be preserved and not destroyed during the lifetime of the person ever. Upon the demise of the patient where there are no court cases pending, the records can be removed from active status and turned to inactive status. Health service providers (HSPs) are free to decide when to make a record inactive; however, it is preferable to follow the "three (3)-year rule," where all records of a deceased are made inactive 3 years after death. These guidelines pertain to government hospitals only.

Protected Health Information (PHI) would refer to any individually identifiable information whether oral or recorded in any form or medium that (1) is created or received by a stakeholder and (2) relates to past, present, or future physical or mental health conditions of an individual;

(3) the provision of healthcare to the individual; or (4) past, present, or future payment for healthcare to an individual. Patients will have the sufficient privileges to inspect and view their medical records without any time limit. Patient's privileges to amend data shall be limited to correction of errors in the recorded patient/medical details within 30 days. Patients can demand from a healthcare provider a copy of their medical records which should be provided within 30 days of receipt of communication of request. The existing Indian laws including Information Technology (IT) Act 2000 and their amendments from time to time would prevail.

CONCLUSION

Medical records are the best defense against medicolegal litigation. It is well established that poor record means poor defense and no record means no defense. So when medical record is incomplete or lost, it may cost a much for defense. Somebody has rightly said that dance like no one is watching, chart like it may one day be read aloud in a deposition. So it is vital for every medical personnel not only chart with due diligence but also preserve the medical record. Always remember most of the time litigation is filed with medical records that are in hand with patients that OPD prescriptions, discharge card, referral letter, and investigations so that there will never be a chance to review it and some of the vital documents may be hidden in oblique motives. So it is prudent to prepare these documents with maximum care and always get a receipt while issuing them. To remove all the doubts all doctors should preserve medical record for at least 3 years as per Medical Council Guidelines and daily case register, etc., for 6 years as per Income Tax rules. Electronic recordkeeping is somewhat gray area and more clarity should be sought by medical professionals. Always better be safe than sorry in maintaining medical records. Records will always remember even if doctor and patient forget it.

KEY LEARNING POINTS

- Records and documents can be "friends or foes" in the hours of crisis.
- Documents are the property of the hospital.
- The records/documents can be physical, electronic or audio-visual.
- The documents which are confidential shall be handed over to other relatives with the permission of the patient.
- The documents shall be preserved for the recommended period as mentioned in the article.
- As per NMC guidelines they should be given to the patient/relatives in 72 hours.

BIBLIOGRAPHY

1. AIR 1996 BOMBAY 198, (1996) 2 ALLMR 1 (BOM). [online] Available from https://www.aironline.in/legal-judgements/AIR%201996%20BOMBAY%20198 [Last accessed July, 2024].
2. Huffman EK. Medical Record Management, 9th edition. Berwyn, Illinois: Physicians' Record Company; 1990.
3. Wilkins A. (2011). How a pair of astrologers helped invent modern medical record-keeping. [online] available at https://gizmodo.com/how-a-pair-of-astrologers-helped-invent-modern-medical-5850286 [Last accessed July, 2024].

8

CHAPTER

Consent and Consent Forms

Aarti Avinash Kinikar, Rahul Madhav Dawre, Alka Kuthe

INTRODUCTION

Informed consent and its implications in the medical profession are continuously evolving. Earlier the medical profession was covering the points revolving around and treating patients. In today's time, the healthcare worker has to consider other points viz., moral issues, ethical issues, and the legal code and judiciary system which was earlier under the cover while treating the patients. Consent has a chief role to play in the welfare and health of the patient and to provide transparency in treatment and other spheres viz., legal and ethical code of conduct. The medical profession is trending toward consumer and service provider models, due to which there is disharmony between the two parties. "Free consent" is the bridge to reduce disharmony and promote the quality of care for the patient and as well for treating physician. Each country has its own set of protocols for consent with a few minute differences. The main aim and purpose of free consent are to provide the best available treatment for the patient and to promote the best clinical practices for healthcare professionals.

HISTORY OF CONSENT

The term informed consent first came into use in the year 1957, but its value and further discussion on the vitality of consent began in the mid-70s. As the idea of informed consent evolved, the discussion of appropriate guidelines moved increasingly from a narrow focus on the physician's or researcher's obligation to disclose information to the quality of a patient's or subject's understanding of information and the right to authorize or refuse a biomedical intervention.

Till the mid-20s-first century, medical management and treatment were purely based on trust and Hippocratic Corpus, i.e., beneficence and nonmaleficence. After the World War II, a lot of laws were reformed to save the right of human beings as patients or study subjects. It includes the Nuremberg code of 1947, the Declaration of Helsinki (1964), and section 13 of the Indian Contract Act (ICA) 1974. These acts made a drastic change in the field of human research and medical management. As the medical field is turning into a multimillion industry and the doctor-patient relationship is inclined toward the service provider-consumer relationship.

As per the Right to Health subsection, the charters of the human rights subsection in the National Human Right Commission dated 30th August, 2018 clearly state that every patient has the right to informed consent. This right is endorsed by MCI Code of Ethics Section 7.16,

Annexure 8 of standards for Hospital level 1 by National Clinical Establishments Council set up as per Clinical Establishment Act 2010, the Consumer Protection Act, 1986 and the Drugs and Cosmetic Act 1940, Rules 2016 on informed consent.

- It covers the right to get informed consent before any high-risk medical/surgical treatment/operation.
- It also mentions the hospital's role in the appropriate implication of these rules and regulations in their hospital.
- It came into existence after the Consumer Protection Act (COPRA).

DEFINITION AND TYPES OF CONSENT

Section 13 of the ICA defines consent as "Two or more persons are said to be in consent when they agree upon the same thing in the same sense *(consensus-ad-idem)*" **(Fig. 8.1)**.

Free Consent

Under section 14 of the ICA, "Consent is said to be free when it is not caused by coercion, undue influence, fraud, misrepresentation, or mistake."

Explanation of the aforementioned points in detail is given in the following text:

- *Coercion*: Under section 15 of the ICA, "Coercion" is the committing, or threatening to commit, any act forbidden by the Indian Penal Code (IPC) (45 of 1860) or the unlawful detaining, or threatening to detain, any property, to the prejudice of any person whatever, to cause any person to agree.
- *Undue influence*: Under section 16 of the ICA, where the relations subsisting between the parties are such that one of the parties is in a position to dominate the will of the other and uses that position to obtain an unfair advantage over the other.
- *Fraud (Section 17)*: "Fraud" means and includes any of the following acts committed by a party to a contract, or with his connivance, or by his agent, with intent to deceive another party thereto of his agent, or to induce him to enter into the contract: (1) the suggestion, as a fact, of that which is not true, by one who does not believe it to be true; (2) the active concealment of a fact by one having knowledge or belief of the fact; (3) a promise made without any intention of performing it; (4) any other act fitted to deceive; and (5) any such act or omission as the law specially declares to be fraudulent.

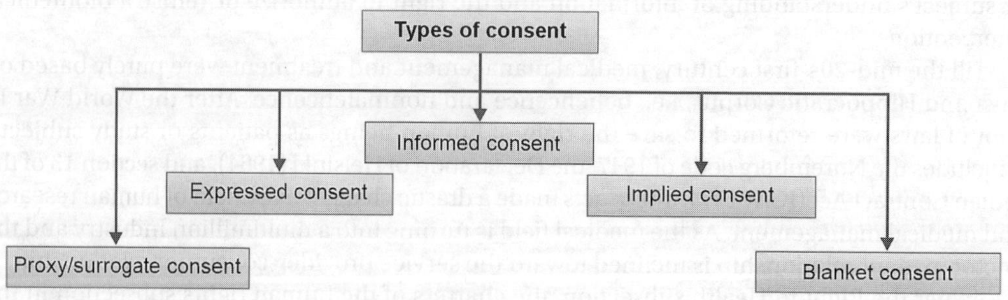

Fig. 8.1: Types of consent.

- *Misrepresentation (Section 18)*: "Causing, however innocently, a party to an agreement to make a mistake as to the substance of the thing which is the subject of the agreement."
- *Mistake of fact (Section 20)*: "Where both the parties to an agreement are under a mistake as to a matter of fact essential to the agreement, the agreement is void." A party cannot be allowed to get any relief on the ground that he had done some particular act in ignorance of the law. The mistake may be bilateral mistakes where both parties to an agreement are under mistake as a matter of fact. The mistake must relate to a matter of fact essential to the agreement.

Section 90 IPC states that Consent is void if given under fear of injury, or under a misconception of fact, and if the person doing the act knows, or has reason to believe, that the consent was given in consequence of such fear or misconception; or Consent of an insane person: If the consent is given by a person who, from unsoundness of mind, or intoxication, is unable to understand the nature and consequence of that to which he gives his consent; or Consent of the child: Unless the contrary appears from the context if the consent is given by a person who is under 12 years of age.

IMPLIED CONSENT

This is the most common and most widely used consent in all fields including medical and surgical branches. The implied consent is not objective, invisible, and not documented, even then it is admissible and valid in a court of law. It is also known as *Implicit Consent*. For example, when a patient enters the dental clinic and sits on the dental chair, his consent is implied for examination, diagnosis, and consultation. In the same way, if a patient visits a physician/surgeon for consultation for his/her illness/ailment. He/she is giving implied consent to take history and do a physical examination including inspection, palpation, percussion, and auscultation. In the same way for doing breath analysis for sobriety implied consent is sufficient to use a breath analyzer. Implied consent is given from the time of entry into the outpatient department or consultant office by the virtue of body language or gesture.

EXPRESS CONSENT

It is also known as *Explicit Consent*. The terms used in the consent must be clear, concerned with the issue and fully explicit language. It could be written or oral. Both types of consent are valid in law.

- *Oral consent*: This type of consent may be used for a minor procedure. Earlier it was necessary to have a witness during this consent, the witness may be any third person from a hospital or a relative. But the reproducibility of expressed oral consent is difficult considering the memory of third party and no documented proof. If the same consent is recorded with the help of audio-visual aid, the consent will become permanent and easily reproducible. In this case, the consent is valid and presentable in a court of law.
- *Written consent:* This consent is easily reproducible and is permanent. It is valid in a court of law.

For the examination of gynecological, ear-nose-throat (ENT), and general surgery patients per vaginum, per aural, and rectal examination, respectively, oral express consent is sufficient and written consent is not required. But, for the internal or physical examination, it is prudent to keep a female nurse or relative for the female patient during the time of examination. For the phlebotomist, the same consent is pertinent even though includes the collection of the blood sample. The collection of blood samples is a trivial procedure and is not considered life-threatening. Hence, the procedure of blood sample collection does not require written express consent. Though express consent is sufficient for physical examination, written informed consent for any procedure/minor surgery is a must and should be taken.

INFORMED CONSENT

Informed consent was used in 1957 in California. The doctrine of informed consent is based on the sound mind of the patient to think or decide whether to continue treatment or not. The concept of informed consent implies an objective test of the doctor to advise the patient of the advantages and disadvantages of undergoing the proposed treatment and more particularly to advise the patient of the risk involved. Here the doctor explains to the patient-relevant details regarding the nature of his disease, the various investigation and diagnostic procedures involved, the course and alternatives to the treatment proposed, the risk involved, and the prognosis and approximate expenditure for the same.

Anticipatory Consent

It is preferred to know the complication or major side effects of any surgical procedure and may require any further add-on surgery in any predefined surgical procedure. If the add-on surgery is known, a doctor can counsel the patient regarding the same and can take consent in advance to proceed with the required add-on procedure, if the complication arises rather than discussing and taking second consent.

For example:

- If a laparoscopic appendicectomy is planned in a case which is grand para with a history of three times lower segment cesarean section (LSCS) for delivery, during laparoscopic appendicectomy, the surgeon found multiple adhesions for which the surgeon needs to do open laparotomy and appendicectomy. In such cases, anticipatory consent is taken.

Intraoperative Consent

If the patient developed or had unforeseen or rarer complications during the surgery which is life-threatening and may cause further damage, another modality, i.e., another surgery which is not taken in the consent before surgery is necessary to save the patient's life. In these cases, intraoperative consent is essential and must be taken.

- In a case of grand para with a history of previous LSCS for delivery is again planned for LSCS for the second delivery. The consent for LSCS is taken prior, but during surgery, the surgeon noted profuse bleeding and the team of surgeons decided to go ahead with a total hysterectomy as a life-saving procedure. In this case, intraoperative consent is taken.

The difference between informed and expressed consent is discussed in **Table 8.1**.

Table 8.1: Difference between expressed and informed consent.

Points	*Express consent*	*Informed consent*
Type	General consent	Specific consent
Risk involved	Absent or minimal	Mild to severe
Discussion	Minimal to absent	In-depth—procedure, side effects, complications, etc.
Example	For taking blood pressure, drawing blood samples, etc.	For surgical procedure

PROXY CONSENT OR SURROGATE CONSENT

If the patient is not in the state of giving consent, in that case, the legal guardian/spouse/kin/major descendant, gives consent. It should be remembered that it is valid only in cases where the operation/mentioned surgery/treatment is of utmost necessity and could not be waited till the patient get conscious or medically fit to give consent. The decision of hysterectomy in nonindicated cases and nonemergency situations cannot be taken by the husband or legal guardians.

BLANKET CONSENT

The consent obtained to the effect that the patient is willing to undergo any type of treatment including surgeries without mentioning any procedure taken before admitting the patient is termed as blank consent. Such consents, however, have no legal validity as they do not mention any specific procedure, or it is possible complication.

Who Should or Can Take Consent?

The responsibility of taking consent lies with the treating physician/surgeon at the time of procedure or surgery. The best knowledge regarding the patient's condition lies with the treating physician/surgeon. The witness must be present during the counseling session regarding disease disclosure and discussion of available possible treatment modalities and the signing of the consent form. The subordinate doctors/nurses may only give add-on points from general points to specific points related to the mentioned procedure/surgery.

Who Can Give Informed Consent?

Patients with both the following points are fulfilled:
- A person or patient of >18 years.
- A person is mentally sound at the time of consent.

Conditions in Which Informed Consent is Required

- Minor or major invasive diagnostic or therapeutic surgical procedure/intervention;
- Chemotherapy, radiotherapy, and brachytherapy;

- Invasive radiological and investigational procedures;
- Medical research;
- Medical reports and sharing of patient's medical information where there is a chance of breach in doctor–patient confidentiality.

Conditions Where Patients' Valid Written Informed Consent is Not Required

In the following cases, legally authorized representatives are required to sign the consent form.
- *Minors*: Patients below eighteen (18) years old.
- *Mentally incompetent*: Patients who are permanently or temporarily incompetent due to psychiatric illness or are mentally challenged.
- *Impaired judgment*: Patients with permanent or temporary impairment, e.g., impaired judgment caused by some medications, substance abuse or severe hemodynamically unstable.

Conditions Where the Criteria for Consent may be Waived Off

In an emergency

It is not uncommon to get a patient in casualty in an unconscious state, under sedation or shock, or in other life-threatening situations. In these cases, he/she is unable to understand the condition and give legally valid consent for further diagnosis and treatment or surgery if required. And most of the time, there is no legal guardian or relative with the patients. Under these circumstances, a physician/surgeon can evade all the prerequisites for procuring valid consent and do whatever is necessary to save a life of a patient, child, or adult from permanent disability. Even though when parents or legal guardians are present at the casualty and the doctor is alone and to the best of his knowledge, the consent-taking process is time-consuming and life-threatening, he can take decisions for the continuation of treatment/surgery. The second in command, i.e., another doctor or staff nurse can inform the condition of the patient to parents/legal guardians.

However, such emergency treatment/surgery should be restricted only to the problems necessary. Anything else that could be performed later electively should be deferred. If during the emergency process, some coincidental and nonurgent problem is encountered, it should be dealt with later with other consent being obtained. For example, a sterilization procedure should not be performed during an emergency lifesaving laparotomy for ruptured tubal pregnancy.

If patient is minor

The question that arises here is what is meant by the word minor? The definition of minor is not given in any law or science books, but the definition of major as per the Indian Majority Act, 1875 is as follows:
- *Definition:* Age of majority of persons domiciled in India:
  - Every person domiciled in India shall attain the age of majority on his completing the age of 18 years and not before.
  - In computing the age of any person, the day on which he was born is to be included as a whole day and he shall be deemed to have attained majority at the beginning of the 18th anniversary of that day.

The second question that remains is if the child above 12 years is mature enough to give valid consent. The Indian law states that under section 90 a child below 12 years of age cannot be considered mature enough to give valid consent. As per the law section 89 IPC, the legal guardian/parents can give valid consent on the behalf of a minor patient. The rule for valid consent is not clear in law. The deduction of section 89 and section 90 of the IPC suggests that a child <12 years cannot give consent, but a child >12 years can give consent. This gray zone of 12–18 years is not clear in the law. As per the National Health Survey (NHS), in the United Kingdom, the age for consent is 16 years and over. The Children's Act 2005 South Africa mentions that children over 12 years of age can consent for the same provided they have the maturity "to understand the benefits, risks, social, and other implications of the treatment." Otherwise, the legal guardian or parents will give valid consent for medical or surgical treatment. In India, as per the Indian Council of Medical Research (ICMR) ethical guidelines, the legal age for consent is mentioned as 18 years and above.

If the patient is mentally challenged

The mentally challenged person criteria include the following:
- Legal age >18 years of age.
- He/she is unable to understand the effect and consequences of the disease, its treatment, and related complications *per se*.

  In the aforementioned case, consent must be taken from parents or legal guardians.

The third-party consent

It is taken from any family member such as spouse, grandparents, or in-laws in the family even when the patient is major with normal mental health. Such type of consent is invalid in a court of law. As per the law, in Standards for Female and Male Sterilization Services-2005, the spouse's consent is not required for male or female sterilization but is desirable.

Consent for research

As per the ICMR ethical guidelines, written valid consent is necessary for all types of research. The age criteria are the same as mentioned in previous sections. But assent is required in the age group of 7–18 years, in addition to consent from the parents/legal guardian. The research study should be explained to children between 7 and 18 years in easy language and with understandable content. The researcher cannot research if the child refused the assent for the study. There is a provision of waiver of assent where the available intervention is anticipated to benefit the child but would be available only if the child participates in the study, waiver of assent could be allowed **(Table 8.2)**.

Table 8.2: Difference between the consent and assent.

Point	*In assent*	*In consent*
Used as verb	It means to agree with an opinion	It implies willingness or granting permission for something to happen
Used as noun	It means agreement	It suggests permission/approval given by individual
Definition	The agreement is given by minors or people incapable of giving implied consent	The individual voluntarily agrees to the request by another person
In research activities	Agreeing to participate in a research study	Legally entered an agreement to participate in a research study
As per law	Not valid; not binding	Valid and binding

Doctrine of therapeutic privilege

It is also known as a *therapeutic exception*. The therapeutic privilege is used by doctors in medical/surgical situations where the doctor believes that disclosure of the information to the patient at that juncture may do more harm or may possess serious health-related consequences. In these scenarios, the doctor can withhold the disclosure of information to be given to the patient. For example, if the patient is a case of angina pectoris and is emotionally unstable. The doctor can withhold the disclosure of some information that the doctor may feel will precipitate angina and could be life-threatening. But it is the responsibility of the doctor to inform the same information to the spouse/kin/parents, or legal guardian and take written consent paper of the reason for withholding information to the patient. The information should be disclosed as soon as the patient is emotionally or mentally stable to handle the information.

Doctrine of loco parentis

It is a Latin term meaning "in the place of parents." It applies to schools, boarding schools, orphanages, nursing homes, etc. It gives the responsibility to these institutions to take decisions for medical treatment in the absence of parents. Once the parents reach the hospital, the patient's responsibility will return to the parents. Hence, it is the doctor's responsibility to retake the signature of the parents on the consent form whether the procedure is to be performed or already performed for the sake of the patient life at that moment.

ADVANCE DIRECTIVES

It is a lawfully valid and permitted document which is prepared in advance to designate as an individual(s) viz., spouse, kin, a close friend, or any other person to whom the executor willingly gives authority to speak on his behalf if the executor/patient is not in a condition to decide for himself/herself. At the need for any major medical decisions to take such as which healthcare option could be taken or whether the treatment should be continued or not. It contains directions for CPR, artificial nutrition, maintenance on a ventilator, blood transfusions, etc., at the terminal stage of illness.

As per the landmark judgment passed by the Hon'ble Constitution Bench of four Judges of the Supreme Court of India titled "Common Cause versus Union of India, 2018 (5) SCC 1," the advance medical directives are legal in India.

It needs to be clear that the advance medical directive is not equivalent to euthanasia **(Table 8.3)**.

Table 8.3: Difference between the advance medical directives and euthanasia.

Advance medical directives	*Euthanasia*
It is a refusal to take treatment even if it is lifesaving	Actively give some medicine or drug to kill a patient
For this written valid consent is a must and submit to the magistrate in advance	No guideline
Legally valid in India	Illegal in India

Refusal to Give Consent for Treatment/Surgery

As per the Human Rights Act, the patient may take the decisions for his/her own body. The mentally competent adult can take the decision not to take medical advice, treatment, and surgical intervention or select an alternative mode of treatment even if the disease is life-threatening. The doctor cannot refuse to acknowledge the patient's demands. For example, if the mentally capable adult diabetic patient desires not to take an insulin injection, the doctor cannot force the patient to take the insulin injection, if the patient can take a decision. Refusal should not be merely the absence of consent. The patient needs to sign a written valid consent of refusal of treatment. The doctor can refer or discharge this case from his hospital. In the case of a minor or mentally challenged patient, if the parents or legal guardian refuses to take treatment, the court can overrule the case and give instructions to the physician or hospital to continue treatment.

PREPRINTED CONSENT FORMS

Majority of hospitals use dummy consent forms. These forms may be preprinted, in English or in the local language, simple to understand, and covers most of the points of consent forms. However, one consent form cannot be ideal or covers all the points of medical/surgical treatment or its related risks or complications in it. Even if the fill-in-the-blank format is used for consent forms, it is difficult to justify the means of a valid consent form. Hence, it is preferable to write separate consent for each case, handwritten, in a language in which the patient/legal guardian/spouse is comfortable.

Points to be Covered in Valid Consent Form

- Local language and English language
- Date and time of consent
- Name of patient
- Name of witness/spouse/legal guardian
- If the spouse or legal guardian, their relation with the patient and the contact number
- Name of the hospital with the address
- Points of free consent
- Working diagnosis
- Medical/surgical procedure required (in short—but should cover the majority of the required information—sometimes may require a rough diagram to make the patient or legal guardian understand the procedure)
- Name of leading doctors involved in medical/surgical procedures.
- Date and time of medical/surgical procedure
- Inadvertent/related complications if any may occur and their percentage
- Side effects/aftereffects of medical/surgical procedure
- Signature of a doctor, patient/spouse/relative and one witness
- Left-hand thumb imprint if spouse/relative and one witness is illiterate

May or May Not Include in the Consent Form

- Expected benefits after the procedure
- Alternative treatment modality if any is available
- Consequences of not taking medical/surgical treatment/procedure
- Cost of treatment/surgery, if applicable

Conditions Where Informed Consent is NOT Required from Patient

- Medicolegal case bought by the police under section IPC 53 Criminal Penal Code (Punishments to which offenders are liable under the provisions of this Code are—death; imprisonment for life, etc.).
- Examination under court orders
- Prisoners (new)
- If the patient is incompetent to give valid consent
  - Due to minor age
  - The patient is mentally challenged.
  - Emergency—unconscious, intoxicated due to drug/alcohol, sedatives, etc.

FEW CASES RELATED TO CONSENT IN INDIAN JUDICIARY

Case 1

Issue: Not taking consent for surgery from the patient in the nonemergency case.

Court verdict: The treating surgeon shall refund the operation and hospital fees with interest at the rate of 10% per annum from the date of payment till the date of repayment, i.e., the respondent shall pay to the appellant a sum of INR 25,000 as compensation with interest thereon at the rate of 10% per annum from November 19, 2003 (the date of the order of Commission) till the date of payment. The appellant will also be entitled to costs of INR 5,000 from the respondent.

Case 2

Issue: Blanket consent for surgery.

Court verdict: The court affirmed the consent is not taken appropriately.

Case 3

Issue: Hysterectomy done without consent.

Court verdict: The treating surgeon has done what is required to save the life of the patient. The case was dismissed.

Case 4

Issue: Complications of surgery not explained to the patient.

Court verdict: The treating surgeon has to inform all the complications of surgery to the patient. The doctor was made liable to pay a sum of INR 3.5 lakhs to the patient as compensation for negligence.

Case 5

Issue: No negative consent for surgery on case paper.

Court verdict: The treating surgeon has to take positive as well as negative consent on paper. The court dismissed the doctor's plea. The doctor was made liable to pay the patient as compensation for negligence.

Case 6

Issue: No proper consent for surgery on case paper.

Court verdict: The court dismissed all allegations against the surgeons. The court stated that uniform use of this preprinted and fixed "informed consent cum undertaking" form on the part of the opposite party no. 1 (hospital) was unfair trade practice within the meaning of section 2(1)(r) of the Act 1986 and deem it just and appropriate to impose a cost of INR 10 lakhs on the opposite party no. 1 (hospital), to be deposited with the Consumer Legal Aid Account of this Commission within 4 weeks of the pronouncement of the reasoned judgment, and to direct the opposite party no. 1 (hospital) to discontinue its said unfair trade practice with immediate effect.

Consent is an evolving process, it started from verbal consent to written informed consent, and now in many places, audio visual aided consent is accepted.

CONCLUSION

There are many instances where doctors worldwide have failed to comply with the informed consent standard, resulting in a loss in the judiciary system, even after providing the clinically professional standard of care. The importance and weightage of informed consent are huge. It is prudent for healthcare professionals to understand free consent and expand the knowledge and practices related to it.

KEY LEARNING POINTS

- In today's world, it is essential and mandatory to take written consent in the presence of an unbiased witness before any medical or surgical procedure.
- Any consent will not be considered free consent if the person is terrified to say "NO" or not in the state to understand the meaning of either "YES" or "NO."
- There are limitations for third party consent.
- Assent is a must for clinical research on 7–18 years in spite of consent from legal guardians/parents.

BIBLIOGRAPHY

1. CAG of India. The Indian Contract Act, 1972. [online] Available from https://www.cag.gov.in/uploads/media/Indian-Contract-Act-1872-20200816140128.pdf. [Last accessed August, 2024].
2. CaseMine™. Vinod Khanna vs. G. Stone Urology and Laparoscopy Hospital and 2 Ors. [online] Available from https://www.casemine.com/judgement/in/5f03ab2c9fca1957d423d004. [Last accessed August, 2024].
3. Council for International Organizations of Medical Sciences. (2016). International ethical guidelines for health-related research involving humans. [online] Available from https://cioms.ch/wp-content/uploads/2017/01/WEB-CIOMS-EthicalGuidelines.pdf. [Last accessed August, 2024].
4. Dik BJ, Doenges TJ. (2019). Declaration of Helsinki. [online] Available from https://www.britannica.com/topic/Declaration-of-Helsinki. [Last accessed August, 2024].
5. Encyclopedia.com. (2022). Informed Consent: I. History of Informed Consent. [online] Available from <https://www.encyclopedia.com>. [Last accessed August, 2024].
6. Indian Council of Medical Research-2017. National Ethical Guidelines For Biomedical And Health Research Involving Human Participants. [online] Available from https://ethics.ncdirindia.org/asset/pdf/ICMR_National_Ethical_Guidelines.pdf. [Last accessed August, 2024].
7. Ministry of Law and Justice. Indian Majority Act-1975. [online] Available from The Majority Act, 1875 |Legislative Department | Ministry of Law and Justice | GoI. [Last accessed August, 2024].
8. Mitscherlich A, Mielke F. The Nuremberg Code (1947). In: Mitscherlich A, Mielke F (Eds). Doctors of infamy: the story of the Nazi medical crimes. New York: Schuman; 1949. pp. xxiii-xxv.
9. National Human Rights Commission India. Annual Report-2018. [online] Available from https://nhrc.nic.in/sites/default/files/Annual%20Report%202018-29_final.pdf. [Last accessed August, 2024].
10. NHRC. (2022). Annual Report-2017-2018 of National Human rights commission India. [online] Available from Annual Reports | National Human Rights Commission India (nhrc.nic.in). [Last accessed August, 2024].

9

CHAPTER

Medical Negligence

Devaraj V Raichur

INTRODUCTION

"Medical negligence" is an expression used to describe actions or omissions by medical practitioners, during their profession, unduly causing damage to the patients. It is not defined in any of the Indian statutes. Worldwide, and in India, the laws relating to medical negligence are becoming progressively well-defined through various judgments over years. An understanding of the issue is helpful to medical practitioners in the context of increasing litigations and compensations.

WHAT IS NEGLIGENCE?

In *Blyth* vs. *The Company of Proprietors of the Birmingham Waterworks,* Baron Alderson J, observed:

> *"Negligence is the omission to do something which a reasonable man, guided upon those considerations which ordinarily regulate the conduct of human affairs, would do, or doing something which a prudent and reasonable man would not do."*
>
> Over the years this has been considered the definition of negligence.

He further went on to highlight the importance of *foreseeability* in considering if an action is negligent, in the following words:

> *"Such a state of circumstances (of the case) constitutes a contingency against which no reasonable man can provide. The result was an accident, for which the defendants cannot be held liable."*

The *contextual nature* of what constitutes negligence was addressed by the Supreme Court of India in *Municipal Corporation of Greater Bombay* vs. *Laxman Iyer*:

> *"Negligence means either subjectively a careless state of mind, or objectively careless conduct. Negligence is not an absolute term but is a relative one; it is rather a comparative term. No absolute standard can be fixed and no mathematically exact formula can be laid down by which negligence or lack of it can be infallibly measured in a given case. What constitutes negligence varies under different conditions and in determining whether negligence exists in a particular case, or whether a mere act or course of conduct amounts to negligence, all the attending and surrounding facts and circumstances*

have to be taken into account. To determine whether an act would be or would not be negligent, it is relevant to determine if any reasonable man would foresee that the act would cause damage or not. The omission to do what the law obligates or even the failure to do anything in a manner, mode, or method envisaged by law would equally and per se constitute negligence in the part of such persons. If the answer is in the affirmative, it is a negligent act."

In *Spring Meadows Hospital* vs. *Harjol Ahluwalia,* the Supreme Court held that judgment errors do not always infer negligence.

Further, it is noted that negligence does not always mean absolute carelessness but want of such a degree of care as is required in particular circumstances.

THE ELEMENTS OF NEGLIGENCE

For an act or omission to be considered as negligence by the court, the four elements that must be present are: (1) duty, (2) breach of the duty, (3) damage, and (4) direct causation of the damage.

For any act or omission by the doctor to be considered as medical negligence, all the following essential elements need to be present: (1) duty of care (doctor-patient relationship), (2) dereliction (or breach) in the duty, (3) reasonably foreseeable damage resulting to the patient, and (4) direct causation of the damage by the breach in the duty.

If one or more of the elements are missing, it would not be legally relevant.

Duty of Care

In *Dr Laxman Balkrishna Joshi* vs. *Dr Trimbark Babu Godbole and Anr.* and *AS Mittal* vs. *State of UP*, it was observed by the Supreme Court of India that a doctor owes to his patient the duties of care in: (1) deciding whether to undertake the case, (2) deciding what treatment to give, and (3) the administration of the treatment. A breach of any of the aforementioned duties may give a cause of action for negligence. The practitioner must bring to task a reasonable degree of skill and knowledge and must exercise a reasonable degree of care. Neither the very highest degree nor a very low degree of care and competence judged in the light of the particular circumstances of each case is what the law requires.

Thus, in any situation where a doctor-patient relationship is established, there is a duty of care by the physician to the patient.

Dereliction (or Breach) in Duty

The medical practitioner is expected to have proper qualifications and skills. He must be registered with the appropriate authority. The practitioner must practice a level of care appropriate to the situation and reasonable degree of skill. If such behavior is lacking, it could constitute an element for considering medical negligence.

In *Indian Medical Association* vs. *VP Shantha,* the Supreme Court held:

"...The approach of the courts is to require that professional men should possess a certain minimum degree of competence and that they should exercise reasonable care in the discharge of their duties. In general, a professional man owes to his client a duty

in tort as well as in contract to exercise reasonable care in giving advice or performing services."

If there is no breach of duty on the part of the medical practitioner, there is no medical negligence though the patient suffered damage. In *Dr Ganesh Prasad and Anr.* vs. *Lal Janamajay Nath Shahdeo, I,* the National Commission held that where proper treatment is given and death occurred due to the process of disease and its complication, it cannot be held that doctors and hospital are negligent.

Reasonably Foreseeable Damage and Direct Causation

It was observed in *King* vs. *Phillips* that a question of negligence arises only when there is a direct harm to the plaintiff by the misconduct and the harm should be foreseeable.

As we saw earlier, from the observations of Baron Alderson (Judge) in *Blyth* vs. *the Company of Proprietors of the Birmingham Waterworks,* it is clear that damage is an essential element of negligence. In the context of negligence, damages to the patient that are accidental in nature cannot be considered for medical negligence. For considering medical negligence, the patient must have suffered a damage which is clearly identifiable and recognized by law as that which could be foreseen by a reasonably competent practitioner. Further, damage as a natural consequence of a recognized and professionally accepted form of management cannot be considered for medical negligence; this applies to the medical/surgical procedures, in the presence of a real and valid consent. It is worth noting here that the concept of real and valid consent has been considered to be appropriate for the current Indian context, in *Samira Kohli* vs. *Prabha Manchanda Dr and Anr.*, in preference over the concept of informed consent as in *Canterbury* vs. *Spence.*

Apart from the damage, to consider medical negligence, it must be shown by the complainant that the breach in the duty of care is the direct and proximate cause of the damage suffered by the patient.

BURDEN OF PROOF

In general, the burden of proof lies with the complainant. The complainant has to produce evidences to prove that all the elements of medical negligence are fulfilled.

However, in case of *res ipsa loquitur*, the onus of proof shifts to the defendant (medical practitioner), who has to prove that damage did not occur from his conduct (breach of duty of care). Further, in negligence per se, no further proof of negligence is required.

RES IPSA LOQUITUR

If it is improbable that the damage complained of could have resulted without the act or omission of the medical practitioner, the maxim of *res ipsa loquitur* (from the Latin, meaning "*the thing speaks for itself*") is used.

The National Commission in *Dr G Vivekananda Verma* vs. *Chinta Bhramaramba and Ors.,* held, "The petitioner surgeon gave anesthesia himself and has not shown how "anoxic encephalopathy" occurred and whether immediate action was taken to avoid the complication and whether timely treatment was imparted to the patient to avoid anoxic encephalopathy. From the records of the Swatantra Hospital and NIIMS it is seen that the patient died due to anoxic encephalopathy suffered during tonsillectomy. We agree with the findings of the state commission that there is deficiency in service and negligence by the petitioner. It is clear that the doctrine of *res ipsa loquitur* applies in the present case."

The National Commission in *Dr Ravishankar vs. Jery K Thomas and Anr.,* observed that it has no option but to deduce that it was a clear case of medical negligence on the part of the appellant (doctor), and held that he was liable, for leaving behind ribbon gauze in the right side of the nose after a septoplasty resulting in several complications.

NEGLIGENCE PER SE

Negligence per se, according to *Black's Law Dictionary,* is *"Negligence established as a matter of law, so that breach of the duty is not a jury question."* Negligence per se usually arises from a statutory violation. It is also termed as legal negligence.

Where a person is guilty of negligence per se, no further proof is needed.

The Supreme Court held, *"A person who does not have knowledge of a particular system of medicine but practices in that system is a quack,"* while the Court was dealing with the absence of basic qualifications of a homeopathic doctor to practice allopathy, in *Poonam Verma* vs. *Ashwin Patel and Ors.*

TESTS OF MEDICAL NEGLIGENCE: BOLAM TEST AND BOLITHO TEST

Bolam Test

The principle of the test for medical negligence laid in *Bolam* vs. *Friern Hospital Management Committee* is being followed in India. In that case, McNair J, observed:

> *"...A doctor is not negligent if he has acted in accordance with a practice accepted as proper by a responsible body of medical men skilled in that particular art... Putting it the other way round, a doctor is not negligent if he is acting in accordance with such a practice, merely because there is a body of opinion that takes a contrary view. At the same time, that does not mean that a medical man can obstinately and pig-headedly carry on with some old technique if it has been proved to be contrary to what is really substantially the whole of informed medical opinion."*

In *Achutrao Haribhau Khodwa* vs. *State of Maharashtra,* the Supreme Court held:

> *"The skill of medical practitioners differs from doctor to doctor. The nature of the profession is such that there may be more than one course of treatment which may be advisable for treating a patient. Courts would indeed be slow in attributing negligence on the part of a doctor if he has performed his duties to the best of his ability and with due care and caution. Medical opinion may differ with regard to the course of action to be taken by a doctor treating a patient, but as long as a doctor acts in a manner which is acceptable to the medical profession and the court finds that he has attended on the patient with due care, skill, and diligence and if the patient still does not survive or suffers a permanent ailment, it would be difficult to hold the doctor to be guilty of negligence.*

In cases where the doctors act carelessly and in a manner which is not expected of a medical practitioner, then in such a case an action in torts would be maintainable."

In *Jacob Mathew* vs. *State of Punjab*, the Supreme Court laid down Bolam test as the most efficient measure of testing medical negligence and said that by this standard, a professional may be held liable for negligence on one of the two findings:

1. Either he was not possessed of the requisite skill which he professed to have possessed; or
2. He did not exercise, with reasonable competence in the given case, the skill which he did possess.

Poonam Verma vs. *Ashwin Patel and Ors., State of Haryana and others* vs. *Smt Santra JT 2000 (5) SC 34,* and *Suresh Gupta (Dr)* vs. *Government of NCT of Delhi* are some of the many other examples where Bolam test has been held good in India.

Bolitho Test

As we saw earlier, the commonly used test in India to prove that a medical practitioner failed to meet the required standard of care is the Bolam test. The Bolitho test, which resulted from the 1996 court case of *Bolitho* vs. *City and Hackney health authorities,* is a modification of the Bolam test. According to the Bolam test no doctor can be found guilty of negligence if they have acted in accordance with a responsible body of medical opinion. The Bolitho test clarifies that "a responsible body" to be one whose opinion had a "logical basis."

While the Bolitho test has received considerable judicial endorsement in England, it has been brought up in the Indian Supreme Court on only two occasions.

In *Vinitha Ashok* vs. *Lakshmi Hospital,* the Supreme Court clarified:

"...A doctor will be liable for negligence in respect of diagnosis and treatment in spite of a body of professional opinion approving his conduct where it has not been established to the court's satisfaction that such opinion relied on is reasonable or responsible. If it can be demonstrated that the professional opinion is not capable of withstanding the logical analysis, the court would be entitled to hold that the body of opinion is not reasonable or responsible."

It was stated in *Samira Kohli* vs. *Prabha Manchanda Dr and Anr. 1 (2008) CPJ 56 (SC),* where the court clearly pointed out, "A beginning has been made in Bolitho vs. City and Hackney HA 1998 1 AC 232 and Pearce vs. United Bristol Healthcare NHS Trust 1998 (48) BMLR 118. We have however, consciously preferred the "real consent" concept evolved in Bolam..."

However, in the recent years, at least some of the legal luminaries have expressed the need to redefine the test for medical negligence in India.

In *V Kishan Rao* vs. *Nikhil Super Speciality Hospital and Anr.*, Justice AK Ganguly addressed the Supreme Court observed:

"Even though Bolam test was accepted by this Court as providing the standard norms in cases of medical negligence, in the country of its origin, it is questioned on various grounds. It has been found that the inherent danger in Bolam test is that if the Courts defer too readily to expert evidence medical standards would obviously decline."

CRIMINAL MEDICAL NEGLIGENCE

As with negligence in general, medical negligence too has possibility of criminal liability. As a rule, for criminal liability there needs to be *mens rea* (criminal intent; literal meaning, "guilty mind"). Negligence is an exception to this rule. Deaths, hurts, and grievous hurts caused by rash and negligent acts by the offender are punishable under the *Bharatiya Nyaya Sanhita*, 2023 (BNS).

While civil liability may lead to paying compensation, a criminal liability under Section 106(1), and Section 125(a) and 125(b) of the BNS is punishable with imprisonment of either description (simple or rigorous) or with fine or with both; the offence is cognizable, bailable, triable by Magistrate of the first class and noncompoundable. The BNS sections are as follows:

- 106. Causing death by negligence. (1) Whoever causes death of any person by doing any rash or negligent act not amounting to culpable homicide, shall be punished with imprisonment of either description for a term which may extend to 5 years, and shall also be liable to fine; and if such act is done by a registered medical practitioner while performing medical procedure, he shall be punished with imprisonment of either description for a term which may extend to 2 years, and shall also be liable to fine.
  Explanation: For the purposes of this sub-section, "registered medical practitioner" means a medical practitioner who possesses any medical qualification recognized under the National Medical Commission Act, 2019 (30 of 2019) and whose name has been entered in the National Medical Register or a State Medical Register under that Act.
  The offence is cognizable, bailable, triable by Magistrate of the first class and noncompoundable.
- 125. Act endangering life or personal safety of others. Whoever does any act so rashly or negligently as to endanger human life or the personal safety of others, shall be punished with imprisonment of either description for a term which may extend to 3 months or with fine which may extend to ₹2,500, or with both, but (a) where hurt is caused, shall be punished with imprisonment of either description for a term which may extend to 6 months, or with fine which may extend to ₹5,000, or with both; (b) where grievous hurt is caused, shall be punished with imprisonment of either description for a term which may extend to 3 years, or with fine which may extend to ₹10,000, or with both.
  The offence is cognizable, bailable, triable by any Magistrate and compoundable by the person to whom hurt is caused with the permission of the court.

The Supreme Court in *Syed Akbar* vs. *State of Karnataka* held that negligence required to be proved in a criminal case must be gross and not based on just an error of judgment. Further, it observed that there is a marked difference in the standard of proof in cases of civil negligence and those of criminal negligence. In a case of civil negligence, the allegation can be proved by the doctrine of preponderance of probability, but the charge of criminal negligence has to be proved beyond reasonable doubt. Where negligence is an essential ingredient of the offence, the negligence to be established by the prosecution must be culpable or gross and not the negligence merely based upon an error of judgment.

In *Dr Suresh Gupta* vs. *Government of NCT of Delhi and Anr.*, the Supreme Court held that the threshold of negligence required establishing criminal liability for a doctor or surgeon is kept being so high that it may be termed as "gross negligence" or "recklessness." It is not just a matter of not providing the appropriate care, attention, and skill. As noted earlier, judgment errors do not always infer negligence. "When a patient's death results merely from an error of judgment or an accident, no criminal liability should be attached to it. Mere inadvertence or some degree of want of adequate care might lead to civil liability but not criminal liability."

CONCLUSION

In conclusion, litigations claiming medical negligence and compensations given by the courts are on the rise. The medical fraternity needs to get acquainted with what the law requires of them. Knowledge on what constitutes medical negligence and what could be used to defend a litigation is helpful. Distinguishing civil and criminal liability is important. Bolam test is the standard test to prove medical negligence in India. Bolitho test is increasingly being relied upon as a test for establishing medical negligence in England and some Indian legal experts consider it could be a better test for India, too.

KEY LEARNING POINTS

- Litigations claiming medical negligence and the compensation given are rising.
- The essential elements for liability under medical negligence constitute: Duty of care, dereliction (breach) of the duty, damage happening to the patient that is foreseeable, and direct and proximate causation of the damage; all these elements must be proven to claim medical negligence.
- Burden of proof is with the complainant.
- In *res ipsa loquitur* the onus of proof shifts to the defender (medical practitioner) and in negligence *per se*, no further proof is necessary.
- Civil liability may lead to paying compensation and criminal liability could result in imprisonment or/ and fine.

BIBLIOGRAPHY

1. *A.S. Mittal v. State of U.P.* AIR 1989 SC 1570.
2. *Achutrao Haribhau Khodwa v. State of Maharashtra* (1996) 2 SCC 634.
3. Black HC. Black's Law Dictionary. In: Garner BA (Ed). Black's Law Dictionary, 9th edition. Minesota: West Publishing Co.; 2009. p. 1135.
4. *Blyth v. The Company of Proprietors of The Birmingham Waterworks [1856] EWHC Exch J65 (06 February 1856).*
5. *Bolam v. Friern Hospital Management Committee* (1957) 1 WLR 582 : (1957) 2 All ER 118.
6. *Bolitho v. City and Hackney health authorities* (1998) 1 AC 232.
7. *Canterbury v. Spence* 464 F.2d. 772, 782 D.C. Cir. 1972.
8. Chandra MS, Bada Math S. Progress in Medicine: Compensation and medical negligence in India: Does the system need a quick fix or an overhaul? Ann Indian Acad Neurol. 2016;19(Suppl 1):S21-7.
9. *Dr. G. Vivekananda Verma vs Chinta Bharamaramba and Ors.* III (2006) CPJ 104 (NC).
10. *Dr. Ganesh Prasad and Anr. v. Lal Janamajay Nath Shahdeo, I* (2006) CPJ 117 (NC).
11. *Dr. Laxman Balkrishna Joshi vs. Dr. Trimbark Babu Godbole and Anr.* AIR 1969 SC 128.
12. *Dr. Ravishankar vs. Jery K. Thomas and Anr.* II (2006) CPJ 138 (NC).
13. *Indian Medical Assn. v. V.P. Shantha* (1995) 6 SCC 651.
14. *Jacob Mathew v. State of Punjab*, 2005 6 SCC 1.
15. *King v. Phillips* [1953] 1 QB 429.
16. Municipal Corpn. Of Greater Bombay v Laxman Iyer, 2003 (8) SCC 731

17. *Poonam Verma vs. Ashwin Patel and Ors.* (1996) 4 SCC 322.
18. *Samira Kohli vs. Prabha Manchanda Dr. & Anr.* 1 (2008) CPJ 56 (SC).
19. Spring Meadows Hospital v. Harjol Ahluwalia (1998) 4 SCC 39.
20. *State of Haryana and others v. Smt. Santra J.T.* 2000(5) SC 34.
21. *Suresh Gupta (Dr) v. Govt. of NCT of Delhi* (2004) 6 SCC 422.
22. *Syed Akbar v. State of Karnataka* (1980) 1 SCC 30.
23. The Indian Penal Code, 1860.
24. *V. Kishan Rao v. Nikhil Super Speciality Hospital & Anr.* [2010] 5 S.C.R. 1
25. *Vinitha Ashok v. Lakshmi Hospital* (2001) 8 SCC 731.

10

CHAPTER

Errors in Medical Practice

Sushil Kumar, Deepshikha, Kumar Diwakar

INTRODUCTION

Any incorrect action or statement has the potential to harm patients and have medicolegal repercussions in the practice of medicine. Although errors should not occur, they inevitably do because, as Alexander Pope famously put it, "*to err is human.*" It is our responsibility to minimize errors as much as possible. We can develop methods to prevent errors by having a deeper understanding of errors and how they happen. The use of technology plays a major role in this. According to the severity of the injury they cause, the location where they occur, or other factors, medical errors have been classified in a variety of ways over time. This chapter describes the numerous types of medical errors, as well as their causes, prevention, and remedies.

DEFINITIONS

Medical Error

Medical error is the failure of a planned activity to be accomplished as intended (i.e., an execution error) or the implementation of an incorrect plan to accomplish an objective (i.e., a planning error). Errors can be brought on by an act of commission or omission that has the potential to produce an unanticipated outcome or omission and they frequently reveal flaws in the delivery of healthcare systems. Medical errors fall into two primary categories.

Errors of Omission

Error of omission happens as a result of inaction. This is a healthcare provider's failure to take action that would have prevented a patient from suffering severe health compromise, long-term disability, or even death. This idea is often explained as a medical professional not performing in a reasonable prudent way in the given circumstances. Examples include failing to request diagnostic tests to make a diagnosis or failing to administer a patient a proven drug that is essential to stabilize or treat their condition.

Errors of the Commission

Error of the commission occurs because of the improper action taken. It involves medical professionals acting in a way that altered the patient's outcome. Examples include mistakes made when prescribing (incorrect prescription), dispensing, and administering (wrong dose, wrong time, and wrong manner).

Errors can also be divided into two broad groups:

1. *Active error*: Events that happen right before an incident or accident are called active errors. This is the actual incident that produces the harm or a catastrophe. These are the conducts of those operating closely with patients on the front lines, such as doctors and nurses. Performing surgery on the incorrect person or limb, for instance.
2. *Latent error*: They are inherent flaws in the system and include errors in the design of systems or processes, issues with the setup or upkeep of equipment, and inadequate organizational structures.

When a latent error occurs in combination with an active human error, some type of event manifests in the patient. The active human error triggers the hidden latent error, resulting in an adverse event.

Every catastrophic failure has a systemic flaw (latent error) at its root that is brought on by an act of commission or omission (active error) by personnel directly involved in patient care.

Adverse Event

Adverse event is a kind of injury that, often, is brought on by error in medical or surgical care and necessitates medical attention as opposed to a complication(s) of disease. Medical management encompasses all facets of care, including diagnosis, treatment, failure to diagnose or treat, and the processes and tools used to administer care. Adverse events may be preventable or nonpreventable. Preventable adverse event is caused by an error or other type of systems or equipment failure and thus can be attributed to medical error. During medical treatment, an adverse event could happen unintended or as a side effect. Unintentional injury, extended hospital stays, or physical disabilities brought on by the administration of treatment in medical or surgical patients are examples of adverse occurrences. Complications brought on by extended hospitalization or by aspects of the healthcare system itself might also be considered adverse events. All adverse events may not be the result of negligence or errors.

Negligence

Negligence is failure to provide the standard of care that a competent, average healthcare practitioner would provide in the same situation when caring for the patient in question. For instance, the medical professional might have neglected to review the pathology report, which resulted in the cancer being undetected or the surgeon might have left an instrument or sponge inside the patient.

Negligent Adverse Events

An adverse event that occurred as a result of negligence or a healthcare worker's failure to perform as per the standard of care is negligent adverse event. Examples include a patient who experienced a neurological deficit after surgery in which the surgeon accidentally cut a nerve, which was outside the range of the procedure's typical problems.

Near Miss

Near miss is an unsafe incident or circumstance involving a patient that, because of early intervention or some other factor, did not take place and therefore potential harm was prevented. It is advisable to take these into account in reporting so that, even though no error occurred, there is still potential to identify issues in the system for improvement through the improvement in the system.

Never Event

Errors that ought never to happen to any patient are known as never events. These major adverse occurrences are easily recognizable, quantifiable, and typically avoidable. One example is surgery performed on the incorrect limb.

Sentinel Event

Sentinel event is defined as any unforeseen circumstance that results in serious, temporary, or permanent or psychological harm or patient death that is not directly related to the illness or progression of the disease. This is the result of serious mismanagement or neglect toward the patients on the part of healthcare providers. Sentinel instances must always be investigated to determine the cause and action should be taken to prevent future occurrences. All never events are sentinel events. In addition, events that can lead to loss of reputation or loss of business are also considered sentinel events.

Following are some examples of sentinel events:
- Burn injury to neonates kept under warmer
- Bilirubin encephalopathy in hospitalized neonates
- Lost guidewire while putting central venous catheter
- Wrong patients or wrong site surgery
- Abduction of child from hospital
- Injury to finger or other body parts by rats in hospitalized patients
- Transfusion reaction due to unmatched blood products
- Intrapartum maternal death
- Death of full-term infant in utero
- Rape or physical harm to the hospitalized patients

The investigation must be conducted after sentinel events to determine the root cause. To determine the cause, there are two approaches. These are:
1. Root cause analysis (RCA)
2. Failure mode and effects analysis (FMEA)

Root Cause Analysis

Root cause analysis is used to identify the root cause of an error, to identify a preventative strategy, and then implement the strategy going forward to stop reoccurring problems. As an illustration, a doctor might administer azithromycin to a patient who is allergic to erythromycin. Patient experienced anaphylactic shock and passed away. To prevent a repeat of this incident, an investigation should be done to determine the cause and a training session on drug interactions should be given to all relevant healthcare workers.

There are five basic tools for RCA, though there are more complicated tools also.

1. Pareto
2. Five why analysis
3. Fish bone diagram
4. Scatter plot
5. Process mapping that leads to failure mode analysis

Details of the methods can be found in various quality improvement guideline books.

Failure Mode and Effects Analysis

Failure mode and effects analysis is a systematic and proactive strategy for evaluating a process' potential points of failure as well as the repercussions of those failures. Even if a healthcare provider is careful, an error may still happen, according to failure mode and effect analysis. It serves as error-catching safety nets. Failure mode analysis essentially involves breaking down the process into small steps and identifying possible slip ups. Example of a failure mode and effect analysis: Physician prescribes medication; nurse confirms order; pharmacist verifies and dispenses medication; nurse again verifies pharmacist's accuracy; and finally, nurse administers medication to patients.

PREVALENCE

Having an actual prevalence of medical errors is quite challenging. The primary factors are underreporting, a fear-based stigma, and a lack of registry systems in the majority of nations around the globe. The Institute of Medicine (IOM) published a report titled "To Err is Human: Building a Safer Health System" on November 29, 1999. The world learned about medical error for the first time with the publication of this report. According to this analysis, 44,000–98,000 Americans per year pass away as a result of medical mistakes that may have been avoided. Prior to that, Brennan et al. examined the medical records of 30,121 patients admitted to 51 acute care hospitals in New York in 1984 and found that 3.7% of those patients experienced some sort of adverse event at the time of discharge. As much as 237 million medical errors occur at some point in England. On August 26, 2019, the World Health Organization (WHO) noted that the chance of dying when traveling by air is one in three million, compared to one in 300 when obtaining medical care. According to a Johns Hopkins study, after heart attacks and cancer, medical errors are the third most common cause of mortality in the United States.

According to a Harvard research, India experiences 5.2 million medical errors per year. A lot of medical errors happen in India, as they do in other developing nations, because there are not enough qualified doctors and nurses to monitor clinical outcomes, according to data from the British Medical Journal.

CAUSES OF MEDICAL ERROR

Multiple factors have been associated with medical practice error. Doctors, nurses, other medical professionals, and the system itself might be responsible for this. It could be the result of inattention, a lack of knowledge, or lack of expertise. Environmental factors, such as a heavy workload, ongoing duty hours, and insufficient sleep, may be involved. The skewed ratio of patients to doctors and nurses increases the likelihood of errors. The complexity of medical knowledge and the unpredictability of clinical forecasts can occasionally result in errors. According to a recent Johns Hopkins study, medical errors are most frequently caused by inadequate communication between doctors, nurses, and patients. A study demonstrated that long working hours, a lack of expertise, poor supervision, and complex cases are common causes of error. The system itself is another significant factor in medical mistakes. Errors may occur due to a lack of a patient safety policy, administrative leadership, or commitment to reducing medical errors.

REPORTING OF MEDICAL ERROR

The current state of patient safety calls for the reporting of medical errors. Actions to prevent an error cannot be taken without knowledge of the error. Therefore, reporting a medical error is currently considered to be one of the world's top endeavors by the majority of countries. Medical errors are often grossly underreported by anywhere between 50 and 96%. The explanation for this underreporting may be because healthcare professionals are not motivated to report errors or are not knowledgeable of how to recognize them. The most frequent reason for underreporting is fear of the consequences. Other contributing factors include a lack of confidentiality, a fear of being held accountable, a fear of being seen as incompetent, a concern of losing one's position within an organization, a worry of a decline in appraisal, a fear of how patients and family members would react, and a fear of receiving negative feedback from peers.

Increased error reporting is very challenging to achieve without a workplace culture being free from fear. Top leadership has to understand and take lead in this. The reported error should be investigated to determine its root cause and suggestions should be made so that future occurrences of the same issue can be avoided. Healthcare workers are encouraged to disclose errors using nonpunitive approaches. Patients should be encouraged to report errors as well. Some errors will not be discovered by doctors unless patients report them in some cases. Error should be taken into account because it compromises patient safety as well as the physician's psychology by causing them to feel less confident, frustrated, and angry.

Every healthcare organization ought to have a robust protocol and reporting system in place. Now in greater numbers than ever before, anonymous reporting systems are being developed on a global scale to promote the reporting of medical errors.

MEDICAL ERRORS IN DIFFERENT SITUATIONS

Medication Errors

A medication error is defined by National Coordinating Council for Medication Error Reporting and Prevention (NCCERP) as "any preventable event that may cause or lead to inappropriate medication use or patient harm while the medication is in the control of the healthcare professional, patient, or consumer. Such events may be related to professional practice, healthcare products, procedures, and systems, including prescribing; order communication; product labeling, packaging, and nomenclature; compounding; dispensing;

distribution; administration; education; monitoring; and use." The council also provides various recommendations on each aspect of medication to prevent errors. Medication errors can be broadly classified into prescribing errors, dispensing errors, and administration errors. Prescription errors were found to be the most prevalent, as was the case in many previous research, according to a study from Ahmedabad. Antibiotics were the most frequently associated class of drugs with errors. Patients of extreme ages, those taking several medicines, an excessive workload and staff weariness, issues with medicine storage, medications that look alike or sound alike, and high-risk medications are all common causes of medication errors.

Prevention of Medication Errors

Together, doctors, nurses, pharmacists, and other medical personnel should work to prescribe, administer, and supervise the entire process. Every step should be verified again (double check). Prescription and dispensing errors can be decreased by adopting technology, such as electronic medical records (EMRs) and computerized physician order entry (CPOE). Look-alike and sound-alike medicines should be tagged and stored separately with staff awareness. The availability of high-risk medications should be checked regularly, as should the routine disposal of expired medications. Drug labels on the tubing and tubing separators should be applied to patients receiving numerous infusions.

Surgical Errors

Despite protocols and numerous inspections, surgical errors frequently occur. Common examples of surgical errors include operating on the wrong body part, making an incision in the incorrect location, accidentally severing a nerve, and leaving a gauge or instrument within the patient. In addition to these, mistakes can happen before surgery, during anesthesia, and during postoperative care. In patients who had surgery, mistakes occurred at a rate of 3%, of which 54% were avoidable. Before beginning a surgery, the lead surgeon will typically double check all the specifics, but there are numerous individuals involved and something can go wrong at any point.

Prevention of Surgical Errors

The ability to perform surgery requires a team's performance with good coordination and open communication among all members, including surgeons, nurses, anesthetists, and other essential staff. This includes decision-making at the preoperative, intraoperative, and postoperative levels as well as technical skills of surgeons and nurses. Written protocols are created for operating rooms, particularly those involving document cross-checking, verifying the location of surgery, and accounting for sponges and tools. A surgical plan is established beforehand. Regular checks should be made to ensure protocol adherence. However, protocols only address a minor portion of error management. Surgeons should occasionally take special courses and training to hone their technical and decision-making abilities. Simulators can help students overcome their learning curves.

Diagnostic Errors

Correct and timely diagnosis is a global priority in patient safety as its absence leads to serious preventable health issues including death. A United States of America (USA)-based

IOM report defines diagnostic errors as "failure to establish an accurate and timely explanation of the patient's health problem or communicate that explanation to the patient." These mistakes are viewed as lost opportunities, where doing things differently would have produced desired results. This chance can be lost by the patient, the system, the care team (e.g., the laboratory performing the tests or paramedical staff handling samples), the patient (e.g., delayed follow-up and noncompliance to tests), the system, or even the doctor. However, missed opportunities are not usually the source of delayed or incorrect diagnoses and missed opportunities are not always harmful. Common pediatric disorders that resulted in claims owing to diagnostic mistakes were described in a systematic review of medicolegal cases. These included pneumonia, sepsis, meningitis, appendicitis, gastroenteritis, and malignancy.

Prevention of Diagnostic Errors

The literature has identified eight intervention areas as follows:

1. Improving diagnostic reasoning
2. Government policies to strengthen primary care
3. Patient awareness
4. Utilization of information technology
5. Diagnostic error identification and reporting system
6. Improving access to good quality tools and high-end tests
7. Optimizing diagnostic strategies in primary healthcare setups
8. Develop feedback systems for clinicians about their diagnosis

Equipment Errors

By increasing effectiveness, reducing expense, delivering excellent care, and ensuring patient safety, devices and equipment are very helpful in providing healthcare services to patients. However, they play a key role in medical mistakes. These mistakes may be the result of user error or technical problems with the machine. Technical issues that lead to errors include things such as inadequate maintenance, low-quality devices with poor design, and accuracy. User errors are brought on by a lack of expertise, inadequate training, poor calibration maintenance, and improper instruction.

Prevention of Equipment Errors

All medical professionals should be aware about and appropriately trained in the use of various instruments and devices. Documenting proper maintenance should be done. Every device must adhere to the required quality and safety standards. When making improvements, a device error reporting system might be quite beneficial.

Errors in Communication

Verbal Errors

Verbal communication between healthcare professionals and patients, as well as between healthcare professionals themselves, has the potential of errors.

A verbal order is any prescription for medication that is given verbally, either in person or over the phone. In addition, verbal communication involves requesting diagnostic tests or any other action for which a written request is not made. It is advisable to utilize verbal directions only in dire circumstances because these circumstances increase the likelihood of misinterpretation resulting in errors. Errors in verbal instructions can be caused by several things, including weariness, background noise, medicine names that are similar, and language barriers.

When communicating a patient's sickness and the best course of treatment with relatives and asking for their agreement, there is a risk of misinterpretation owing to a lack of comprehension or insufficient contact, which can lead to mistakes and neglect.

Prevention of verbal communication errors

While giving verbal orders on some treatments between doctors and their subordinates, there should be a read-back system. When discussing critical reports, the read-back mechanism should be available as well. One of the most important factors in creating a trustworthy and positive environment in hospitals is communication between patients and healthcare professionals. There should be a system in place to periodically train healthcare professionals in soft skills. Patients should be given enough time and opportunities to ask questions as they are being briefed on their health status, future management strategy, complications, and prognosis. This will cut the number of medical errors. Encourage patients to inquire about new tests, unexpected diagnostic procedures, drugs, and the proper surgical site in order to make them active partners in preventing medical errors.

Written Errors

The use of nonstandard abbreviations and illegible handwriting are frequent errors in medical prescriptions that result in incorrect medication administration. A limitation is failing to object to improperly written directions. Incorrect labeling of samples or specimens also results in written errors aside from prescriptions.

Prevention of written errors

Writing effective prescriptions ought to be practiced. Avoid using symbols such as @ or > in your text. All capital letters should be used when writing the generic names of medications. Never shorten the names of medications, such as writing ADR for adrenaline or MS for morphine sulphate. It is preferable to write a zero before the decimal when writing pharmacological doses in decimals, e.g., 0.1 mg rather than .1 mg. A following zero should also be avoided, e.g., 0.1 mg rather than 0.10 mg. The process of identifying patients, writing prescriptions, determining dosages, and administering medications have to be double checked. In the event of confusion, staff members should be encouraged to double check and query written directives.

Errors during Acute Intervention

Medical mistakes are more likely to occur in situations involving cardiac arrest, intubation, or other acute life-threatening occurrences. The likelihood of severe errors increases with hasty decision-making and the immediate need for life-saving medications and treatments, particularly in the absence of documented orders. An example would be administering a high-risk medicine inadvertently or utilizing an Ambu bag improperly connected to an oxygen source.

Prevention of Errors in Acute Intervention

We all know that a code blue emergency can happen at any time, anywhere in the hospital. In order to reduce errors during acute intervention, a critical response team, also known as a code blue team, should be developed to manage this kind of crisis. The team should receive frequent training and be put to test with mock drills. When it is necessary, critical response teams bring expertise to the patient's bedside.

When deteriorating patients' end-of-life care plans are discussed with the patient and family at the time of admission, team efficacy is increased. Family meetings can lead to the identification of objectives that enhance end-of-life care and prevent unnecessary procedures.

Other strategies include using simulation to teach the team and creating standardized carts with all the instruments and high-risk medications the team will need.

Healthcare-associated Infection

Infections that occur more than 48 hours after a patient is admitted to the hospital are known as healthcare-associated infections (HAIs). Each infection has a unique incubation period; thus, it is important to keep this in mind when labeling HAI and building a temporal relationship between infections and hospitalization. Healthcare provider occupational infections are included in HAI. One of the most frequent problems among hospitalized patients and a source of concern for medical professionals is HAI. Morbidity, mortality, duration of hospital stays, the financial burden on families and the healthcare system, and dissatisfaction—all rise as a result. It affects 3.2% of hospitalized patients in the USA, 6.5% of hospitalized patients in European state, and a substantially greater percentage of patients in the rest of the world.

There are mainly four types of HAI. These are:

1. Catheter-related blood stream infection (CRBSI)
2. Catheter-related urinary tract infection (CAUTI)
3. Surgical site soft tissue infection (SSI)
4. Ventilator-associated pneumonia (VAP)

Prevention of Healthcare-associated Infections

Effective method of prevention and control of HAI should be the one of the prime concerns of any healthcare providers and for patients' safety. Any healthcare provider should have written guidelines for preventions and control of infection, antimicrobial policy, surveillance policy, disinfection policy, isolation policy, and policy for infection of an outbreak of infections.

Prevention of CRBSI: Wise decision of site selection of insertion of central line should be done to minimize contamination, expert person, with all universal aseptic precautions, should insert the central line. Trained nurses should take care of proper dressing and change of dressing of line should be done. Monitoring of central line for phlebitis, daily monitoring for need of central line, limitation of lumen, and early removal when not needed are some interventions which limit the CRBSI.

Prevention of CAUTI: Daily assessment of need of urinary catheter and removal of it as soon as possible is the best step to decrease CAUTI. It should be inserted with all universal aseptic precautions by expert hand.

Prevention of SSI: There are three measures which help in prevention of SSI: (1) Preoperative measure—it includes preoperative reduction of modifiable risk factors of infection such as making patients euglycemic, cessation of smoking, administration of preoperative antibiotics, and decolonization of specific pathogens. (2) Operative—it includes maintaining optimal perfusion of site to prevent hypoxia, and maintain euglycemia and euthermia. (3) Postoperative—it includes appropriate dressing of sites and administration of antibiotics.

Prevention of VAP: There are VAP care bundle that prevent the VAP which include head end elevation of bed up to 30°–45°, oral care with 1% chlorhexidine with aseptic method, sedation interruption as per hospital policy, peptic ulcer prophylaxis, and deep vein thrombosis prophylaxis.

DISCLOSURE OF MEDICAL ERROR

Medical error disclosure refers to the process in which a healthcare provider communicates with a patient, their family, or a designated representative to acknowledge an error that has occurred in the course of care. This involves explaining the details of the error, its consequences, and how it relates to the patient's health outcomes in a way that is clear and relevant to the patient's understanding. The goal of this communication is to promote transparency, build trust, and enhance the overall safety culture in healthcare settings. Medical personnel have an ethical duty to inform patients when an error has been made. It should be done at the appropriate time and in the appropriate situation and they should be fairly compensated for the injury they have suffered. A medical error that was not promptly communicated to the patient by the practitioner has been demonstrated to increase the likelihood of litigation. An unreported medical error that harms a patient may be considered negligent. Additionally, revealing errors to the medical community aids in the development of preventative measures. Hospitals and other organizations might greatly benefit from the data on reported errors in order to develop procedures and rules that would reduce mistakes and, consequently, neglect. A study on residents working at a tertiary care hospital in south India found that the majority of doctors cited punishment as a significant factor in underreporting errors and stressed the importance of a confidential reporting system for better reporting. They also advocated disclosing information to patients after speaking with colleagues.

There is a lack of formal training to doctors and nurses on how to disclose medical errors to patients. In recent times, workshops are being conducted with patient simulation to train medical professionals on the art of disclosing medical errors. Doctors and nurses do not receive enough formal training on how to inform patients of medical errors. In order to teach medical practitioners the art of revealing medical errors, workshops including patient simulation are being conducted.

CONCLUSION

The incidence of errors has gone down compared to the past due to extensive research on them and the development of standardized procedures and practices for their prevention, yet they still happen. The prevention of medical errors requires a collaborative effort by physicians, pharmacists, and nurses. Checks can be conducted at various levels, including communication, documentation, action, such as the administration of drugs or surgery, and personnel. All healthcare professionals need to be aware of potential patient harm and legal issues. Establishing an error reporting system that is effective and helps to reduce errors requires a supportive atmosphere with effective communication.

KEY LEARNING POINTS

- Medical errors are an inherent component of the work of healthcare professionals. Most of them can be avoided, but they must acknowledge that errors will inevitably happen.
- Retrospective analysis of errors reveal gaps in our knowledge and the actions as well as deficiencies in the infrastructure and policies of the institution.
- Every method should be used with the utmost care to prevent common medical errors. To check compliance and strengthen the system, routine audits must be performed.
- Our ethical duty to disclose medical errors to patients should not be ignored and errors should not be covered up.
- All healthcare facilities should develop a reliable anonymous error reporting mechanism to prevent judging and harsh punishment.
- Healthcare workers should be encouraged to report errors and formally trained to handle medical error disclosure.

BIBLIOGRAPHY

1. Aashita Sah A, Khan ZH, Khokhar A. Basic concept of patient safety in healthcare delivery. Int J Curr Res. 2018;10(08):72926-32.
2. Aljabari S, Kadhim Z. Common Barriers to Reporting Medical Errors. ScientificWorldJournal. 2021;2021:6494889.
3. Amir S, Vaswani VR, Vaswani R. Knowledge, attitude, practice about disclosure of medical errors among residents of a tertiary care hospital, Dakshina Kannada. Int J Health Sci Res. 2017;7(7):45-52.
4. Barach P, Small SD. Reporting and preventing medical mishaps: Lessons from non-medical near miss reporting systems. BMJ. 2000;320(7237):759-63.
5. Baraiya K, Thummar K. Medication error: A systematic review and comparison of reporting system in USA, UK and India. World J Pharm Pharmaceut Sci. 2020;9(8):1011-30.
6. Bari A, Khan RA, Rathore AW. Medical errors; causes, consequences, emotional response and resulting behavioral change. Pak J Med Sci. 2016;32(3):523-8.
7. Brennan TA, Leape LL, Laird NM, et al. Incidence of adverse events and negligence in hospitalized patients. N Engl J Med. 1991;324:370-6.
8. Carver N, Gupta V, Hipskind JE. Medical Error. In: StatPearls [Internet]. Treasure Island (FL): StatPearls Publishing; 2023.
9. Cheragi MA, Manoocheri H, Mohammadnejad E, et al. Types and causes of medication errors from nurse's viewpoint. Iran J Nurs Midwifery Res. 2013;18(3):228-31.
10. Hiatt HH, Barnes BA, Brennan TA, et al. A study of medical injury and medical malpractice. An overview. N Engl J Med. 1989;321(7):480-4.
11. Hines S, Kynoch K, Khalil H. Effectiveness of interventions to prevent medication errors: An umbrella systematic review protocol. JBI Database System Rev Implement Rep. 2018;16(2):291-6.
12. Holden RJ, Karsh BT. A review of medical error reporting system design considerations and a proposed cross-level systems research framework. Hum Factors. 2007;49(2):257-76.
13. Hyman WA. Errors in the use of medical equipment. In: Bogner MS (Ed). Human Error in Medicine, 1st edition. Boca Raton: CRC press; 1994.

14. Kellogg KM, Hettinger Z, Shah M, et al. Our current approach to root cause analysis: Is it contributing to our failure to improve patient safety? BMJ Qual Saf. 2017;26(5):381-7.
15. Kohn LT, Corrigan JM, Donaldson MS; Institute of Medicine (US) Committee on Quality of Health Care in America (Eds). To Err is Human: Building a Safer Health System. Washington, DC: National Academy Press, Institute of Medicine; 1999.
16. Leape LL, Lawthers AG, Brennan TA, et al. Preventing medical injury. QRB Qual Rev Bull. 1993;19:144-9.
17. Mansour R, Ammar K, Al-Tabba A, et al. Disclosure of medical errors: physicians' knowledge, attitudes and practices (KAP) in an oncology center. BMC Med Ethics. 2020;21:74.
18. Ministry of health and family welfare (MoHFW). (2020). National guidelines on infection prevention and control in healthcare facilities. [online] Available from https://www.mohfw.gov.in/pdf/National%20Guidelines%20for%20IPC%20in%20HCF%20-%20final%281%29.pdf [Last accessed May, 2024].
19. Moghaddasi H. Verbal Orders in Medicine: Challenges; Problems and Solution. JOJ Nurse Health Care. 2017;1(5):555575.
20. National Coordinating Council for Medication Error Reporting and Prevention (NCC MERP). (2016). About Medication Errors. [online] Available from https://www.nccmerp.org/about-medication-errors [Last accessed May, 2024].
21. Patel N, Desai M, Shah S, et al. A study of medication errors in a tertiary care hospital. Perspect Clin Res. 2016;7(4):168-73.
22. Patra KP, De Jesus O. Sentinel Event. In: StatPearls [Internet]. Treasure Island (FL): StatPearls Publishing; 2023.
23. Reason J (Ed). Human Error. Cambridge: Cambridge University Press; 1990.
24. Rekha B, Saurabh B. Evaluation of Prevalence of Medication Errors in a Multispecialty Teaching Hospital, Dehradun (Uttarakhand), India. Indian J Pharm Pract. 2013;6(1):19-24.
25. Rodziewicz TL, Houseman B, Hipskind JE. Medical Error Reduction and Prevention. In: StatPearls [Internet]. Treasure Island (FL): StatPearls Publishing; 2023.
26. Sarker SK, Vincent C. Errors in surgery. Int J Surg. 2005;3(1):75-81.
27. Sikora A, Zahra F. Nosocomial Infections. In: StatPearls [Internet]. Treasure Island (FL): StatPearls Publishing; 2023.
28. Singh H, Naik AD, Rao R, et al. Reducing diagnostic errors through effective communication: Harnessing the power of information technology. J Gen Intern Med. 2008;23(4):489-94.
29. Singh H, Schiff GD, Graber ML, et al. The global burden of diagnostic errors in primary care. BMJ Qual Saf. 2017;26(6):484-94.
30. Tase A, Buckle P, Ni MZ, et al. Medical device error and failure reporting: Learning from the car industry. J Patient Saf Risk Manag. 2021;26(3):251604352110082.
31. Thomas EJ, Brennan TA. Errors and adverse events in medicine: an overview. In: Williams J, Vincent C (Eds). Clinical Risk Management: Enhancing Patient Safety, 2nd edition. London: BMJ Publishing. 2001. pp. 31-43.
32. van Tilburg CM, Leistikow IP, Rademaker CM, et al. Health Care Failure Mode and Effect Analysis: a useful proactive risk analysis in a pediatric oncology ward. Qual Saf Health Care. 2006;15(1):58-63.
33. Wallace E, Lowry J, Smith SM, et al. The epidemiology of malpractice claims in primary care: a systematic review. BMJ Open. 2013;3(7):e002929.
34. Welsh D, Zephyr D, Pfeifle AL, et al. Development of the barriers to error disclosure assessment tool. J Patient Safe. 2017.
35. World Health Organization. Diagnostic Errors: Technical Series on Safer Primary Care. Geneva: World Health Organization; 2016.
36. Wu AW, Christensen JF, McPhee SJ. Errors in medical practice. In: Feldman MD, Christensen JF, Satterfield JM (Eds). Behavioral Medicine: A Guide for Clinical Practice, 4th edition. New York: McGraw Hill; 2014.

11

CHAPTER

Criminal Liability

VP Singh, Charu Mittal, Ishita Banerjee

INTRODUCTION

The law understands that in the context of the relationship between a doctor and patient, there is the establishment of a contract with the agreement to provide services, even if it has not been signed in a document; in the latter case, the contract is called "tacit". But this relationship can also be extracontractual when no previous agreement exists, for example, when the patient reaches a hospital or emergency room and is attended to by the doctor on duty or in the case of assistance to a victim on the road. Because of this relationship, contractual or extracontractual, it creates obligations. In any case, the primary physician's duties include care and safety of patients. The medical practitioners are well aware about the civil liability incurred upon them in case of any harm to the patient due to medical negligence. However, the concept of criminal liability in medical profession is not very clear to most of the medical professionals. It is extremely important to understand the concept of criminal liability and the safeguards available, so as to practice safely and confidently.

VISUALIZE A REAL-LIFE SCENARIO!

After a busy shift in the emergency ward when a patient, Mr. X, is admitted, the attending doctor reaches to a quick decision that the patient is sadly in the process of dying and that intervention would be futile. The family members are upset with that decision. Patient Mr. X dies shortly thereafter.

Three months later, the doctor receives a request from the police to attend a formal investigation under caution. The family has obtained evidence to suggest that Mr. X's disease was treatable, and that the decision not to treat was negligent, basic medical tests were not undertaken and the independent expert providing that evidence considers the doctor's decision fell below reasonable care.

While such scenario is uncommon, it does arise from time to time. The effect on the individual doctor subjected to these investigations is catastrophic, they are faced with criminal charges which may result in a custodial sentence and would, in any event, endanger their registration and livelihood.

RELEVANT PROVISIONS OF INDIAN PENAL CODE 1860/*BHARATIYA NYAYA SANHITA* 2023 (TABLE 11.1)

Table 11.1: Relevant Provisions of Indian Penal Code 1860/*Bharatiya Nyaya Sanhita* 2023.

IPC	*BNS*	
Sec 52	**2(11)**	Nothing is said to be done or believed in **"good faith"** which is done or believed without due care and attention
Sec 80	**18**	**Accident in doing a lawful act:** Nothing is an offence which is done by accident or misfortune, and without any criminal intention or knowledge in the doing of a lawful act in a lawful manner by lawful means and with proper care and caution
Sec 81	**19**	**Act likely to cause harm, but done without criminal intent, and to prevent other harm:** Nothing is an offence, if it be done without any criminal intention to cause harm, and in good faith for the purpose of preventing or avoiding other harm to person or property
Sec 87	**25**	**Act not intended and not known to be likely to cause death or grievous hurt, done by consent:** Which is not known by the doer to be likely to cause death or grievous hurt, is an offence by reason of any harm which it may cause, or be intended by the doer to cause, to any person, above 18 years of age, who has given consent; or by reason of any harm which it may be known by the doer to be likely to cause to any such person who has consented to take the risk of that harm
Sec 88	**26**	**Act not intended to cause death, done by consent in good faith for person's benefit:** It is an offence by reason of any harm which it may cause, or be intended by the doer to cause, or be known by the doer to be likely to cause, to any person for whose benefit it is done in good faith, and who has given a consent, to suffer that harm, or to take the risk of that harm ***Illustration*:** A, a surgeon, knowing that a particular operation is likely to cause the death of Z, who suffers under the painful complaint, but not intending to cause Z's death, and intending, in good faith, Z's benefit, performs that operation on Z, with Z's consent. A has committed no offence
Sec 90	**28**	**Consent known to be given under fear or misconception:** A consent is not such a consent as is intended by any section of this *Sanhita*: (a) If the consent is given by a person under fear of injury, or under a misconception of fact, and if the person doing the act knows, or has reason to believe, that the consent was given in consequence of such fear or misconception; or (b) If the consent is given by a person who, from unsoundness of mind, or intoxication, is unable to understand the nature and consequence of consent; or (c) Unless the contrary appears from the context, if the consent is given by a person who is under 12 years of age

Continued

Continued

IPC	*BNS*	
Sec 91	**29**	**Exclusion of acts which are offences independently of harm caused:** The exceptions in sections 25, 26, and 27 do not extend to acts which are offences independently of any harm which they may cause, or be intended to cause, or be known to be likely to cause, to the person giving the consent, or on whose behalf the consent is given ***Illustration:*** Causing miscarriage (unless caused in good faith for the purpose of saving the life of the woman) is an offence independently of any harm which it may cause or be intended to cause to the woman. Therefore, it is not an offence "by reason of such harm"; and the consent of the woman or of her guardian to the causing of such miscarriage does not justify the act
Sec 92	**30**	**Act done in good faith for benefit of a person without consent:** To a person for whose benefit it is done in good faith, even without that person's consent, or if that person is incapable of giving consent, and has no guardian or other person in lawful charge of him from whom it is possible to obtain consent in time for the thing to be done with benefit: Provided that this exception shall not extend to— (a) The intentional causing of death, or the attempting to cause death; (b) The doing of anything which the person doing it knows to be likely to cause death, or the curing of any grievous disease or infirmity; (c) The voluntary causing of hurt, or to the attempting to cause hurt, for any purpose other than the preventing of death or hurt; ***Illustrations:*** (1) Z is thrown from his horse, and is insensible. A, a surgeon, finds that Z requires to be trepanned. A, not intending Z's death, but in good faith, for Z's benefit, performs the trepan before Z recovers his power of judging for himself. A has committed no offence (3) A, a surgeon, sees a child suffer an accident which is likely to prove fatal unless an operation be immediately performed. There is no time to apply to the child's guardian. A performs the operation in spite of the entreaties of the child, intending, in good faith, the child's benefit. A has committed no offence
Sec 93	**31**	**No communication made in good faith is an offence** by reason of any harm to the person to whom it is made, if it is made for the benefit of that person ***Illustration:*** A, a surgeon, in good faith, communicates to a patient his opinion that he cannot live. The patient dies in consequence of the shock. A has committed no offence, though he knew it to be likely that the communication might cause the patient's death
Sec 304A	**106(1)**	**Causing death by negligence:** By doing any rash or negligent act not amounting to culpable homicide, shall be punished with imprisonment of either description for a term which may extend to 5 years, and shall also be liable to fine; and if such act is done by a registered medical practitioner while performing medical procedure, he shall be punished with imprisonment of either description for a term which may extend to 2 years, and shall also be liable to fine **Explanation:** For the purposes of this sub-section, "registered medical practitioner" means a medical practitioner who possesses any medical qualification recognized under the National Medical Commission Act, 2019 and whose name has been entered in the National Medical Register or a State Medical Register under that Act

Continued

Continued

IPC	*BNS*	
Sec 337	**125(a)**	**Act endangering life or personal safety of others:** Rashly or negligently as to endanger human life or the personal safety of others, shall be punished with imprisonment of either description for a term which may extend to three months or with fine which may extend to ₹2,500, or with both, but— (a) Where hurt is caused, shall be punished with imprisonment of either description for a term which may extend to 6 months, or with fine which may extend to ₹5,000, or with both
Sec 338	**125(b)**	**Causing grievous hurt by act endangering life or personal safety of others:** (b) Where grievous hurt is caused, shall be punished with imprisonment of either description for a term which may extend to 3 years, or with fine which may extend to ₹10,000, or with both

CRIMINAL NEGLIGENCE

There can be an allegation of criminal negligence against the doctor if a patient dies during an operation or other kind of treatment; if it can be proved that the death was the result of malicious intention, or gross negligence.

In the Santra case, the Supreme Court has pointed out that liability in civil law is based upon the amount of damages incurred; in criminal law, the amount and degree of negligence is a factor in determining liability. However, certain elements must be established to determine criminal liability in any particular case, the motive of the offence, the magnitude of the offence, and the character of the offender.

In an important decision in the case of *Dr. Laxman Balkrishna Joshi vs. Dr. Trimbak Bapu Godbole*, the Supreme Court held that if a doctor has adopted a practice that is considered "proper" by a reasonable body of medical professionals who are skilled in that particular field, he or she will not be held negligent only because something went wrong.

In *Poonam Verma vs. Ashwin Patel*, the Supreme Court has distinguished between negligence, rashness, and recklessness. A person who is rash knows the consequences but foolishly thinks that they will not occur as a result of her/his act. A reckless person knows the consequences but does not care whether or not they result from her/his act. Any conduct falling short of recklessness and deliberate wrongdoing should not be the subject of criminal liability.

Thus, a doctor cannot be held criminally responsible for a patient's death unless it is shown that he/she was negligent or incompetent, with such disregard for the life and safety of the patient that it amounted to a crime against the State.

Section 80 and Section 88 of the Indian Penal Code (IPC) contain defenses for doctors accused of criminal liability. Under section (U/S) 80 (accident in doing a lawful act) nothing is an offence that is done by accident or misfortune and without any criminal intention or knowledge in the doing of a lawful act in a lawful manner by lawful means and with proper care and caution. According to Section 88, a person cannot be accused of an offence if she/he performs an act in good faith for the other's benefit, does not intend to cause harm even if there is a risk, and the patient has explicitly or implicitly given consent.

What is Criminal Negligence as Per Law?

Criminal negligence is largely a matter of degree; it is incapable of a precise definition. To prove whether or not it exists is like chasing a mirage. It requires that any of the following to be established in a case of criminal medical negligence.

"*Gross Lack of competency or gross inattention, or wanton indifferences to the patient's safety, which may arise from gross ignorance of the science of medicine and surgery or through gross negligence, either in the application and selection of remedies, lack of proper skill in the use of instruments and failure to give proper attention to the patient.*"

In UK the case of *R v Adomako* (1995) set down the test for gross negligence manslaughter. The defendant was a locum anesthetist at an operation to correct a detached retina. He failed to notice that a tube had become dislodged during the course of the operation which resulted in the patient being deprived of oxygen. The patient suffered a cardiac arrest and died. The defendant was convicted of manslaughter and appealed to the House of Lords on the basis that gross negligence was not the correct test for involuntary manslaughter. The House of Lords dismissed his appeal and held that gross negligence is the correct test.

To be convicted of gross negligence manslaughter, a doctor must have breached a duty of care owed by them to the patient causing death and the breach of the standard of care must be "*so grossly negligent as to justify a criminal conviction.*" The standard of care demanded of the doctor is the standard of the reasonably skilled and experienced doctor in the doctor's particular field of medicine. It is ultimately a question of fact for the jury to determine whether the standard of care provided was so badly negligent that it can properly be condemned as criminal.

In *R v Prentice and R v Sullman* (1993) two junior doctors were acquitted of manslaughter on appeal after they wrongly injected vincristine intrathecally into the patient's spine when the cytotoxic drug should have been administered intravenously. This resulted in the patient's death. It was held that the question for the jury to answer in relation to a charge of gross negligence manslaughter was whether, in the case of each doctor, the jury was sure that the failure to ascertain the correct mode of administering the drug was negligent to the point of criminality. The jury should be directed to have regard to all of the circumstances of the case. The case ultimately turned upon the fact that there were many mitigating circumstances in the case, and the jury found that although the doctors had acted negligently, they had not acted grossly negligently.

In India, a doctor may be liable in a civil case for negligence but mere carelessness or want of due attention and skill cannot be described as so reckless or grossly negligent as to make her/him criminally liable. The courts held that this distinction was necessary so that the hazards of medical professionals being exposed to civil liability may not unreasonably extend to criminal liability and expose them to the risk of imprisonment for alleged criminal negligence.

Dr. Suresh Gupta vs. Government of NCT of Delhi and Anr. (2004) Supreme Court of India

The doctor (a plastic surgeon) was accused on the charge U/S 304-A of the IPC for causing death of his patient. The patient was operated by him for removing his nasal deformity. Cardiac arrest occurred on table, resuscitative measures were started and patient shifted to tertiary center. Postmortem report was very categorical and clear and it was clearly mentioned that death was due to complication of aspiration of blood during the operation. Allegation was leveled of not introducing a cuffed endotracheal tube of proper size so as to prevent aspiration of blood from the wound in the respiratory passage.

Comments by Court

Operation was conducted by both the accused persons: Surgeon and anesthetist (latter passed away before judgment). It is also clear from the material on record that deceased was young man of 38 years having no cardiac problem at all, due to incision at wrong part blood seeped into the respiratory passage and because of that patient immediately collapsed and died. Where a patient dies due to the negligent medical treatment of the doctor, the doctor can be made liable in civil law for paying compensation and damages in tort and at the same time, if the degree of negligence is so gross and his act was reckless as to endanger the life of the patient, he would also be made criminally liable for offence U/S 304-A of IPC. Mere lack of proper care, precaution, and attention or inadvertence might create civil liability but not a criminal one. No case of recklessness or gross negligence has been made out against the doctor to compel him to face the trial for offence U/S 304-A of the IPC.

Thus, in the above case the Supreme Court distinguished between an error of judgment and culpable negligence. It held that criminal prosecution of doctors without adequate medical opinion pointing to their guilt would do great disservice to the community. A doctor cannot be tried for culpable or criminal negligence in all cases of medical mishaps or misfortunes. Hence, the complaint against the doctor must show negligence or rashness of such a degree as to indicate a mental state that can be described as totally apathetic toward the patient. Such gross negligence alone is punishable. The complainant must prove the allegation against the doctor by citing the best evidence available in medical science and by presenting expert opinion.

In some situations, the complainant can invoke the principle of *res ipsa loquitur* or "the thing speaks for itself." The National Consumer Disputes Redressal Commission (NCDRC) applied this principle in *Dr. Janak Kantimathi Nathan vs. Murlidhar Eknath Masane*. The 13-year-old son of the complainant was under treatment for epilepsy and as his condition had worsened, the opinion of a neurophysician was taken, who changed the medicines despite which the child did not improve, and also developed skin rash with one of the drugs. He was hospitalized and administered some injections by duty doctor following which he became unconscious and in spite of shifting to intensive care unit (ICU) after 2 days he passed away. The attending doctor (defendant) did not attend to him over the weekend and had two visits during hospitalization during which he stated that child was sleeping. Father filed a complaint of negligence against treating doctor as well as the hospital. NCDRC upheld decision of State Commission against hospital and treating doctor as negligent in providing adequate and appropriate care. The principle of *res ipsa loquitur* comes into operation only when there is proof that the occurrence was unexpected, that the accident could not have happened without negligence and lapses on the part of the treating doctor, and that the circumstances conclusively show that the doctor and not any other person was negligent.

Burden of Proof!

The burden of proof of negligence, carelessness, or insufficiency generally lies with the complainant. The law requires a higher standard of evidence than otherwise, to support an allegation of negligence against a doctor. In cases of medical negligence, the patient must establish her/his claim against the doctor.

In *Calcutta Medical Research Institute* vs. *Bimalesh Chatterjee*, it was held that the onus of proving negligence and the resultant deficiency in service was clearly on the complainant. In *Kanhaiya Kumar Singh* vs. *Park Medicare and Research Centre*, it was held that negligence has to be established and cannot be presumed. Even after adopting all medical procedures as prescribed, a qualified doctor may commit an error.

What Criminal Negligence Means for a Doctor?

In case of allegation of criminal negligence, the physician should be able to prove that he used reasonable and ordinary care in the treatment of his patient to the best of his judgment. He is, however, not liable for an error of judgment. The issue of fixing criminal liability was decided in the Supreme Court in the case of *Jacob Mathew* vs. *State of Punjab*. No doctor turned up for about 20–25 minutes. Then, Dr. Jacob Mathew and Dr. Allen Joseph came to the patient's room. An oxygen cylinder was brought and connected to patient's mouth but breathing problem increased further. The cylinder was found to be empty. Another doctor came who declared that the patient was dead. It was alleged that death occurred due to the carelessness of doctors and nurses, nonavailability of oxygen cylinder and an empty cylinder was fixed on the mouth, and his breathing was totally stopped.

Case was filed U/S 304-A IPC (related to criminal complaints). Defense stated that deceased was suffering from cancer in terminal stage and was not being admitted by any hospital in the country. His sons requested the hospital authorities that even on compassionate grounds their father may be admitted in the hospital. The patient was treated with utmost care and caution and every effort was made by all the attending staff to give appropriate medical treatment to the patient but what was ordained to happen, did happen.

A private complaint of rashness or negligence against a doctor may not be entertained without prima facie evidence in the form of a credible opinion of another competent doctor supporting the charge. In addition, the investigating officer should give an independent opinion, preferably that of a government doctor. Finally, a doctor may be arrested only if the investigating officer believes that she/he would not be available for prosecution unless arrested.

Thus, when a first information report (FIR) is filed against a doctor for the death of a patient who was under his treatment, under the IPC Section 304-A the doctor can be arrested only after negligence is proved in the opinion of an expert committee which analyses the medical aspects of the case and circumstances. Up till now, Indian Courts have been very careful not to hold qualified doctors criminally liable for patients' deaths that are the result of a mere mistake of judgment in the selection and application of remedies and when the death resulted merely from an error of judgment or an inadvertent death.

Charges of Criminal Negligence against Doctor Under Section 338 IPC

As seen earlier, section 338 relates to causing grievous hurt by act endangering life or personal safety of others. It is to be kept in mind that the crime as mentioned in section 338 IPC requires proof that the appellant caused the patient's condition to the acute stage as illustrated by the judgment in following case.

Dr. PB Desai vs. State of Maharashtra

The patient was suffering from cancer for which she was under medical treatment since 1977. In 1987, she was treated in Sloan Kettering Memorial Hospital in New York. However, it did not yield any positive results. The doctors in that hospital declared her beyond surgical treatment and she was sent back to India. Treating doctor started administering the medication prescribed by the doctors in USA. Within a few days, the patient started suffering from vaginal bleeding, because of which her doctor advised hospitalization. After a few days of hospitalization, for the vaginal bleeding, opinion of the appellant was taken, who advised exploratory laparotomy (surgery), in order to ascertain whether the patient's uterus can or cannot be removed in order to stop the vaginal bleeding. Operation was started by her treating doctor who found intra-abdominal conditions inoperable and took an opinion from the appellant on table who advised closure in view of inoperability. Patient developed fistula few days later and was kept hospitalized for 3 months. She passed away after about 1 year.

In court main allegation against the appellant was that he did not take personal care and attention by performing the operation himself in spite of contractual agreement for operation. It was alleged that the very advice of the appellant for surgical operation, even when the doctors at USA had opined to the contrary, was inappropriate. It was, thus alleged that the aforesaid acts of omission and commission amounted to professional misconduct as well as offence punishable U/S 338 of the IPC. This was upheld by High Court and doctor filed an appeal in Supreme Court.

Comments by Apex Court

The decision of the appellant advising exploratory laparotomy was not an act of negligence, much less wanton negligence. Failure to act on the part of the appellant, in conducting surgical procedure, and not taking care thereafter as well, established his negligence in tort law, i.e., in civil domain. It could have been wanton negligence only if the doctor had faltered and acted in rash and gross negligent manner in performing that procedure. At the same time, his act of omission, afterward, in not doing the surgery himself and remaining absent from the scene and neglecting the patient, even thereafter, when she was suffering the consequences of fistula, is an act of negligence and is definitely blameworthy (though that is not the part of criminal charge). However, we are of the opinion that the omission is not of a kind which has given rise to criminal liability under the given circumstances. The appellant's omission in not rendering complete and undivided legally owed duty to patient and not performing the procedure himself has not made any difference. It was not the cause of the patient's death which was undoubtedly because of the acute chronic cancer condition. In such a scenario, it is enough to keep off the clutches of criminal law. The negligent conduct in the nature of omission of the appellant is not so gross as to entail criminal liability on the appellant U/S 338 of the IPC. For the aforesaid reasons, we have no option but to conclude that though the conduct of the appellant constituted not only professional misconduct for which adequate penalty has been meted out to him by the Medical Council, and the negligence on his part also amounts to actionable wrong in tort, it does not transcend into the criminal liability, and in no case makes him liable for offence U/S 338, IPC as the ingredients of that provision have not been satisfied.

The *Bharatiya Nyaya Sanhita* Act (BNS) and *Bhartiya Nagrik Suraksha Sanhita* Act (BNNS) have been enacted, accepted in 2023 and have replaced the Indian Penal Code (IPC). The main differences between the IPC and the new BNS are enumerated in the following **Table 11.2.**

Table 11.2: Criminal liability for deaths due to medical negligence.

	Old Criminal Laws IPC/CrPC	***New Criminal Laws BNS/BNSS***
Causing deaths due to medical negligence	No dedicated section for deaths due to Medical Negligence—Extrapolated from Section 304A of IPC	Dedicated section for deaths due to Medical Negligence—Section 106 subsection 1 of BNS
Section invoked	Section 304A of IPC • Bailable offence	Section 106(1) of BNS • Bailable offence
Crime committed	Causing deaths due to rash and negligent act	Causing deaths due to rash and negligent act with special mention of RMP
Degree of rashness/ negligence	Not defined	Not defined
Punishment	Up to 2 years jail term OR fine	Up to 2 years jail term AND ALSO fine
Registered Medical Practitioner (RMP)	No mention	Defined as a medical practitioner who possesses any medical qualification recognized under the National Medical Commission Act 2019 and whose name has been entered in the Nation Medical Register or a State Medical Register under the Act
Specific situation of causing death due to rash and negligent act	No mention	While doing a medical procedure
Culpable homicide not amounting to murder	Section 304 IPC • Non-bailable offence	Section 105 BNS • Non-bailable offence
Murder	Section 302 IPC • Non-bailable offence	Section 103 BNS • Non bailable offence
Sections that protect doctors for acts done in good faith	Section 88 IPC Section 80 IPC Section 81 IPC Section 87, 88, 89 IPC Section 92, 93 IPC	Section 26 BNS Section 18 BNS Section 19 BNS Section 25, 26, 27 BNS Section 30, 31 BNS
Preliminary enquiry	No mention	Section 173(3) BNSS • For punishment with jail term 3 years or more than 3 years but less than 7 years • A timeline of 14 days has been fixed
Sanction from sanctioning authority before prosecuting government servant	Section 197 CrPC	Section 218 BNSS • A timeline of 120 days has been fixed beyond which sanction would deemed to have been given
Causing hurt and grievous hurt	Section 319–326 IPC	Section 114–118 BNS
Definition of grievous hurt	Duration of bodily pain of 20 days	Duration of bodily pain reduced to 15 days to qualify grievous hurt

Continued

Continued

	Old Criminal Laws IPC/CrPC	***New Criminal Laws BNS/BNSS***
Causing grievous hurt resulting in vegetative state or permanent disability	No mention	Section 117(3) BNS
Making a false document	Section 464–466 IPC	Section 335–337 BNS
Cheating	Section 415–420 IPC	Section 318, 319 BNS

CONCLUSION

In medicolegal matters too, prevention is still the best medicine. Good medical practice and a good doctor-patient relationship are still the best ways to minimize lawsuits and their repercussions. Properly qualified and medically well-trained doctors also need to have some knowledge of pertinent legal terminology, judicial mechanisms in lawsuits, and ethical procedures, but should not take defense initiatives without prior advice and consultation of a medicolegal consultant and a lawyer well versed with medicolegal issues. Adequate information of relevant laws coupled with adherence to proper and ethical medical practice is usually sufficient to safeguard a doctor against frivolous complaints.

KEY LEARNING POINTS

- Accept only those patients for whom you are qualified and competent to treat. Refer others to relevant specialists without wasting any time.
- Properly document the complaints, investigations, and advice in every case.
- Attend a patient to best of one's ability once a doctor–patient relationship has been established or make documented alternative arrangements when unavailable.
- Counsel and document clearly and honestly about treatment options and potential difficulties in the clinical situation.
- If different modes of treatment are available, make a short notation of these options in patient's papers after the discussion, mentioning choice taken by patient/relatives.
- Suggest a second opinion and document this advice when dealing with an unusual or difficult case, especially in an aggressive patient or relatives.
- Never overstep one's qualifications and involve colleagues of other specialties as indicated.
- Communicate frankly with relatives regarding the management, especially in critical cases.
- Document if there is any failure to follow instructions appropriately.
- Ensure well-equipped indoor facilities and proper staff for monitoring as well as providing timely and correct treatment as advised.
- Visit the patient regularly and communicate about the condition with patient and/or relatives.
- In surgical cases notes of surgeon and anesthetist must not contradict each other especially in cases of mishaps.
- Provide option of timely referral in critical cases and document willingness or refusal.
- If possible, enquire about patient even after referral. This maintains confidence of patient and relatives in the referring doctor.

BIBLIOGRAPHY

1. A. Sikri. Dr. PB Desai vs. State of Maharashtra and Anr. Supreme court of India, Criminal Appeal No. 1432/2013, (Arising out of SLP (Crl.) No. 9568, 2012.
2. Calcutta Medical Research Institute vs. Bimalesh Chatterjee I (1999) CPJ 13 (NC).
3. Criminal Appeal nos 144-145 of 2004. Jacob Mathew vs. State of Punjab, (2005) 6 SCC 1.
4. Dr Janak Kantimathi Nathan vs. Murlidhar Eknath Masane 2002 (2) CPR 138.
5. Dr Laxman Balkrishna Joshi vs. Dr Trimbak Bapu Godbole AIR 1969 (SC)128.
6. Dr. Suresh Gupta vs. Govt. of NCT of Delhi and Anr on 4 August, 2004, Supreme Court of India.
7. House of Lords decision in R vs. Adomako (1994) 3 All ER 79.
8. Kanhaiya Kumar Singh vs. Park Medicare and Research Centre III (1999) CPJ 9 (NC).
9. Mondaq. When will a Doctor's negligent acts or Omissions attract Criminal Liability? [online] Available from https://www.mondaq.com/uk/healthcare/189340/when-will-a-doctors-negligent-acts-or-omissions-attract-criminal-liability. [Last accessed August, 2024].
10. Murthy KK. Medical negligence and the law. Indian J Med Ethics. 2007;4(3):116-8.
11. Poonam Verma vs. Ashwin Patel (1996) 4 SCC 332.
12. R vs. Prentice and R vs. Sullman (1993) 4 All ER 935.
13. State of Haryana vs. Smt. Santra (2000) 5 SCC 182:: AIR 2000 SC 3335.
14. The Indian Penal Code, 1860. Act No. 45 of 1860 (6th October, 1860).

CHAPTER

12 Difficult Situations in Practice

Girish Kumthekar

INTRODUCTION

All hospitals, one or the other day, face anticipated or unexpected difficult situations. The difficult situations can diffuse easily or may take a bad turn. When these problems arise in small individual proprietary hospitals or small-to-medium multispecialty hospitals, the situation and circumstances are different, and we will delve more into this sector. The big or multispecialty corporate hospitals have a different and faceless channel to settle these matters and no one is personally involved. However, in a small proprietary hospital, the consultant is directly across the table and must tackle the situations that may prove to be a nightmare.

The difficult situations one can face are as follows:

- Emergency patient from a road accident
- Patient's ailment not related to specialty
- Shifting a critically ill patient
- Sudden death and mob violence
- Brought dead
- Settlement of bills or recovery of dues

EMERGENCY ACCIDENT ADMISSION

This is a relatively mild situation wherein road accident victims are brought to the nearest hospital.

After a Supreme Court (SC) judgment (Parmanand Katara v. Union of India), you are duty-bound to treat the victim of an accident. It is expected from doctor or hospital that at least first aid must be given and if necessary, stabilize the patient with the available resources and guide the kins of the victim to shift to a proper hospital and counsel them accordingly. Please remember that in such situations, one is not expected to give extraordinary treatment or do some heroic efforts but must try to give the maximum possible support and shift the patient promptly to an appropriate clinical care facility.

PATIENT'S AILMENT NOT RELATED TO SPECIALTY

If the patient does not belong to your specialty, unless you are confident that an on-call specialist will be able to come on time and handle the patient, do not venture into this just to keep admission with you. You may lose the golden hour in such a situation and put yourself in trouble.

Whenever you are treating such a patient, take sufficient time to talk to the relatives or concerned person in detail about the situation, need for further action, and referral. If you are giving preliminary treatment and injectables, explain everything to the relatives and document everything. It may so happen that you will get unnecessary blame that death is caused by the medications you have given. Counseling of the relatives and chronological documentation of events are absolutely necessary in such cases.

SHIFTING A CRITICALLY ILL PATIENT

One more not-difficult-but-tricky situation wherein a critically ill patient is admitted, or becomes critical during treatment, or the infrastructure is not adequate to treat such patient, it is in the best interest of the patient and treating doctors to shift the patient to a tertiary care center. There are two things to be settled here:

1. Convince the relatives and counsel them for referral.
2. Do this without damage to one's own image and ego.

The first one is simple and relatives usually get convinced but the second part is image and ego. This is where one must compromise. Identify your own and hospital's limitations and shift the patient. Anticipate the problem in advance and shift the patient in time so that further allegations can be avoided. Learn to say "NO" to relatives and more importantly to yourself.

In this situation, it is prudent to give correct options to relatives. Never compel them for admission to a specific center. It is wise to call for an ambulance as a help to relatives. The ambulance must be well equipped to handle such patients during transfer. Give a referral chit to the concerned center explaining the necessity, provisional diagnosis, and treatment given. Keep a copy of the referral chit for your record and if the patient is on life support, accompany the patient or ask your clinical assistant doctor to accompany. This requirement of accompanying doctor is specifically enumerated by SC in one of the judgments.

SUDDEN DEATH

Sudden is defined as happening quickly and without any warning while sudden death is defined as instantaneous and unexpected death not caused by violence.

The important ingredient here is "not caused by violence". Unexpected death occurring during the course of treatment is sudden death. The sudden death could be caused during ward treatment or on an operation table. We have to deal with these two deaths differently.

Death in a Ward or Room During the Course of Treatment

We are not going to deal with causes of death in detail as this is not the purpose of this chapter.

However, just to enumerate, the causes of sudden death may be the following:

- Hemorrhagic shock
- Neurogenic shock
- Cardiogenic shock
- Endotoxic shock
- Anaphylactic shock
- *Other causes:*
  - *Embolism:* Amniotic fluid, air, or thrombus
  - *Anesthesia complications:* Mendelson's syndrome
- *More than one factor such as*:
  - Hemorrhagic and endotoxic shock
  - Hemorrhagic and neurogenic shock

Such death is usually postoperative or due to an undesired response or turn in the health of a patient being treated in a ward or room. Such death usually happens when the treating physician and nursing staff are not around and is invariably witnessed by the family member or attendant of the deceased. Sudden death itself constitutes a shock to the family. It is equally shocking to the treating doctor. Intense efforts are usually made by treating doctors or nursing staff on the site with available resources. In small nursing homes, this is the time when certain deficiencies are noticed by the bystanders or the relatives of the deceased. Usually, there is shouting, loud orders by the doctors, commotion, and a lot of hurry and worry in the body language of all those who are trying to resuscitate the ailing patient. This all is witnessed by the relatives of the patient and when death is declared, the efforts go unnoticed and it is only the deficiencies that are pointed out.

The gravity of this situation can be diluted by the following:

- Keep all resuscitative measures ready 24 × 7. These include emergency drug tray with drugs within expiry date, resuscitation equipment, oxygen cylinder if there is no central oxygen, tubes, defibrillator, and pulse oximeter.
- All the relatives and bystanders must be asked politely to leave the ward or room.
- Inform the seriousness of the health and give assurance that all measures are being taken to revive the patient.
- Break the bad news in a highly polite and dignified way. By dignified way means doctor is not supposed to show extreme emotions like crying in front of the relatives. The doctor must keep his composure and show confidence. He must share sorrow with the relatives but only professionally. This may appear odd to begin with but one must remember, the more extreme emotions you show the relatives become more suspicious.

After the death is declared, all the responsible relatives must be called upon to share information. At this point, remember to call out only responsible relatives and talk to them in a separate room, preferably in your consulting room. The relatives must be taken into confidence, the situation explained and if the cause of death is obvious, it must be explained properly. If there is doubt on the cause of death, medicolegal (ML)/clinical postmortem examination must be done. It takes a lot of effort to convince the relatives about the necessity of postmortem, but it is worth taking the efforts than to land in trouble later. If you feel postmortem is a must and relatives are not giving consent, you can take help of the police and get it done.

Intraoperative Death in Operation Theater or Immediate Postoperative Death in Recovery Room and Mob Violence

This really is a very difficult situation, particularly in elective operation, more so for the gynecologists where majority of the operations are elective and performed on a healthy patient. Most of the times, the patient enters the operation theater (OT) in good physical and mental condition and a lifeless body is brought out on a gurney. This is really shocking to relatives who are not prepared for such an eventuality. The story is different in high-risk cases, accidents, and complicated surgeries wherein the relatives are prepared for eventuality one way or the other.

The anticipated reactions of the relatives to such sudden death are:

- Anger and anguish
- *Immediate explanation:* Relatives demand immediate explanation on the spot, which is not possible for the doctors and the agitation and suspicion in the minds of relatives aggravates.
- Financial waver and immediate compensation
- *Immediate police action:* This usually is demanded by the so-called leaders of that particular area or community. They pressurize the police to register crime and arrest the doctor immediately. However, after SC's "Jacob Mathew judgment", which has prescribed a procedure to arrest a doctor, State governments have issued a directive to police, which are followed in most incidents.
- Verbal or physical abuse and immediate retaliation with destruction of property

Immediate reactions of the treating doctor that should be avoided:

- *Run away from the situation*: Never do this. It will only make things worse.
- *Immediate cover-up and unnecessary explanations:* This should be avoided. The doctors should not face multiple relatives immediately and start giving explanations to each and everyone. The paramedical staff should also be told to remain silent and avoid different versions of the situation. One should keep his nerves, take a break for a few minutes after exhaustive resuscitative efforts have failed, organize the things in OT, pool all the empty vials used during resuscitative measures, and collect all the papers and take them into your custody (this is to prevent unauthorized copying of the papers without knowledge of anybody). Later, one should call only the responsible relatives separately into the counseling or consulting room and explain the situation.
- *Settle the matter as early as possible by political or financial means*: This is the most common practice adopted by doctors but this should be avoided under any circumstances as this sets a precedence for future mischief mongers and political leaders.
- *Fight the situation overconfidently*: This is to be avoided not only verbally but even with body language. Dismissing the relatives, not giving a proper explanation, or challenging them by any means aggravates the situation further.
- *Retaliate the abuse by abusive language*: This possibly is the worst thing a doctor can do. The dictum is that relatives may abuse in any language, you cannot reply in the same

language as your abusive language shall be capitalized immediately and more and more abuses will start getting hurled at you. This also increases the tension in the atmosphere and temperatures start getting very high. Many times, relatives do it on purpose just to provoke you and capitalize on it later on.

Probable actions the relatives may take in such a situation:

- Manhandle the doctor and destruction of the property and hospital equipment.
- Threaten the doctor.
- Lodge a criminal complaint.
- Insist on arrest of the doctor (we have some solace from this after SC directives).
- Invite the media to spread the news (though very traumatic situation, just do not worry, the publicity does not affect your reputation in a long run and remember public memory is less than 24 hours).
- Demand for money (this probably is the ulterior motive of relatives).
  These situations are self-explanatory and we have to deal with them instinctively.

What a Doctor Should Do?

- *Call colleagues and seniors for help*: This probably works more than anything else. Prepare a task force on the platform of organizations like Indian Medical Association (IMA) or Specialty society. All seniors and colleagues from all specialties should rush to the troubled spot at the shortest notice. This diffuses the situation very fast. There may be many people in the mob who happen to be patients of one or the other doctor from the task force and such senior consultant can diffuse the situation and mediate on behalf of the treating doctor.
- If the situation is going out of hands, call the police.
- Different visitors or relatives at different times may ask explanation afresh. This should be avoided and an explanation must be given only once and only to responsible relatives.
- Involve only the responsible persons from the aggrieved family.
- Involvement of local politician is quite controversial and depends on the situation. Personally, we do not recommend it as you put yourself in a vulnerable position later on when the politician demands his pound of flesh. But in the past many doctors have benefitted after getting help from politicians.
- Be a patient listener to the allegations and abuses.
- Discuss the problem with colleagues who have come in to help and prepare a logical sequence of events.
- Take time to prepare the case paper and put proper notes.
- Cooperate with the legal arm.
- In case, a cause of death can be given, certify the death.
- Ideally, ML postmortem is a must. It substantiates your diagnosis and actions.

Breaking the News

Breaking the bad news should be handled very carefully. Each case deserves to be handled by its merits. The various ways in which the bad news can be broken are as follows:

- *Immediate:* Sometimes it is necessary to declare death immediately. This method has both its pros and cons. It can bring around immediate violent reaction as stated earlier. Sometimes immediate declaration reflects transparency and relatives do not grumble much. This all is circumstantial and a doctor must use his/her utmost management skills.

- *After cover-up*: Cover-up does not mean manipulations or fabrications. It means the place where the patient has died, in OT or ward, there is a lot of mess around like maybe a pool of blood or blood-stained sponges, etc. This should be cleaned and tidy up. Preserve all material in an orderly manner so that your efforts can be accounted for. The procedure of keeping the patient on artificial means and pretending that the patient is alive does not work in the true sense. It is a common practice to keep the patient on a ventilator and break the news slowly after intensifying the situation step by step. The problem here is many of the bystanders and witnessing relatives are wise enough to realize that things have gone wrong. They feel that extensions and pretensions are a drama for other causes (mostly financial) and then they retaliate.
- *Conveniently by another person may be a staff nurse or servants*: This probably is the simplest way but sometimes agitated relatives are not happy, and they want a direct interaction with the doctor. Though not an everyday situation in small hospitals, the staff must be well briefed and trained to break the news if delegated to do so.
- *After asking all the responsible relatives to gather and then explain in the presence of colleagues*: This probably is the safest way to break the news. This should be done preferably in your own consulting room. Remember that your consulting room is the most comfortable place for such thing. You happen to be the most powerful person in your own consulting room. Sit comfortably on your chair, ask your colleagues to sit by your side, and ask the relative to sit across the table. This creates a wall of power between you and relatives and keeps you safe. Never go directly toward the mob. This makes you vulnerable and may precipitate direct manhandling.

Medicolegal Aspects of Sudden Death

- Sudden death is treated as an accidental death and it requires a very high degree of negligence to prove that it was caused by a negligent and rash act.
- It invites the Indian Penal Code (IPC) section 304A/304 or BNS Sections 106 (1)/105, which means death caused due to rash and negligent acts by several persons with a common intention.
- It is a cognizable and bailable offense. Bail can be granted by the investigating officer, no court is needed.
- On request of the doctor, or in case of medicolegal case, custody of the human remains is taken by the police and shifted for postmortem.
- The investigating officer can demand copies of all documents and charts related to the case. It is not necessary to provide them immediately. You can ask for some time. Complete the papers to the last detail and provide the officer with Xerox copies. In fact, never hand over original papers to the authorities. You may lose your defense forever.

Most of the time, in cases of mob violence and difficult situations after sudden death, the demand of the agitating relatives of the deceased is to file a case and arrest the doctor immediately. Fortunately for us, the Honorable SC in its judgment directed the Central/State governments to frame statutory rules or executive instructions as regards prosecution against doctors (Jacob Matthews vs. State of Punjab delivered on 5th August, 2005). Until governments prepare such statutory rules, the Honorable SC has given directives that govern the prosecution of doctors for offenses of which criminal rashness or criminal negligence is an ingredient. Remember these directives are to be followed only when the death has occurred during the course of treatment.

The Honorable SC says that:

- A private complaint may not be entertained unless the complainant has produced prima facie evidence before the Court in the form of a credible opinion given by another competent doctor to support the charge of rashness or negligence on the part of the accused doctor.
- The investigating officer should, before proceeding against the doctor accused of rash or negligent act or omission, obtain an independent and competent medical opinion preferably from a doctor in government service qualified in that branch of medical practice who can normally be expected to give an impartial and unbiased opinion.
- A doctor accused of rashness or negligence, may not be arrested in a routine manner (simply because a charge has been leveled against him/her). Unless his/her arrest is necessary for furthering the investigation or for collecting evidence or unless the investigating officer feels satisfied that the doctor proceeded against would not make himself/herself available to face the prosecution unless arrested, the arrest may be withheld.

The directives are self-explanatory and whenever there is imminent arrest, one can use the copy of this judgment and ask the police officer to abide by the directives.

Other legal actions a doctor can face after such a mishap are:

- Action under the Consumer Protection Act
- Action in civil court for compensation.

We are not going to go into details of these actions but in a recent judgment, the Honorable SC has again given us a great relief. The Court has said in its judgment that a case against doctors should not be admitted immediately by consumer court or civil court. Instead, the courts should serve notice to the concerned doctor and ask for an explanation or expert opinion from the competent medical board at the district place. If not satisfied with the reply or the recommendation of the competent board, the court may proceed to admit a complaint.

Recent amendments in the Code of Criminal Procedure (CrPC) are also a great relief as arrest can be avoided as per provisions.

BROUGHT DEAD

This situation is faced mainly by pediatricians, general practitioners, or general hospitals. The dilemma faced by attending physician is what to do in such cases. The doctor must see the patient anyway and declare the death. The question arises as to death certificate, cause of death, information to the police, and what records to keep. These are the few directives that may not be foolproof but may help to resolve the dilemma.

- Always attend the brought dead patient in your outpatient department (OPD) or emergency room (ER) (do not admit directly). Do not delegate the nursing staff or clinical assistants to attend the brought-in dead body and declare death and push the relatives to take away the body.
- Prepare an OPD case paper only with your OPD number and date and timing of arrival of the deceased. Put in detail the names of accompanying persons, their relation with the

deceased, and at least two identification marks of each of them and take their signatures. Have two witnesses with you to sign, preferably other bystanders or relatives of the deceased. Avoid your own staff as witness.

- Write down the history given by the relatives verbatim.
- Record at least two identification marks of the dead body.
- Declare the death after careful examination and auscultation for at least 5 minutes and if possible, electrocardiograph (ECG) recording may be taken.
- In case of any suspicion, do not hesitate to inform the police and ask them to take necessary action.
- In case the deceased is known and under your treatment for a terminal illness, you may give a death certificate.
- Keep your OPD record carefully. The investigating officer may ask for a copy or you may have to attend court as a witness in case of eventuality.

The message is do not avoid attending brought dead cases, be careful with records and examination and cooperate with law whenever necessary.

SETTLEMENT OF BILLS AND RECOVERY OF BILLS

This is again a very difficult situation, and to tackle this situation you need more social, managerial, and manipulative skills rather than medical knowledge. Taking regular advance equivalent to the expected bill on that day is probably the best policy. But when it comes to sudden death or unexpected complications that drain the resources of patient and relatives, the situation arises. Doctors, currently, are at the receiving end of the society for many reasons. They never understand the use of intellectual property and its encashment and always feel that we are taking money unnecessarily. This misconception needs to be removed and it will take time.

So far, as the legal aspect of the recovery and nonpayment of bills is considered, we really have very few options, which are as follows:

- Forgo the bill and forget it once and for all.
- Take an advance cheque for the remaining amount so that some legal option remains with us.
- Reduce the bill, give concessions, etc.
- Use mediators or request acquaintances from both parties to mediate.
- File a civil suit for recovery of the bill which requires an advocate, court fees, and a long waiting period—not really advisable.
- In case, there are previous dues of bill from such patient, you have a right to refuse to see and treat such patient. Exercise this right if necessary.

Ultimately, it is the skill you develop over the years of practice as to how to recover dues or settle the bill.

The doctors should not use harsh words and should never give ultimatums to patient. Stopping or discontinuing treatment for nonpayment of bills as well as keeping the patient waiting, at the door of OT before the operation starts, or asking for advance during the course of surgery is not a good practice. Things work until they are straight forward but once something goes wrong, they bounce back upon you.

Ultimately, all these difficult situations are going to stay and we must learn to live with them, tackle them as nicely as possible, and reduce our stress. My usual advice to my colleagues is, "instead *of losing sleep over how to increase footfall at the door of hospital, try to give good care to the patients who have come to you and enjoy a sound sleep*".

CONCLUSION

From the above discussion, one may get scared as to how to practice in future. But these situations do come up very infrequently in a lifetime. The seniors will realize that in decades of practice they have rarely come across such situations. When you face it, it is really very traumatizing. To certain extent, such write-ups help you in tackling such situations, but remember ultimately, it is the situation and your communication skills, your temperament, and the help you get all matter. A few key points to be repeated in conclusion are as follows.

- Try to use your skills to your comfort level. You must know when to stop and define your boundaries. You are not supposed to do something extraordinary or heroic unless the situation demands. Otherwise, routine management is good enough.
- Proper communication and counseling are very important. One must give sufficient time to each and every patient and such communication must be documented well.
- Try to be reasonable in practice. Remember, you are not God and near to God. You are just a simple human being entitled to do something different with human life because of your knowledge, training, and experience. It is important to believe, *"you do not cure patients; you only help them to get cured with the help of your knowledge and armamentarium"*.
- Never hesitate to call for help. Prepare your own group as quick responders.
- Always work within the frame of established laws and cooperate with the legal arms as and when necessary.
- Record keeping, be it audio, video, or black and white; it is of utmost importance.

KEY LEARNING POINTS

- Every hospital and every practitioner is going to face difficult situations at least once in a lifetime.
- Be ready to face such situations with all your armamentarium like infrastructure, manpower, documentation, and above all help.
- Share your experience with others and learn from others' experience to subjugate the situation.
- Being totally submissive or overconfident and arrogant is equally damaging.
- Do not hesitate to call for help from colleagues and seniors and at times from police and other legal help.
- Never give importance to adverse publicity and damage to reputation. Remember, public memory is very short and things become normal the second day.
- It is not advisable to get depressed due to the incident, just treat it as collateral damage and proceed in life.
- Always have adequate insurance and indemnity.
- Prepare a uniform statement about the situation and always stick to it.
- Acquire adequate legal knowledge and remain updated.
- Comply with the legal requirements such as registration with authorities, pollution control board, and renew all the licenses in time.
- Keep your medical knowledge updated and use it as and when required.
- Proper communication with the patient and relatives is of utmost importance and spare a definite time for counseling, consent, and other documentation.

BIBLIOGRAPHY

1. Institute of Medicine and Law. (2022). Supreme Court's comment on medicine and negligence. Dr Martin D'Souza versus Mohammad Ishfak AIR 2002. [online] Available from https://www.mlcd.in/notes/details.aspx?id=ELykR3kQPf0%3D [Last accessed May, 2024].
2. Supreme Court of India. (2005). Case no: Appeal (crl.) 144-145 of 2004. Jacob Mathews versus the State of Punjab. [online] Available from https://main.sci.gov.in/jonew/judis/27088.pdf [Last accessed May, 2024].

SECTION

3

Legal Procedures

Section Editor: NL Sridhar

Section Outline

13

CHAPTER

How to Defend a Case?

Mahesh Baldwa, Amit Padvi, Namita Padvi

"The best way to defend yourself is to preempt prosecuting you in court of law."

INTRODUCTION

According to a study by the American Medical Association 42% of doctors had faced a malpractice claim at some point in their careers. The same report also found that 65% of medical malpractice claims are dropped, dismissed, or withdrawn. So, being sued for malpractice certainly does not mean that the doctor did anything wrong or will be held liable for medical negligence. We don't have statistics related to India but may be similar if not worse than western countries.

ARE CONSUMER CASES DECREASING RECENTLY IN INDIA?

In the year 2018 a total of 3241 cases of medical negligence cases had been filed in India while in the year 2019 only 2638 cases of medical negligence cases, which is 18.61%. At the level of National Consumer Commission, i.e., 435 medical negligence cases filed in 2019 as compared to 2018 with only 433 medical negligence cases. In all State Commissions 566 medical negligence cases have been filed in year 2019 as compared to 861 medical negligence cases in the year 2018, which is (295; 34.26% less in year 2019), whereas in all District Commissions only 1637 medical negligence cases filed in the year 2019 as compared to year 2018 reported 1946 medical negligence cases. There was a decrease of 309 (15.88%) cases at the level of District Commissions in the year 2019 as compared to 2018.

TYPES OF MEDICAL NEGLIGENCE

Medical negligence can occur in different ways. The medical profession has its own ethical parameters and code of conduct. However, negligence by doctors has to be determined by judges who are not trained in medical science. They rely on experts' opinion and decide on the basis of basic principles of reasonableness and prudence. There is often a thin dividing line between the three levels of negligence; lata culpa, gross neglect; levis culpa, ordinary neglect; and levissima culpa, slight neglect [Smt. Madhubala vs Govt. of NCT of Delhi and Ors. 2005]. The level of negligence depends on the entire context—which includes the place, the time, the individuals involved, and the level of complications. The difference between medical negligence and medical error is well-settled, and the principles are well-founded being clearly laid down in numerous cases by the Supreme Court [Kirplani & Ors. 2009]. Thus, there is a need to appreciate this differentiation by the society so that doctors do not get indicted for impractical reasons.

Some other types of alleged negligence is complications of disease, drug and surgery is dubbed as medical negligence.

- *Potential litigant*: A reasonable doctor should consider every patient as a potential litigant. It is to keep a doctor in constant awareness to stick to a prescribed standard of care and avoid any adventurous attempt. A doctor should not ignore any allegation in any form (oral or written) and should be able to handle allegations with clear and firmness in an intelligent and sympathetic manner.

Complaint not maintainable though this point was not raised in lower courts—"Karta' of Joint Hindu Family" cannot be said to be availing services of medical practitioner in respect of pregnancy of his sister-in-law Jaganarayan Lal vs. Doctor Smt. Girija Tiwari (SC), 2021(3) Apex Court Judgments (SC) 467: 2021(3) MadWN (Civil) 366, Civil Appeal No. 2539 of 2011. D/d. 15.9.2021.

Consumer Protection Act, 1986, Section 2(1)(b)—Deficiency in service regarding treatment to pregnant sister-in-law—Dismissal of complaint filed by brother-in-law as "Karta of Joint Hindu family—Held, appellant 'Karta' of Joint Hindu Family cannot be said to be availing services of medical practitioner in respect of pregnancy of his sister-in-law. Concept of Joint Hindu Family does not extend to treatment of pregnant sister-in-law—No objection regarding maintainability of complaint raised either before State Commission or National Commission, but such issue of maintainability of complaint goes to root of case and nonmaintainable on bare assertions of complaint alone. Hence, complaint not maintainable.

LOCUS STANDI OF PERSON FILING CASE

The questions of locus standi of the complainant to file and maintain a complaint against the doctor is also very important particularly in Consumer Protection Act and other acts. It is held that when wife and son of deceased patient are alive, a consumer complaint filed by the brother of deceased is not maintainable (Parimal Kumar Acharya vs. Dr. Tapan Kumar Chakraborty, 2005 (1) Consumer Protection Reporter 474). Similarly, a consumer complaint filed by wife of deceased alleging negligence of doctor in treatment of her deceased husband, filed after her remarriage is not maintainable (2005 (1) Consumer Protection Reporter 493/(2005 (1) CPJ 792 (Shantha V. Gowda versus Kempegowda Institute of Medical Sciences and others). However, in Dr. PB Lal versus Suresh Chandra Roy (2006(2)CPR 1). Bihar State Consumer Disputes Redressal Commissioner has held that complaint of husband in respect of loss of eye-sight of wife is maintainable on the ground that not only the victim but also beneficiary of services is entitled to file such complaint. There is, therefore, no strait-jacket formula of law or principle to find out locus standi of a complainant. It has to be ascertained from the facts of each case. As a result, it is necessary to verify locus standi of the complainant to file such a complaint with reference to the facts of the case and to take appropriate defense/plea in the written statement/say of the doctors.

2015-Two Judge Supreme Court

Complainant not maintainable without sanction of Government as per Criminal Procedure Code, 1973 Section 197—Prosecution of Public Servant.

Dr. Manorama Tiwari v. Surendra Nath Rai (2JJSC), Criminal Appeal No. 1193 of 2015 (Arising out of S.L.P. (Crl) No. 9386 of 2012). D/d. 10.9.2015.

Miss Tapsi Rai, aged 14 years underwent surgery in Maharani Government Hospital, Jagdalpur, Bastar. The operation necessitated due to pain developed by the patient in the abdomen, was performed by the appellants, namely, Dr. (Smt.) Manorama Tiwari, Dr. B.R. Kawdo and Dr. Pradeep Pandey. Consent to operate was taken from the respondent. However, even after surgery, the condition of the patient did not improve, and she died on the same day. Accused were medical officers in Government Hospital. They performed surgery on a patient who died—Complaint under Section 304A IPC against the medical officers making allegations of negligence—Complainant not maintainable without sanction of Government as per Criminal Procedure Code, 1973 Section 197—Prosecution of Public Servant—No one can take such proceedings without such sanction.

High Court has erred in law in dismissing the criminal revision filed by the appellants and affirming the order of the Magistrate rejecting their application as to maintainability of the criminal complaint without sanction from the State Government. In our opinion, it is a clear case where appellants were discharging their public duties, as they were performing surgery on the patient in the Government Hospital. It is not disputed that the appellants were the Medical Officers in the Government Hospital. As such, the criminal prosecution of the appellants initiated by the respondent (complainant) is not maintainable without the sanction from the State Government. Matajog Dubey vs. H.C. Bhari, AIR 1956 Supreme Court 44. Even Guidelines for prosecution of medical negligence reiterated in Jacob Mathews 2005(3) RCR (Criminal) 836, relied.

AGAINST GOVERNMENT SERVANT CRIMINAL CASE

The omission complained of due to which offence is stated to have been committed, was intrinsically connected with discharge of official duty of the appellant, as such the protection under Section 197 CrPC from prosecution without sanction of the competent authority, is available to the appellant.

The accused (Doctor) did not provide an official vehicle to shift patient from Primary Health Centre to District Hospital. It is omission of accused connected with performance of official duties—Accused could not be prosecuted without sanction—1955 (1) SCR 1177 : 1955 (2) SCR 925 : 2009 (3) RCR (Criminal) 835 : 2009 (5) Recent Apex Judgment (RAJ) 110 Relied.

The right approach to the import of these words lies between these two extremes. While on the one hand, it is not every offence committed by a public servant while engaged in the performance of his official duty, which is entitled to the protection of Section 197(1), an act constituting an offence, directly and reasonably connected with his official duty will require sanction for prosecution under the said provision. As pointed out by Ramaswami, J. in Baijnath vs. State of M.P., AIR 1966 Supreme Court 220.

It is the quality of the act that is important, and if it falls within the scope and range of its official duties the protection contemplated by Section 197 of the Criminal Procedure Code will be attracted.

In sum, the sine qua non for the applicability of this section is that the offence charged, be it one of commission or omission, must be one which has been committed by the public servant either in his official capacity or under color of the office held by him "(emphasis in original)".

In view of the aforesaid discussion, it is clear that the omission complained of due to which offence is stated to have been committed, was intrinsically connected with discharge of official duty of the appellant, as such the protection under Section 197 CrPC from prosecution without sanction of the competent authority, is available to the appellant. Thus, he could not have been prosecuted without sanction. It would be for the competent authority to consider the question of grant of sanction in accordance with law. In case sanction is granted only then the appellant can be prosecuted and not otherwise. Resultantly, the impugned orders are set aside, the appeal is allowed.

DEFENDING CRIMINAL COURT CASE

Any act or omission which is prohibited by law and is punishable by law is a crime. The punishment for such crime is decided by following procedures of criminal trial. The criminal trials in India are well-established statutory, administrative and judicial framework. The whole criminal law consists of three main acts:

1. Indian Penal Code, 1860 {1}
2. Code of Criminal Procedure, 1973{2}
3. Indian Evidence Act, 1872. {3}

Dictum in criminal cases:

1. Unless proved negligent the doctor is not negligent
2. Medical board opinion is must for pursuing medical negligence case in criminal court by prosecution as per supreme court three judge bench in Jacob Mathew v. State of Punjab,(2005) 6 SCC 1 {4} and same is also followed in Martin F. D'Souza v. Mohd. Ishfaq (2009) 3 SCC 1, {5}V Kishan Rao v. Nikhil Super Speciality Hospital (2010) 5 SCC 513 {6}
3. Deny all allegations from beginning till end of the criminal trial as accused
4. Wait patiently till prosecution establishes the case of negligence
5. Attend each and every date in court of law to keep everything under control

Warrant Cases where allegation is murdering a patient—very unusual for doctor to get such kind of criminal case

According to Section 2(x) of Code of Criminal Procedure, 1973 a warrant case is one which relates to offenses punishable with death, imprisonment for life or imprisonment for a term exceeding two years. The trial in warrant cases starts either by the filing of FIR in a police station or by filing a complaint before a Magistrate. Later, if the Magistrate is satisfied that the offense is punishable for more than two years, he sends the case to the sessions court for trial. The process of sending it to session's court is called "committing it to session's court".

The important features of a warrant case are:

- Charges must be mentioned in a warrant case
- Personal appearance of accused is mandatory
- A warrant case cannot be converted into a summons case
- The accused can examine and cross-examine the witnesses more than once.
- The Magistrate should ensure that the provisions of Section 207 are.

- Section 207 of CrPC 1973, includes the supply of copies such as police report, FIR, statements recorded or any other relevant document to the accused.

The stages of trial in warrant cases are given from Section 238 to Section 250 of the Code of Criminal Procedure, 1973. Different Stages of Criminal Trial in a Warrant Case when instituted by the police report:

- *First information report*: Under Section 154 of the Code of Criminal Procedure, a FIR or First Information Report is registered. FIR puts the case into motion. A FIR is information given by someone (aggrieved) to the police relating to the commitment of an offense.
- *Investigation:* The next step after the filing of FIR is the investigation by the investigating officer. A conclusion is made by the investigating officer by examining facts and circumstances, collecting evidence, examining various persons and taking their statements in writing and all the other steps necessary for completing the investigation and then that conclusion is filed to the Magistrate as a police report.
- *Charges*: If, after considering the police report and other important documents, the accused is not discharged then the court frames charges under which he is to be trialled. In a warrant case, the charges should be framed in writing.
- *Plea of guilty*: Section 241 of the Code of Criminal Procedure, 1973 talks about the plea of guilty, after framing of the charges the accused is given an opportunity to plead guilty, and the responsibility lies with the judge to ensure that the plea of guilt was voluntarily made. The judge may upon its discretion convict the accused.
- *Prosecution evidence*: After the charges are framed, and the accused pleads guilty, then the court requires the prosecution to produce evidence to prove the guilt of the accused. The prosecution is required to support their evidence with statements from its witnesses. This process is called "examination in chief". The Magistrate has the power to issue summons to any person as a witness or orders him to produce any document.
- *Statement of the accused*: Section 313 of the Criminal Procedure Code gives an opportunity to the accused to be heard and explain the facts and circumstances of the case. The statements of the accused are not recorded under oath and can be used against him in the trial.
- *Defence evidence*: An opportunity is given to the accused in a case where he is not being acquitted to produce so as to defend his case. The defense can produce both oral and documentary evidence. In India, since the burden of proof is on the prosecution the defense, in general, is not required to give any defense evidence.
- *Judgement*: The final decision of the court with reasons given in support of the acquittal or conviction of the accused is known as judgement. In case the accused is acquitted, prosecution is given time to appeal against the order of the court. When the person is convicted, then both sides are invited to give arguments on the punishment which is to be awarded. This is usually done when the person is convicted of an offense whose punishment is life imprisonment or capital punishment.

Stages of Criminal Trial in a Warrant Case when Private Complaint institutes case—this is common against doctor under s. 304A or 337 or 338 of Indian penal court.

EXAMINATION OF COMPLAINANT AND ITS WITNESSES

On the filing of the complaint, the court will examine the complainant and its witnesses on the same day or any other day to decide whether any offense is made against the accused person or not.

Magistrate may order an inquiry

After examination of the complainant, the Magistrate may order an inquiry into the matter and submit a report for the same.

If sufficient evidence is found

After examination of the complaint and the investigation report, the court may come to a conclusion whether the complaint is genuine or whether the prosecution has sufficient evidence against the accused or not.

If sufficient evidence is not found

If the court does not find any sufficient material through which he can convict the accused, then the court will dismiss the complaint and record its reason for dismissal.

After examination of the complaint and the inquiry report, if the court thinks that the prosecution has a genuine case and there are sufficient material and evidence with the prosecution to charge the accused then the Magistrate may issue a warrant or a summon depending on the facts and circumstances. This is described as below.

SUMMON CASES

According to Section 2(w) of Code of Criminal Procedure, 1973, Those cases in which an offense is punishable with an imprisonment of fewer than two years is a summon case. A summon case doesn't require the method of preparing the evidence. Nevertheless, a summon case can be converted into a warrant case by the Magistrate if after looking into the case he thinks that the case is not a summon case.

Important Points about Summons Case

- A summons case can be converted into a warrant case.
- The person accused need not be present personally.
- The person accused should be informed about the charges orally. No need for framing the charges in writing.
- The accused gets only one opportunity to cross-examine the witnesses.
- The different stages of criminal trial in a summon case are given from Section 251 to Section 259 of the Code of Criminal procedure.

Stages of Criminal Trial in a Summons Case

- *Pretrial*: In the pretrial stage, the process such as filing of FIR and investigation is conducted.
- *Charges*: In summons trials, charges are not framed in writing. The accused appears before the court or is brought before the court then the Magistrate would orally state the facts of the offense, he is answerable.
- *Plea of guilty*: The Magistrate after stating the facts of the offense will ask the accused if he pleads guilty or has any defense to support his case. If the accused pleads guilty, the Magistrate records the statement in the words of the accused as far as possible and may convict him on his discretion.
- *Plea of guilty and absence of the accused*: In cases, where the accused wants to plead guilty without appearing in the court, the accused is supposed to send ₹1,000/- by post or through

a messenger (lawyer) to the Magistrate. The absentee should also send a letter containing acceptance of guilt and the amount of fine provided in the summons. The Magistrate can on his discretion convict the accused.

- *Prosecution and defense evidence*: In summons case, the procedure followed is very simple and elaborate procedures are eliminated. If the accused does not plead guilty, then the process of trial starts. The prosecution and the defense are asked to present evidence in support of their cases. The Magistrate is also empowered to take the statement of the accused.
- *Judgement*: When the sentence is pronounced in a summons case, the parties need not argue on the amount of punishment given. The sentence is the sole discretion of the judge. If the accused is acquitted, the prosecution has the right to appeal. This right to appeal is also extended to the accused.

SUMMARY TRIAL

Cases which generally take only one or two hearings to decide the matter come under this category. The summary trials are reserved for small offenses to reduce the burden on courts and to save time and money. Those cases in which an offense is punishable with an imprisonment of not more than six months can be tried in a summary way. The point worth noting is that, if the case is being tried in a summary way, a person cannot be awarded a punishment of imprisonment for more than three months.

The trial procedure is provided from Section 260 to Section 265 of the Code of Criminal Procedure.

Stages of Criminal Trial in Summary Cases

- The procedure followed in the summary trial is similar to summons-case.
- Imprisonment up to 3 months can be passed.
- In the judgement of a summary trial, the judge should record the substance of the evidence and a brief statement of the finding of the court with reasons.
- Out-of-court settlement for criminal cases is known as compounding
- Section 320 of CrPC allows settling cases outside court and it is known as compounding of criminal cases. The list of cases outside Section 320 of CrPC does not allow settling cases outside court. Cases where death or grievous injury has occurred compounding is not allowed.
- Abatement of proceedings on the death of the accused.

Death of the Accused in Criminal Case

The ultimate object of the criminal proceedings is to punish the accused on his conviction of any offence. Therefore, the criminal proceedings abate on the death of the accused, as their continuance thereafter will be infructuous and meaningless.

Plea Bargaining

Provisions relating to plea bargaining in Indian criminal justice system are provided in Chapter XXI-A-Section 265 B CrPC which was added by Criminal Law (Amendment) Act 2005 (2 of 2006) which came into force on 5.7.2006. Plea bargaining is a pretrial negotiation between the accused and the prosecution where the accused agrees to plead guilty in exchange for certain concessions by the prosecution. It is a bargain where a defendant pleads guilty to a lesser charge and the prosecutors in return drop more serious charges. It is not available for all types of crime, e.g., a person cannot claim plea bargaining after committing heinous crimes or for the crimes which are punishable with death or life imprisonment.

Q. Are procedures in the consumer court and other civil courts like civil judge, special civil judge, and permanent lok Adalat save and except criminal court which is described above?
Ans: Yes, most of the procedures in civil courts follow civil procedure code in limited or unlimited form. Consumer courts are one of the special kinds of civil court. The main difference between civil courts and criminal courts is remedy sought by complainant. If complainant wants you to be jailed then he/she will seek criminal courts otherwise for monetary compensation shall seek civil or consumer courts.

SETTLING OUT OF THE COURT: STATUS

- 2018, A study by the Harvard University last year showed that nearly 500,000 deaths occur in India annually due to medical errors triggered by lack of practical knowledge among the doctors and nurses to handle patients when brought to the hospital.
- In 2017, 43 lakhs such cases are pending in various consumer courts in the country
- Only 15% of medical negligence cases are genuine.

Q. No. 1. Is out-of-court settlement legal?
Ans: *Civil*: One can opt for out-of-court settlement in all civil cases. S. 89 of CPC 1899 The Indian Arbitration Act enabled it. In 2002, Alternative Dispute Resolution (ADR) mechanism in Section 89 of CPC.

ADR has emerged as a significant movement in these countries and has not only helped reduce cost and time taken for resolution of disputes, but also in providing a congenial atmosphere and a less formal and less complicated.

ADR—OUTSIDE COURT SETTLEMENT

■ Advantage

Out-of-court settlement success rate range from ~90% cases, fast speed, low cost, things are with in control of parties, no fault ascribed, formal relationship maintained—bitterness between parties, confidentiality maintained, amicable settlement, courts agree to consent terms filed by parties.

■ Disadvantage

Failure is in 10–15% cases further legal action continues

■ Types of Alternate Dispute Resolution

- Negotiation—involves people in disputes communicating directly via patient's relatives.
- Mediation is when an impartial person (a mediator) known to both parties appointed by authority of parties themselves, usually an impartial doctor.

- Conciliation—known in society as impartial common person from who suo moto assumes role of conciliator to end dispute impartially between two conflicting parties informally, usually, a social worker, politician.
- Facilitation known in society as impartial common person from who suo moto assumes role of facilitator sees to disputes impartially between more than two conflicting parties informally, usually a person from impartial police person, CMO, senior bureaucrat.
- Arbitration—is a formal process appoint independent third person (the arbitrator) and are bound by arbitrator's decision. Arbitration is a formal process and can follow similar procedures to court proceedings where witnesses can be called, and evidence can be presented to argue the parties' respective cases.
- Except for arbitration, people involved in dispute resolution come to their own agreement. Mediators, facilitators and conciliators can give information and advice, but do not impose a decision about how the dispute should be resolved.

Who will pay for an out-of-court settlement?

Usually parties themselves pay as per agreed terms and conditions if case in pre-litigation stage. Will indemnity policy cover out-of-court settlement?

1. If it is mentioned in professional indemnity policy to cover out-of-court settlement.
2. Out-of-court settlement terms and conditions known as consent terms approved by court. This is covered by indemnity insurance policy.

Status of out-of-court settlement

Generally, an out-of-court settlement allows one party to pay a sum of money to the other and in return the other party will close their lawsuit. Mainly, a settlement is a lawfully binding agreement which ends the case exclusive of going to court.

CASE LAW ON FIR

[While registration of FIR is mandatory, arrest of the accused immediately on registration of FIR is not at all mandatory.]

Registration of FIR is mandatory under Section 154 of the Code, if the information discloses commission of a cognizable offence and no preliminary injury is permissible in such a situation.

Mediation under CPA 2019

Mediation under section 74, 75, 76, 77, 78, 79, 80, 81 of Consumer Protection Act 2019 {7} Mediation is allowed for medical negligence except for death and grievous injury.

CASE LAW

Hysterectomy operation of the patient conducted in hospital having no I.C.U. facility—Death of patient. It is medical negligence, also other observations for speedy disposal of consumer cases by out-of-court settlement, etc., were made.

Bijoy Sinha Roy (D) vs. Biswanath Das, (2 JJ, SC) Civil Appeal Nos. 4761 of 2009. D/d. 30.8.2017. In a case where hysterectomy operation of the patient conducted in hospital having no I.C.U. facility—Death of patient—It is medical negligence 5 lakhs awarded other observation in above judgement were Providing speedy remedy to a consumer—Consider use of video conferencing facility for examining expert witnesses wherever necessary

To achieve the object of providing speedy remedy to a consumer steps can be taken of the Act. The National Commission has administrative control over all the State Commissions. Thus, the National Commission is competent to introduce monitoring mechanism for speedy disposal. It is well known that matters are pending at different levels for sufficiently long period which defeats the very object and purpose of the Act. We request the National Commission to consider this aspect and formulate an appropriate action plan. In this regard, we may refer to a recent decision in Hussain v. State of U.P., 2017(2) RCR (Criminal) 312 : 2017(2) Recent Apex Judgments (R.A.J.) 357 : (2017) 5 SCC 702 by which directions for action plans have been issued. The National Commission may also consider use of video conferencing facility for examining expert witnesses wherever necessary see observations in Krishna Veni 2017(2) RCR (Civil) 358: 2017(2) Recent Apex Judgments (R.A.J.) 373: (2017) 4 SCC 150.

Section 89 has been added to CPC—use ADR—settlement of disputes outside the Court.

The other aspect relates to use of ADR. By Act 46 of 1999, Section 89 has been added to CPC laying down mechanism for settlement of disputes outside the Court. Even though strictly speaking, the said provision is applicable only to civil courts, there is no reason to exclude its applicability to Consumer Fora having regard to the object of the said provision and the object of the consumer protection law. Accordingly, we are of the view that the said provision ought to be duly invoked by the Consumer Fora. We request the National Commission to issue appropriate directions in this regard see observations of this Court on the issue of remedy of mediation in Salem Advocate Bar Association, T.N. v. UOI 2002(4) RCR (Civil) 786 : (2003) 1 SCC 49, para 9-10; Salem Advocate Bar Association, T.N. v. UOI 2005(3) RCR (Civil) 530 : (2005) 6 SCC 344, para 53; Afcons Infrastructure Ltd. v. Cherian Varkey Construction Company Pvt. Ltd. (2010) 8 SCC 24, para 28, 43-45; Moti Ram (dead) through Lrs. v. Ashok Kumar 2011(1) RCR (Civil) 332: (2011) 1 SCC 466; Vikram Bakshi & Ors. v. Sonia Khosla (Dead) by Legal Representatives 2014(3) Recent Apex Judgments (R.A.J.) 542 : (2014) 15 SCC 80

Coordinate with the National Legal Services Authority and the State Legal Services Authorities

It will be open to the National Commission and the State Commission to coordinate with the National Legal Services Authority and the State Legal Services Authorities under the Legal Services Authority Act, 1987.

Following Questions and Answers are Made to Understand Simplified Way Civil and Consumer Alleged Medical Negligence Cases be Dealt

In most instances, multiple defendant medical providers are named where the plaintiff uses the "shotgun" approach, where the plaintiff will name any and all potential individuals, institutions, or business entities that may or may not have played a direct or indirect role in the care of the patient during the time the alleged injury occurred.

OUTSIDE COURT SETTLEMENT PRIOR TO RECEIVING NOTICE

Q. No. 1. Should the doctor yield to demand of asking money for alleged negligence when you feel that you were not at all negligent?

Ans: No, This will just postpone a problem. The reason being such patient's is more likely to take you through legal process once you pay them.

Q. No. 2. Should the doctor yield to demand of asking money for alleged negligence if you feel that you were negligent?

Ans: Depends upon facts and circumstance of attitude of relatives. If attitude is perceived to be favorable then get a "memorandum of out-of-court settlement for accord and satisfaction" be drafted and signed by following a proper procedure. Take lawyers or medicolegal advisor's help in drafting and executing the procedure. It is not recommended for bad attitude patient's relatives.

CASE LAW

Out-of-court settlement—court agreed

K.T. Manickaraj v. M/s. Apollo Hospital Enterprises Ltd., (NCDRC)(New Delhi), Consumer Case No. 133 of 2008. D/d. 24.3.2021.

Terms of Memorandum of Agreement shows that ex-gratia payment of ₹45 lakhs received by Complainants were full and final settlement and not any installment for compensation as alleged by Complainants—nothing on record to prove that Opposite Parties promised to pay ₹2 Crores for patient—therefore, complaint dismissed.

RECEIVING LEGAL NOTICE AND REPLYING IT

Q. No. 3. Should one receive a legal notice sent by lawyer?

Ans: Yes, as doctor has an opportunity to answer, can focus on planning future defense if case is filed in any court.

Q. No. 4. Should one reply legal notice himself or through lawyer?

Ans: Yes, doctor should reply legal notice through lawyer in consultation with medicolegal advisor's mind.

Q. No. 5. Why doctor should reply legal notice through lawyer in consultation with medico-legal advisor's mind?

Ans: Lawyer cannot differentiate and give the required flavor that doctor gave treatment diligently, prudently with due care and caution. Lawyer's reply is mechanical denying alleged negligence. Lawyers usually have no detail knowledge of medicine. Lawyers are not able to explain inherent and unavoidable medical complications. Medical Complications are ubiquitous. Lawyers cannot understand intricate mechanisms involved in body medical physiology and underlying medical pathology. This lands Lawyers to draw half backed conclusions in cases of alleged medical negligence. Most lawyers wish to depend upon procedural aspects of law restricting them to the law of limitation, law of alibi, law of evidence. Lawyers hardly touch upon medical facts to defend the case. Lawyers land their doctor clients in an odious situation of presenting the case alien to medical fraternity. Lawyer working in tandem with Medicolegal advisor can bring forth medical facts in legal notice reply facts circumstances which led to death, disability, transfer or increased expenses or hardships to relatives more convincingly for which doctor was not responsible.

OUTSIDE COURT SETTLEMENT AFTER RECEIVING NOTICE BY NEGOTIATIONS

Q. No. 6. Should doctor yield legal notice demand of asking money for alleged negligence by negotiations with patient's lawyer or your own lawyer?

Ans: Chances of success are remote yet explore the possibility. But guiding principles are same as described above for "outside court settlement".

POST NOTICE: SLEEP OVER THE MATTER OR BE PROACTIVE

Q. No. 7. What is the usual advice of Lawyer in post notice period?

Ans: Lawyers say that wait till the next legal move of the patient. Lawyers attitude is do not take till trouble actually troubles doctor then only take trouble in hurry to address the trouble leaves no time for doctor to gather the evidence which is vital to the alleged medical negligence case.

Q. No. 8. Should one be proactive in preparing defense?

Ans: Medicolegal advice is "Yes", because a forewarned doctor is forearmed in gathering evidence. In medical negligence case, it is very time consuming to collect required evidence. Hurriedly collected scientific medical literature, evidence of affidavits of eyewitness and expert witness are less useful if not corroborated with pleadings in written statement, affidavit of evidence and rejoinders.

NATURE OF EVIDENCE

Q. No. 9. What is the nature of evidence courts require?

Ans: Courts require evidence for diligence, prudence, care and caution in the alleged medical negligence case. Case papers explaining the process of disease, treatment and surgery, complications and their timely treatment needs to be properly explained as part of documentary evidence.

PRUDENCE

Q. No. 10. What is the evidence of prudence of doctor?

Ans: To prove doctors prudence in court evidence showing doctors qualifications, experience, competence and skills is required.

QUALIFICATIONS

Q. No. 11. What is the evidence of qualifications?

Ans: To prove prudence based on doctors' qualifications in court as evidence, only submit ethics and registration board of National Medical Council Act-2019 recognized qualifications and say on the basis of that you have treated the case.

Q. No. 12. How to plead prudence when postgraduate qualification which is not recognized?

Ans: To prove prudence when postgraduate qualification which are not recognized by Medical Council of India or State Medical Council you have to prepare your evidence of prudence based MBBS qualifications only. Avoid writing on your letterhead words Expert or specialist or "*Daksha*" or "*Tagya*" or "*Visheshagya*" so as to avoid negligence per se observation of court. Instead, such doctors should safely plead and write on their letterhead's words like "Advisor" or "Counselor" or "Trained" or "Experienced" "*Salahagar*" or "*Anubhavi*". Never plead or claim that you are by virtue of qualification and expert or specialist or super-specialist in the field if your degree is not NMC or SMC recognized. Claiming in court that your qualified postgraduate specialist/expert if your degree is not MCI recognized may put you in gross legal trouble. Practicing medicine in the field of that any specialty on the basis of experience and training is allowed but do not plead or claim to possess the unrecognized qualification in the court of law in medical negligence case. If possible, attach MBBS, MD, DM, Mch marksheets and transcripts.

WHEN EXPERIENCE IS CONSIDERED SKILL

Q. No. 13. What is the evidence of experience?

Ans: To prove prudence based on doctors' experience in court as evidence, submit work experience certificates of medical colleges, medical institutes, and attendance of medical workshop certificates. Prepare a good Biodata with number of surgeries/procedures done.

COMPETENCE

Q. No. 14. What is the evidence of MBBS doctor's field of competence?

Ans: To prove prudence of field of competence of MBBS doctors in court as evidence, MBBS person should submit and I, II and III MBBS marksheets from medical college showing study, knowledge, competence and skill in conducting the treatment given in alleged medical negligence. MBBS person should submit transcript from medical college. Also prepare a good Biodata with number of surgeries/procedures done. Submit attendance of medical workshop certificates. One has to say very clearly that on the basis MBBS qualifications, one has treated the case, and one is not claiming to have treated the case in the capacity of a qualified specialist/ expert in that specialty.

Q. No. 15. Can MBBS doctor plead that one is competent to do give care to any diseases belonging to medical specialty usually given by qualified specialist in field possessing postgraduate diploma or degree?

Ans: Yes, there is no legal bar in conducting the treatment if one is competent to conduct treatment in cases belonging to any medical specialty as long as one does not claim to be qualified specialist in that field of senility. MBBS should not claim through signboards and letterheads that he is a qualified specialist in that medical field.

PRUDENCE OF SKILL

Q. No. 16. How to plead with prudence of skill?

Ans: The prudence of skill is a combination of qualifications, work experience and competence, which should be reflected in Biodata of doctor and case paper showing conduct of treatment of case to be in a peer approved way. Collected scientific medical literature, evidence of affidavits of eyewitness and expert witness are less useful if not corroborated with pleadings in written statement, affidavit of evidence and rejoinders. Attach a work logbook of surgeries performed, and anesthesia given for surgical and anesthesia specialist.

RECEIVE OR REFUSE NOTICE

Q. No. 17. Should you receive or refuse notice from any courts?

Receive summons from any courts and never refuse summons. Not defending yourself/hospital/nursing home properly in a case of alleged negligence shall enable the court to pass ex-parte order of negligence and compensation against you. That will send wrong message to other doctors, press and media precedent that doctors are generally negligent and not law abiding. This will cause spiraling of premiums of professional indemnity insurance by insurance companies and the medical professionals resorting to defensive practice.

TIME GIVEN FOR FILING WRITTEN STATEMENT

Q. No. 18. In how many days one should prepare and file to answer complaints?

Ans: Usually within 30 and if allowed 45 days or date is specified in the summons.

Q. No. 19. What is the legal name for answer/reply to complaint?

Ans: Legal name for answer/reply of any complaint is written version or written statement (WS) of opposite party (OP) or respondent.

STUDY OF COMPLAINT

Q. No. 20. How to read title of complaint with a view to reply Complaint?

Ans: Title of complaint contains name of court, place, name of complainant and opposite parties (OPs) and their addresses. While one reads complaint one will find that it starts with the name of court and place where it is situated. It should have the territorial jurisdiction over place where you practice. Under the new Consumer Protection Act, 2019 (new CPA) the complainant can file anywhere, where he/she resides. Read the name of complainant whether he is patient himself, guardian, parent, any organization or legal heir. If it does not fall into that category then, challenge. Then read the name of OP or all OP's and see whether you are sued in your own name or in the name of Hospital/Nursing Home. You have to see whether it is beneficial to reply separately or jointly. If you have, individual medical indemnity policy replies separately. If you have additional Hospital/Establishment error and Omission policy then reply jointly. See whether insurance party is named as OP or not? If not then make an application to add insurance company a party. Also see who else treated this patient and if possible and necessary make an application to add their names as OP.

Q. No. 21. How to read typical initial 6 to 8 paragraphs of complaint with a view to reply?
Ans: Paragraphs no. 1 of complaint usually describes the age, occupation and income or earning capabilities of the patient. Paragraphs no. 2 of complaint usually describes what patient was suffering from and laymen diagnosis and in complainant's view what treatment was required to be given. Paragraphs no. 3 of C, usually describes, doctors capabilities/in-capabilities of leaving mob while doing surgery, infrastructure and promises made to patient. Paragraphs no. 4 of complaint usually describes, what payment was made? Paragraphs no. 5 of complaint usually describes whether doctor issued receipts and for some he did not issue receipts. Paragraphs no. 6 of complaint usually makes a point blank blunt allegation of negligence in conducting treatment, diagnosis or investigations, anesthesia, operation or procedure. Paragraphs no. 7 of complaint describes if patient is transferred to some other hospital then that event, those doctor's views and money spent here. Paragraphs no. 8 of complaint is about the nurses/staff/assistants or any such related issue.

Q. No. 22. How to read typical middle 6 to 8 paragraphs of complaint with a view to reply?
Ans: Paragraphs no. 9 to 12 of complaint will describe in laymen details about doctors' capabilities/in-capabilities, infrastructure, promises made to patient by repeating same thing again and again irritatingly. Paragraphs no. 13 to 18 of complaint will describe in laymen details about alleged negligence in conducting treatment, diagnosis or investigations, anesthesia, operation or procedure by repeating same thing again and again. Paragraphs no. 19 to 22 of complaint will describe in laymen details about transferred to some other hospital then that event, those doctor's views and money spent there, by repeating same thing again and again.

Q. No. 23. How to read typical penultimate 3 to 6 paragraphs with a view to reply?
Ans: Paragraphs no. 22 to 25 of complaint will describe in laymen correlation between negligence and loss suffered in details by repeating same thing again and again Paragraphs no. 25 to 27 of complaint will describe jurisdiction, cause of action and fees paid with petition under new Consumer Protection Act-2019. Complainant can file complaint in any territorial jurisdiction where he/she says or works for gain.

Q. No. 24. How to read typical prayer clause paragraphs with a view to reply?
Ans: Summarize alleged negligence causing damages and financial hardships. If it is consumer courts they usually will asks compensation of 100 lakhs (now reduced to < 50 lakhs from 30-12-2022) in District court or more than 100 lakhs to 1000 lakhs (now reduced to 50 lakhs to 2 crores from 30-12-2022) in state commission. The national commission demand is ₹10 crores (now reduced to ₹2 crores and above from 30-12-2022).

SUMMARY AND CLASSIFICATION OF ALLEGATIONS

Q. No. 25. How to classify the allegations with a view to reply?
Ans: Usually allegations are related to mean that doctor is not qualified, there was inadequate infrastructure, nurses and staff members are not qualified did not attend, doctor delayed in diagnosing or misdiagnosis or delay in investigating or treating the patient. Doctor was not present during emergency. Consent was not obtained. There was overcharging. Transfer to higher center delayed. A plethora of derogatory words are used against the medical profession, doctors, nurses and staff members. Sometimes allegations of unnecessary investigations and treatment are used. Excessive irrational compensation is asked in complaint.

WRITTEN STATEMENT (WS) UNDER NEW CPA-2019 OR ANY OTHER COURT

Q. No. 26. How to reply initial 6 to 8 paragraphs of complaint in written statement (WS) of doctor/opposite party (OP)?

Ans: Reply to Paragraphs no. 1 of complaint that patient did not inform/misinformed you about occupation and income or earning capabilities. Patient is not a consumer. Reply to Paragraphs no. 2 of complaint ignoring what patient has described what patient was suffering from and laymen his diagnosis and in his about treatment and write what you have written in your case paper. Reply to Paragraphs no. 3 of complaint agreeing to your capabilities as per what degrees medical council registration shows and deny in-capabilities in qualification, knowledge, experience, skill, infrastructure by attaching required certificates to prove the same. Deny any promises or guarantee and warranty with respect to the 100% success or end results of treatment made to patient party, as professionals do not guarantee cure. Make a note of hiding previous illnesses. Reply to Paragraphs no. 4 of complaint; deny if payment made was less and describe actual payment made and ask complainant to produce receipts in court. Reply to Paragraphs no. 5 of complaint deny, not issuing receipts. Reply to Paragraphs no. 6 of complaint deny point blank blunt all allegations of negligence in conducting treatment, diagnosis or investigations, anesthesia, operation or procedure and say it was conducted diligently, prudently with due care and caution. Reply to Paragraphs no. 7 of complaint that patient is transferred to some other hospital diligently, prudently with due care and caution and give reason for transfer. Deny if you do not agree with doctor's views or confirm it. Deny money spent there and say you are not responsible for same as you did everything diligently, prudently with due care and caution. Reply to Paragraphs no. 8 of complaint about the staff/assistants that they worked under your direct supervision and directions, and they are individually for any action/inactions as you were deciding authority on conduct of all aspects related to patient.

Q. No. 27. How to reply to middle 6 to 8 paragraphs of complaint?

Ans: Reply by saying Paragraphs no. 9 to 12 of complaint is repetition of allegations doctors capabilities/in-capabilities, infrastructure, promises made to patient by repeating same thing again and again irritatingly and same is already replied in earlier paragraphs. Reply to Paragraphs no. 13 to 18 of complaint by denying all allegations and saying it is laymen view and details about alleged negligence in conducting treatment, diagnosis or investigations, anesthesia, failed operation or procedure by repeating same thing again and again, which is replied earlier. Reply to Paragraphs no. 19 to 22 of complaint deny allegations by saying, it is laymen details about transfer and your conduct of transfer is described in earlier para. Deny all allegations based on other hospital doctor's views. Deny allegations about money spent there and say it is being unnecessarily repeated describing same wrong things again and again. Don't forget to include willingness for mediation and file separate application for same.

Q. No. 28. How to reply to penultimate 3to 6 paragraphs of complaint?

Ans: Reply Paragraphs no. 22 to 25 of complaint by saying that it is laymen correlation between negligence and loss suffered and enclose scientific literature and affidavit of expert from other doctors supporting your view. Reply to Paragraphs no. 25 to 27 of complaint and say whether jurisdiction, cause of action and fees paid with petition are correct or incorrect. In case it is incorrect then one has to move separate miscellaneous application to lodge objection to jurisdiction, cause of action.

Q. No. 29. How to reply to prayer clause paragraphs of complaint?

Ans: Deny alleged negligence causing damages and financial hardships point blank. Deny having incurred any liability of paying anything to complaint. All you say that alleged negligence is wrong and denied since you did everything diligently, prudently with due care and caution which is evident from certificates of qualification, experience, skill and competence, photographs show infrastructure, scientific literature shows complications which can occur leading to death or disability and same is also. With reference to the contents of alleged prayer clause is based on mere allegations without any admissible evidence under the Indian Evidence Act. Say that this is highly inflated claim. Section 34(1) of CPA 2019 clearly states that the complainant has right to claim only what is actually paid for goods or services rendered to complainant. One should be excluding mental and physical trauma, which are notional and cannot be quantified in terms of money.

CASE LAWS ON INFLATED CLAIMS

1. Ramesh Kumar v. Dr. Akhil Saxena & Ors., Civil Appeal No. 7984 of 2016, the Hon'ble Supreme Court upheld the dismissal of Consumer Complaint No. 351/2012 as inflated claim observed by this Commission for 6 crores 30 lakhs- remanded back- bench hunting not allowed.
2. Chanchali Narendra v. Continental Hospitals, (NCDRC)—Consumer Case No. 2447 of 2019. D/d. 18.6.2020, consent form mention of only pain as side effects, but CT Cisternography test patient party's assumption that there was a leak at the site of lumber puncture was not acceptable to court, Complaint is vague, apart from being grossly inflated amount of ₹3 crores, dismissed.

SYNOPSIS OR HOW TO SUMMARIZE WRITTEN STATEMENT (WS)

Q. No. 30. How to reply by classifying the allegations of complaint and replying in summary way?

Ans: Deny allegations are related to mean that doctors are not qualified, there was inadequate infrastructure by certificates of qualification, experience, skill and competence, photographs, deny staff members did not attend supported by affidavit of eyewitness, deny that doctor conducted delayed in diagnosing or misdiagnosis or delay in investigating or treating the patient on the basis of case papers. Deny that doctor was not present during emergency supported by affidavit of eyewitnesses. Deny Consent was not obtained by showing consent. Deny overcharging by enclosing carbon copy of actual bill. Transfer to higher center delayed. Deny plethora of derogatory words that are used against medical profession, doctors, nurses and staff members by threatening to take legal action separately for these remarks. Deny allegations of unnecessary investigations and treatments using scientific literature and affidavit from an expert witness. Prove that the compensation asked is excessive and irrational of complaint and in any case you are not liable as you conducted everything diligently, prudently with due care and caution as described above.

Q. No. 31. What general precautions should one take to reply by classifying the allegations of complaint and replying in summary way?

Ans: First and foremost, denying all allegations of negligence and deficiency in service needs to be emphasized. Whatever pleas in defense are raised they should be supported by evidence in the first instance of mentioning specifically in reply to the complaint. Subsequent new explanation/pleas during hearing of the case are liable to be rejected.

LEGAL TECHNICAL DEFENCES

Q. No. 32. What is Legal technical defenses for doctors/hospitals in preparing WS defense?

Ans: Legal technical defenses for doctors/hospitals are:

a. Cause of action
b. Pecuniary/territorial jurisdiction

c. Non-joinder or mis-joinder of proper and necessary parties
d. Free service given
e. No locus standi as legal representative (LR)
f. Case subjudice civil/criminal court
g. The compensation claimed is highly inflated or exaggerated
h. The complaint is time-barred
i. The complaint is frivolous and vexatious
j. CC has complicated issues involved; requiring recording of evidence of experts, hence, complaint case should be filed in a civil court.
k. Doctor is dead, i.e., action personalis moritur cum persona
l. In case, there is indemnity insurance or hospital error and omission policy make insurance company a party to suit. File miscellaneous application to add them to array of respondents.

BURDEN OF PROOF

The court has held the opinion that medical negligence has to be established and cannot be presumed. In cases of medical negligence, the patient must establish her/his claim against the doctor as in Kanhaiya Kumar Singh vs. Park Medicare and Research Centre III, CPJ 9 (NC) 1999. The burden of proof is correspondingly greater on the person who alleges negligence against a doctor. A doctor can be held liable for negligence only if one can prove that she/he is guilty of a failure that no doctor with ordinary skills would be guilty of if acting with reasonable care. The burden of proof of negligence, carelessness, or insufficiency generally lies with the complainant. The law requires a higher standard of evidence than otherwise to support an allegation of negligence against a doctor. In Bimalesh Chatterjee case, it was held that the onus of proving negligence and the resultant deficiency in service was clearly on the complainant as in Calcutta Medical Research Institute vs. Bimalesh Chatterjee I. CPJ 13 (NC) 1999. When the damage is too remote, it is not considered as an immediate result of medical negligence.

CASE LAW

In absence of proof of payment made by complainant to OP as consideration for services obtained, complainant does not fall within purview of consumer—Complaint was also barred by limitation and no application for condonation of delay was filed—Revision Petition dismissed.

B. Kasi Reddy v. Dr. T. Viswarupachari (NCDRC)(New Delhi),2015(2) C.P.R. 497 : 2015(66) R.C.R.(Civil) 220,Revision Petition No. 1431 of 2014. (Against the Order dated 29/01/2014 in Appeal No. 364/2013 of the State Commission Andhra Pradesh). D/d. 15.4.2015.

Accidental injury—Complainant met with an accident and sustained injury to his right leg-Complications developed after treatment due to negligence of OP. In a number of cases free services are rendered by private hospitals to known and needy persons. In absence of proof of payment made by complainant to OP as consideration for services obtained, complainant does not fall within purview of consumer. Complaint was also barred by limitation and no application for condonation of delay was filed—Revision Petition dismissed.

Condonation of delay—Constitution Bench judgment where delay beyond period of 30 + 15 day (45 days) cannot be condoned by NCDRC applies prospectively.

Rejection of application for condonation of delay in filing written statement in view of Constitution Bench judgment of Supreme Court in case reported in New India Assurance Company Limited v. Hilli Multipurpose Cold Storage Private Limited, (2020) 5 SCC 757,where delay beyond period of 30 + 15 day (45 days) cannot be condoned by NCDRC—Held, application for condonation of delay filed prior to judgment of Constitution Bench and judgment was to operate prospectively. Delay only for 7 days for which valid explanation given and with consent of parties, therefore, condonation of delay of 7 days in filing reply on payment of cost of ₹25,000/-.

Non-joinder or mis-joinder of proper and necessary parties
Cataract surgery—no negligence , non-joinder of necessary party
Mr. Balkar Singh vs. Dr. Siddharth Sain (Delhi SCDRC) Complaint Case No. 459 of 2013. D/d. 25.07.2022.

Cataract surgery—no negligence. It is clear from the record that the opposite party was working with the Medfort Hospital and the hospital, being an employer of the opposite party, is vicariously liable for the acts of his employees. Once an allegation is made that the patient was admitted in a particular hospital and evidence is produced to satisfy that he suffered complications because of lack of proper care and negligence, then the burden lies on the hospital to justify that there was no negligence on the part of the treating doctor/or hospital. Since the hospital is a necessary party in the present case and the same has not been made party in the present complaint, the present complaint is dismissed for non-joinder of necessary party.

FACTUAL DEFENCE

Q. No. 33. What is Factual defense for doctors/hospitals in preparing a written statement (WS) defense?

Ans: Factual defense are:

a. Prepare factual matrix supported by case paper/discharge summary record of patient
b. Detailed Biodata of doctor supported by qualifications, experience, training, experience, expertise, certificates/appreciation certificates/awards/attendance at various updates, conferences, workshops
c. Photographs showing infrastructure of OT, ICU, special state of art gadgetry
d. Affidavit of eyewitness.

AFFIDAVITS OF EXPERT DOCTORS AND SCIENTIFIC LITERATURE

Q. No. 34. What is defense by supplying affidavits of expert doctors and scientific literature in preparing WS defense?

Ans: Annex 5 to 10 affidavits of expert doctors to state that you conducted everything diligently, prudently with due care and caution. Also annex 5 to 10 scientific literature to show you conducted everything diligently, prudently with due care and caution as per standard text book way. If available, in case of death, if medical board was set up by police then its favorable report or favorable postmortem report or favorable civil surgeon report is valuable. In case of death due to poisoning, favorable forensic laboratory report. In case of alleged disability in available then submit any favorable disability certificate or report. In case of transfer next hospital case records, discharge card to be submitted if favorable.

OTHER RESIDUAL DEFENCES

Q. No. 35. What are other residual defenses to be written in WS defense?

Ans: They are:

a. Complainant not coming to the court with clean hands, i.e., he has suppressed material facts, e.g., previous illness, treatment, etc.
b. There are inconsistencies between notices sent directly or through a lawyer/consumer groups and the complaint made in the court. The inconsistencies should be specifically pointed out.

c. Circumstances of the case, viz., there was, emergency, lack of facilities (e.g., rural area), no one to give history of patient's illness, etc.
d. Burden of proof of duty of care, breach of that duty; causation, damage, etc., is on the complainant
e. Claim against doctor/hospital usually fails if it can be proved that there was a break in the chain of causation (novus actus interveniens). This is where an act by a third party supersedes the original negligent act of the OP/doctor/defendant. The court must decide whether the original act of the defendant was responsible for the damage or if the intervening act constitutes a novus actus interveniens, that is, the second act caused the damage. The second act could be an intervening act by a third party or an intervening act by the claimant himself.
f. Consultation/treatment taken by patient from other doctors/other systems of medicine simultaneously. This will subdue/dilute the alleged negligence of OP as many other reasons for occurrence of damage make it impossible to pinpoint at OP.
g. Contributory negligence—As in all other defenses, this defense must be pleaded in the first instance showing how exactly it contributed to damage caused by alleged medical negligence.

CASE LAW

Contributory negligence of not following up: Mrs. Baljeet Kaur v. Dhaliwal Hospital, (PSCDRC) (Chandigarh), First Appeal Nos. 562 and 573 of 2015. D/d. 5.6.2017. Post-surgery complications—Deficiency in service—Bile leakage—Complainant never visited OP No. 1 after removal of her stitches—No medical literature provided by complainant nor any expert witness is examined to prove fact that renal dysfunction was an outcome of this bile leakage—Complainant herself has not visited OPs after removal of her stitches and follow up—OPs cannot be held medically negligent—Moreover, no doctor can assure recovery of patient from any complication. Impugned order set aside—Complaint dismissed.

BASICS OF RULES OF DRAFTING OF REPLY

Q. No. 36. What are other usual basics of rules of drafting of reply/defense by or on behalf of the doctor/hospital?

Ans: The very purpose of defense drafting is to create a record, which makes part and parcel of proceedings in court and helpful even when case is lost and one needs to appeal. Since you cannot add / alter /amend or take a new plea in appeal court. Defense should be in writing which should contain plea about the doctor's/hospital's denial/clarification/explaining cause and effect relationship in reply to the complaint.

It is necessary to reply to the complaint para-wise and the allegations need denial or explanation, and your comments should be written down para-wise against each of the allegations narrated in complaint.

Defense (reply) is legal opportunity to narrate or state in written format to reply each of the allegations made by the complainant as well as provides one's own version of the matters under dispute. A basic legal and fundamental purpose of the defense is that, when read in tandem or conjunction with the complaint, it should make clear those disputed points on which parties are not in agreeing to.

The most important rule in drafting a defense is to ensure that every material allegation in the complaint is properly answered and dealt with supporting evidence as an annexure.

DEALING WITH AN ALLEGATION AGAINST THE DOCTOR/HOSPITAL

Q. No. 37. What are dealing with an allegation against the doctor/hospital?

You have to admit and reply on statement in your favor. You have to deny all unfavorable statements and allegations with explanation with evidence to show the defendant's side of the story is wrong, false, vexatious, motivated to extract money.

Sometimes the defendant has no evidence to rebut the allegation with the help of medical record then look whether it can be supported by affidavit of eyewitness or affidavit of expert witness. Court takes it for granted that if any allegation, which is neither denied nor admitted in your answer, is, deemed to have been admitted as evidence without proof. The best way to make sure that nothing is admitted by above said legal dictum of court presumption of guilt since allegation is neither denied nor admitted; is by dealing with each of the complainant's allegations one by one in para-wise manner. The defendant's response to the allegations made by the complainant gives proper picture of whole event on larger canvass with respect to case. Court is prompted to works with broad framework of the defense with respect to complaint. It gives court not only fair idea about disputes between the parties. Whenever a single paragraph contains more than one allegation, each must be specifically admitted or denied. When the allegation is denied, there is need to give elaborate explanation with evidence in that paragraph.

In some cases, a paragraph may appear to consist of one allegation while in fact containing a central allegation and one or more subordinate allegations. Therefore, it is essential that while dealing with a paragraph of the complainant, subordinate allegations should not be given a pass or overlooked. Simply admitting allegations in the paragraph would therefore admit subordinate allegations that the defendant should deny or traverse it diligently.

The defendant should not deny and traverse any indirect or implied allegations in the complainant's paragraphs with specific reply with evidence. But where a single paragraph of the complaint contains multiple and complicated allegations, the appropriate reply/answer or response may be a conclusion of admissions, non-admissions and/or denials or to traverse the paragraph by a combination of non-admissions and denials with proper evidence. It should also be particularly noted that in drafting the reply, the proper approach is to deny or traverse both the fact and statement or narrations causing damage and its extent since they are not supported by disability certificate or expert witness by complainant.

PLEADING ADDITIONAL FACTS BY DOCTOR/HOSPITAL

Q. No. 38. What are pleading additional facts by doctor/hospital?

Ans: An important function of the defense is to plead additional facts, which fill gaps and explain and clarify or correct cause and effect relationship based on theory of percentage of complications or death occurring while treating the illness. All errors in the complainant's account of the events alleged to have given rise to a cause of action should be accepted/denied or explained. It should be in conformity with reply to the notice received, all the allegations made therein should be rebutted in as short a language as possible reserving therein the right to take further appropriate defense after the filing of complaint.

PROCEDURAL DEFENCES/ACTION TAKEN BY DOCTOR/HOSPITAL

Q. No. 39. What are the procedural defenses/action to be taken by doctor/hospital?

Ans: As mentioned above once again take objection to the pecuniary, territorial jurisdiction of the Any Court as also that the complaint raises complicated questions of fact and law and/or requires leading of voluminous evidence should be raised if applicable.

SWORN VERIFICATIONS REQUIRED FOR

Q. No. 40. How a written statement (WS) should be properly verified and sworn.

Q. No. 41. Written statement should be properly verified and sworn in front of notary or registrar of court concerned

Q. No. 42. How all affidavits of eye or expert witness are properly verified and sworn.

Ans: The affidavits of eye or expert witness should be properly verified and sworn in front of notary or registrar of court concerned. Expert witness on letterhead has less value and liable for cross-examination more often than sworn affidavit.

FILE OBJECTION FOR THE COMPLAINT WITHOUT AFFIDAVIT

Q. No. 43. How to file objection for the complaint without affidavit and which has not been properly verified, sworn or attested.

Ans: Move a miscellaneous application to file objection for the complaint without affidavit and which has not been properly verified, sworn or attested by notary and prayer clause should ask for dismissal with cost.

APPLICATION FOR CROSS-EXAMINATION OF THE WITNESSES

Q. No. 44. How to file application for cross-examination of the witnesses, and re-butt the evidence of the complainant?

Ans: Move a separate miscellaneous application for cross-examination the witnesses of the complaint and prayer clause should ask for dismissal with cost if they do not arrange for cross examination.

Q. No. 45. How to file application, objections for additional pleas to be raised after receipt of complaint in rejoinder?

Ans: Doctor has to file application objections for additional pleas to be raised after receipt of complaint in rejoinder by complainant. Move a separate miscellaneous application for objecting to additional pleas to be raised after receipt of complainant's cross-objection in rejoinder then prayer clause should ask for dismissal with cost if they do not arrange for cross-examination.

AFFIDAVIT OF EVIDENCE

Q. No. 46. How to file affidavit of evidence?

Ans: Submit affidavit of expert witness and file a list of expert witnesses with affidavit of evidence. Expert evidence could be rebuttal of complainant's evidence in the form of affidavits by doctors willing to give evidence in defense. Also submit relevant medical literature.

CASE LAW

Two judge Supreme Court

Commission/Forum cannot be utilized to collect evidence on behalf of complainant

Mukesh Tyagi v. Fortis Escorts Heart Institute, Civil Appeal Nos. 4390-4391 of 2019. D/d. 8.4.2019.

Appellant alleging medical negligence sought direction for constitution of medical board by AIIMS to report on treatment afforded to deceased on basis of records—Burden of proving medical negligence lies on appellant—Forum cannot be utilized to collect evidence on behalf of complainant.

Burden of proof—Appellant complained medical negligence on part of respondents before NCDRC—At interim stage appellant sought direction for constitution of medical board by AIIMS to report on treatment afforded to deceased on basis of records of case—NCDRC rejected application though granting opportunity to appellant to produce his own evidence in support of complaint—Order of NCDRC granting liberty to appellant to do so and hence, declining to entertain application is unexceptionable—Burden of proving medical negligence lies on appellant—Forum cannot be utilized to collect evidence on behalf of complainant—appeal dismissed.

WRITTEN ARGUMENTS

Q. No. 47. How to file written arguments?

Ans: Written arguments should classify disputed and undisputed points. Then put medical scientific explanation of complication leading to disability and death supported by affidavits of expert witness, relevant literature and case laws. Important case laws for doctors are:

1. Supreme Court of India In Dr. Harish Kumar Khurana v. Joginder Singh Civil Appeal No.7380 of 2009. D/d. 7.9.2021. No Medical negligence, where treatment is not successful or patient dies during surgery, it cannot be automatically assumed that medical professional was negligent. Overruled NCDRC who applied res ipsa loquitur to pay compensation.
2. Supreme Court of India Indian Medical Association v/s V.P Shantha, (1995) 6 SCC 657 specifies what cases of obvious medical negligence can only be filed under CPA 2019
3. Supreme Court of India Jacob Mathew vs. State of Punjab (2005) 6 SSC 1 says medical board opinion required before admitting medical negligence case
4. Supreme Court of India Ins. Malhotra (Ms) Vs. Dr. A Kriplani and others 2009(4) SCC 705, complications does not mean its negligence
5. Supreme Court of India State of Punjab vs. Shiv Ram and Ors. (AIR 2005 SC 3280)—failure of surgery does not mean its negligence
6. Supreme Court of India Kusum Sharma and Another vs Batra Hospital and Medical Research Centre and Others (2010) 3 SCC 480, complications does not mean its negligence. It has given eleven guideline for negligence

APPEAL

Q. No. 48. How to file an Appeal?

Ans: Appeal must be filed after a complaint is decided against a doctor/hospital within the time limit, within forty five days of passing of the order from district commission to state commission or from state commission to national commission within 30 days, from national commission to Supreme Court within 30 days.

CASE LAW

Appeal As Barred By Limitation

J.P. Hospital v. Jatinder Pal Singh, (NCDRC), Revision Petition No. 3882 of 2017 in Appeal No. 742 of 2017. D/d. 05.02.2018.

Complaint filed before Dist. Forum alleging deficiency in service—Complaint partly allowed—State Commission dismissed appeal as barred by limitation—hence, present revision—Plea taken by petitioners to effect that they were assured by Insurance Company that against order passed by Dist. Forum on 12.1.2017 an appeal would be filed by them and Petitioners could join them in said Appeal but subsequently Insurance Company retracted from its stated stand, is clearly an after-thought—Having been held guilty of medical negligence, it was for petitioners to contest said finding against them, if they were aggrieved by order by Dist. Forum, and not depend on Insurance Company for protecting their interest—Petitioners failed to make out any cause, much less a "sufficient cause" for condonation of inordinate delay in filing the appeal—Delay not condoned.

CROSS APPEAL

Q. No. 49. What is cross Appeal?

Ans: Both the parties are dissatisfied with lower court decision so complainant and OP both file appeal within the time limit, within forty five days or thirty days of passing of the order from district to state commission or from state commission to national commission or from national commission to Supreme Court respectively. This is known as cross appeal and both the appeal are together.

REVIEW/REVISION PETITION

Q. No. 50. What is review/revision petition?

Ans: Only review is allowed for order passed by same commission. Revision petitions are not allowed under new CPA 2019. Only appeals are allowed.

EXECUTION PETITION

Q. No. 51. What is execution petition?

Ans: Usually if the order is not complied by OP then complainant can file an execution petition in consumer courts. This enforcement is known as execution petition. Proceedings are separately taken up and both the parties have to attend the hearing on appointed day and time. The only way to halt execution proceedings is obtain stay of higher court on the lower court order.

MISCELLANEOUS APPLICATION

Q. No. 52. What is miscellaneous application?

Ans: Matters related to errors in name of parties, not with in proper jurisdiction, not with in limitation period of 2 years under CPA 2019, section 69, execution of orders, grant of stay on orders of lower court , interim relief's, removal of name from array of opposite party or adding name of extra OP or insurance company. All the matters, which are not, covered above need a miscellaneous application.

DURATION OF PROCEEDINGS

Q. No. 53. How much time for disposal of case in consumer courts is prescribed?

Ans: Prescribed time limit is 90 days in cases allegations of deficiency in service and five months where goods require testing in appropriate laboratory. File an application to decide within 90 days. That CPA 2019, section 38 and sub-section (7) states that every complaint before District Commission shall be disposed of as expeditiously as possible and endeavor shall be made to decide the complaint within a period of three months from the date of receipt of notice by opposite party where the complaint does not require analysis or testing of commodities and within five months if it requires analysis or testing of commodities, hence as per section 38 (7) if any compensation is granted against OP, he shall not be liable to pay any interest beyond the period of three months for the procedure and laxity in the judicial proceeding by way of adjournments after adjournments. That, three judges bench of Supreme Court under article 141 of constitution of India in Dr. J.J. Merchant and Ors. v/s Shrinath Chaturvedi (2002) 6 SCC 635 supports section 38.

Q. No. 54. Are fees prescribed for filing complaint and appeal?

Ans: Fifty percent of award to the lower court needs to be deposited before filing appeal.

COURT FEES

Q. No. 55. How much fee for complaint in court and how much for appeal is prescribed?

Ans: no fees up to claim for ₹5 lakhs, rest of the amount up to ₹2 crores have slabs of minimal amount of money in few thousand for complainant for filing appeals for complainants no fees but respondent has to deposit half of decretal amount.

INFORM INSURANCE COMPANY

Q. No. 56. How to inform insurance company?

Ans: In case there is an indemnity or hospital error and omission insurance policy in existence the doctor/hospital should inform the insurance company in writing immediately on a complaint being lodged by a patient with a copy of the complaint and notice received from the court.

Frivolous Litigations

Inderjeet Kaur Kalsi vs. Nct Of Delhi &Anr. on 27 November, 2013, https://indiankanoon.org/doc/103374589/

Before parting with this case, I consider it necessary to pen down that one of the reasons for over-flowing of court dockets is the frivolous litigation in which the Courts are engaged by the litigants and which is dragged as long as possible. Even if these litigants ultimately loose the case, they become the real victors and have the last laugh. This class of people who perpetuate illegal acts by obtaining stays and injunctions from the Courts must be made to pay the sufferer not only the entire illegal gains made by them as costs to the person deprived of his right and also must be burdened with exemplary costs. Faith of people in judiciary can only be sustained if the persons on the right side of the law do not feel that even if they keep fighting for justice in the Court and ultimately win, they would turn out to be a fool since winning a case after 20 or 30 years would make wrong doer as real gainer, who had reaped the benefits for all those years. Thus, it becomes the duty of the Courts to see that such wrong doers are discouraged at every step and even if they succeed in prolonging the litigation due to their money power, ultimately they must suffer the costs of all these years long litigation. Despite settled legal positions, the obvious wrong doers, use one after another tier of judicial review mechanism as a gamble, knowing fully well that dice is always loaded in their favor, since even if they lose, the time gained is the real gain. This situation must be redeemed by the Courts.

FACTUAL DEFENSES

1. A doctor must mention his qualifications, training, experience, expertise, etc. Support with relevant documents.
2. Doctor should mention his hospital's infrastructure facilities, special facilities, back-up support with documents.
3. Written evidence of consent of the patient/relative/attendant to assumption of inherent and special risks in the treatment.
4. Any Proof that complainant has not come to the court with clean hands, i.e., he has suppressed material facts, e.g., previous illness, treatment, etc.
5. Inconsistence between notices sent directly or through consumer groups and the complaint made in the court.
6. Written evidence of consent of the patient/relative/attendant to assumption of inherent and special risks in the treatment.
7. Circumstances of the case; viz., emergency situation existed, lack of facilities (e.g., rural area), no responsible person accompanying the patient, no one to give history of patient's illness, etc.

8. Burden of proof of: (i) duty of care; (ii) breach of that duty; (iii) causation; (iv) damage, etc., is on the complainant.
9. Proof that treating doctor/hospital had sufficient knowledge, skill, care and infrastructure (Rely/quote standard textbooks with attested photocopies).
10. Proof that there was consultation/treatment by patient from other doctor/other systems of medicine simultaneously.
11. Any other reasons/more than one reason/for occurrence of damage.
12. Any proof of contributory negligence, i.e., patient was brought late, in critical condition, complication existed beforehand, treatment was not adhered to, was lost to follow-up, etc.

TECHNICAL DEFENSES

Proof that the medical service rendered was free of charge (now, this is applicable in certain situations only).

CASE LAW

It is only where the hospital provides medical services free of charge across board to all patients, it would stand outside purview of the Consumer Protection Act.

Three judge bench Supreme Court of India, Union of India v. N. K. Srivastav Civil Appeal No. 2823 of 2020 (Arising out of Special Leave Petition (C) No. 28056 of 2017). D/d. 23.7.2020.

Old Consumer Protection Act, 1986 Section 2(1)(O) Consumer forum—Jurisdiction—It is only where hospital provides medical services free of charge across board to all patients it would stand outside purview of the Act—Hospital which renders free services to certain category of patients, while providing for services which are charged to bulk of others would not lie outside purview of jurisdiction of Consumer fora.

1. Concurrent adjudication in another court.
2. If the court does not have pecuniary/territorial jurisdiction.
3. If the complaint is time-barred.
4. A Plea that since complicated issues are involved, which require recording of evidence of experts, hence case should be relegated to a civil court. But such a plea must be used at the beginning of the trial.
5. Inform your insurance company in writing with a copy of the complaint.

PREVENTION BY PROFESSIONAL INDEMNITY

Insurance cover is important otherwise doctors in small towns will become bankrupt.

The compensation amount awarded are in crores highest being ₹11.5 crores till now. Profession indemnity insurance is a must for every practicing doctor because it not only covers the claims of compensation awarded against doctor/hospital but also provides a sense of security to doctors that even if some negligence is proved the insurance company will take care of it. Hence, for survival and continuity of practice indemnity has become mandatory. Get clarification about details about different premium rates of insurance in case of individual insurance, doctor/nursing home/hospital with qualified staff and unqualified but trained staff because when the insurance company is paying the compensation it usually makes such enquiries. The insurance companies not only pay the compensation to other party but also arrange for the legal help from advocates. But please be aware; there are reports that they sometimes join hands with other party for monetary gains justifying themselves that it's the insurance company, not the doctor, who has to pay the compensation. Here we must understand that only the money paid as compensation is not everything because our reputation and financial standing is also is at stake.

What can be the **role of professional association** like IMA: These bodies can play a major role in resumption of harmonious relations between doctor community and patients. With the help of media they can arrange seminars inviting doctors and common public where public can discuss their grievances and doubts with the doctors. This will establish an atmosphere of transparency and will improve trust and faith of the patients for doctors they can establish their own grievances cell where complaints of patients can be addressed and if the concerned doctors have really erred then some sort of out-of-court settlement can be arranged. They can arrange TV shows and talk shows to discuss various issues, which confuse public hence leading to mistrust and anger. IMA keeps informing parents about various medical issues through its website. These efforts will go a long way in improving doctor-patient relationships.

Avoid medical malpractice stress syndrome

Medical malpractice lawsuits are not quick. It could take years after years, on and on after alleged incident for a malpractice case gets resolved in court of law. Malpractice cases have to go through a long process including written statement, evidence, documentation, consent, medical literature, expert witness discovery of additional evidence. While in the midst of a malpractice case, one needs to stay focused on other important areas of your life. Life is to live. Move ahead in spite of case against you. The friends, family support system needs to be mobilized and obsessing over the case should be avoided. The medical malpractice stress syndrome is real. It is experienced to some degree by all physicians who are sued. Potential side effects as a result of being named a malpractice defendant include anxiety, helplessness, and humiliation to name a view. A deeply emotional response is common and understandable, given the recriminations and cognitive dissonance that is often associated with malpractice litigation. Malpractice cases routinely take years to litigate; it is a marathon, not a sprint. Prepare yourself mentally for a prolonged, slow-moving process.

CONCLUSION

The doctors we trust shouldn't cause harm, or make existing injuries or illnesses worse. And, if they do, we would like to hold them accountable for the damage. At the same time, good doctors shouldn't be punished for harm they didn't cause. While these ideas sound simple enough, in actual practice it is more complex. There are several defenses available to medical professionals accused of malpractice. Doctor may argue that his care was in line with the standards upheld in the medical profession, or that the patient's injuries weren't the result of a medical error. Contributory negligence, medical professionals aren't the only ones to blame for an injury. If a medical professional can show that the injury would not have occurred had it not been for a negligent act by the patient, he or she may have a valid defense against a malpractice claim.

Respectable Minority Principle—Sometimes medical professionals decide to pursue a new or more radical form of treatment in order to effectively treat a patient. While the decision may place the doctor outside of the medical mainstream, he/she could have a valid defense to a medical malpractice claim if a respectable minority of medical professionals supports the line of treatment. Of course, the doctor must first inform the patient about the risks involved. This is Bolams law. Good Samaritan means if a doctor aids someone in an emergency situation, he/she will be protected from civil liability should anything go wrong during the rescue. Generally, however, a medical professional who voluntarily aids someone owes that person the same duty of care and treatment as that of a reasonably competent physician under the same or similar circumstances. Statute of Limitations places time limits on when an action can be brought for medical malpractice usually 2 or 3 years from cause of action except the "discovery rule," which holds that the statute of limitations period doesn't begin until an injury is actually discovered. If the medical professional can show that the patient discovered the injury at a certain point and that the statute of limitations has since run, the case may be dismissed.

KEY LEARNING POINTS

- Outside court settlement prior to receiving notice when you feel that you were not at all negligent.
- Reply to legal notice.
- One should discourage outside court settlement after receiving notice.
- Don't sleep over the matter after receiving legal notice.
- Courts require evidence for diligence, prudence, care and caution in the alleged medical negligence case. Case papers explaining the process of disease, treatment and surgery, complications and their timely treatment needs to be properly explained as part of documentary evidence.

BIBLIOGRAPHY

1. Afcons Infrastructure Ltd. v. Cherian Varkey Construction Company Pvt. Ltd. (2010) 8 SCC 24, para 28, 43-45.
2. Alternate Dispute Redressal Act 46 of 1999.
3. B. Kasi Reddy v. Dr. T. Viswarupachari (NCDRC)(New Delhi),2015(2) C.P.R. 497 : 2015(66) R.C.R.(Civil) 220, Revision Petition No. 1431 of 2014. (Against the Order dated 29/01/2014 in Appeal No. 364/2013 of the State Commission Andhra Pradesh). D/d. 15.4.2015.
4. Baldwa M., Baldwa V. Padvi N. Baldwa S, Legal Issues in Critical Care, Published by CBS Publishers & Distributors Pvt Ltd, India, 2022,ISBN : 978-93-90709-13-7.
5. Baldwa M., Baldwa V. Padvi N. Baldwa S, Legal Issues in Medical Practice, Published by CBS Publishers & Distributors Pvt Ltd, India, 2018, ISBN 10: 938647834XISBN 13: 9789386478344.
6. Bijoy Sinha Roy (D) v. Biswanath Das, (2 JJ,SC) Civil Appeal Nos. 4761 of 2009. D/d. 30.8.2017.
7. Calcutta Medical Research Institute vs. Bimalesh Chatterjee I. CPJ 13 (NC) 1999.
8. Chanchali Narendra v. Continental Hospitals, (NCDRC)-Consumer Case No. 2447 of 2019. D/d. 18.6.2020.
9. Code of Criminal Procedure, 1973.
10. Consumer Protection Act 2019.
11. Dr. Harish Kumar Khurana v. Joginder Singh Civil Appeal No.7380 of 2009. D/d. 7.9.2021.
12. Dr. J.J. Merchant & Ors. v/s Shrinath Chaturvedi (2002) 6 SCC 635.
13. Hussain v. State of U.P., 2017(2) RCR (Criminal) 312 : 2017(2) Recent Apex Judgments (R.A.J.) 357 : (2017) 5 SCC 702.
14. Indian Evidence Act, 1872.
15. Indian Medical Association v/s V.P Shantha, (1995) 6 SCC 657.
16. Indian Penal Code, 1860.
17. Ins. Malhotra (Ms) Vs. Dr. A Kriplani & others 2009(4) SCC 705.
18. J.P. Hospital v. Jatinder Pal Singh, (NCDRC), Revision Petition No. 3882 of 2017 in Appeal No. 742 of 2017. D/d. 05.02.2018.
19. Jacob Mathew v. State of Punjab, (2005) 6 SCC 1.
20. Jacob Mathew vs. State of Punjab (2005) 6 SSC 1.
21. K.T. Manickaraj v. M/s. Apollo Hospital Enterprises Ltd., (NCDRC)(New Delhi), Consumer Case No. 133 of 2008. D/d. 24.3.2021.
22. Kanhaiya Kumar Singh vs. Park Medicare and Research Centre III, CPJ 9 (NC) 1999.

23. Krishna Veni 2017(2) RCR (Civil) 358 : 2017(2) Recent Apex Judgments (R.A.J.) 373 : (2017) 4 SCC 150.
24. Kusum Sharma and Another vs Batra Hospital and Medical Research Centre and Others (2010) 3 SCC 480.
25. Martin F. D'Souza v. Mohd. Ishfaq (2009) 3 SCC 1.
26. Moti Ram (dead) through Lrs. v. Ashok Kumar 2011(1) RCR (Civil) 332 : (2011) 1 SCC 466; Vikram Bakshi & Ors. v. Sonia Khosla (Dead) by Legal.
27. Mrs. Baljeet Kaur v. Dhaliwal Hospital, (PSCDRC)(Chandigarh), First Appeal Nos. 562 and 573 of 2015. D/d. 5.6.2017.
28. Ramesh Kumar v. Dr. Akhil Saxena & Ors., Civil Appeal No. 7984 of 2016.
29. Salem Advocate Bar Association, T.N. v. UOI 2002(4) RCR (Civil) 786 : (2003) 1 SCC 49, para 9-10; Salem Advocate Bar Association, T.N. v. UOI 2005(3) RCR (Civil) 530 : (2005) 6 SCC 344, para 53.
30. State of Punjab vs. Shiv Ram & Ors. (AIR 2005 SC 3280).
31. The National Legal Services Authority and the State Legal Services Authorities under the Legal Services Authority Act, 1987.
32. Union of India v. N.K. Srivastav Civil Appeal No. 2823 of 2020 (Arising out of Special Leave Petition (C) No. 28056 of 2017). D/d. 23.7.2020.
33. V Kishan Rao v. Nikhil Super Speciality Hospital (2010) 5 SCC 513.

14 CHAPTER Specific Legal Issues

Mahesh Baldwa, Namita Padvi, Amit Padvi

"Judicial misconduct breaks down the very fibre of what is necessary for functional judiciary is to be fair and impartial."

INTRODUCTION

The matters pending before court of law legally termed as sub-judice, should not be tried in other jurisdictions of court of law, judicial impropriety, willful judicial impropriety, legal hierarchy, beyond jurisdiction happens when a lower court does not follow judge made law pronounced under article 141 of Constitution of India 1950.

SUB-JUDICE

Sub-judice is a Latin phrase which originates from Roman law, which had a very heavy influence on the development of the Western legal system. In Latin, it means that it is "under a judge. A case that is before the bar for determination, rather than one being settled out of court," currently under trial or being considered by a judge or court. The term may be used synonymously with "the present case" or "the case at bar" by some lawyers. In England and Wales, New Zealand, Australia, India, and Canada it is generally considered inappropriate to comment publicly on cases *sub-judice*, which can be an offence in itself, leading to contempt of court proceedings.

In the United States, there are First Amendment concerns about stifling the right of free speech which prevents such tight restrictions on comments *sub-judice*. However, State Rules of Professional Conduct governing attorneys often place restrictions on the out-of-court statements, an attorney may make regarding an ongoing case. In the thalidomide case in the 1970s in the UK, comment in a newspaper article about the defendant company being negligent was held to be *sub-judice*.

Sub-judice and Right to Information—2005

Provisions of Section 8(1), (h) Right to Information (RTI)-2005 can be applied only if the matter is under investigation or the disclosure of information would impede the process of investigation. In the present case, the investigation has already been completed and has also acted on the basis of the investigation report. Therefore, provisions of Section 8(1) (h) are not applicable. In so far as the matter being *sub-judice* is concerned, the Central Information Commission has, time and again, held that a matter being under *sub-judice* is not a ground to deny the information unless covered under any other exempted provisions of the RTI Act-2005.

The Justifications for the *Sub-judice* Rule

The *sub-judice* rule exists primarily to protect those individuals participating in legal proceedings from being influenced by public discussion, most often in the traditional media. A subsidiary aspect is concerned with the administration of justice as a whole—in this case the *sub-judice* rule seeks to prohibit publications which, while not influencing the outcome of a trial, have the tendency to prejudice issues at stake in it or to embarrass the court involved, and so impede the administration of justice. There is, thus, an obvious relationship between the *sub-judice* rule and the rules of evidence. The sub-judice rule supports the rules of evidence by attempting to ensure that inadmissible evidence, and material which while admissible is not admitted into evidence, is excluded.

Case Laws Related to *Sub-judice*

In Bhanamal Gulzarilal Pvt. Ltd. versus Union of India and others preferred vide Revision Petition No. 61 of 1990. Decided on 9th November, 1990, reported in 1986-94 Consumer II 9O (NC) the Hon'ble National Commission held:

"The mere fact that a Writ Petition has been filed by the opposite party before the Allahabad High Court challenging the order passed by the District Forum and an interim order of stay had been passed by the High Court in the said Writ Petition which is pending before the High Court did not constitute any valid justification for the State Commission to summarily dispose of the appeal without dealing with it on the merits. The proper procedure to be adopted by the State Commission was to postpone the hearing and disposal of the appeal until after the final disposal of the Writ Petition by the High Court the Order of the State Commission disposing of the appeal by merely stating that a Writ Petition had been filed before the High Court and an interim stay has been issued is therefore manifestly illegal and without jurisdiction. The said order is hereby set aside and the appeal is remanded to the State Commission, UP with the direction that it should be heard and decided after the Writ Petition before the High Court is finally disposed of by the High Court."

In the case of Dr Sameer P Deshpande versus Mahaveer J Jain Maharashtra state consumer said "We find that the contention raised by authorized representative for the petitioners that the defense of the petitioners herein in the criminal court will be prejudice if the petitioners are required to file their written versions before the Consumer Forum is valid particularly in the light of observations of the Hon'ble Supreme Court in the case reported in AIR-1998-SC-2118 (in the matters of) Kusheshwar Dubey versus M/s. Bharat Coking Coal Ltd. and Others. In view of this, we allow both these revision petitions and set aside the order passed by the District Forum and direct that further hearing of these two consumer complaints against the petitioners herein shall be stayed till the evidence of the prosecution is over in Criminal Complaint No. 668/PS/11 and Criminal Complaint No. 518/PS/11 (both filed in the court of Metropolitan Magistrate, Kurla). However, it is hereby made clear that once the prosecution evidence in Criminal Complaint No. 668/PS/11 is over, the Petitioner shall immediately inform to the District Forum and the District Forum may proceed for hearing of Consumer Complaint No. 301 of 2011 without any further delay. Likewise, once the prosecution evidence in Criminal Complaint No. 518/PS/11 is over, the Petitioner shall immediately inform to the District Forum and the District Forum may proceed for hearing of Consumer Complaint No. 302 of 2011 without any further delay. With these directions, both these revision petitions stand disposed of. Order accordingly pronounced and dictated on 16 September, 2014.

SUB-JUDICE MATTERS OPERATE AS HEREUNDER

In the case of Samar Nath Mukherjee versus Dr Saroj Ghosh (WBSCDRC), Case No. 162/O of 1998. D/d. 11.8.2000.

- The complainant has not produced any scrap of paper to show that in fact any amount has been paid to the nursing home or to the attending physicians for the service rendered by them. Therefore, we have no hesitation to hold that the contention raised by the opposite party is well-founded and we see no reason to reject the same.
- The second ground of objection is that the complainant has lodged a complaint with the learned Additional Chief Judicial Magistrate, Sealdah and a specific case has been started. The police have submitted chargesheet upon completion of investigation and the trial is proceeding. It is not disputed that the evidence of the complainant is being recorded. In view of the circumstances, learned counsel for the respondent submits that the present case should not be proceeded with. We find substance in this objection. It appears that with regard to the same subject-matter involving identical issues a criminal case awaits decision. Accordingly, we think that it would not be appropriate for this commission to conduct a concurred adjudication of those issues covering the subject-matter in the instant case under a summary proceeding under the Act when they are already pending adjudication before a criminal court. Accordingly, we are constrained to hold that this complaint is untenable as the said matter is sub-judice before the competent criminal court. In view of the discussion aforesaid we uphold both the contentions raised by the learned counsel for the opposite party and hold that the present complaint cannot be entertained and is as such liable to be dismissed.

Media Trial/Pre-judgement of a Case *Sub-judice*

Serious view on Nilesh Navalakha versus Union of India (Bombay) (DB) Public Interest Litigation (St) No. 92252 of 2020 with Interim Application No. 95156 of 2020, with Criminal Appellate Jurisdiction Public Interest Litigation (St) No. 1774 of 2020, with Civil PIL-CJ-LD-VC-No.40 of 2020, With Original Side Public Interest Litigation (L) No. 3145 of 2020, with Criminal Public Interest Litigation (St) No. 2339 of 2020. D/d. 18.01.2021.

In relation to the self-regulatory framework, it is submitted that the News Broadcasting Standards Regulations provide for a Code of Conduct under which the authority (NBSA) would entertain complaints and take actions. The maximum fine to be imposed by the authority is ₹1,00,000 and in addition to this power, for the reasons to be recorded in writing, it may warn, admonish, censure, express disapproval against and/or impose a fine upon the broadcaster and/or recommend to the concerned authority for suspension/ revocation of license of such broadcaster. It is submitted that the "Code of Ethics and Broadcasting Standards" also makes no provision in regard to contempt of court or media trial or a pre-judgement. There are specific guidelines covering reportage as issued by the News Broadcasters Association (NBA). In paragraph 3.3 it is provided that "Reports on crime should not amount to pre-judging or pre-deciding a matter that is or is likely to be sub-judice". In paragraph 3.4 of these guidelines, it is provided that "No publicity should be given to the accused or witnesses that may interfere in the administration of justice or be prejudicial to a fair trial." It is submitted that despite the statutory and self-regulatory framework, in regard to the ongoing criminal investigation into the death of the actor, certain TV channels for the past few months were conducting a persistent media trial and have been running programs/hashtags calling for the arrest of the actress. It is submitted that the record establishes that no action whatsoever has been taken against such TV channels/broadcasts either by the UOI or by the news broadcasters. Such persistent inaction in the face of repeated broadcasts over a number of months, must result in a conclusion of total abdication of their duty/obligation by the UOI/EMMC (Union of India/Electronic Media Monitoring Centre) and by the NBA to stop such offending broadcasts. It is submitted that it is a misapprehension that such media trial or a prejudgment during the pendency of a criminal investigation, does not affect the administration of justice and does not constitute contempt of court. In either of these situations, it is felt just and necessary that this court clarifies and directs that such media trial/pre-judgement, during a pending criminal investigation, or the pendency of a criminal proceeding, affects the administration of justice, constitutes contempt of court and is covered by the prohibition contained in section 5 of the Cable Television Networks (CTVN) Act read with rule 6(f) of the CTVN Rules. The government be accordingly directed to take steps under section 20(3) of the CTVN Act to prohibit the transmission or retransmission of such programs and/or broadcasts.

The Hon'ble National Commission in the case of Electronics Corporation of India versus A Prasada Rao preferred vide Revision Petition NO. 5 of 1989 decided on 14th September, 1989 - 1986-94 held (five-judge bench) held as here under:

"This Revision Petition cannot be entertained by us at this stage since the identical matter: is admittedly *sub-judice* before the High Court of Andhra Pradesh in Writ Petition No. 10412 of 1989. The Revision Petition will stand dismissed on this preliminary ground leaving it open to the petitioner to approach this, Commission afresh, at a later stage. So advised and if the law permits the petitioner so to do."

In a similar case in Viswalakshmi Sasidharan and Others versus The Branch Manager, Syndicate Bank reported in [I (1996) CPJ I (NC)] the Hon'ble National Commission held as here under:

"This petition has to fail on the short ground that a suit in respect of the same matter is pending between these parties in the District Court, Jaipur and it is open to the petitioner to raise in the said suit all the contentions that he has raised before this Commission. We have already held in a number of cases that when a matter is *sub-judice* before a competent Civil Court, this Commission will not entertain a petition in respect of the identical subject-matter. On this limited ground, this petition is dismissed."

JUDICIAL IMPROPRIETY

In the case of Kumar and Another versus State of UP and five others decided on 2 November, 2020, the Hon'ble Supreme Court held as here under:

We cannot help but disapprove the approach of the High Court for reasons already noticed in Dwarikesh Sugar Industries Ltd. versus Prem Heavy Engineering Works (P) Ltd and another, 1997 (6) SCC 450, observing:

"When a position, in law, is well settled as a result of judicial pronouncement of this court, it would amount to judicial impropriety to say the least, for the subordinate courts including the High Courts to ignore the settled decisions and then to pass a judicial order which is clearly contrary to the settled legal position. Such judicial adventurism cannot be permitted and we strongly deprecate the tendency of the subordinate courts in not applying the settled principles and in passing whimsical orders which necessarily has the effect of granting wrongful and unwarranted relief to one of the parties. It is time that this tendency stops."

In the case of Simarjeet Singh Bains versus The State of Punjab and Another decided on 23 July, 2021 it was categorically held that the phrase "*Judicial* Impropriety" is nowhere defined. However, in a broader perspective, it can be held to be an act of a *judicial* officer which violates law or..................

Elangovan versus Arulmighu Tharakeswara Swamy... on 11 December, 2020.

"(I) When a position, in law, is well settled as a result of judicial pronouncement of this Court, it would amount to judicial impropriety to say the least, for the subordinate Courts to ignore the settled decisions rendered by High Courts and the Supreme Court and then to pass a judicial order which is clearly contrary to the settled legal position. Such judicial adventurism should be avoided.

Supriya Devi versus State of Bihar (Patna), Criminal Writ Jurisdiction Case No. 3293 of 2018. D/d. 13.8.2019.

Since I have already held that the FIR of the case in question was instituted on the basis of an illegal order passed by the learned Chief Judicial Magistrate, in the opinion of this Court, allowing the prosecution to continue further on the basis of such an FIR would certainly result in injustice and would prevent promotion of justice. It would also amount to promoting judicial impropriety as no subordinate court including the High Court can ignore the settled decision of the Supreme Court and then pass a judicial order contrary to the settled legal position.

Sanjay Pathak versus State of Bihar (Patna), Criminal Writ Jurisdiction Case No. 1145 of 2019. D/d. 14.8.2019. Since I have already held that the FIR of the case in question was instituted on the basis of an illegal order passed by the learned Chief Judicial Magistrate, in the opinion of this Court, allowing the prosecution to continue further on the basis of such an FIR would certainly result in injustice and would prevent promotion of justice. It would also amount to promoting judicial impropriety as no subordinate court including the High Court can ignore the settled decision of the Supreme Court and then pass a judicial order contrary to the settled legal position.

Tapas Paul versus Biplab Kumar Chowdhury (Calcutta) (DB), AST 352 of 2014 with ASTA 254 of 2014, with AST 355 of 2014, with ASTA 255 of 2014. D/d. 13.8.2014. The learned Trial Court had no occasion to consider the submissions advanced on behalf of the appellants not only assailing the impugned judgment but also on merits including maintainability of the writ petition. We are hearing an appeal against the ad interim order. The writ petition is still pending. Confining ourselves to the impugned order we are, unable to endorse the view of the learned Trial Court that the private respondent No. 7 could be booked under Sections 115, 141, 153A, and 509 of the Indian Penal Code. In expressing our dissent, we wish to point out the caution sounded, in the case of State of Bihar versus JAC Saldanha reported in 1980(1) SCC 554, in dealing with criminal matters "relevant facts may be stated with circumspection, as the case is sub-judice because any overt or covert expression of opinion on the facts in controversy awaiting adjudication may be censored as judicial impropriety."

Jagtar Ram versus Union of India, (Himachal Pradesh) (DB) Civil Writ Petition No. 6333 of 2021. D/d. 03.12.2021. There has to be zero tolerance on the part of the court when it gets down to decide cases of unauthorized encroachments, obstructions, and illegal constructions, violation of statutory plans and schemes. Therefore, even on the ground of sympathy, the court cannot come to the rescue of the petitioner or else such direction would be blatant violation of the orders of the Hon'ble Supreme Court and grant of any relief to the petitioner is not only impermissible, but would even amount to judicial impropriety, blatant and scant respect for the orders of the Hon'ble Supreme Court which otherwise are binding upon this court under Article 141 of the Constitution of India.

Sanjay Gaur versus Bank of Baroda (Rajasthan), SB Civil Writ Petition No. 5019 of 2020. D/d. 29.11.2021.

We cannot help but disapprove the approach of the High Court for reasons already noticed in Dwarikesh Sugar Industries Ltd. versus Prem Heavy Engineering Works (P) Ltd., observing: (SCC p. 463, para 32).

"When a position, in law, is well settled as a result of judicial pronouncement of this Court, it would amount to judicial impropriety to say the least, for the subordinate courts including the High Courts to ignore the settled decisions and then to pass a judicial order which is clearly contrary to the settled legal position. Such judicial adventurism cannot be permitted and we strongly deprecate the tendency of the subordinate courts in not applying the settled principles and in passing whimsical orders which necessarily has the effect of granting wrongful and unwarranted relief to one of the parties. It is time that this tendency stops."

"The impugned orders are therefore contrary to the law laid down by this Court under Article 141 of the Constitution and unsustainable. They are, therefore, set aside and the appeal is allowed."

In, M/S. Utility Builders and Leasing (P) Ltd, versus Mohd. Ali Beg And *M/s.* Utility Builders and Leasing (P) Ltd. versus Mrs. Ishrat Kazrani Revision Petition No. 21 and 22 of 1992 Decided on 1st September, 1992-1986-99 Consumer 3820 (NC). The Hon'ble National commission has held:

"The main question arising out of these cases is identical with the one pending before the Supreme Court in the appeal preferred against the decision of this Commission; In MM Sood versus Lucknow Development Authority, 1986-95 Consumer 149 (NC) (RA. No. 10 of 1990). Hence, propriety demands that the hearing of these cases should be postponed until the Supreme Court renders its final decision in that appeal particularly since the operation of order in that case has been stayed by Supreme Court. These petitions are accordingly adjourned sine die."

Again, in Regional Manager, APIIC and another Petitioners versus AN Raju Respondent and AN Raju Petitioner versus Regional Manager, APIIC and another Respondents Revision 1986-99 Consumer 3838 (NS) Petition Nos. 18 and 24 of 1992 Decided on 20th August, 1992 the Hon'ble National Commission held:

"The question arising in this case is identical with the one pending before the Supreme Court in the appeal preferred against the decision of this Commission in Lucknow Development Authority versus MM Sood, 1986-95 Consumer 149 (NC) (F. A. No. 10 of 1990). Propriety demands that the hearing of this case should be postponed until the Supreme Court renders its final decision."

WILLFUL JUDICIAL IMPROPRIETY

"Willful judicial impropriety" occurs if the Bench ventures to interpret the matter when it has judicial notice that the matter is seized with the same issue in higher court in hierarchy.

In, *M/s* D. Navinchandra and Co., Bombay versus Union of India and others, 1987 (3) SCC 66, Mukherji, J (as His Lordship then was) speaking for a three-judge bench of the Apex Court stated the law in the following terms:

"Generally legal positions laid down by the court would be binding on all concerned even though some of them have not been made parties nor were served normally notice of such proceedings."

In Food Corporation and Another versus Yadav Engineer and Contractor reported in 1982 (2) sec 499 the Supreme Court held:

"It may be pointed out here that the Divisional Bench decision of the Madhya Pradesh High Court which was in terms binding on the learned Judge of the High Court, and it was specifically submitted to us that even though the attention of the learned Judge was invited, he neither referred to it nor distinguished it. Times without number this Court has observed that considerations of judicial propriety and decorum require that if a learned Single Judge hearing a matter is inclined to take the view contrary to the earlier decision of a Division Bench of the same High Court, it would be judicial impropriety to ignore that decision but after referring to the binding decision he may direct that the papers be placed before the Chief Justice of the High Court to enable him to constitute a larger Bench to examine the question. Judicial committee demands that a binding decision to which attention has been drawn should neither be ignored nor overlooked (see Mahadeolal Kanodia versus Administrator-General of WB Shri Bhagwan versus Ram Chand and State of Gujarat versus Ramprakash P Puri).

Ajay Kumar Bhuyan versus State of Orissa, (SC)

2003(1) SCT 368: 2003(1) SCC 707: 2002(Sup4) SCR 464: 2002(8) SLR 9: 2003 LIC 78: 2003 SCC (L&S) 124: 2002(8) Supreme 531: 2002 AIR (SCW) 4866: 2003(1) PLJR 203: 2003(1) JLJR 203, Civil Appeal Nos. 3978-3979 of 1998. D/d. 3.12.2002.

Constitution of India, Articles 141, 142, and 215 - Judgments and precedents - Binding force of Supreme Court judgments - All the High Courts and subordinate courts as also the Tribunals must follow the already settled principles of law - Giving comments on settled judicial principles is nothing but judicial indiscipline and judicial adventurism which cannot be tolerated.

So much said regarding Courts would apply with equal, if not more, force to Administrative Tribunals and it is beyond comprehension as to how an Administrative Tribunal could have hazarded a decision like the one rendered on 22.10.1990, which both in law and for all purposes must be treated as "non est," and at any rate not binding upon the Bench of the Tribunal.

JUDICIAL HIERARCHY

The term means that all quasi-judicial Forums/Tribunal are accountable and subordinate to the High Court of the State which in turn to Hon'ble Supreme Court under article 141 of Constitution of India.

Beyond Jurisdiction of National Commission to go into validity of discharge/retirement under Armed Forces Tribunal Act, 2007.

Cpl. Ashish Kumar Chauhan (Retd) versus Commanding Officer (NCDRC), Consumer Case No. 647 of 2017. D/d. 27.8.2021.

Discharge from service —Complaint before National Commission—Jurisdiction of National Commission to go into validity of discharge/retirement of complainant barred under Armed Forces Tribunal Act, 2007.

Enhancement of compensation to ₹2.5 crore in addition to original compensation of ₹95,03,00,000—Complainant watchman in Food Corporation of India and while on duty under "Operation Parakram," complainant was admitted to Opposite Party Hospital—Complainant developed HIV infection after blood transfusion and his disease was made "non-attributable to service" per Medical Board—Part of complaint is for compensation, alleging medical negligence, violation of human right and defamation not covered under term service matters as such complaint not barred under Armed Forces Tribunal Act, 2007—No Expert Opinion to effect that at time of blood transfusion in body of complainant, staff of Opposite Party committed any negligence—No record relating to treatment of complaint of June-July 2002 is still in custody of opposite parties—No adverse inference can be drawn against Opposite Parties that they withheld material evidence in their possession—Allegation that opponents continuously harassed Complainant for more than 14 years, adopted unreasonable, unjustified as not complaint against any opponent made during service period. Thus, jurisdiction of National Commission to go into validity of discharge/retirement of complainant barred under Armed Forces Tribunal Act, 2007. Hence, complaint dismissed.

DO'S AND DON'TS

- The sub-judice rule exists primarily to protect litigants.
- RTI-2005 is applicable to government medical establishment.
- Provisions of Section 8(1), (h) RTI-2005 can be applied only if the matter is under investigation.
- Provisions of Section 8(1) (h) are not applicable; the investigation has already been completed and has also acted on the basis of the investigation report.
- "Willful judicial impropriety" when subordinate judiciary ventures to interpret the matter when it has judicial notice that the matter is seized with the same issue in higher court in hierarchy.

SUMMARY AND CONCLUSION

The *sub-judice* rule exists primarily to protect litigants from two simultaneous litigations on same cause of action. RTI-2005 is applicable to government medical establishment only. "Willful judicial impropriety" when subordinate judiciary ventures to interpret the matter when it has judicial notice that the matter is seized with the same issue in higher court in hierarchy.

KEY LEARNING POINTS

- The doctors should use defense of sub-judice if matter is in multiple courts.
- Judicial impropriety happens when under article 141 many a times the supreme court judgments are not followed by lower judiciary particularly with respect to law of limitation, res ipsa loquitur maxim, hence an application to that effect should be filed in the court to follow supreme court precedents.
- Willful judicial impropriety happens when lower judicial hierarchy is put to notice that judicial impropriety hence pleaded. It needs to be pleaded by miscellaneous application quoting supreme court judgments which are not followed by lower judiciary hierarchy particularly with respect to law of limitation, Res ipsa loquitur maxim, contributory negligence, quantum of compensation, etc. So, special application to that effect should be filed in the court to follow Supreme Court precedents otherwise it may amount to willful judicial impropriety.

BIBLIOGRAPHY

1. Baldwa M, Baldwa V, Padvi N, et al. Legal Issues in Critical Care, 1st edition. New Delhi: CBS Publishers and Distributors Private Limited; 2022.
2. Baldwa M, Baldwa V, Padvi N, et al. Legal Issues in Medical Practice, 1st edition. New Delhi: CBS Publishers and Distributors Private Limited; 2018.
3. Bhanamal Gulzarilal Pvt. Ltd. Petitioner versus Union of India and others Respondents Revision Petition No. 61 of 1990. Decided on 9th November, 1990, 1986-94 CONSUMER II 9O(NS).
4. Cpl. Ashish Kumar Chauhan (Retd) versus Commanding Officer (NCDRC), Consumer Case No. 647 of 2017. D/d. 27.8.2021.
5. Dwarikesh Sugar Industries Ltd. versus Prem Heavy Engineering Works (P) Ltd., observing: (SCC p. 463, para 32).
6. Electronics Corporation of India versus A Prasada Rao Revision Petition NO. 5 of 1989 Decided on 14th September, 1989 - 1986-94 CONSUMER 1218 (NS) held (5-Judge Bench).
7. Food Corporation and Another versus Yadav Engineer and Contractor 1982 (2) sec 499.
8. Jagtar Ram versus Union of India (Himachal Pradesh) (DB) Civil Writ Petition No. 6333 of 2021. D/d. 03.12.2021.
9. MM Sood versus Lucknow Development Authority, 1986-95 CONSUMER 149 (NS) (RA. No.10 of 1990).
10. M/S. Utility Builders and Leasing (P) Ltd, versus Mohd. Ali Beg and M/s. Utility Builders and Leasing (P) Ltd. versus Mrs. Ishrat Kazrani Revision Petition No. 21 and 22 of 1992 Decided on 1st September, 1992 - 1986-99 CONSUMER 3820 (NS).
11. M/s D. Navinchandra and Co., Bombay versus Union of India and others, 1987 (3) SCC 66.
12. Nilesh Navalakha versus Union of India (Bombay) (DB) Public Interest Litigation (St) No. 92252 of 2020 With Interim Application No. 95156 of 2020, with Criminal Appellate Jurisdiction Public Interest Litigation (St) No.1774 of 2020, with Civil PIL-CJ-LD-VC-No.40 of 2020, with Original Side Public Interest Litigation (L) No.3145 of 2020, with Criminal Public Interest Litigation (St) No. 2339 of 2020. D/d. 18.01.2021.
13. Regional Manager, APIIC and another Petitioners versus AN Raju Respondent and AN Raju Petitioner versus Regional Manager, APIIC and another Respondents Revision 1986-99 CONSUMER 3838 (NS) Petition Nos. 18 and 24 of 1992 Decided on 20th August, 1992.
14. Right to Information Act; 2005.
15. Samar Nath Mukherjee versus Dr. Saroj Ghosh (WBSCDRC), Case No. 162/O of 1998. D/d. 11.8.2000.
16. Sanjay Gaur versus Bank of Baroda (Rajasthan), SB Civil Writ Petition No. 5019 of 2020. D/d. 29.11.2021.
17. Sanjay Pathak versus State of Bihar (Patna), Criminal Writ Jurisdiction Case No 1145 of 2019 (Arising Out of PS. Case No.–308, Year–2016, Thana–Gardanibag District-Patna). D/d. 14.8.2019.
18. Southern Field Ventures Pvt. Ltd versus Federal Bank Ltd (Kerala) (DB) WA No. 696 of 2021 (Against the Judgment In WP(C) 8210/2021 of High Court of Kerala Dated 29.3.2021). D/d. 29.11.2021.
19. State of Bihar versus JAC Saldanha reported in 1980 (1) SCC 554.
20. Supriya Devi versus State of Bihar (Patna), Criminal Writ Jurisdiction Case No.3293 of 2018 (Arising Out of PS. Case No.–85, Year–2018, Thana–Vishnupad, District–Gaya). D/d. 13.8.2019.
21. Tapas Paul versus Biplab Kumar Chowdhury (Calcutta) (DB), AST 352 of 2014 with ASTA 254 of 2014 with AST 355 of 2014 with ASTA 255 of 2014. D/d. 13.8.2014.13.
22. The Constitution of India; 1950.
23. Viswalakshmi Sasidharan and Others versus the Branch Manager, Syndicate Bank [I (1996) CPJ I (NC)] the Hon'ble National Commission held.

14.1 Vicarious Liability

Neeraj Nagpal

INTRODUCTION

Vicarious liability is a legal principle which holds one person or party responsible for the actions of another person. Specifically, it is the liability that an employer may have for the actions of their employees. Under the concept of vicarious liability, an employer can be held responsible for the negligent or wrongful actions of an employee that occur within the scope of the employees duties. For example, if an employee causes an accident while driving a company vehicle during duty hours, the employer may be held responsible for any resulting damages or injuries.

VICARIOUS LIABILITY IN MEDICINE

In medical profession the concept of vicarious liability has wide ramifications. This liability extends to the hospital/employer for the wrongs or negligent acts of its employees, irrespective of whether the employment is permanent, temporary, casual, paid or honorary, whole time or part time as in the case of visiting physicians or surgeons. It is now well settled that the hospital is also vicariously liable for the acts of its doctors. The concept is based on the fact that the employer or principal has a greater ability to control and influence the behavior of their employees. The hospital should, therefore, bear the responsibility for any harm caused by those employees in the course of their employment.

The employer being held responsible for the driver of ambulance causing an accident, the helper pushing a trolley or wheelchair and causing a fall with resulting injury, the Resident Medical Officer not attending to a patient in time, Burn injury from cautery or warm water bag, unattended post anesthesia patient found dead from aspiration or even medical negligence of doctors employed by the hospital are all examples of vicarious liability of a hospital in various situations. Hospitals at times make wrong claims of availability of certain facilities such as 24 hours emergency services when they lack even the most basic amenities like a doctor being available round the clock, essential equipment in working order, and ventilator and other intensive care facilities, etc., and this construes direct negligence on part of hospital. If a hospital gives advertisement which claims guaranteed results for operative procedures or treatment of certain diseases and then do not give desired outcome to those who are attracted by those advertisements, this would also amount to negligence even though the surgeon performing the procedure or the treating physician may only be a visiting consultant.

Medical education and training also occurs within healthcare facilities and the hospital is vicariously liable for negligence of its residents/trainees. The issue of whether, in India, the head of a unit or the consultant should be held responsible for negligence of a resident doctor who is under his charge is something that has vexed medicolegal scholars and remains to be answered definitively. Medical trainees are supposed to be supervised while undergoing their undergraduate as well as postgraduate training and hence the liability of the supervisor in case of injury to the patient needs to be explored and carefully and definitively answered. Appropriating vicarious liability between hospitals who hires the resident doctor or the visiting consultant on whose direction he works is another problem area. Hospitals have tried to escape liability by claiming that the resident was a "borrowed servant" of the visiting consultant for the duration of the task in question. The challenge for the judicial system would be to give justice to a patient harmed due to negligence but not simultaneously stifle the clinical training of resident doctors which is so essential for society.

LAW ON VICARIOUS LIABILITY IN MEDICAL NEGLIGENCE IN INDIA

It is settled law in India that the hospital is vicariously liable for the acts of its doctors. This was enunciated clearly in the case of Savita Garg versus National Heart Institute, decided by the Supreme Court (SC). The same view was also upheld in Balram Prasad's case where it was held that AMRI hospital was liable vicariously for actions of its doctors and should pay the entire compensation except for the small fraction specifically imposed on doctors. In the case of "Spring Meadows Hospital versus Harjol Ahluwalia, it was held by the honorable Supreme Court that whenever a gross medical mistake is made it will always result in findings of negligence by the court. Use of wrong drug or wrong gas during anesthesia would lead to the imposition of liability. A consultant could also be held negligent if he delegates the responsibility to his junior while being fully aware that the junior was not properly trained and incapable of performing the task properly.

Similarly in the case of Achutrao Haribhau Khodwa versus State of Maharashtra, the SC has held unequivocally that the state (employer) would be vicariously liable for the damages which may become payable on account of negligence of its doctors or other employees. Even the Government which establishes and administers hospitals through its Department of Health, are also held vicariously liable along with the individual hospital for negligent actions of their employees (V Krishna Kumar vs. State of Tamil Nadu).

Honorable Supreme Court in case of Smt. Santra versus State of Haryana and Others, held that the contention that the State is not vicariously liable for the negligence of it officers in performing the sterilization operation cannot be accepted in view of the law already settled by Supreme Court in *N Nagendra Rao and Company versus State of AP*, and in *Common Cause, A Registered Society versus Union of India and Others.*

A hospital can be held to be vicariously liable for injury caused to the patients by the negligence of their staff on numerous grounds. Various High Courts have reiterated this view over time. Kerala High Court in Joseph @ Pappachan versus Dr George Moonjerly, held that those who run hospital are in law under the same duty as the doctors they employ. When hospitals accept a patient for treatment, they must use reasonable care and skill to ease him of his ailment... "The hospital authorities cannot, of course, do it by themselves; they have no ears to listen to the stethoscope, and no hands to hold the surgeon's scalpel. They must do it by the staff which they employ; and if their staff are negligent in giving treatment, they are just as liable for that negligence as anyone else who employs other to do his duties for him".

In the case of Aparna Dutta versus Apollo Hospitals Enterprises Ltd., the Madras High Court held that medical services were being provided by the hospital. It is up to the hospital as to under what terms it employs the doctors and surgeons and because of this the hospital will remain liable. The hospital is expected to provide proper medical services and stating that there is no master-servant relationship between the hospital, and the surgeon who performed the operation will not absolve the hospital of its liability. If negligence is established, then to say that the surgeon was not employed by the hospital would not be a valid defense.

In case of S Bhanupriya versus State of Tamil Nadu forceps was used to deliver a child and this caused perineal tears including tear in rectum. Patient had to undergo multiple surgeries to recover from the complications. The Madras HC held that Government is vicariously responsible for negligence on part of the Government Hospital not having referred the patient to medical college and compensation was awarded.

However, in case titled Dr MK Gourikutty, and etc., versus MK Madhavan and Others a patient had died following sterilization done postpartum, and the Court decided that not only the State Government had to pay the compensation awarded due to vicarious liability but also the anesthesiologists and other staff.

In Punjab State versus Surinder Kaur, the Punjab and Haryana High court decided that... since the doctor was working in a government hospital and was performing the duty while he/she was under the employment of the State hence it was the State that would be held vicariously liable. It is for the State to determine the liability of the erring doctors and recover it from them. This would be their internal affair but as far as the patient is concerned, she should be paid the compensation by the State Government.

In the case of Thangapandi versus Director of Primary Health Services and Others decided by the Madurai Bench of Madras High Court, patient had delivered at Primary Health Center by staff nurse and midwife and developed postpartum hemorrhage (PPH). No doctor was available. She was later taken to Government Hospital where she was declared brought dead. The vicarious liability of Director Health Services was held.

The National Consumer Redressal Commission in case of Smt. Rekha Gupta versus Bombay Hospital Trust and Another, observed that "It is the hospital who has to own up for the conduct of its employees whatever may be the rules under which they have been employed". The defense that the hospital only provided its infrastructure and provided the support staff such as nurses and other paramedical staff and technicians and that it cannot by itself recommend or perform any operation or amputation, is not sufficient to escape liability. The commission observed that hospital raises all bills including the doctors fee and deducts a commission while paying to the consultant. Such arguments were deemed to be superficial by the court. As per the decision the hospital authorities are responsible not only for actions of their nurses, doctors, and other staff, who are its employees but also for the other visiting consultants, and surgeons, who may be practicing independently but also admit/operate in the hospital. It is inconsequential whether the said surgeons/consultants are permanent or temporary, contractual resident or visiting consultants, and may be working in the hospital full time or part time.

The National Commission in the case of SP Aggarwal versus Sanjay Gandhi PG Institute also held that "In view of the fact that several doctors and paramedical staff of the appellant institute were involved in treatment, it is the institute which has to be held vicariously liable to compensate the complainant."

In case of Sheela Srivastava versus Rajiv Gandhi Cancer Institute and Research Centre and others, National Consumer Disputes Redressal Commission decided that "... vicarious liability extends to the primary liability of the hospital for the wrongs or negligent acts of its servants, irrespective of whether their employment is permanent or temporary or casual paid or honorary, whole time or part time as in the case of visiting physicians or surgeons. By now it is well settled that the hospital is also vicariously liable for the acts of its doctors."

A hospital was also penalized for a wrong depiction of qualifications of doctor to give the impression that she is a qualified gynecologist by adding MD (Gynecology) against her name. Her qualifications was considered equivalent to MBBS (Bachelor of Medicine, Bachelor of

Surgery) as per rules of Medical Council of India (MCI) and it was construed as negligence that the hospital created an impression that the doctor possessed postgraduate (PG) degree in gynecology whereas the doctor had actually trained in Germany and the postgraduate training in Obstetrics and Gynecology done by her there was not recognized by the MCI.

The National Consumer Disputes Redressal Commission (NCDRC) in Kamala R Bhat versus Manipal North Side Hospital and Another decided on a case where sigmoid colon perforation had occurred during surgery for hernia and later this resulted in death. The court concluded that the hospital has failed to establish that it is not vicariously liable for the acts of its doctor. The hospital failed to submit evidence establishing that the doctor was not under its control and not acting as its agent in providing care to the patient. Therefore, hospital is vicariously liable for the negligence of the surgeon.

To be held to be vicariously liable for injury certain criteria need to be met:
- The injury should have occurred while the employee was on duty.
- The injury should have been caused by an activity the employee was hired to perform.
- The employer benefited in some way from the activity the employee was performing at the time of the injury.

LEGAL PRINCIPLE

The term "vicarious liability" is assigned when one person, who by himself is blameless, but held liable for another person's mischief/mistake. Vicarious liability is justified by two Latin maxims—"*respondeat superior*" meaning "let the master answer" and "*qui facit per alium facit per se*" which means that "He who acts through another acts himself". Vicarious liability is imposed on hospital/employer based on principle of "respondeat superior" which also means that an employer is liable for the negligent act or omission of an employee if the act or omission has been done within the course and scope of his employment. Control of the employer over the employee and manner in which he exerts such control on the way the employee works, is what determines the employer-employee relationship.

Vicarious liability has been justified for the following reasons:
- It is considered that the master has the "deepest pockets". The wealth of an employer is much more than that of an employee and any compensation awarded to the employee may simply be beyond his capacity to pay. Also, an employer has access to resources via insurance. These reasons at least in some cases have had an unconscious influence on the development of the legal principle of vicarious liability.
- Vicarious liability creates a financial interest which encourages the employer to train his employees and inculcate safe working practices. This helps in accident prevention and leads to less chances of injury to others.
- As the employer hires employees to run his business and hence makes a profit from the activities of his employees. Consequently, he should also bear any losses if any that those activities may cause.

There are, however, certain exceptions to "respondeat superior" principle. If someone is employed as an independent contractor, which means that the person is hired to perform a certain task and the employer has no control on how he performs that task. In contrast to regular employees who are subject to day-to-day control by their employer, independent contractors generally have independent businesses or are independent professionals, and are hired solely to perform certain specific task, and are paid "for the task assigned". They generally have "sole control over the means and methods of accomplishing the work".

The fact that physicians/surgeons exercise independent medical judgment in the treatment of their patients is used as a factor showing the absence of control by hospitals. This "sole control" is, however, only one factor and other issues also come into play to determine whether an employed physician is an employee or an independent contractor. There are circumstances when even though the employer hires an independent contractor, an employer would still be responsible for the actionable negligence of the independent contractor. Generally, this is referred to as "ostensible agency," and "apparent authority." Here one party (hospital) shows the other party (visiting consultant) as its agent without actually giving him authority or power of independent decision making. The basis of imposing liability on the employer is because the employer has done something to imply that the independent contractor is its employee. For example, if hospital advertises names of doctors in its hoardings who may be only visiting consultants and attracts patients to the establishment in their name. Also whether patient was informed that treating doctor is not an employee and had come just to perform a procedure and would not be available thereafter would then matter.

CAN VICARIOUS LIABILITY EXTEND TO CRIMINAL NEGLIGENCE?

Section 34 of the Indian Penal Code, 1860 provides that when a criminal act is done by several persons in furtherance of the common intention of all, each of such persons is liable for that act in the same manner as if it were done by him alone. While the notion of vicarious responsibility is a civil concept, it has recently gained widespread acceptance in criminal law as well. In context of criminal law, vicarious liability appropriates guilt to a person for wrongful acts and deeds committed by someone else. This doctrine is considered to be fundamentally flawed under criminal law because it is based on principles of respondent superior which is concerned with distributing loss caused by tortious act. However, every case resolved under criminal law for vicarious culpability should be led by fundamental logic and clear evidence in order to characterize the case as just, fair, and equal.

SUMMARY/CONCLUSION

Extending the concept of vicarious liability from motor accidents to medical profession is fraught with dangers. In India a hospital or the employer (government or private) is vicariously liable for actions of their workers in tort. What is unclear is whether liability for criminal negligence of an individual would be assigned to his employer. However, can be concluded that depending on the quantum of damage or loss sustained out of such negligence or wrongdoing and considering the circumstances related there to, the liability will be burdened against the principal or employer accordingly. Also, the vicarious liability of the supervisor/consultant/unit head for the negligence of the resident trainee are vexatious issues which require clarity in India.

KEY LEARNING POINTS

- A hospital is responsible and liable for wrongful actions of its nurses, doctors, staff in the line of duty.
- Government/Individual/Trust/Corporate owners would be responsible and liable besides the individual hospital for negligence of its employees within their line of duty.
- Action or omission should have occurred while the employee was on duty and while doing the job he was hired to do.
- Claiming that the doctor was a visiting consultant does not absolve the hospital of its vicarious liability.

BIBLIOGRAPHY

1. Achutrao Haribhau Khodwa versus State of Maharashtra (1996) 2 SCC 634.
2. Alswanger versus Smego, 257 Conn. 58, 67–68, 776. A.2d 444 (2001).
3. Aparna Dutta versus Apollo Hospitals Enterprises Ltd. [2002 ACJ 954 (Madras HC).
4. Bhanupriya versus State of Tamil Nadu, WP No 26460 of 2007.
5. Common Cause, A Registered Society versus Union of India and Others. (1999) 6 SCC 667.
6. Dr MK Gourikutty and etc. versus MK Madhavan and Others [AIR 2001 Kerala HC (DB) 398].
7. Dr Balram Prasad versus Dr Kunal Saha (2014) 1 SCC 384.
8. Dr Sr Louie and Another versus Kannolil Pathumma and Another NCDRC [1993 (1) CPR 422 (NCDRC)].
9. Joseph @ Pappachan versus Dr George Moonjerly [1994 (1) KLJ 782 (Kerala HC)].
10. Kamala R. Bhat versus Manipal North Side Hospital and Another, on 31 March, 2016 Appeal no 192 of 2005 NCDRC.
11. N Nagendra Rao and Co. versus State of AP, (1994) 6 SCC 205.
12. Punjab State versus Surinder Kaur [2001 ACJ 1266 (P&H-HC)].
13. SP Aggarwal versus Sanjay Gandhi PG Institute 2010(2) CPJ 212.
14. Savita Garg versus National Heart Institute (2004) 8 SCC 56.
15. Sheela Srivastava versus Rajiv Gandhi Cancer Institute and Research Centre and 5 Others 2018 (3) CPR 384.
16. Smt. Rekha Gupta versus Bombay Hospital Trust and Another. [2003 (2) CPJ 160 (NCDRC)].
17. Smt. Santra versus State of Haryana & Others [(2005) 5 SCC 182].
18. Spring Meadows Hospital versus Harjol Ahluwalia [(1998) 4 SCC 39].
19. Thangapandi versus Director of Primary Health Services and Others, Madurai Bench of Madras High Court 10/12/2010 (2011) 1 MLJ 1329.
20. Thornton RG. Responsibility for the acts of others. Proc (Baylor Univ Med Cent). 2010;23(3):313-5.

14.2 Ratio Decidendi and Obiter Dicta

Sudhir Mishra

INTRODUCTION

Doctors and medical students confront ethical and legal issues in clinical practice every day, though they may not be aware of them at all times. Many of these never become the focus of attention because they are dealt with unconsciously and for the most part the doctor practising good medicine will be acting morally and within the law. But this cannot be assumed. It is also increasingly expected that doctors should be able to explain and justify their decisions to patients, parents, other relatives, other health professionals, media, regulators and in some situations the courts. To do this doctors need to be both clinically competent, ethically sensitive and should have the understanding of the law. This chapter is meant to emphasize on two parts of the doctrine of precedent "ratio decidendi" and "obiter dicta". Doctrine of precedent essentially means that a court should decide similar cases on similar legal principles.

DEFINITION

Law created by the courts known as *common law* is based on *precedent* which is recorded in court reports. Each case report sets out the facts of a case, the rationale and legal issues to reach a decision. To clarify further, decision made by one court in relation to a particular issue can become binding on judges considering the same issues at a later date. This is called *precedent.* Such precedents are only set by judges in senior courts and apply to the courts equal to or below them. *Precedent* has a very important role in common law. The concept of *precedent* also attempts to ensure consistency in the law while also allowing for the law to develop over time. To understand how precedent works familiarity with two legal concepts *ratio decidendi* and *obiter dictum* is needed.

Ratio decidendi is a Latin phrase implying *"the reasons for the decision"*—the principles a judge uses in making his decisions (judgment). Afterwards these principles become binding and are followed by courts lower in the hierarchy, if a case with facts sufficiently similar is presented to them. To further simplify the facts the decision or judgement of a judge may fall into two parts: the *ratio decidendi* (reason for the decision) and *obiter dictum* (something said by the way). The *ratio decidendi* of a case is the principle of law on which a decision is based. When a judge delivers judgement in a case, he outlines the facts which he finds have been proved on the evidence. Then he applies the law to those facts and arrives at a decision, for which he gives the reason. This reason is called the *ratio decidendi.* It also refers to that the part of the judgement which is delivered at the end of a case explaining the reasons for the decision.

Obiter dicta in Latin means *"other things said"*. Although similar to ratio decidendi, it does not form a binding precedent. It becomes a persuasive precedent and a judge in a later case may or may not follow it as it is not binding. However, they may consider it when making their decision. These statements, made by a judge, in the course of giving his reasons for a decision, are not necessary elements of the reasons for judgment. That means that the judge could have given the same decision without making the statements. Under the common law, obiter dicta are not binding on courts in subsequent cases.

Examples:

1. *Indian Medical Association vs. V.P. Shantha and Ors on 13 November, 1995*: Where Supreme Court held that services provided by healthcare providers do fall under the purview of consumer protection act is an example of ratio decendi. Also, the observation that hospitals where all patients (and not particular patient) are treated free of cost are exempt, is also an example of ratio decendi.
2. *Briody v St Helen's and Knowsley AHA (2001)*: Ms Bridoy lost her baby during the delivery and also her uterus had to be removed. The negligence charge was upheld.

   This deprived her of a chance to have a baby of her own. She desperately wanted a family through surrogacy for which she appealed to court for recovery of cost from negligent team. The court of appeal did not agree and ruled that it was not appropriate for her to recover the costs of surrogacy. This is an example of ratio decidendi as this decision binds any court of appeal or lower court for cases of similar nature. The judge also stated that in her view the cost of other treatment such as in vitro fertilization (IVF) using donor eggs would also not be recoverable as damages from the negligent team. This statement was obiter dictum and not binding but may be used by lawyers to support their argument should such a case arise.
3. *R v Howe (1987)*, Howe and Bannister were driven with a person by M where they killed M. Howe tried to defend himself with the argument that they were *under duress* as they feared that M will kill him if he did not do as directed by M. It was decided by the House of Lords that *duress could not be used as a defence* against a murder charge (ratio decidendi). The Lords also stated that duress cannot be used as a defense against attempted murder (obiter dicta).

   In R v Gotts (1992), a defendant charged with attempted murder tried to defend himself using duress. Here the obiter statement from Howe was used as a persuasive precedent and consequently he was found guilty.
4. A couple go out to shop, leaving their dog in the car. For some unknown reason, the dog got excited and started jumping around. The dog was not sick or was not in an uncomfortable environment. By jumping around the dog shatters the rear glass window and a shard of glass flies off, hits the eye of a passer-by. This eye was removed due to injury.

   Is the couple liable to pay compensation for the man's eye? The court did not agree. The court said that they should only be liable, if they caused harm by doing something that could be reasonably foreseen as likely to cause harm. We are not liable if we fail to guard against "fantastic possibilities" that happen to occur. The couple therefore did not have to pay compensation (the *ratio decidendi*). It can simply be expressed simply as: Where harm is caused by an incident which is unforeseeable, the defendants were not liable.

   It is interesting to note that in the case above about the dog, one judge said that if you knew your dog had an excitable tendency or went mad in cars, then you would be liable if it caused someone harm in a predictable way (*obiter dictum*).

   Res ipsa loquitur is only a rule of evidence and operates in the domain of civil law, especially in cases of torts and helps in determining the onus of proof in actions relating to negligence. It cannot be pressed in service for determining per se the liability for negligence within the domain of criminal law. Res ipsa loquitur has, if at all, a limited application in trial on a charge of criminal negligence.

An example of ratio decidendi from the case is "A private complaint may not be entertained unless the complainant has produced prima facie evidence before the court in the form of a credible opinion given by another competent doctor to support the charge of rashness or negligence on the part of the accused doctor".

The *ratio decidendi* of a case must never be confused with *obiter dictum*. What lays down the law is the *ratio decidendi* and not the *obiter dictum* no matter how celebrated or how renowned the judge is. What is binding as a precedent is the ratio and not the obiter. It is, however, important to note that where an *obiter dictum* in one case has been adopted and becomes *ratio decidendi* in a latter case, such obiter dictum will be taken to have acquired the force of ratio decidendi and would therefore become binding. [Afro Continental Nigeria Ltd. V Joseph Ayantuyi and Ors V. Governor of Ondo state and 2 Ors (1995) 12 SCNJ 1].

CONCLUSION

Ratio decidendi is a law or guideline laid down by the highest (or higher) courts which act as precedent and are binding on lower courts for further judgments in similar situations, unless the laws are created by parliament contrary to the judgment.

Obiter dictum is the observations made by the courts in the course of judgments which are nonbinding on lower courts but may be used as principle for argument in lower court. If a higher court delivers a judgment based on these principles, it becomes ration decidendi and becomes binding on lower courts.

KEY LEARNING POINTS

- Courts work on law and precedents.
- Precedents set by higher courts and followed by the lower courts in future, if a similar situation is placed before them.
- Ratio decidendi is "reason for decision" in a particular judgment based on which law is applied. It is binding on lower courts as precedent.
- "Obiter dicta" is other observations made during the course of judgment. They also form the precedent except that they are not binding on lower court for future judgements.

BIBLIOGRAPHY

1. Stewart C, Kerridge I, Parker M. The Australian Medico-legal Handbook. Churchill Livingstone, Elsevier Publication: Australia; 2008. pp. 24-5.
2. Corfield L, Granne I, Latimer-Saye W. ABC of Medical Law. BMJ. Willey-Blackwell Publishing: Oxford; 2009. pp. 1-29.
3. Ratio Decidendi: The legal principles behind the court decisions. http://www.lawmentor.co.uk/glossary/R/ratio-decidendi/ [Assessed on 19/04/2014].
4. Anthony VanDuzer J. Law of Partnerships and Corporations. 3rd Revised edition. Irwin Law Publishers: Toronto; 2009.
5. Indian Medical Association vs V.P. Shantha & Ors on 13 November, 1995. 1996 AIR 550, 1995 SCC (6) 651.
6. Bamgbose and Olatokunbo John. Digest of Judgments of the Supreme Court of Nigeria: Vols 1 and 2, Safari books publishers, 2014, Onireke Ibadan.
7. Jacob Mathew vs State of Punjab & Anr on 5 August, 2005. Appeal (crl.) 144-145 of 2004.

15

CHAPTER

Important Case Laws

Rajendra Borkar, CM Chhajer, Satish Tiwari

INTRODUCTION

There are many cases related to medicolegal issues involving doctor–patient relationships. In the present era of deteriorating doctor–patient relationships, the patient or relatives always feel that unexpected outcome is due to deficiency in duty by the doctor or hospital staff. The internet or media leaves no stone unturned in adding fuel to the fire by circulating unscientific or biased information. The court cases for negligence in care and treatment are increasing by leaps and bounds. As far as the medical services were concerned, different courts had different rulings till Supreme Court in November 1995 by its ruling in the following case included medical services in Consumer Protection Act (CPA) under section 2 (I) (o) of CPA 1986. We will also discuss some other important cases in this chapter.

INDIAN MEDICAL ASSOCIATION VS. VP SHANTHA 1996 SC 550, 1995 SCC (6) 651

The honorable Supreme Court made the following observation:

The Act seeks to protect the interest of consumers as a class. Medical service rendered by a practitioner can't be judged on the basis of any fixed norms. It is true that a requirement about a member having adequate knowledge or experience in dealing with the problems relating to medicine is absent. It will be for the parties to place the necessary material and the knowledge and the experience which the members will have in the fields indicated in the Act would enable them to arrive at their findings on the basis of that material.

Hospitals where some are charged and some are treated free cannot be excluded because it will mean that, higher standard and better quality for those who pay and inferior quality for those who avail free of cost.

Success and failure are beyond professional people's control. Hence, only a minimum degree of competence and reasonable care is required. The trend is toward narrowing of immunity to professionals. Medical practitioners are not immune from claims for damages.

In cases of insurance policies, the patient is the beneficiary. The service cannot be said to be free of cost though the payment is made by insurance company. Similarly payments made by employer for the employee also don't mean free service and such cases fall within the ambit of the Act.

SC CIVIL APPEAL NO. 2646-49 OF 09 DECIDED ON 14/5/24

The National Consumer Distress Redressal Commission in 2007 held that the Advocates/Lawyers are under the Consumer Protection Act. In this case the following submissions were made in SC:

The Advocates Act, 61 lays down professionals stands for compliance and determining the professional misconduct. The legal profession is noble profession and not business/trade. Hence, applying CPA to advocates will open floodgate of unnecessary litigations leading to speculative/ vexatious claims. There are inherent complexities in legal issues which lacks definitive answers. Multiple parties with conflict of interests are involved and the outcome depends upon:

1. Lawyer's skill and knowledge
2. Strategies by opposing counsel
3. Decision of Judges

There are no universal standard of care in law. They have Duty to Court, Client, Colleague and Opponent. A *vakalatnama* is filed for Advocate as client's agent representing on his behalf (not service provider) and hence, not under CPA. But, services given outside court like; drafting notice, legal guidance etc are covered under CPA.

The analysis of this includes:

The protections of consumer interests are against the trader/manufacturers. There were many shortcomings in 1986 Act—hence re-enacted in 2019. The disposal of cases was delayed. In present scenario there are many changes in international trade/e-commerce and new forms of unfair trade practices and misleading advertisements.

The professional can't be businessman/traders and clients/patients can't be consumers. The profession involves some learning/science/mental skill, etc., and requires advanced/ special knowledge/training/proficiency. The professionals have to perform skill, specialized and mental work, have moral principle beyond general duty and the professional associations regulate standard code/conduct, have high status in the community. The success can't be achieved in each and every case as some factors are beyond professional's control. Hence, professionals can't be equated at par with trader/businessman.

There is nothing on record to suggest that the Parliamentary legislature ever intended to include the Professions/Professionals within the purview of CP Act. We are of the opinion that the three judge bench in IMA v. V P Shanta deserves to be revisited by a larger bench. We therefore refer the matter to Hon. Chief Justice of India for his Lordship consideration.

THE HIGH COURT OF BOMBAY PIL NO. 58 OF 2021

Civil Appellate Jurisdiction in Medicos Legal Action Group vs. Union of India held as follows: According to the court this is a thoroughly misconceived Public Interest Litigation, and we have no doubt that it deserves outright Dismissal. The petitioning Trust seeks declaration from this Court that services performed by healthcare service providers are not included within the purview of the Consumer Protection Act, 2019. According to petitioners, the parliamentary debates on the Consumer Protection Bill, 2018 led to exclusion of "healthcare" from the definition of the term "service". We see no reason to hold that merely because of enactment of the 2019 Act upon repeal of the 1986 Act as well as the parliamentary debates referred to, the efficacy of the law laid down in the decision in Indian Medical Association (Supra) as a binding precedent would stand eroded. Despite not taking a rigid view, we are of the clear opinion that the contention raised by the learned counsel for the petitioning Trust, of the Hon'ble Minister having made certain statements in course of parliamentary debates that preceded the 2019 Act, is of little relevance. If at all the Parliament while repealing and replacing the 1986 Act with the 2019 Act had intended to give a meaning to the term "service" different from the one given by the Supreme Court, such intention ought to have been reflected in clear words by a specific exclusion of "health care" from the purview of the 2019 Act. We, therefore, hold that mere repeal of the 1986 Act by the 2019 Act, without anything more, would not result in exclusion of "health care" services. The petitioning Trust shall pay, as costs, ₹50,000/- to the Maharashtra State Legal Services Authority.

POONAM VARMA VS. ASHWIN PATEL (AIR 1996 SC 2111)

This important case deals with **crosspathy**. In this case, the honorable Supreme Court observed that:

The right to practice, in any particular system of medicine, is dependent upon registration which is permissible only if qualification, and that too, a recognized qualification, is possessed by a person in that system. If registered under Homeopathy, he was under a statutory duty not to enter the field of any other system of medicine. He is liable to be prosecuted under Sec. 15 (3) of the Medical Council Act of 1956.

A practitioner or medical practitioner means a person who is engaged in the practice of modern scientific medicine in any of its branches including surgery and obstetrics, but not including veterinary medicine or surgery or the Ayurvedic, Unani, Homeopathic, or Biochemic system of medicine.

According to the Medical Council Act and Bombay Homeopathic Practitioners Act, there is mutual exclusion for right to practice in any particular system of medicine. The practice is dependent upon registration, which is permissible only if qualification, and that too, a recognized qualification, is possessed by a person in that system. A person cannot claim to treat the patients by drugs of another system, which he might not have studied at any stage. Anatomy and physiology may be common to all systems of medicines, but so far as the study of drug is concerned, the pharmacology of all the systems is entirely different. Therefore, a person having studied one particular system of medicine cannot claim deep and complete knowledge about the drugs of the other system of medicine.

A person who doesn't have knowledge of a particular system of medicine but practices in that system is a quack and a mere pretender to medical knowledge or skill, or to put it differently, a charlatan.

DR MUKHTIAR CHAND VS. STATE OF PUNJAB (8/10/1998)

It was categorically held that: The question relates not only to the right to practice medical profession but also to the right to life which includes health and well-being. A medical practitioner, registered with the Board of Ayurvedic and Unani System, Punjab, and was practicing modern system of medicines was served with an order of the district drugs inspector, prohibiting him from keeping in his possession any allopathic drug and further issuing general direction to the chemists not to issue allopathic drugs to any patient on the prescription of the said doctor.

The right of practitioners of Indian medicine to practice modern scientific system of medicine (Allopathic) is protected under Section 17(3) (b) of Indian Medicine Central Council Act, 1970 of the medical systems that in vogue in India, Ayurveda is being practiced throughout India, but Sidha is practiced in South India. These systems differ very little both in theory and practice. The Indian Medical Degrees Act, 1916 ("1916 Act") was enacted to ban conferring of degrees or issuing of certificates, license etc. to practice western medical science, by persons or authorities other than those specified in the schedule and notified by state governments.

From the discussion what emerges is that drugs can be sold or supplied by pharmacist or druggist only on the prescription of a "registered medical practitioner" who can also store them for treatment. Now the notifications issued by the Punjab Government on October 29, 1967 and the circular by the Rajasthan Government on July 26, 1982, it has already been pointed out that for purposes of clause (iii) of Rule 2(ee), what is required is not the qualification in modern system but a declaration by a state government that a person is practicing modern system and that they are registered in a medical register of the state (other than a register for the registration of homeopathic practitioner).

The right to practice any profession or any occupation trade or business is a fundamental right guaranteed under Article 19(1) (g). However this right is subject to any law relating to the professional or technical qualifications necessary for practicing any profession. Regulatory measures on the exercise of this right both with regard to standard of professional qualifications and professional conduct, have been applied, keeping in view not only the right of the practitioners but also the right to life and proper health care of persons who need care and treatment.

Persons holding "recognized medical qualification" cannot be denied registration in any State Medical Register. Further, with regard to rural areas, the prohibition to practice allopathic medicine under that Act did not apply provided a person had commenced practice in any village in the rural area prior to 1912. It can be observed that if any state law relating to registration of medical practitioners permits practice of allopathic medicine on the basis of a degree in integrated medicines, the bar in Section 15(2)(b) of the 1956 Act will not apply. Subject to the other provisions contained in this Act, any medical qualification included in the Second, Third or Fourth Schedule shall be sufficient qualification for enrolment on any State Register of Indian Medicine.

The central register of Indian medicine has to be maintained by the central council under Section 23 of that Act. The prohibition contained in Section 15(2) and the punishment provided in Section 15(3) of the 1956 Act would apply only to persons practicing allopathic system of medicine without obtaining the registration but does not apply to practitioners of Indian medicine. Section 15(2)(b) requires that only those who are registered on State Medical Register alone can practice allopathic medicine and secondly, the prohibition is directed against every person who is not registered on any State Medical Register and all such persons are precluded from practicing allopathic medicine. A degree holder in integrated courses is imparted not only the theoretical knowledge of modern medicine but also training there under, is the claim. The arguments proceed that persons who registered under the 1970 Act and have done integrated courses, are entitled to practice allopathic medicine. In our view, all that the definition of 'Indian Medicine' and the clarifications issued by the central council enable such practitioners of Indian medicine is to make use of the modern advances in various sciences such as Radiology (X-ray), complete blood picture report, lipids report, ECG, etc. for purposes of practicing in their own system. However, if any State Act recognized the qualification of integrated course as sufficient qualification for registration in the State Medical Register of that State, the prohibition of Section

15(2)(b) will not be attracted. The right to practice a system of medicine is derived from the Act under which a medical practitioner is registered.

SPRING MEADOWS HOSPITAL VS. HARJOT AHLUWALIA (AIR 1998 SC 1801)

This important case deals with *delegation of duties* to the juniors or paramedical staff. The Hon. SC observed that:

Medical organizations who in the garb of doing service to the humanity have continued commercial activities and have been mercilessly extracting money from helpless patients and their family members and yet don't provide the necessary services. The relationship between the doctor and the patient is not always equally balanced. There has been growing awareness in the public mind to bring the negligence of such doctors to light. *Both the minor child and the parents are consumers,* and compensation may be awarded to both.

DR SURESH GUPTA VS. GOVT. OF NCT OF DELHI (2004) 6 SCC 422

This is one of the judgments in which SC has highlighted and discussed the ambiguity related to criminal liability on the doctors. The court held that, the legal position is almost firmly established that where a patient dies due to the negligent treatment of the doctor, the doctor can be made liable in civil law for paying compensation and damages and at the same time, if the degree of negligence is so gross and his Act was so reckless as to endanger the life of the patient, he would also be made criminally liable for offense under Sec. 304-A IPC. Every careless Act of the medical man can't be termed as "criminal" it can be termed "criminal" only when the medical man exhibits a gross lack of competence or inaction and wanton indifference to his patient's safety, and which is found to have arisen from gross ignorance or gross negligence. Where a patient's death results merely from error or judgment or an accident; no criminal liability should be attached to it. Mere inadvertence or some degree of want of adequate care and caution might create civil liability but would not suffice to hold him criminally liable. In various kinds of medical treatment and surgical operation, likelihood of an accident or misfortune leading to death can't be ruled out. A patient willingly takes such a risk. This is part of doctor–patient relationship and mutual trust between them.

DR JACOB MATHEWS VS. STATE OF PUNJAB (2005) CPJ SC 9

In this landmark judgment, the Hon. SC has discussed the criminal liability and negligence of medical practitioners. The important issue before the court was; whether a different standard is applicable for recording a finding of negligence when a professional, in particular, a doctor is to be held guilty of negligence? The essential ingredient of "*Mens Rea*" can't be excluded from consideration when the charge consists of criminal negligence. The recklessness is not located in a desire to cause harm; it resides in the reckless state of mind when there is intention to cause harm and an utter disregard for the possible consequences. A physician would not assure the patient of full recovery in every case. A surgeon can't and doesn't guarantee that the result of surgery would invariably be beneficial, much less to the extent of 100%. The standard to be applied for judging would be that of an ordinary competent person exercising ordinary skill in that profession. This has to be judged in the light of knowledge available at the time (of the incident), and not at the date of trial. The law does not require of a professional man that he be a paragon combining the qualities of polymath and prophet. No sensible professional would intentionally commit an Act or omission, which would result in loss or injury to the patient as the professional reputation of the person is at stake. He doesn't gain anything by acting with negligence or by omitting to do an Act. Many incidences involve a contribution from more than one person, and the tendency is to blame the last identifiable element in the chain of causation—the person holding the "smoking gun".

Indiscriminate prosecution of medical professionals for criminal negligence is counter-productive and does no service or good to the society. Many a complainant prefers recourse to the criminal process as a tool for pressurizing the medical professional for extracting uncalled for or unjust compensation. Such malicious proceedings have to be guarded against. There is a need for protecting doctors from frivolous/unjust prosecution.

THE HON. SC IN SAMIRA KOHLI V. DR PRABHA MANCHANDA I (2008) CPJ 56 (SC)

It was elaborately discussed regarding consent and exceeding consent. The court observed that the patient's consent is to be obtained before commencing treatment and the consent should be real and valid. Additional or unauthorized surgery may be beneficial, saving time, expenses, pain and suffering, etc. but it cannot be a ground for defense or negligence in cases of assault/battery. The patient was admitted for diagnostic Laparoscopy. There was no consent for removal of reproductive organs, neither there was emergency nor life threatening (Principle of necessity). The patient was neither minor nor mentally challenged/incapacitated. The appellant was temporarily unconscious and hence the respondent ought to have waited till appellant regains consciousness and give consent. The mother's consent can't be considered valid in absence of emergency. The doctor should communicate all inherent and potential hazards of the proposed treatment, the alternatives to treatment, if any, and the likely effect if patient remained untreated. Thus, there is "Real Consent Concept" (more accepted in UK) or "Reasonably Prudent Patient Test" (preferred in USA, Canada, and Australia, etc.).

These stringent standards of disclosure are subjected to only two exceptions:

1. Where there was a genuine emergency, e.g., the patient was unconscious; and
2. Where the information would be harmful to the patient, e.g., where it might cause psychological damage, or where the patient would become so emotionally distraught as to prevent a rational decision.

In India, majority of citizens requiring medical care and treatment fall below the poverty line. Most of them are illiterate or semiliterate. They cannot comprehend medical terms, concepts, and treatment procedures. They don't have access to effective but costly diagnostic procedures. What choice do these poor patient have? Any treatment, of whatever degree, is a boon or a favor, for them. The stark reality is that for a vast majority, the concept of informed consent or any form of consent, and choice in treatment, has no meaning or relevance.

But unfortunately, all doctors in government hospitals are not paragons of service, nor fortunately, all private hospitals/doctors are commercial minded. There are many doctors in government hospitals who don't care about patient and unscrupulously insists upon 'unofficial' payment for free treatment or insist upon private consultations. On the other hand, many private hospitals/doctors give the best treatment without exploitation, at a reasonable cost, and charging a fee, which is reasonable recompense for the service rendered. Of course, some doctors, both in private or in government service, look at patients not as persons who should be relieved from pain and suffering by prompt and proper treatment at an affordable cost, but as potential income-providers/customers who can be exploited by prolonged or radical diagnostic and treatment procedures. It is this minority who bring a bad name to the entire profession. We will be very happy if what we have observed is an overstatement, but our intuition tells us that it is an understatement.

The principles of Consent can be summarized as follows:

- The consent should be real and valid and on the basis of adequate information.
- Information should enable the patient to make a balanced judgment. The doctor should disclose; (i) the nature/procedure of treatment along with purpose, benefits, and effects, (ii) the alternatives if any, (iii) an outline of the substantial risks and, (iv) adverse consequences of refusing treatment. The surgeon need not warn the patient of remote risks, any more than an anesthetist need warn the patient that a certain small number of those anesthetized will suffer cardiac arrest or never recover consciousness. In hysterectomy although the surgeon will tell the patient that it is proposed to remove her uterus and perhaps her ovaries and describe what that will mean for her future well-being (sterility, premature menopause), she need not be warned of the possibility of damage to the ureter, vesico-vaginal fistula, fatal hemorrhage or anesthetic death.
- Consent given only for a diagnostic procedure can't be considered as consent for therapeutic treatment. Consent given for a specific treatment will not be valid for conducting some other treatment.
- There can be a common consent for diagnostic and operative procedures where they are contemplated. There can also be a common consent for a particular surgical procedure and an additional/further procedure that may become necessary during the course of surgery.
- The "Real Consent Concept" evolved in *Bolam and Sidaway* is preferable to the "Reasonably Prudent Patient Test" concept in Canterbury. While the latter can be the concept for the future but not for the present.

VINOD KHANNA VS. RG STONE HOSPITAL NC 428 OF 2018

A patient with Immunocompromised state was taken for surgery to drain abscess and prostatectomy. The postoperative period was marked by the patient passing urine from the rectum. A compensation of ₹ 1.8 crore was demanded after 8 years of cause of action in 2010. According to experts a Fistula; a known Complication, heals with time. The Medical Board also found no negligence. But, the National Commission (NC) observed that the Consent forms had blank spaces, and handwritten entries and sign. The Commission held that the complaint is frivolous/bereft of merit and ill-conceived but, the consent forms and the consent taken is not proper. The pre-printed consent forms are administrative arbitrariness and one-sided high handedness, and to be unfair and deceptive. We don't find any deficiency in service or negligence. But, use of pre-printed forms is unfair trade practice; hence, rupees 10 lakh were to be paid to the Consumer Legal Aid Account of NC. This decision of NC was stayed by honorable Supreme Court.

MARTIN F. D'SOUZA VS. MOHD. ISHFAQ, SC IN CA NO. 3541 OF 2002

The law, like medicine, is an inexact science. One cannot predict with certainty the outcome of many cases. It depends on the particular facts and circumstances of the case, and also the personal notions of the Judge concerned who is hearing the case. Before dealing with these principles two things have to be kept in mind:

1. Judges are not experts in medical science, rather they are laymen. Moreover, judges have to usually rely on testimonies of other doctors which may not necessarily in all cases be objective, since like in all professions and services, doctors too sometimes have a tendency to support their colleagues charged with medical negligence. The testimony may also be difficult to understand, particularly in complicated matters, for a layman in medical matters like a judge; and
2. A balance has to be struck in such cases. While doctors who cause death or agony due to negligence should certainly be penalized, it must also be remembered that like all professionals' doctors too can make errors of judgment but if they are punished for this no doctor can practice his vocation with equanimity.

GENERAL PRINCIPLES RELATING TO MEDICAL NEGLIGENCE

The deviation from normal practice is not necessarily negligence. To establish liability, it must be shown: (1) that there is a usual and normal practice; (2) that the defendant has not adopted it; and (3) that the course in fact adopted is one no professional man of ordinary skill would have taken had he been acting with ordinary care. An error of judgment may or may not be negligent. At times, the professional is confronted with making a choice between the devil and the deep sea and has to choose the lesser evil. There may be a few cases where an exceptionally brilliant doctor performs an operation or prescribes a treatment which has never been tried before to save the life of a patient when no known method of treatment is available. Science advances by experimentation, but experiments sometime end in failure, e.g., the operation on the Iranian twin sisters who were joined at the head since birth or the first heart transplant by Dr Barnard in South Africa. However, in such cases it is advisable for the doctor to explain the situation to the patient and take his written consent. Discretion being the better part of velour, a medical professional would feel better advised to leave a terminal patient to his own fate in the case of emergency where the chance of success may be 10% (or so), rather than taking the risk of making a last-ditch effort toward saving the subject and facing a criminal prosecution if his effort fails. Such timidity forced upon a doctor would be a disservice to society.

Precautions which doctor/hospital/nursing home should take:

- Current practices, infrastructure, paramedical, and other staff, hygiene and sterility should be observed strictly.
- No prescription should ordinarily be given without actual examination. The tendency to give prescriptions over the telephone, except in an acute emergency, should be avoided.
- A doctor should not merely go by the version of the patient but should also make his own analysis including tests and investigations where necessary.
- A doctor should not experiment unless necessary and even then, he should ordinarily get a written consent.

- An expert should be consulted in case of doubt. The patient was diagnosed as having "Mild Lateral Wall Ischemia". The doctor prescribed medicine for gastroenteritis, but he expired. It was held that the doctor was negligent as he should have advised consulting a cardiologist in writing.
- Full record of the diagnosis treatment, etc., should be maintained.
- The medical profession is a noble profession, and it should not be brought down to the level of a simple business or commerce. The truth of the matter, sadly, is that today in India many doctors (though not all) have become totally money-minded and have forgotten their Hippocratic Oath. Since most people in India are poor the consequence is that for them proper medical treatment is next to impossible, and hence they have to rely on quacks. The law is a watchdog, and not a bloodhound, and as long as doctors do their duty with reasonable care, they will not be held liable even if their treatment was unsuccessful.

Considering the facts of the case we cannot hold that the appellant was guilty of negligence. Dr Soonawalla is an eminent doctor of India of international repute, and he would not have ordinarily referred a patient to an incompetent doctor. This is one factor which goes in favor of the appellant. A patient who does not listen to his doctor's advice often has to face the adverse consequences.

We have carefully perused the judgment of the NC and we regret that we are unable to concur with the views expressed therein. The Commission, which consists of laymen in the field of medicine, has sought to substitute its own views over that of medical experts, and has practically acted as super specialists. All doctors cannot be fitted into a straight-jacketed formula, and cannot be penalized for departing from that formula.

While this court has no sympathy for doctors who are negligent, it must also be said that frivolous complaints against doctors have increased by leaps and bounds particularly after the medical profession was placed within the purview of the CPA. In cases of head injuries earlier the doctor who was first approached would start giving first aid and apply stitches. However, now what is often seen is that doctors out of fear of facing legal proceedings do not give first aid, and instead tell him to proceed to the hospital by which time the patient may develop other complications.

Hence, Courts/Consumer Fora should keep the above factors in mind when deciding cases related to medical negligence, and not take a view which would be in fact a disservice to the public. It may be mentioned that the All India Institute of Sciences has been doing outstanding research in stem cell therapy for the last 8 years or so for treating patients suffering from paralysis, terminal cardiac condition, and parkinsonism, etc., though not yet with very notable success. This does not mean that the work of stem cell therapy should stop, otherwise science cannot progress.

We, therefore, direct that whenever a complaint is received against a doctor or hospital by the Consumer Fora (whether District, State, or National) or by the Criminal Court then before issuing notice to the doctor or hospital the Consumer Forum or Criminal Court should first refer the matter to a competent doctor or committee of doctors, specialized in the field relating to which the medical negligence is attributed, and only after that doctor or committee reports that there is a prima facie case of negligence should notice be then issued. We further warn the police officials not to arrest or harass doctors unless the facts clearly come within the parameters laid down in Jacob Mathew's case; otherwise the policemen will themselves have to face legal action. Extraordinary situations require extraordinary remedies. Life is surely more important than side effects. For example, many antitubercular drugs (e.g., streptomycin) can cause impairment of hearing. Does this mean that TB patients should be allowed to die and not be given the antitubercular drug because it impairs the hearing? Surely, the answer will be negative.

The courts and Consumer Fora are not experts in medical science, and must not substitute their own views over that of specialists. The entire medical fraternity cannot be blamed or branded as lacking in integrity or competence just because of some bad apples. It must be remembered that sometimes despite their best efforts the treatment fails.

THE STEROID CASE

In Malay Kumar vs. Dr Sukumar Mukherjee and Dr Kunal Saha vs. Dr Sukumar Mukherjee (SC Aug 2009), the Hon. SC has discussed the various issues related to negligence, civil liability, and criminal liability. The Court observed that for the use of steroid in TEN there are different opinions (Cleavage of opinion). We refer to them as the pro-steroid group and anti-steroid group. The question is as to whether the treatment was in accordance with the medical protocol. We are also cognizant of the fact that, once the initial burden has been discharged by the complainant by making out a case of negligence on the part of the hospital or the doctor concerned, the onus then shifts on to the hospital or to the attending doctors and it is for the hospital to satisfy the Court that there was no lack of care or diligence. The hospitals are institutions; people expect better and efficient service; if the hospital fails to discharge their duties through their doctors, it is the hospital which has to justify and not impleading a particular doctor will not absolve the hospital of its responsibilities. In this case, however, instead of prescribing to a quick acting steroid, the prescription of a long-acting steroid without foreseeing its implications is certainly an Act of negligence. Furthermore, after prescribing a steroid, the effect of immune-suppression, ought to have been foreseen. No doctor has the right to use the drug beyond the maximum recommended dose.

It is also of some great significance that the concerned doctors took recourse to the blame game. It is generally expected that very senior doctors would behave responsibly, and they are entitled to take any defense which is available to them, but they should not resort to mudslinging. It is to be noted that the doctrine of cumulative effect is not available in criminal law. In this connection, I deem it proper to quote a remark of Lord Denning MR in White House vs. Jordan... Take heed of what has happened in the United States. 'Medical malpractice' cases there are very worrying, especially as they are tried by juries who have sympathy for the patient and none for the doctor who is insured. The doctors insure but the premiums become very high; and these have to be passed on in fees to the patients. Experienced practitioners are known to have refused to treat patients for fear of being accused of negligence. Young men are even deterred from entering the profession because of the risks involved. In the interests of all, we must avoid such consequences in England. Not only must we avoid excessive damages. We must say and say firmly, that in a professional man, an error of judgment is not negligence..". Keeping all the above facts in mind the civil negligence was held and the criminal negligence charges were dismissed.

KUSUM SHARMA VS. BATRA HOSPITAL (SC 10TH FEB, 2010)

In this case, the SC has discussed many previous national and international cases before finalizing the principles of medical negligence.

Brief facts are as under:

It was found that there was a smooth surface mass and surgery became imperative. On test, the tumor was found to be malignant. According to the appellants, considerable pain, inconvenience, and anxiety were caused even after surgery. After another expert consultation a second surgery was carried out. The appellants alleged that the informed consent was completely lacking. The appellants also alleged that there was nothing on record to conclusively establish malignancy of the tumor before the operation was undertaken. The appellants also had the grievance that they were not told about the possible complications of the operation. According to the appellants, the "anterior" approach adopted was not the correct approach. Surgery should have been done by "posterior" approach.

The medical texts quoted above discuss of both approaches for adrenalectomy. Nowhere the appellant has been able to support her contention that posterior approach was the only possible and proper approach and respondent was negligent in adopting the anterior approach. Dr Shukla, Additional Professor at AIIMS and a well-known surgeon stated in unequivocal terms in response to a specific question that for malignant tumors, by and large, we prefer anterior approach. Dr Nandi, Professor and Head of Gastrointestinal Surgery at AIIMS also supported "anterior" approach and confirmed and reconfirmed adoption of "anterior" approach in view of inherent advantages of the approach.

In view of the medical literature and the evidence of eminent doctors of AIIMS, the National Commission did not find any merit in the allegations leveled.

It is also mentioned that the conduct of the deceased was negligent when he was discharged. The doctors specifically advised him "Regular Follow Up" which the deceased failed to attend. The Fitness Certificate issued also bore the endorsement "he would need prolonged and regular follow up". However, the deceased did not make any effort and was totally negligent.

The risk involved in the operation was explained to the petitioner, her husband, and their relative and they agreed after due consultation with their family doctor. During surgery the tail of the pancreas was traumatized during retraction as the patient was extremely obese. The damage to the pancreas was repaired immediately. The histopathology report recorded the tumor being malignant. Since cases of adrenal cancer have a very poor prognosis, six slides were sent to Sir Ganga Ram Hospital for confirmation. The histopathology report from Sir Ganga Ram Hospital also indicated cancer.

In the discharge summary prepared initially, it was recorded specifically that the mass was malignant. However, the appellants had requested to delete all references about cancer as her husband was likely to read the same. She apprehended that in such an event her husband would become mentally disturbed. Having regard to the apprehension expressed by the appellant, respondents prepared a fresh discharge summary which did not contain any reference to cancer. The diagnosis of cancer was not an afterthought. The diagnosis was considered after two histopathological reports.

Moreover, it seems that by American law a failure to warn the patient of dangers of treatment is not, in itself, negligence. In one case, it has been said that you judge it by the conduct of the man on the top of a Clapham omnibus. He is an ordinary man. However, in situations that involve the use of some special skill or competence, then the test for negligence is not based on the standard of the man on the Clapham omnibus, because that man does not possess or profess to have that special skill.

Negligence has many manifestations: It may be active negligence, collateral negligence, comparative negligence, concurrent negligence, continued negligence, criminal negligence, gross negligence, hazardous negligence, active and passive negligence, wilful or reckless negligence, or negligence *per se*.

Negligence *per-se* is defined in Black's Law Dictionary as:
Conduct, whether of action or omission, which may be declared and treated as negligence without any argument or proof as to the particular surrounding circumstances, either because it is in violation of a statute or valid municipal ordinance, or because it is so palpably opposed to the dictates of common prudence that it can be said without hesitation or doubt that no careful person would have been guilty of it.

A professional deserves total protection. The Indian Penal Code has taken care to ensure that people who act in good faith should not be punished. Sections 88, 92 and 370 of the **Indian Penal Code** give adequate protection to the professional and particularly medical professionals.

The Privy Council in John Oni Akerele vs. The King AIR 1943 PC 72 dealt with a case where a doctor was accused of manslaughter, reckless and negligent act and was convicted. His conviction was set aside, and it was held:

- That a doctor is not criminally responsible unless his negligence or incompetence went beyond a mere matter of compensation between subjects and showed such disregard for life and safety as to amount to a crime against the state.
- That, the degree of negligence required is gross, and that neither a jury nor a court can transform negligence of a lesser degree into gross negligence merely by giving it that appellation.
- While deciding whether the medical professional is guilty of negligence following well-known principles must be kept in view:
    - Negligence is the breach of a duty exercised by omission which a reasonable man, guided by those considerations which ordinarily regulate the conduct of human affairs, would do, or doing something which a prudent and reasonable man would not do.
    - In the realm of diagnosis and treatment there is scope for genuine difference of opinion and one professional doctor is clearly not negligent merely because his conclusion differs from that of others.
    - The medical professional is often called upon to adopt a procedure which involves higher risk, but which he honestly believes is providing greater chances of success rather than a procedure involving lesser risk but higher chances of failure.
    - The practitioners at times also have to be saved from such a class of complainants who use criminal process as a tool for pressurizing the professionals/hospitals particularly private hospitals or clinics for extracting uncalled for compensation.

In our view, the aforementioned principles must be kept in view while deciding the cases of negligence. We should not be understood to have held that doctors can never be prosecuted for negligence. It is imperative that the doctors must be able to perform their duties with a free mind. The appeal being devoid of any merit is dismissed.

CA NO. 1386/2001 BETWEEN MS. MALHOTRA VS. DR KRIPLANI MARCH 24, 2009

The Hon. SC in an appeal filed vide observed as follows: This appeal arises out of order of the NC. Brief facts are:
After the operation Priya was removed to the recovery room where she allegedly told the appellant by gestures that she was having severe pain in the chest and breathing difficulty. The postmortem report revealed the cause of death was due to peritonitis with renal failure.

The appellant filed police complaint and also before the Medical Council. The appellant could not lead the evidence of any expert in support. On consideration of the entire material on record, the commission dismissed the complaint.

The learned counsel for the appellant contended that the order of the commission is bad on facts and in law as the same is passed without proper appreciation of the evidence made in examination-in-chief before the commission which has gone un-rebutted and uncontroverted as she has not been cross-examined by the respondents. The learned counsel also contended that the appellant, despite her sincere efforts, could not get the assistance of expert doctors in support of her complaint, the commission in the interest of the appellant could have on its own summoned expert doctors from some government institutions to ascertain whether proper and necessary medical treatment was given or the doctors of Bombay Hospital were, in any manner, negligent and careless.

On opening the abdomen, it was noticed that the patient had active miliary tuberculosis. It was also noticed that the intestines were perforated. It was conclusively proved by the post-mortem examination that the sutured intestines had healed and had not developed any leak. The doctors-respondents who were involved in the treatment have established that the course of treatment pursued by them was in no way contradictory or against the treatment. Doctors had informed the patient and relatives well in time that condition was critical, and kidney transplantation could not be done.

In the backdrop of the factual situation of the present case, we have examined the principles of law laid down by this Court in Jacob Mathew vs. State of Punjab. There is a marked tendency to look for a human factor to blame for an untoward event, a tendency which is closely linked with the desire to punish. For a medical accident or failure, the responsibility may lie with the medical practitioner, and equally it may not. The purpose of holding a professional liable for his act, if negligent, is to make life safer and to eliminate the possibility of recurrence of negligence in future. To hold in favor of existence of negligence, associated with the action or inaction of a medical professional, requires an in-depth understanding of the working of a professional as also the nature of the job and of errors committed by chance, which do not necessarily involve the element of culpability.

A medical practitioner faced with an emergency ordinarily tries his best to redeem the patient out. He does not gain anything by acting with negligence or by omitting to do an act. A surgeon with shaky hands under fear of legal action can't perform a successful operation and a quivering physician can't administer the end-dose of medicine. If the hands be trembling with the dangling fear of facing a criminal prosecution in the event of failure for whatever reason.

Finally, on our independent examination of the entire material on record discussed hereinabove, we find that the Commission has properly and rightly appreciated the entire factual and legal aspects and there is no infirmity or perversity in the findings recorded which warrants any interference in this appeal. We, thus, find no merit and substance in the submissions made on behalf of the appellant.

THE HON. SC KISHAN RAO VS. NIKHIL SUPER SPECIALTY HOSPI, (8 MAR 2010) CIVIL APPEAL NO. 2641 OF 2010

It observed as follows:

The State Commission had concluded that there was no negligence. All possible care was taken; no expert opinion was produced, hence dismissed.

The appellant alleged that the tests did not show that his wife was suffering from malaria. Also it was alleged that wife was not responding, the complainant had seen some particles in the saline bottle. Patient in spite of repeated resuscitative measure patient could not be revived, declared dead.

The District Forum ordered that the complainant is entitled to compensation. The forum relied on the evidence of Dr Venkateswar Rao who categorically deposed "I have not treated the case for malaria fever". However, the death certificate disclosed that the patient died due to "cardio-respiratory arrest and malaria". The forum came to the conclusion that the patient was subjected to wrong treatment and was awarded compensation and other directions.

The State Forum found that the complainant failed to establish any negligence, and the findings of the District Forum were overturned. In the order of the State Commission, there is a casual reference to the effect that "there is also no expert opinion to state that the line of treatment adopted is wrong or negligent".

In the opinion of this court, before forming an opinion that expert evidence is necessary, the Fora under the act must come to a conclusion that the case is complicated enough to require the opinion of an expert or that the facts of the case are such that it cannot be resolved by the members of the Fora without the assistance of expert opinion. This Court makes it clear that in these matters no mechanical approach can be followed by these Fora. Each case has to be judged on its own facts. If a decision is taken that in all cases medical negligence has to be proved on the basis of expert evidence, in that event the efficacy of the remedy provided under this act will be unnecessarily burdened and in many cases such a remedy would be illusory.

Even though Bolam test "has not been uprooted" it has come under some criticism as has been noted in Jackson & Powell on Professional Negligence (Sweet & Maxwell), Fifth edition, 2002. In the context of such jurisprudential thinking, time has come for this court also to reconsider the parameters set down in Bolam test as a guide to decide cases on negligence and especially in view of Article 21 of Constitution which encompasses within its guarantee, a right to medical treatment and care. In England, the Bolam test is now considered merely a "rule of practice or of evidence. It is not a rule of law". However, as in the larger Bench of this court in Jacob Mathew vs. State of Punjab, Chief Justice Lahoti has accepted Bolam test as correctly laying down the standards for judging cases of medical negligence. We follow the same and refuse to depart from it.

Chief Justice, this Lordship held that to constitute negligence in criminal law the essential ingredient of "*mens rea*" cannot be excluded. This fundamental distinction pointed out in the unanimous three Judge Bench decision in Mathew (supra) was unfortunately not followed in the subsequent two Judge Bench of this Court in Martin F. D'Souza.

In Mathew, the direction for consulting the opinion of another doctor before proceeding with criminal investigation was confined only in cases of criminal complaint and not in respect of cases before the Consumer Fora. This distinction has been accepted in the judgment of this court in Malay Kumar Ganguly.

About the requirement of expert evidence, this court made it clear in Indian Medical Association that before the Fora under the Act both simple and complicated cases may come. The Act preserves the right of the consumer to approach the civil court in complicated cases of medical negligence for necessary relief. However, this Court held that cases in which complicated questions do not arise, the Forum can give redressal to consumers on the basis of a summary trial on affidavits. A careful reading makes the following position clear:

- There may be simple cases of negligence where expert evidence is not required.
- Those cases should be decided by the Fora on the basis of the procedure prescribed under the said Act.

- In complicated cases the parties have a right to go to the Civil Court.
- That right of the parties to go to Civil Court is preserved under Section 3.

The decision in Indian Medical Association has been further explained and reiterated in another three judge Bench decision in Dr Merchant vs. Shrinath Chaturvedi reported in (2002) 6 SCC 635. The three Judge Bench in Dr Merchant accepted the position that it has to be left to the discretion of Commission "to examine experts if required in an appropriate matter.

In PGI Chandigarh vs. Jaspal Singh, (2009) 7 SCC 330, also the Court held that mismatch in transfusion of blood resulting in death of the patient, after 40 days, is a case of medical negligence. Though the learned Judges have not used the expression *res ipsa loquitur* but a case of mismatch blood transfusion is one of *res ipsa loquitur*.

In a case where negligence is evident, the principle of *res ipsa loquitur* operates and the complainant does not have to prove anything. If the general directions in D'Souza are to be followed, then the doctrine of *res ipsa loquitur* would be redundant.

When a judgment is rendered by ignoring the provisions of the governing statute and earlier larger bench decision such decisions are rendered "Per incuriam". "Per incuriam" are decisions given in ignorance or forgetfulness of some inconsistent statutory provision or of some authority binding on the court concerned, so that some part of the decision or some step in the reasoning on which it is based, is found, on that account to be demonstrably wrong.

This Court, however, makes it clear that before the consumer Fora if any of the parties wants to adduce expert evidence, the members of the Fora by applying their mind to the facts and circumstances and the materials on record can allow the parties to adduce such evidence if it is appropriate to do so. These questions are to be judged on the facts of each case and there cannot be a mechanical or strait jacket approach. When the Fora finds that expert evidence is required, the Fora must keep in mind that an expert witness normally discharges two functions. The first duty of the expert is to explain the technical issues as clearly as possible so that it can be understood by a common man. The other function is to assist the Fora in deciding whether the acts of the practitioners or the hospital constitute negligence.

This Court further holds that State Commission and the NC fell into an error by opining to the contrary. This Court is constrained to set aside the orders passed by the State and the NC and restores the order passed by the District Forum.

THE TAMIL NADU SIDDHA MED GRADUATES ASSO, VS. SMT. LETIKA SARAN, I.P.S.

Preferred vide **Cont.P.No.775 of 2010** Dated **23.7.2010** observed.

Contempt Petition was filed alleging violation of the order of this Court passed in W.P.No.10746 of 2006 and W.P.No.9648 of 2006. The specific order was to the following effect:

There will be an order of interim injunction restraining the respondent from interfering with the professional practice of members of the association who hold valid registration certificate issued by the council to practice as registered Siddha medical practitioners as prescribed under Section 2(1) (e) of the Indian Medicine Central Council Act, 1970 as well as, as per the notifications issued under the said Act.

The grievance is that subsequent to the said order, the Principal Secretary to Government in his communication addressed to DG of police with a copy marked to the registrar of TN Homeopathy Medical Council enclosed a further communication wherein he made it clear that Institutionally qualified practitioners of Ayurveda, Siddha, and Unani who are registered in the Tamil Nadu Board of Indian Medicine are eligible to practice in the respective system with Allopathy based on the training and teaching they had in the course and that they cannot exclusively do the practice in Allopathy. In the very same communication, a further direction was issued to the following effect:

I, therefore, request you to instruct the police officers in the districts not to intervene with the practice of registered practitioners of Siddha, Ayurveda, Unani, and Naturopathy who are registered in the TN Siddha Medical Council and TN Board of Indian Medicine. If any of these doctors are exclusively doing practice in Allopathy, names of these doctors may be intimated to the council and the government for taking action against them under the TN Sidha System of Medicine (Development and Registration of Practitioners) Act 1997 and TN Board of Indian Medicine Rules.

In the reference cited, the government have stated that the police department in the course of their action against the Quacks has inspected the clinics run by the registered medical practitioners in Siddha, Ayurveda, Homeopathy, and Unani and arrested some of them as they had practiced Allopathy. The Government has informed that as per section 17(3) B of the Indian Medicine Central Council Act, 1970 the institutionally qualified practitioners of Siddha, Ayurveda, and Unani, Homeopathy are eligible to practice respective systems with modern scientific medicine including surgery and Gynecology Obstetrics, Anesthesiology, ENT and Ophthalmology, etc. based on the training and teaching.

Hence, all Commissioners of Police/IG of Police, DIG of Police, and SP are requested to instruct the police officers in the cities and districts not to intervene with the practice of registered practitioners of Siddha, Ayurveda, Unani, Homeopathy, and Naturopathy.

In the light of the said circular, it is imperative that no proceedings can be initiated against any of those registered practitioners, who are eligible to practice irrespective of the respective system also with modern medicine including surgery and gynecology Obstetrics, Anesthesiology, ENT and Ophthalmology, etc. If any action has been taken against such medical practitioners referred to above, it is needless to state that, such action should be dropped forthwith pending further orders in the writ petition.

The Hon. SC in Civil Appeal no. 1337 of 2007, Ayurvedic Doctor's Asso. vs. State of Maharashtra held that these appeals challenge the final judgment of the Bombay HC dismissing the petitions while granting the limited relief to petitioners who hold degree/diploma in electropathy or homoeoelectropathy. It was made clear that those who hold degree/diploma in Electropathy or homoeoelectropathy may practice in electropathy or electrotherapy without registration as medical practitioners but they would not be entitled to practice as or claim to be medical practitioners, doctors etc. and they were also not entitled to use any title, like Dr or any abbreviations prefixing or suffixing their names which may indicate that they are doctors or medical practitioners. Three categories of persons filed the writ petitioners before the High Court. They are as follows:

- The persons who hold either, degree/diploma of Vaidya Visharad or Ayurved Ratna or equivalent degree awarded by Hindi Sahitya Sammelan Prayag or Allahabad and other institutions whose degree and diplomas are not recognized in Schedule II of the Indian Medical Central Council Act, 1970
- The persons who claim to be practicing in Ayurved on the basis of long experience
- The persons who claim to hold degrees/diplomas in electropathy or homoeoelectropathy.

Stand of the appellants is that they were registered under the Bihar Development of Ayurvedic and Unani Systems of Medicine Act, 1951 (the "Bihar Act"). Their names were entered as registered practitioners. Though they did not hold any degree or diploma or certificate of any recognized institution they possess sufficient knowledge and skill requisite for practice of medicines, surgery and have acquired a certain amount of eminence in the medical science and also fulfill the conditions imposed by the regulations made by the Bihar Council of Ayurvedic and Unani Medicines (the "Council"). They were practicing mostly in rural places of Maharashtra. Undisputedly, the names of the appellants have been entered in the registers. The Indian Medicine Central Council Act, (the "Central Act") was introduced in 1970. Prior to that the Maharashtra Medical Practitioners Act, 1961 (the "Maharashtra Act") was in force. The appellants claim that they belong to the third category as enumerated in the Schedule.

It is submitted that Section 17 of the Central Act is of considerable relevance. Section 17 (1) refers to possession of medical qualifications included in Second, Third, and Fourth Schedules for enrolment in the State Register of Indian Medicine. It is pointed out that merely because the appellant does not possess the requisite qualification that cannot in any way disentitle them from practicing as same would be violative of Article 19 (1) (g) of the Constitution of India. Under Section 29 of the Central Act, a person whose name is included in the Central Register is entitled as a matter of right to practice in any part of India. Since the names of the appellants find place in the Bihar State Registers they are, as a matter of right, entitled to be included in the Central Register. It is submitted that the restriction imposed under the Central Act from practicing, unless names appear in the Central Register will be violative of Article 14. It is pointed out that the Central Government also felt the need for giving protection to persons like the appellants and recommendations were made.

Learned counsel for the respondent-state on the other hand submitted that there was no question of any right to practice. As contended, the educational qualifications prescribed are regulatory measures and they are reasonable restrictions.

BIHAR ACT

Persons entitled to be registered: Every person possessing any of the qualifications specified in the schedule shall subject to the provisions contained in this Act, and on payment of the prescribed fees be entitled to have his name entered in the register subject to such conditions as the council may impose.

MAHARASHTRA ACT

"Registered practitioner" means a practitioner whose name is for the time being entered in the register.

Registration of Practitioners

- As soon as may be after the appointed day, the registrar shall prepare and maintain thereafter a register of practitioners of Indian Medicine for the state.
- The register shall be divided into three parts, namely:
  - Part I containing the names of practitioners who possess any of the qualifications specified in the Schedule.
  - Part II containing the names of practitioners, whose names were included before the 1st day of October 1976.

- Part III containing the names of practitioners, who on the 30th September 1976 were enlisted practitioners and who are on that day deemed to have become registered practitioners under Section 18.

Every registered practitioner shall be given a certificate of registration in the form prescribed by rules. The practitioner shall display the certificate of registration in a conspicuous place in his dispensary, clinic or place of practice.

Section 33: Prohibition of Medical Practice by Persons Not Registered

Notwithstanding anything contained in any law for the time being in force or in any judgment, decree, or order of any Court, no person other than a medical practitioner whose name is entered in:

- The register maintained under this Act; or
- The register or the list prepared and maintained under the Bombay Homoeopathic and Biochemic Practitioners Act, 1959 (Bom. XII of 1960) or under any other law for the time being in force in relation to the qualifications and registration of Homoeopathic or Biochemic Practitioners in any part of the State; or
- The register prepared and maintained under the Maharashtra Medical Council Act, 1965; (Mah XLVI of 1965), or
- The Indian Medical Register prepared and maintained under the Indian Medical Council Act, 1956 (CII of 1956).

Section 37: Liberty to Practice in Rural Areas

Notwithstanding anything contained in this Chapter, a person may practice medicine in any rural area:

- If he has commenced practice in any village in the said area prior to a date on which a practitioner registered under the Bombay Medical Act, 1912 or under the Bombay Medical Practitioners' Act, 1938, (or any law corresponding thereto) or under the Bombay Homoeopathic Act, 1951, (or other law in relation to the qualifications and registration of Homoeopathic or Biochemic Practitioners) for the time being in force, has commenced, and is in regular practice of medicine in that village, and
- So long as he continues to practice in that village as his principal place of practice.

CENTRAL ACT

"Central Register of Indian Medicine" means the register maintained by the Central Council under this Act.

So far as the claim that once the name is included in the register of a particular State there is a right to practice in any part of the country is not tenable on the face of Section 29 of the Central Act. The right to practice is restricted in the sense that only if the name finds place in the Central Register, then the question of practicing in any part of the country arise.

The conditions under Section 23 of the Central Act are cumulative. Since the appellants undisputedly do not possess recognized qualifications as defined in Section 2(1)(h) their names cannot be included in the Central Register. As a consequence, they cannot practice in any part of India because of non-inclusion of their names in the Central Register. It is for the State to see that there is a need for having qualifications in terms of Second and Fourth Schedule. In terms of Article 19(6) of the Constitution, reasonable restriction can always be put on the exercise of right under Article 19(g).

As far as the degrees and diplomas of non-recognized institutions are concerned, this Court had the occasion to deal with the issue in Delhi Pradesh Registered Medical Practitioners vs. Director of Health, Delhi Services [1997 (11) SCC 687]. It was interalia observed as follows.

"We are, however, unable to accept such contention. Sub-section (3) of Section 17 of the Indian Medicine Central Council Act, 1970, only envisages that where before the enactment of the said Indian Medicine Central Act, 1970 on the basis of requisite qualification which was then recognized, a person got himself registered as practitioner in the disciplines contemplated under the said Act or in the absence of any requirement for registration such person had been practicing for 5 years or intended to be registered and was also entitled to be registered, the right of such person to practice in the discipline concerned including the privileges of a registered practitioner stood protected even though such practitioner did not possess requisite qualification under the said Act of 1970. In the Objects and Reasons, it was mentioned.

"The Committee is of the opinion that the existing rights and privileges of practitioners of Indian medicine should be given adequate safeguards. The Committee in order to achieve the object, have added three new paragraphs to sub-section (3) protecting: (i) the rights to practice of those practitioners of Indian medicine who may not, under the proposed legislation, possess a recognized qualification subject to the condition that they are already enrolled on a state Register of Indian medicine on the date of commencement of this Act; (ii) the privileges conferred on the practitioners of Indian Medicine enrolled on a State Register, under any law in force in that State; and (iii) the right to practice in a State of those practitioners who have been practicing Indian medicine in that state for not less than 5 years where no register of Indian medicine was maintained earlier."

We may also indicate here that what constitutes proper education and requisite expertise for a practitioner in Indian medicine, must be left to the proper authority having requisite knowledge in the subject.

Above being the position, the High Court was justified in dismissing the writ petitions. However, the prosecution was lodged in terms of Section 33 for alleged violation of provisions of the Maharashtra Act. Considering the peculiar facts of the case, we direct that the prosecution shall not be continued in respect of the past infractions. However, from today onwards, it is open to the authorities to act as provided in the Statute. The appeals are dismissed subject to the directions relating to the prosecution.

PARMANAND KATARA VS. UNION OF INDIA 28 AUGUST, 1989

The Hon. SC reported in **AIR 2039, SCR (3) 997** held as follows:

The petitioner, a human right activist, concerning the death of a scooterist states that the person was taken to the nearest hospital, but the doctors refused to attend; told that he be taken to hospital, authorized to handle medicolegal cases; and the victim succumbed. The petitioner prayed the directions be issued to the Union of India that every injured citizen should instantaneously be given medical aid to preserve life and thereafter the procedural criminal law should be allowed to operate in order to avoid negligent death, and in the event of breach of such direction, apart from any action that may be taken for negligence, appropriate compensation should be admissible.

It was stated by government that there was no provision in the Indian Penal Code, Criminal Procedure Code, or the Motor Vehicles Act, etc., which prevented doctors from promptly attending seriously injured and accident cases before the arrival of police. The Court held: (1) Article 21 of the Constitution casts the obligation on the State to preserve life; (2) There can be no second opinion that preservation of human life is of paramount importance; (3) Every doctor whether at a government hospital or otherwise has the professional obligation to extend his services with due expertize for protecting life; (4) No law or state action can intervene to avoid/delay the discharge of the paramount obligation cast upon medical profession. The obligation being total, absolute and paramount, laws of procedure whether in statute or otherwise which would interfere with the discharge of this obligation cannot be sustained and must, therefore, give way.

The members of the legal profession, our law courts and everyone concerned will also keep in mind that the medical professional should not be unnecessarily harassed for interrogation or for any other formality and should not be dragged at the police station and it should be avoided as far as possible.

Law courts will not summon a medical professional to give evidence unless the evidence is necessary and even if he is summoned, attempts should be made to see that the people in this profession are not made to wait and waste time unnecessarily.

Obligations to the sick: Though a physician is not bound to treat each and every one asking his services except in emergencies for the sake of humanity and the noble traditions, he should not only be ever ready to respond to the calls of the sick and the injured, but should be mindful of the high character of his mission/responsibility, he should never forget that the health and the lives of those entrusted to his care depend on his skill and attention.

It is also submitted that the formalities under the CrPC or any local laws should not stand in the way of attending an injured. The doctor attending such patients should be indemnified under law from any action by the government/police authorities/any person for not waiting for legal formalities before giving relief as a doctor would be doing his professional duty for which he has taken oath.

Members of the public escorting the injured to the nearest hospital are reluctant to disclose their name or identity as he is detained for eliciting information and may be required to be called for evidence. Similarly, the private practicing doctors are harassed by the police and are, therefore, reluctant to accept the roadside casualty. The Committee under the Chairmanship of the Director-General of health services took the following decisions:

Whenever any medicolegal case is attended by the hospital, the medical officer on duty should inform the duty constable, and should start the required treatment. It will be the duty of the constable to inform the police station concerned or higher police functionaries for further action.

We, therefore, have no hesitation in assuring the persons in the medical profession that these apprehensions, even if have some foundation, should not prevent them from discharging their duty to save a human life and to do all that is necessary. We have no hesitation in saying that it is expected of the members of the legal profession, which is the other honorable profession to honor the persons in the medical profession and see that they are not called to give evidence so long as it is not necessary. It is also expected that where the facts are so clear it is expected that necessary harassment of the members of the medical profession either by way of requests for adjournments or by cross examination should be avoided.

RUNNING CLINIC FROM RESIDENCE NOT A COMMERCIAL ACTIVITY: DELHI HIGH COURT, WEDNESDAY, JULY 04, 2012

Running a clinic from one's residence cannot be labeled a commercial activity, the Delhi High Court has said. Quashing a criminal case against Dr DV Chug, for running a clinic from his house, Justice said. "The professional establishment of a doctor cannot come within the definition of commercial activity. The word 'profession' used to be confined to the three learned professions: Church, Medicine, and Law. There is a fundamental distinction between the professional activities and commercial activities". According to the MCD, running of a doctor's clinic from the residential premises is currently permissible and is not an offence. That the Owner/Occupier of the Property, has changed the use of the property from residential to commercial by running clinic, without written permission of MCD. The learned counsel submitted that the petitioner is now 80 years as on date and the said clinic was closed down 10 years back. Learned counsel has relied upon Dr Devendra M. Surti vs. The State of Gujarat: AIR 1969 SC 63 wherein the Apex Court has observed as under: "Under Section 2(8) of the Act an 'establishment' is defined as meaning 'a shop, commercial establishment, residential hotel, restaurant, eating at house, theatre, or other place of public amusement or entertainment to which this Act applies". It is clear, therefore, that legislature has taken care separately to define each one of the categories of 'the establishments mentioned in Section 2(8) of the Act. It is true that Section 2(4) of the Act has used words of very wide import and grammatically it may include even a consulting room where a doctor examines his patients with the help of a solitary nurse or attendant. But, in our opinion, in the matter of construing the language of Section 2(4) of the Act we must adopt the principle of *noscitur a sociis*. This rule means that, when two or more words which are susceptible to analogous meaning are coupled together, they are understood to be used in their cognate sense. "Associated words take their meaning from one another under the doctrine of *noscitur a sociis*." We are therefore of the opinion that the professional establishment of a doctor cannot come within the definition of Section 2(4) of the Act unless the activity carried out was also commercial in character. The line of demarcation may vary from time to time. It has now, I think, a wider meaning. There is a fundamental distinction therefore between a professional activity and an activity of a commercial character.

Coming to the second submission, after the coming into operation of any of the plans in a zone no person shall use or permit to be used and land or building in that zone otherwise than in conformity with such plan. On the other hand, counsel for MCD has fairly conceded that as on today the running of a doctor's clinic from the residential premises is permissible and is not an offence. More so, in the case Parivar Sewa Sansthan has held that running of "Nursing Home" in residential premises does not come under the commercial activity.

THE HON. SC IN THE CASE OF, STATE OF GUJARAT VS. DR P. A. BHATT

Preferred vide **Civil Appeal Nos. 8553-8557 of 2014 (on April 26, 2023)** observed as follows: A bench of Gujrat High Court held that doctors possessing a degree of BAMS (Bachelor of Ayurved Medicine and Surgery) should be treated at par with the doctors holding MBBS degrees.

The Division Bench of the High Court dismissed all the intra-court appeals holding; (i) that both MBBS and non-MBBS doctors form part of the same cadre and hence no discrimination is permissible within the cadre on the basis of educational qualifications; and (ii) that the non-MBBS doctors were also discharging the same duties and functions discharged by MBBS doctors and were even manning primary health centers independently and that therefore they were entitled to equal pay.

We must remember the fundamental distinction between: (i) the issue of law that equal work entails equal pay; and (ii) the issue of fact as to whether two categories of employees are performing equal work or not?

The recommendations of Tikku Pay Commission for enhancement of the scales of pay were *per se* applicable only to MBBS doctors; *that* the revision of scales of pay in favor of Allopathy doctors was warranted by the perennial shortage of Allopathy doctors; *that* the State Government had to fulfill its Constitutional obligation of providing adequate healthcare infrastructure to the citizens.

It is contended by the learned counsel for the respondents that both Allopathy doctors and AYUSH doctors are appointed to the post of Medical Officer falling in Class-II of Gujarat Medical Services; *that* once persons with different qualifications are appointed to one unified cadre with a common pay scale and governed by one set of rules, then at a later stage, the Government cannot make a classification.

It is thus clear that in the field of rendering professional services at any rate the principle of equal pay for equal work would be inapplicable. In Shyam Babu Verma vs. Union of India, Supreme Court clarified that though *"...the nature of work may be more or less the same, but scale of pay may vary based on academic qualifications or experience which justifies the classification...."* Therefore, it is clear that the classification based upon educational qualification is not violative of Articles 14 and 16 of the Constitution.

In this writ petition filed by them, it was claimed by the respondents herein that they were doing the same work as was done by other medical officers holding MBBS degrees and they also claimed that even as per the job-chart of the General Duty Medical Officers, the duties performed by both categories of doctors are the same. The Government filed an affidavit before the High Court contending *inter alia:*

- While General Hospitals and Government Hospitals come under the Medical Services Department, PHCs, CHCs and Government dispensaries come under the Public Health Department.
- With respect to medical services, doctors with MD/MS or postgraduate degree/diploma are appointed to Class-I specialist cadre.
- Homoeopathy doctors are appointed to Class-III posts;
- Ayurved doctors are appointed to Class-II posts
- There are lot of differences between the duties and responsibilities discharged by both these categories of doctors.

Allopathy doctors are required to perform emergency duties and to provide trauma care. By the very nature of the science that they practice and with the advancement of science and modern medical technology, the emergency duty that Allopathy doctors are capable of performing and the trauma care that they are capable of providing, cannot be performed by Ayurved doctors.

Therefore, we have no doubt that every alternative system of medicine may have its pride of place in history. But today, the practitioners of indigenous systems of medicine do not perform complicated surgical operations. A study of Ayurved does not authorize them to perform these surgeries. Therefore, even while recognizing the importance of Ayurved doctors and the need to promote alternative/indigenous systems of medicine, we cannot be oblivious of the fact that both categories of doctors are certainly not performing equal work to be entitled to equal pay.

THE HIGH COURT GUJARAT IN ASSOCIATION OF PATHOLOGIST VS. SECRETARY, HEALTH DEPT.

Judgment dated 17/09/2010 categorically held as here under:
A prayer was made to ensure that no such laboratory is allowed to operate without qualified pathologists. Pathologists' association preferred the writ with a grievance that unqualified laboratory technicians, claiming to be qualified pathologists, are running various pathological laboratories. Pathologists' association, who are against the practice of laboratory technicians in running pathological laboratory, the learned counsel would contend that all these persons would not possess requisite degree and they cannot be said to be registered qualified pathologists nor they can claim to be laboratory technicians. They are unscrupulous practitioners who are carrying out various tests of pathology and are giving unauthorized diagnosis. On behalf of the aforesaid petitioners, it would be contended that mere possessing of a degree or post graduate degree like MSc (Biochemistry), MSc (Microbiology), etc., would not render the person eligible for registration under the Indian Medical Council Act, 1956 nor they can practice in the pathological field. At the best, they can assist the qualified MBBS pathologists.

Stand of Medical Laboratory Technicians

The Association of Private Pathology Laboratories and other petitioners have taken a similar plea. The syllabus for the trade of medical laboratory technician (pathology) is designed by the Government of India, and the course is offered by several universities. They perform a full range of laboratory tests, and report laboratory findings to pathologists and other physicians. On behalf of the petitioners, the learned counsel would contend that under the law anyone can own a laboratory and there is nothing which restricts setting up of a medical or clinical laboratory to a medical practitioner whose name has been entered in the register maintained under the Indian Medical Council Act or the Gujarat Medical Council Act. A laboratory can be set up even by a company or be run by qualified professionals.

The learned counsel appearing on behalf of the laboratory technicians contended that the recognition of Gujarat Medical Council for running a pathological laboratory is not essential. There is no law in the state of Gujarat nor there any central legislation which insists on additional qualification in pathology as a precondition for owning or running a private laboratory.

Further stand taken by the laboratory technicians is that they do not fall within the purview of the Indian Medical Council Act, 1956 and, therefore, the provisions of the said act are not applicable to the medical laboratory technicians. The said act prohibits a person other than a medical practitioner enrolled in the register maintained under the Act from practicing medicine. It does not prohibit running a medical laboratory.

The work being performed by the technicians cannot be termed as practicing modern scientific medicine. Thus, the work being done by the members of the Association of Medical Laboratory Technicians is essentially a prediagnosis work and the report prepared is an aid in diagnosis and treatment. Therefore, it cannot be said that the members of the association are practicing modern scientific medicine and the bar contained in Section 15(2) would not be attracted to the laboratory technicians.

Discussion and Conclusion

Section 2(f) of the Indian Medical Council Act, 1956, defines "medicine" as modern scientific medicine in all its branches. In Annexure I to the said regulations, the list of higher courses in medical subjects have been listed. Further, the notice to the subsequent paragraph specifically provides that non-medical persons should not be admitted to postgraduate course in Pathology. Further in Group "C" against item No. 10, Clinical Hematology which is a super specialty, it is specifically provided that the candidate must possess the postgraduate degree in Pathology, that means, it talks of a MBBS with Pathology or MD with Biology.

It is also informed that the committee appointed by the state government has also submitted a report which supports the case of the Association of Pathologists. The learned counsel appearing on behalf of the Gujarat Medical Council would rely on a decision of the Madhya Pradesh High Court in the case of Smt. Kamla Patel vs. State of MP, reported in AIR 2007 MP 1925, wherein the Court decided the issue in question and held:

The aforesaid analysis of the provisions of the law prescribing the profession or technical qualifications necessary for the practice of medicine and the law prescribing the qualifications for running a pathology laboratory would show that laboratory technicians registered as a paramedical practitioner under the *Adhiniyam*, 2000, cannot sign or authenticate any pathological test/report or certificate and he can only assist the pathologist registered in the State Medical Register as a medical practitioner in carrying out the technical tests in the Pathology laboratory. In other words, such certificate or test report can only be signed and authenticated by a pathologist having the required qualification such as MBBS, MD or other degrees as mentioned in the Act, 1956.

The Supreme Court in the case of Mukhtiar Chand (Dr) vs. State of Punjab & Haryana, while examining the provisions of Section 15(2) of the Indian Medical Council Act, 1956 held that—a harmonious reading of Section 15 of the 1956 Act and Section 17 of the 1970 Act leads to the conclusion that there is no scope for a person enrolled on the State Register of Indian Medicine or the Central Register of Indian Medicine to practice modern scientific medicine in any of its branches unless that person is also enrolled on a State Medical Register within the meaning of the 1956 Act.

It is a different thing that a pathologist, registered with the Medical Council of India, can take help from a laboratory technician, who has the knowledge to analyze human fluid samples using techniques available, such as manual white blood cell differentials, analysis by a microscope and advanced analytical equipment. We accordingly hold that the laboratory technicians being not pathologists cannot run any laboratory independently. They cannot directly give any report to any patient or any other individual, or to any institution or practicing doctor, without the authentication of the same by the pathologist registered with the medical council. Though it is open to any person or institute to run a pathology laboratory, but no report can be issued without the signature or counter signature of the practicing pathologist recognized by the medical council. The respondents are directed to ensure that no laboratory is run by any unqualified person or institute having no recognized pathologists. However, if such pathological laboratory is run by a pathologist, or if such pathological laboratory engages a pathologist, the respondents may allow such laboratory to run.

THE MUMBAI HIGH COURT (NAGPUR BENCH) IN WRIT PETITION NO.1936 OF 2020 HOSPITALS' ASSOCIATION NAGPUR VS. GOVERNMENT OF MAHARASHTRA

It decided that for Covid Patients treated at any of the Hospital/Nursing homes/Clinics covered under this notification across Maharashtra, rates shall not be more than rates prescribed in Annexure-C. For non-Covid patients' rates will be as per Annexure-A read with Annexure-B. Many Healthcare Providers have agreements/ understandings with various Third-Party Administrators (TPAs) pertaining to package rates for different treatments. Such Healthcare Providers having different package rates for similar treatment with different TPAs shall provide the treatment at the lowest package rate prevailing among different TPAs in its facility. Healthcare Providers shall display at prominent place the details of rates applicable as per this notification. It is the duty of the Healthcare Provider concerned to explain to the patient/ relatives of the patient details of all types of charges. If any of the items mentioned here are used for more than one patient, then the prescribed cost may be divided amongst such patients.

The provisions don't empower the State Government to regulate the recoverable rates by the private hospitals for providing medical services to Non-COVID patients. The fundamental right to practice any profession or to carry on any occupation, trade or business under Article 19(1)(g) of the Constitution includes the right to charge rates, reasonable, proportionate to or commensurate with the nature and quality of the medical treatment and allied services rendered to non-COVID patients, which may differ from hospital to hospital. We hold that the State Legislature is, therefore, not competent either to frame any law in that respect or to issue any notification regulating the rates chargeable by the private hospitals to non-COVID patients.

We, therefore, hold that the impugned directions made applicable to non-COVID patients, cannot be treated to have been issued in exercise of the executive power under Articles 162 and 166 read with Article 13(3)(a) of the Constitution of India. All the Government Hospitals are blocked by COVID-19, as result, the non-COVID patients entitled to free medical treatment in Government Hospitals are required to be admitted in the private hospitals, which are run on commercial basis. It is held that the State Government is not competent to issue impugned directions in respect of non-COVID patients.

■ Some Other Case Laws

The National Consumer Disputes Redressal Commission New Delhi in Revision Petition No. 887 of 2012, 14th May, 2012 held as follows:

The main question which falls for consideration is what is the effect of a medical practitioner, who is an Ayurveda Practitioner but treats the patient in allopathic stream? Late Shri Pandurang Gamare, approached Dr R.R. Singh for the pain below waist in both legs. According to the complaint, the respondent informed that the illness of her husband was serious and may suffer an attack of paralysis. During the night the patient was left under the care of compounder. The compounder was asked to inform the doctor and call him immediately. The compounder did not call the revisionist and himself gave the saline and medicine prescribed. A police complaint was lodged. The act debars the doctors dealing in Ayurveda from indulging in allopathic stream prescribing allopathic drugs. The petitioner was given the benefit of Section 4 of Probation of Offenders Act, 1958 and a compensation in the sum of ₹25,000/- was also awarded.

The complaint filed was dismissed by the District Forum. However, the State Commission reversed the order and directed the petitioner to pay compensation in the sum of ₹ 7 lakhs to the complainant. Aggrieved by that order, the present revision petition has been filed.

Instead of touching the heart of the problem, the learned counsel just skirted it. First of all, the petitioner should not have admitted him in his clinic. He should have advised the patient to move to some renowned hospital. It is difficult to fathom as to how and why drugs like Betnesol, Decadron and Neurobion were prescribed without consulting an allopathic doctor. It is difficult to understand as to how the petitioner switched over to allopathy without any knowledge of the same. His very action smacks of negligence. A Doctor is not supposed to play with the lives of people for his personal gain.

Mumbai, June 13: Observing that doctors are harassed by the authorities under the pretext of not following norms set up for imposing a ban on sex determination tests, the Bombay High Court has quashed a complaint in a lower court against a doctor couple in Maharashtra.

The Court noted that the Additional Director Health Service and appropriate authority has already noticed that in some cases even if flimsy mistakes were committed by doctors, the local appropriate authorities are sealing machines and prosecuting them. "It is also recognized that this kind of action amounts to harassment of medical practitioners", observed Justice AV Nirgude. "In my earlier orders, I have very specifically opined that since the provisions of this Act are very strict, the appropriate authority before taking action against the medical practitioner must act meticulously". Dr Alka Gite and Dr Anant Gite, were charged with offences under Sections 23(1), 25 and 29 of Preconception and Prenatal Diagnostic Techniques Act.

On 16th June, 2011, the appropriate authority visited the clinic, inspected the record and found that the doctors had not filled up Form "F" which is mandatory. A *panchnama* was recorded, "incomplete" forms "F" was seized and two sonography machines were sealed. A notice was also sent to show-cause why action should not be taken against them.

The petitioners replied that they had completely filled up form "F" and had not contravened any provision under the act. The only allegation made against them was that they had not filled up forms "F" completely. In order to verify the correctness of this allegation, the court perused the forms and found that the forms are completely filled up. Only items which were left untouched were item No. 9 and 13. The court noted that item 9 required information regarding history of genetic or medical disease in the family. In no such form in question this information was filled up. Normally, a patient is referred for sonography test to examine the health of the fetus. In this background if the information regarding a patient's genetic disease in the family is not mentioned in item 9, it clearly indicates that there was no genetic medical disease in the family of the patient, the judge noted. "If the form is otherwise completely filled up, the applicants would not have left this item incomplete. The nonfilling of this item thus is not contravention. It is not even lapse or inadvertence".

Item 13 is clearly made applicable wherever laboratory test is recommended. The asterisk mark on the word "recommended" clearly suggests that this item has to be filled up by a laboratory and not by ultrasound clinic. Thus, the allegation that these two items were left incomplete would not attract contravention of Sections 5 or 6 of the Act.

2/9/2013 Mumbai: It is not mandatory for the Maharashtra Medical Council (MMC) to suspend a doctor if a court frames charges against him/her, said the Bombay high court while quashing the suspension of two orthopedic surgeons under the Preconception and Prenatal Diagnostic Techniques Act. Framing of charges by a court does not require the Maharashtra Medical Council to compulsorily suspend a doctor.

A division bench was hearing petitions challenging an MMC's order suspending them for 5 years under Section 23(2) of the Act after a magistrate framed charges against them. Following a sting operation and complaints of sex determination tests being carried out, a civic health officer, seized sonography machines. The doctors said they own the premises and gynecologist Dr Ivan Rocha, who conducted the tests on his portable sonography machine, was a consultant.

The judges observed that the consequences of suspension are "extremely drastic". "If the legislature intended the suspension to continue till the case is disposed of, it would have provided for the same in clear, express terms," the judges noted. MMC's advocate said the doctors were suspended without an inquiry or giving them an opportunity to defend themselves in view of an October 22 ruling that held there was no need for an inquiry to delay action.

The judges said Section 23(2) provides that in the event of charges being framed under the Act, the appropriate authority shall report the same to the MMC for taking necessary action, including suspension of registration. They said the Section does not state that upon reporting the fact of charges being framed, the MMC must suspend the registration, but on the contrary, that it must "initiate the process for considering suspending the registered medical practitioner". They said if the MMC finds that continuation of a doctor on its register is detrimental to public interest, it can issue a suspension order and follow it by an inquiry to consider whether or not to continue the suspension. The HC told the MMC to initiate proceedings to consider whether the registration "ought to be suspended and for what period".

The National Commission in Revision Petition No. 2737 of 2013, held as follows:
The complainant admitted his wife for her delivery was the government hospital, Rajapalayam. The complainant was informed that caesarian delivery to be conducted. The OP instead of attending Thangam attended another delivery. Therefore, the complainant's wife was taken to operation theatre at 11-25 AM who gave birth to a female child and subsequently died at 12:05 PM. Hence, alleging death due to negligence due to delay in the delivery. The district forum dismissed the complaint with observations that the complainant is not a consumer. The state commission held that the complainant is a consumer. The case was remanded back to District Forum for specific clarification as word "ES" mentioned in a case sheet whether "Elective Surgery" or "Emergency Surgery".

"On perusal of the case records, was found that on the date of admission of the complainant, was recorded as DIL, i.e., dangerously ill. But the operation performed belatedly. We are unable to find any reason for any immediate steps taken by the opposite parties when it is noted as DIL. Though they state that surgery was needed the complainant's wife is an Elective one, there is no explanation on the part of the opposite parties about the recording as "Dangerously ill". Thus, irresistibly we reiterate that the opposite parties have utterly failed to prove themselves. Hence, we find no merit in this appeal."

Counsel for the parties heard. The application moved by petitioner for condonation of delay did not specify the sufficient cause for delay. The petitioner explained the delay in "para 3 of application as:

I submit that I was under impression that the government will file an appeal before this Hon'ble Commission. But it did not do so and on the contrary, the medical officer directed me to pay the compensation amount. Therefore, I decided to appeal against the State Commission order. Hence, there is a delay of 60 days in filing the present appeal.

In our view, it is the right time to inform all the government bodies, their agencies and instrumentalities that unless they have reasonable and acceptable explanation for the delay and there was Bonafide effort, there is no need to accept the usual explanation that the file was kept pending for several months/years due to considerable degree of procedural red-tape in the process. The government departments are under a special obligation to ensure that they perform their duties with diligence and commitment. Condonation of delay is an exception and should not be used as an anticipated benefit for government departments. Considering the fact that there was no proper explanation offered by the department for the delay except mentioning of various dates, according to us, the department has miserably failed to give any acceptable and cogent reasons sufficient to condone such a huge delay.

Furthermore, it is necessary to explain that the C.P. Act envisages summary procedure. The Commission cannot adopt an excessive liberal approach which would defeat the very purpose of the C.P. Act. The case is squarely barred by time.

Now, considering the petition on merits; It is quite surprise that the why OP delayed elective cesarean Surgery despite it was recorded as "Dangerously ill" on admission slip. Also, the death of patient within 30 minutes of elective surgery creates many doubts upon the conduct and treatment by OP. As even though it was a Govt. hospital OP should have advised the postmortem for the cause of death. Hence, the entirety appears to be deficiency in service by the OP.

It is a fact that in present days the Hippocratic Oath is at stake; Medical Ethics are being violated by some medical professionals have led to demoralized health services for the poor who lost their precious life....!!

Hence, with all forgoing discussions we are of considered view that, this revision petition sans the merit as well there is huge delay which cannot be condoned. We dismiss this revision petition with modification of orders as the OP is directed to pay ₹50,000/- with interest @ 9% p.a. from the date of filing the complaint. In addition, we impose punitive cost of ₹50,000/- to be paid to complainant.

The Gujarat Medical Council Challenges MCI's Power to Take Punitive Action against Doctors:

September 13, 2013, challenging the administrative powers of apex regulatory body of doctors in India, the Gujarat Medical Council (GMC) has come in full support of Dr Ketan Desai on being appointed as the head of urology despite the fact that suspension of his medical license is still in force. In a categorical letter to the Medical Council of India (MCI), Gujarat Medical Council has questioned the powers of MCI to take disciplinary action not only against Dr Desai but also against any doctor who is registered with any state medical council in India.

The Gujarat government reinstated Dr Desai on which the MCI asked for clarifications from the Gujarat Medical Council. In a staunch reply, the Gujarat Medical Council said, "MCI also does not have the jurisdiction to issue any direction to any State Medical Council for suspending the registration of any medical practitioner enrolled/registered with any State Medical Council".

The situation has led to some confusion over the division of powers between State Medical Councils and the MCI. I understand that in the last two-three cases the Supreme Court and High Courts have interpreted that MCI can take actions against erring doctors, but they were only special cases. It does not make an umbrella rule for every case related to cancellation of license by State Medical Councils. The point has also been established in the Gujarat Medical Council's letter which reads, "In any case it is found to be conclusive position with MCI and continuing to be so till date that registration of a registered medical practitioner shall not be suspended by MCI until a registered medical practitioner is "convicted" by competent court of law."

Giving his opinion on the controversy, a former member of the MCI Board of Governors, "Ideally if MCI has debarred Dr Ketan Desai, Gujarat Medical Council should have respected its decision. It's true that State Medical Councils are separate from Medical Council of India and legally they can reinstate any state registered doctor and also approach MCI over any indiscipline shown by a doctor. But the Gujarat Government should have consulted MCI and its consent should be taken before making such a decision as MCI is national regulating body."

(http://www.indiamedicaltimes.com/2013/09/13/gujarat-medical-council-challenges-mcis-power-to-take-punitive-action-against-doctors/)

The High Court of Kerala, Crl. MC. No. 1394 of 2013 judgment dated **23rd July, 2013** held as hereunder:

This is a petition filed Section 482 of the Code of Criminal Procedure seeking to have final report quashed as far as the petitioner. Smt. Lakshmi Santhosh was carrying at the relevant time. It appears that she felt a slight abdominal pain and therefore, they decided to have a routine checkup. As she was coming out of the hospital, she was informed that she should meet the surgeon also. The surgeon, after the examination, found nothing wrong but he, by way of abundant caution, asked her to consult the gynecologist also. She was administered an ampicillin injection which resulted in causing acute respiratory problems; a condition medically described anaphylactic shock. She was given efcorlin and dexona injection and as the situation did not improve, gave diazepam injection. That worsened the condition into a morbid stage. She was asked to be shifted to hospital which had ventilator facility. A short while thereafter, the doctor informed the relatives that she was no more. During investigation, it was revealed that the doctors who had attended and treated were grossly negligent, the case sheet was not properly maintained, and she was administered medicines without ascertaining her medical history and finally that there was gross negligence in taking necessary steps.

An expert committee of the doctors constituted gave an opinion that the cause of death could be ascertained after the final opinion of the forensic department. The committee formed the opinion that there was no negligence on the part of the doctors who had attended the patient. Subsequently, a medical board was constituted under the Convenorship of Director of Health Services which had opined that there was collective negligence.

After reaching hospital, the patient was taken to the ICU and the petitioner had occasion to see the patient in the ICU. Knowing fully well that the patient would not survive or that the patient was already dead, he chose to inform the relatives of the patient that she would get very well soon. This deliberate false statement by the petitioner shows his complicity.

This case reveals yet another story of carelessness, indifference and callous attitude displayed by the doctors. It is true that several committees were constituted, and all have come to the conclusion that there is no wilful negligence. However, the report of the apex body already made mention of says that there was collective negligence of the doctors. Surprisingly enough, it does not mention about the role played by each of the doctors and the credibility or correctness of the action taken by the respective doctors at the respective moments. The Consumer Disputes Redressal Forum passed order wherein it was found that the first and the second accused herein were negligent and awarded ₹15,00,000/- as compensation.

The fact remains that the death certificate was issued by the petitioner. The materials now before the court show that the petitioner was called at a time when the patient had gone into a morbid condition and there is no material or any report of any committee suggesting that the petitioner had omitted to do something which he could have done to save the petitioner, or he had done something which ought not to have been done. There is nothing to show that the patient could have been managed in such a critical condition by any method except putting the patient on ventilator.

There is an allegation that proper test dose was not taken before ampicillin injection was given. It is surprising to note that the apex body was very casual in its approach and seems to be influenced by the "birds of the same feather syndrome" and was keen to exonerate the doctors who had actually attended to and treated the patient.

The next question that arises for consideration is whether this court will be justified in the facts and circumstances of the case in quashing the proceedings against the petitioner. The power of this court under Section 482 of CrPC is indeed very wide. However, that power is to be exercised only sparingly and in exceptional circumstances. In fact, a perusal of Section 482 of CrPC would show that its scope is considerably limited. The said provision reads as follows: that the power under the said section is to be exercised under three contingencies, they are: (i) to give effect to an order under the Code, (ii) to prevent abuse of the process of court, and (iii) to secure the ends of justice. Among the three, (ii) and (iii) work in both ways. While they deal with the prevention of harassment of innocent persons, they also ensure that a just cause is not thrown out. Even though the power is wide, it is circumscribed by self-imposed restrictions. Normally, the courts will not interfere at the stage of investigation or filing of charge unless there are compelling circumstances. Usually, in matters provided by the Code, the inherent powers are not invoked. One can only say that as per the materials now available, there is nothing to show that the petitioner had contributed in any manner to the death. In fact, the defacto complainant does not seem to have much grievance against him. Her wrath is directed against the first and second accused. One must remember that she is a nurse with vast experience.

Lord Denning said in **Roe vs. Minister of Health (1954) 2 QB 66):** "One final word. These two men have suffered; such a terrible consequence that there is a natural feeling that they should be compensated. However, we should be doing a disservice to the community at large if we are to impose liability on hospitals and doctors for everything that happens to go wrong".

In **Hatcher vs. Black** [(1954) Times, 2nd July] Lord Denning explained the law on the subject of negligence against doctors and hospitals in the following words: "Before I consider the individual facts, In the case of accident on the road, there ought not to be any accident if everyone used proper care; and the same applies in a factory; but in a hospital when a person who is ill goes in for treatment, there is always some risk, 'no matter what care is used'. Every surgical operation involves risks. It would be wrong, and indeed bad law, to say that simply because a misadventure or mishap occurred, the hospital and the doctors are thereby liable. It would be disastrous to the community if it were so. It would means that, a doctor; examining a patient or a surgeon operating at a table instead of getting on with his work, would be forever looking over shoulder to see if someone was coming up with a dagger. His professional reputation is as dear to him as his body, perhaps more so, and an action for negligence can wound his reputation as severely as a dagger can his body, you must not, therefore, find him negligent simply because something happens to go wrong; if, for instance, one of the risks inherent in a operation actually takes place or some complication ensues which lessens or takes away the benefits that were hoped for, or if in a matter of opinion he makes an error of judgment. You should only find him guilty of negligence when he falls short of the standard of a reasonably skillful medical man, in short, when he is deserving of censure for negligence than it is a medical man who is deserving of censure" Equally pertinent are the observations of Lord Denning in Roe's case [(1954)2 QB 66] to the following effect: "It is so easy to be wise after the event and to condemn as negligence that which was only a misadventure. We ought always to be on our guard against it, especially in cases against hospitals and doctors. Medical science has conferred great benefit on mankind, but these benefits are attended by considerable risk. Every surgical operation is attended by risk. We cannot take the benefit without taking the risk. Every advance in technique is also attended by risk. Doctors, like the rest of us, have to learn by experience; and experience often teaches in a hard way. Something goes wrong and shows up a weakness and then it is put right. That is just what happens here. The doctor did not know that there would be undetectable cracks in ampoules, but it was not negligent of him not to know it at that time. We must not look at the 1947 accident with 1954 spectacles".

CONCLUSION

This chapter is based on actual case laws decided by various judicial and quasi-judicial bodies. The conclusions and references are there in each and every case discussed hence, the same is not written again to prevent the repetition. These are the important and landmark judgments related to various issues of medical negligence and health care issues.

KEY LEARNING POINTS

- The doctors or healthcare facilities are included under Consumer Protection Act 2019.
- Avoid cross-pathy and cross-specialty. Practice as per your competence and training.
- Take proper, informed consents. Don't exceed consent.
- Maintain proper records and documents.
- Doctors should be protected from frivolous complaints, especially of criminal negligence. Avoid indiscriminate prosecution.

BIBLIOGRAPHY

1. Dr. Jacob Mathews vs. State Of Punjab III (2005) CPJ SC 9.
2. Samira Kohli vs. Dr Prabha Manchanda I (2008) CPJ 56 (SC).
3. Indian Medical Association vs. V.P. Shantha 1996 SC 550, 1995 SCC (6) 651.
4. SC Civil Appeal No. 2646-49 of 09 decided on 14/5/24.
5. Martin F. D'souza vs. Mohd. Ishfaq, SC in CA no. 3541 of 2002.

16

CHAPTER

Calculation of Compensation

Mahesh Baldwa, Amit Padvi, Namita Padvi

INTRODUCTION

Medicine is an inexact science, yet an art of healing. It is far from exactness of mathematics, physics, and chemistry. The emergence of high compensation awards for medical deficiency claims in India has resulted in apprehensive speculation regarding the result that such remedies may have on the manner in which doctors practice medicine within India and how this process translates into rising costs for the patients. While some argue that an increase in frivolous lawsuits may result, others advocate for stricter regulations in the healthcare sector and believe that substantial compensation will discourage medical negligence. The recent trend of sizable awards in court cases raises concerns about whether this encourages a surge in medical negligence litigation and defensive medicine. Consequently, there is a growing need to reconsider the current approach to addressing medical negligence issues in India.

PARADOX IN CALCULATING COMPENSATION

- When a mass disaster happens, government declares ₹2–10 lakh compensation for dead and ₹50,000/- for injured and disabled.
- Insurance company's premium charges increase with each advancing year for life insurance as mortality risk is high in aged group.
- Insurance company's premium charges increase with each advancing year for inland mediclaim policies.
- Insurance company's premium charges increase with each advancing year for overseas mediclaim policies and stop issuing policies for those aged 70 years and above. Some insurance companies issue overseas mediclaim policies by charging 200–300% above normal charges for that age group.
- In a medical negligence case, individual doctors and hospitals have to pay to one single patient compensation in lakhs and crores.

The Court themselves agreed that it is difficult to calculate compensation for medical negligence cases.

The Supreme Court noted that *"The lack of uniformity and consistency in awarding Compensation has been a matter of grave concern... If different tribunals calculate Compensation differently on the same facts, the litigant, the claimant, the common man will be perplexed, confused, and bewildered. If there is significant divergence and similarities among tribunals in determining the quantum of Compensation on similar facts, it will lead to distrust and dissatisfaction in the system."*

Problem of precedent decisions becoming law is a perpetuating compensation issue.
In India, the judge in the civil court or the consumer court has complete discretion over the compensation amount and hence is bound or forced to consider the impact of the judgment because he/she sets a precedent even in the manner and quantum of damages awarded. The case laws, such as SC, 2 JJ bench in Dr Balram Prasad vs. Kunal Saha 2013(4)CPR 284(SC) and SC, 3 JJ bench in Rajesh vs. Rajvir Singh, (2013) 9 SCC 54, correctly speak about how compensation is inconsistent and is one of the biggest problem that the healthcare sector of India is facing. It is important to consider every case independently because it would be incorrect to not give the facts of every case's situation due importance. However, this increases not only the unpredictability but also the scope of discretion provided to the judge in such situations.

SHOULD THERE BE CAPPING OF CLAIMS?

The *Kunal Saha* case has raised the issues of just and adequate compensation applying *restituo in integrum* and also the efficacy of the quantum of compensation to act as a deterrent. While discussing problems and providing suggestions for these problems, we would often be referring to the *Kunal Saha* case.

- Several countries have capped medical compensation claims. In India, there is no capping on medical negligence claims. This has been marked by awarding Dr Kunal Saha with >11 crores by the honorable Supreme Court. There are two aspects in this claim. The court ordered a compensation of ₹5.96 crore, which with interest crosses ₹11 crore. First aspect is awarding claim of compensation but second aspect of interest is too harsh as medical professionals had no role in delaying court proceeding, which went on for 15 years. Kunal initially lost his fight as both the West Bengal Medical Council and Calcutta High Court dismissed his case against AMRI Hospitals. The NCDRC, however, found the hospital and its doctors guilty of medical negligence and fixed a compensation amount of ₹1.7 crore. Finally, the Supreme Court awarded ₹5.96 crore, which with interest crosses ₹11 crore. The leaders of Indian Medical Association (IMA) headed by famed cardiac surgeon Dr Devi Shetty have now demanded that there should be a maximum limit ("cap") of compensation that any doctor or hospital may pay for causing death of a patient from medical negligence.
- The Indian healthcare system is overburdened by application of "first world regulatory standards with third world infrastructure" making single MBBS doctor clinics extinct and soon small obstetric nursing homes shall perish as the cost of implementing first-world regulatory standards will make them shut shop along with the fear of huge compensations without any cap.
- Even US President Bush is pushing for cap on medical malpractice awards relieve doctors of frivolous lawsuits. Some states in the US have capped damages in medical negligence cases to a maximum of ₹1.5 crore.
- *Preconsent counseling*: Discuss with patient party the capping of compensation in case of rare chance of litigation. Also, discuss that doctor has bought professional indemnity (say, e.g., 50 lakh) and error and omission policy (say, e.g., 50 lakh).
- *In addition to consent, should we make contractual capping of compensation claims?* Author's immediate suggestion is to incorporate in consent/contract forms limiting compensation to

a certain limit (say ₹50 lakh) in case of litigation. These consent/contract documents should be part of pleadings when malpractice litigation is initiated.

- Should compensation be linked to the amount of fee paid by the patient for percentage of disability? In case of death, the amount which should be paid, should also be linked to fee paid.
- Should compensation be linked to the amount of net worth declared by patient taking treatment in consent cum declaration form?

Hence, it is seen several times that even informed consent is legally incomplete; it is time to switch to contract for hiring of medical services to augment informed consent.

Entering in contract for medical services with patient party along with consent for capping the compensation as liquidated damages as opposed to unliquidated damages.

Purpose of Real/Informed Consent

The main purpose of the informed consent process is to protect the patient to uphold autonomy of patient party. Primary purpose of consent is risk disclosures to patient. Consent form by itself is legally incomplete to protect doctor against allegations hurled by patient to seek compensation. Consent protects against patients voluntarily accepting the risks of treatment/surgery (volenti non fit injuria) and who cannot ask for compensation.

Purpose of switching to "contract for hiring of medical services" is to augment informed consent. "Contract for rendering/hiring of medical services" includes consent of patient party along with a number of terms and conditions which are usually not part of consent.

Legal Contract

A contract is a legally binding agreement between two or more parties as per terms of contract, typically involving the medical services. Section 74 of Indian Contract Act (ICA)-1872 governs liquidated damages. Parties at the time of contracting may stipulate an amount in the agreement itself, which shall become payable on the breach of contract, by doctor in favor of patient.

Valid Contract for Hiring/Providing of Medical Services

Valid contracts to be legally enforceable if agreement contains all of the following legal criteria:

- An offer (in the form of proposed surgery/treatment)
- Acceptance by patient party by obtaining valid consent
- Clearly defined terms and conditions (about complications, disabilities, guarantee, warrantee, warnings, and disclaimers)
- Consideration (defined in terms of money and payment schedules)
- Intention to create legal relations (doctor-patient relationship)
- Capacity of the parties (competent to contract)
- Legality of purpose (standard surgery/treatment)
- Description of liquidated damages in case of breach of contract limited to the contractual amount agreed

Compensation Granted Under Tort versus Contract—Which is Bitter?

Consent versus contract for medical services from point of view of restricting compensation in consumer and civil jurisdiction.

Consumer and civil courts usually decide one of the following aspects:

- Deficiency in medical service
- Was there an unfair trade practice?
- Was there any medical negligence?

Hence, one should defend forcefully against alleged medical negligence and try and convert all allegations of negligence to deficiency of service for getting under liquidated damages under law of contract as damages are defined and liquidated within the confines of contracted terms; hence as per terms and conditions of contract, the civil court has to decide. Primary aim should be to convert all allegations of negligence to deficiency of service domain so as to align court granting liquidated compensation as per contract terms and conditions.

Medical negligence under law of torts paves way for the civil court to grant compensation at the court's own discretion as unliquidated with no holds barred on court to grant compensation.

Choice is yours—which bitter pill to swallow—liquidated damages under contract law decided in written contract by capping the compensation or else court shall award unliquidated damages under law of torts.

Compensation calculation is in a vicious circle of uncertainty based on assumption and presumption.

The process of calculating compensation for medical negligence is very uncertain and unpredictable as it varies hugely across different cases, courts, and tribunals resulting in loss of faith on the courts, protracted litigation, and also the frequent appeals and cross appeals.

Why compensation takes into account only few factors such as patient's age, disability, death, and inflation?

Within legal circles, medical negligence is widely recognized as one of the most difficult types of compensation claims for injured plaintiffs. Why that is so? Let us factor it out and break down a few of the concepts and barriers in medical negligence claims. The courts presume the person before taking treatment was having 100% reserve powers in health to fight disease for which he had gone to doctor. It is far from true. The courts do not know medical scientific intricacies and hence avoid factoring out negative aspects of health. The following concept of "reserve power of health" is based on common sense, which any person can understand.

ALTERNATIVE METHOD TO CAP COMPENSATION

This is "Baldwa pleading of negative factors," which is described next.

What is reserve power to fight diseases in human beings?

This is extra power vested in each organ to fight diseases, which is 100% for each organ and system in human body, which operates at full throttle to heal a diseased person when given standard treatment.

Who can be said to have overall 100% "reserve power" to heal?

Legally, let us assume as to which human being can be described to be having 100% "reserve power" to fight diseases when they fall sick. This reserve power is weakened when there are several negative factors. These negative factors operate in certain patients who will have poor outcomes even when standard treatment is given. There is a long list of negative factors that operate in a diseased person. Following is the list that can be easily understood by common persons using common sense without having medical qualifications.

Nine negative factors weakening reserve power must be pleaded separately as and where it is applicable.

Each negative factor is assigned a value of one (1). Following is description of factor:

- *Negative factor 1*: Extremes of age of patient (<5 and >50 years), premature birth
- *Negative factor 2*: Existing comorbidities—unhealthy lifestyle; diabetes mellitus (DM); hypertension (HTN); obesity [body mass index (BMI) > 26 kg/m^2]; tobacco, alcohol, and drug abuse for >1 year in life in any form; malnutrition (BMI < 17 kg/m^2); diseases of abnormal thyroid functions; congenital and acquired diseases; and abnormalities related to central nervous system (CNS), cardiovascular system (CVS), respiratory system (RS), abdominal system (AS); diseases and abnormalities with defective liver function test (LFT) and renal function test (RFT); diseases and abnormalities with defective lipid profile; diseases and abnormalities with defective Hb and iron profile; diseases and abnormalities with defective musculoskeletal system; diseases and abnormalities with defective metabolic disorder; diseases and abnormalities with defective immunological system; diseases and abnormalities related to human immunodeficiency virus (HIV), hepatitis B virus (HBV), and hepatitis C virus (HCV) infections; psychological diseases; diseases and abnormalities due to congenital, familial, genetic diseases, and similar to all previously mentioned concurrent diseases as the list is neither exhaustive nor exclusive.
- *Negative factor 3*: Time period at which the patient is brought for treatment after onset of symptoms; e.g., within 1 week is okay but should be considered brought late after 1 week of illness.
- *Negative factor 4*: Emergency, dying-dying dead (gasping, comatose, and irregular heart rate), critical (vital parameters are on extreme side), serious (extreme pain and suffering, howling, convulsing, breathless, and semiconscious), and similar to all previously mentioned concurrent diseases as the list is neither exhaustive nor exclusive.
- *Negative factor 5*: Brought after taking treatment and doctor shopping with same allopathy or different pathies such as homeopathy, ayurvedic, siddha, and alternative medicines somewhere else.
- *Negative factor 6*: Known complications—it is well recognized that not everyone who has medical treatment gets better to the extent that they had hoped. Some patients will have poor outcomes even with "best," "diligent," and "gold" standard treatment. Complications can arise in surgeries that are not a result of anyone's carelessness or error. This is as per Murphy's law and cascading effect of complications. When known complications in a particular patient occur, these shall manifest 100% in that patient though literature may mention that complication occurs, e.g., 1 in 10 patients.
- *Negative factor 7*: Taking irregular/no treatment; not following or refusing advice; instructions with respect to taking medicines; doing surgery; investigations such as pathological investigations; imaging studies such as X-ray, ultrasonography (USG), computed tomography (CT), magnetic resonance imaging (MRI), and positron emission tomography (PET); blood products refused; referral refused; intensive care unit (ICU) care refused; not taking precautions about food and rest; patient going discharge against medical advice (DAMA) and leave against medical advice (LAMA); keeps doctor shopping; and different pathies shopping.

- *Negative factor 8*: Willful contributory negligence of patient party furthering the illness at any stage
- *Negative factor 9*: Abusive, violent patient party and resorting to mob violence, thus interfering with work of healthcare workers.

How to use of negative factor pleaded might impact the calculation of compensation?
Take any or all nine factors to support deductions with supportive evidence in pleadings to make impact of 10%. Say *each negative* factor has value of one (1) and pleaded forcefully may be able to reduce compensation up to 10%. One has to add all negative factors in pleading with proper scientific evidence. Physicians should understand that by pleading negative factors may help you reduce the liability of paying compensation. Just take a hypothetic example where one has pleaded negative factors and they add up to nine (9). It may work as by multiplying total compensation granted by court with 10 divided by total of negative factors in denominator. Say the total of negative factor is nine. The multiplication factor shall be (10/9). Say ₹100,000 (1 lakh) is awarded by the court of law. Now multiply by 10/9 × 100,000 = ₹10000/= which shall be payable.

Courts take the following factors to grant compensation and none of the above negative factors:
- *Positive factor 1*: Death of patient; medical expenses—resulting from your injuries; travel expenses to and from medical appointments and treatment; domestic assistance—the cost of getting help with home duties; loss of earnings; and consortium (right of association and companionship with one's husband or wife)
- *Positive factor 2*: Disability of patient; medical expenses—resulting from your injuries; travel expenses—to and from medical appointments and treatment; domestic assistance—the cost of getting help with home duties; loss of earnings; pain and suffering; future treatment; consortium (right of association and companionship with one's husband or wife); travel expenses—to and from medical appointments and treatment
- *Positive factor 3*: Inflation, interest on compensation why? When and how to calculate?

CALCULATION OF COMPENSATION AS ON DATE

Old Roman law of "restitutio in integrum" is current coin in compensation.
In the Indian Common law, the basis of computing compensation for any case lies on the legal principle of "restitutio in integrum," which when translated means that the person who is seeking damages due to a wrongful committed him/her is in the position that he/she would have been had the wrong not been committed. This implies that the victim or the family of the victim needs to be compensated for financial loss as well as other losses caused by doctor's or hospital's negligence, future medical expenses, and any pain and suffering that is endured by the victim.

Age-old "Multiplier Method"

In most of the medicolegal cases, the defendants have asserted that the method to determine the compensation which ought to be the "multiplier method" used in Motor Accidents Claims Tribunal (MACT) is applicable for medical negligence cases. In 2 JJ SC, civil appeal No. 4648 OF 2022-Abhimanyu Partap Singh vs Namita Sekhon on July 6, 2022, the multiplier method is most realistic for calculating compensation for road accident victims, says the Supreme Court while enhancing compensation for disability awarded by MACT. The main and principal argument in favor of using such a method is that it at least gives uniformity and predictability. Furthermore, doctors and hospitals will not be compelled and ordered to pay large sums of money to compensate for negligence.

Talking about the history of the multiplier method, it was first created to facilitate awarding compensation in relation to motor vehicle accidents to calculate "no-fault" liability. Therefore, it only stands for the loss of income of the victim only. The sum is calculated according to the "multiplicand," that is, victim's salary minus the amount he spends on himself for the treatment, and the "multiplier", that is, the total number of years that the victim would have earned his salary. The multiplier is calculated by taking into account the average life expectancy, the number of years that the victim will be unemployed, the victim's age, and any other factors concerning the victim's health. The common formula for the calculation of compensation is [(70 – age) × annual income + 30% of for inflation – 1/3 expenses]. Defendants say that this is the figure that will adequately calculate the loss incurred, and therefore this method can be utilized for the calculation of medical negligence cases. However, the argument here is that compensation solely based on the income of the victim is not ethically correct. It simply means that medical negligence causing death or injury to a wealthy person is much more worth when compared to medical negligence that impacted an unemployed individual, homemaker, a child, or a senior citizen. Therefore, being legally unethical, the Supreme Court declined the dependency of calculation of compensation on the multiplier method for medical negligence. In addition, the Supreme Court added other dimensions for the calculation of compensation, which included medical costs incurred by the victim during the litigation, cost of any future medical expenses, compensation toward mental agony and physical pain, and compensation toward loss of litigation and consortium.

Entering in contract for medical services with patient party as described above along with consent for capping the compensation as liquidated damages as opposed to unliquidated damages via third party insurance

Professional indemnity and errors and omissions (E&O) indemnity policy are both third-party insurance policies purchased by the insured doctor (first party) from the insurance company (second party) for protection against the claims of another (third party). Professional indemnity insurance protects you against losses claimed by a third party due to alleged or actual negligence or errors in your professional services or advice. On the other hand, E&O indemnity policy covers the company or an individual against a lawsuit filed by a third party for financial loss during the course of providing services. Professional liability insurance, also known as E&O coverage, is designed to protect your business against claims that professional advice or services you provided caused a customer financial harm due to actual or alleged mistakes or a failure to perform a service.

Other Forms of Insurance to Capping of Compensation

Fixed Amount Third-party Liability versus Indemnity Bases Variable Liability

Indemnification language in a contract is traditionally understood to apply only to third-party claims, which are variable liability insurances based on tort based negligence compensation decided as unliquidated damages by the court.

Fixed Amount Third-party Liability Claim

All patients who are covered under mediclaim automatically policy can be tagged with "Medical Negligence Top-Up Cover"; thus, fixed-amount third-party liability claim could be a new way to give fixed compensation when negligence is alleged by third party causing damages on the lines of railway safety claims. Fixed-amount third-party liability claim is proposed via "Medical Negligence Top-Up Cover" to health insurance policies on lines of railway accident safety insurance. We have statistical data of year 2022; an impressive 265 million healthcare policies (be it under government-assisted *Ayushman Bharat* or purchased by patients themselves) were given in India. While this signifies a significant advancement in healthcare accessibility, a glaring gap remains in the form of "medical negligence coverage." This lack of coverage leaves patients financially vulnerable in the event of alleged medical negligence, often leading to protracted legal battles with low success rates. This initiative would mirror the railways' *Rail* Accident Cover, which offers a ₹10 lakh insurance cover at a nominal premium of less than a rupee. Similarly, the proposed Medical Negligence Top-Up Cover could be offered at a minimal cost, making it accessible to patients with mediclaim policy from *Ayushman Bharat* or bought individually by patient party to cover via alleged "Medical Negligence" causing damage. Thus, introduction of "Medical Negligence Top-Up Cover" annexed to health insurance policies (be it under *Ayushman Bharat* or purchased by patients) presents a significant step toward ensuring the well-being of both patients and healthcare providers. By providing immediate financial relief, reducing the burden of litigation, this initiative will strengthen India's healthcare system, foster a more collaborative healthcare environment, and ultimately benefit all stakeholders. By addressing the concerns of both patients and doctors, "Medical Negligence Top-Up Cover" can contribute to a more supportive, patient-centered, and responsive healthcare system.

No-fault Compulsory Professional Indemnity Issued with Registration to Practice by Respective State Medical Council

Worldwide, most countries have the same legal provisions such as those in India with faster judicial clearance of cases. This is because India has 1.4 billion population with more than 3 crore cases still pending to be heard, amazing! Only two countries have "no-fault" systems. Sweden and New Zealand are maintaining "no-fault" systems. In New Zealand, there is no medical malpractice system but rather a publicly funded accident compensation scheme that bars suing for compensatory damages and separate medical professional accountability processes.

Difficulty in Introducing Reforms Like No-fault

It must be considered that there is nothing more difficult to carry out, or more doubtful of success, or more dangerous to handle, than to initiate a new order of things. Any kind of reform has enemies in all those who profit by the old order system, and only lukewarm defenders in all those who would profit by the new order.

No-fault System

In its strictest form, the term no-fault provides for the payment for patients party for economic losses by producing medical bills incurred to treat complications and lumpsum immediate monetary compensation for disability, death arising out of professional medical treatment or surgery, and restrict the right to sue doctors. Because high-threshold no-fault systems restrict litigation, they tend to reduce costs and delays in paying claims.

By paving way for no-fault professional indemnity, one does not depend upon broad judicial interpretation of medical negligence substituted many a times as *res ipsa loquitur* for a complication or disability, death arising out of medical accident or mishap in treatment or surgery are done away so also Lengthy, unending, seemingly speculative, frustrating court proceedings to all litigants. No fault indemnity insurance eliminates the incentive to inflate claims.

It is always patients who suffer death, disability, and disfigurement due to alleged medical negligence. Though all death, disability, and disfigurement are not due to alleged medical negligence, most of the times, it is patients who suffer from preventable medical error may not indulge in to litigation. Patient party suffers in silence. Hence, all those who receive medical treatment, whether they allege death, disability, or disfigurement due to medical treatment or not, should receive "no-fault" claim from insurance companies. This is a social benefit, which they can choose relinquishing tort remedy under alleged medical negligence law. This will also lead to proactive reporting and learning from errors committed by doctors. "No-fault" medical compensation law should be promulgated to replace medical negligence under law of tort.

Sanity shall prevail to rein fancy, puffed-up compensation claims to get media attention
There is a need to assess using "reserve power" of patient to fight disease "formula" given above so that it may be the way wherein India decides to address medical negligence compensations. Notwithstanding the dread of protective medication, expanding protection premiums, and ascent in costs for patients, it is time that we know about the inequity that the current framework sustains. Systemic deficiencies such as heavy litigation costs, delayed and protracted litigation, and dependence on judicial discretion do not give adequate equity justice to patient as victims and are harming doctors and hospitals as well.

CONCLUSION

Apart from legislative capping of compensation (which currently seems impossible), which shall be incorporated once its time is ripe in India.

No-fault compulsory insurance also can reduce compensation awarded and immediate relief to the affected patient party.

Doctors can incorporate the capping and professional indemnity discussions in preconsent counseling and informed consent.

Apart from consent capping compensation, one can draw a separate contract for medical services in which few lines item-wise should be mentioned as capping of compensation and money value of indemnity insurance purchased by doctor be explicitly disclosed.

Most courts consider the fact that patients reach for treatment to physicians, surgeons, and hospitals in perfect health with 100% reserve power to fight illnesses, which is far from truth. Physician is advised through this article to highlight the condition of patient was not having perfect health with 100% reserve power to fight illnesses in their pleadings. Use of "Baldwa's negative factors in pleadings" as described above with evidence may reduce liability of compensation. There is no dividing line between medical accidents and negligence. All medical accidents are rechristened and negligence using legalized substitution of evidence by using *res ipsa loquitur*. The Court has power to summon, examine, cross-examine, and re-examine experts yet they do not do and use *res ipsa loquitur*. Physician is advised to proactively ask for examination, cross-examination, and re-examination experts by moving applications. Doling out higher and higher compensations for medical negligence has become the norm.

Such higher compensation awarded finds place in print and electronic media immediately. Who can restrain them? It is only left to physicians to ask courts to unearth truth by lawful means. Nation reads more about glamorized medical negligence rather than healing and goodness done by doctors. India is the only nation where press, media, and social media are not interested in keeping citizens healthy. They spread myths and gossips about health. They search for spicy news in their well-being by propagating and highlighting medical negligence. The scarcity of medical doctors as human resources and an enormous urban and rural divide of healthcare services are glamorized rather than chastised. There is poor political will to improve the health and well-being of citizens. The government administration needs to act and put health care resources into proper accessible order, before it passes the point of no return. India needs to upgrade the current arrangement of healthcare, which is getting glamorized in media more for medical negligence rather than for healing. Set the horse in front of the cart of healthcare before it slips out of the hands of governmental agencies.

KEY LEARNING POINTS

- Draw "Contract for hiring of medical services" is to augment informed consent.
- An alternative method to cap compensation is by pleading "Baldwa pleading of negative factors," to reduce compensation awarded by the court of law.
- Entering in contract for medical services with patient party as described above along with consent for capping the compensation as liquidated damages as opposed to unliquidated damages via third party insurance
- Other forms of insurance to capping of compensation—fixed amount third-party liability versus indemnity bases variable liability.
- No-fault compulsory professional indemnity issued with registration to practice by respective state medical council.

BIBLIOGRAPHY

1. ANZIIF. (2022). Clearing up the differences between E&O and PI. [Online] Available from https://anziif.com/professional-development/articles/2022/09/clearing-up-the-differences-between-eo-and-pi [Last accessed May, 2024].
2. Bal BS. An introduction to medical malpractice in the United States. Clin Orthop Relat Res. 2009;467(2):339-47.
3. Baldwa M, Baldwa V, Padvi N, Baldwa S. Legal Issues in Critical Care. India: CBS Publishers & Distributors Pvt Ltd; 2022.
4. Baldwa M, Baldwa V, Padvi N, Baldwa S. Legal Issues in Dermatology. India: CBS Publishers & Distributors Pvt Ltd; 2024.
5. Baldwa M. Factors to be pleaded to reduce compensation awarded by Court of Law. JIMLEA. 2022;10(4):113-20.
6. Bismark M, Paterson R. No-fault compensation in New Zealand: harmonizing injury compensation, provider accountability, and patient safety. Health Aff (Millwood). 2006;25(1):278-83.
7. Bogdan J. Medical malpractice in Sweden and New Zealand: Should their systems be replicated here? Centre for Justice & Democracy. 2011;21.
8. Brennan TA, Studdert DM. (2011). No-Fault Compensation for Medical Injuries. [Online] Available from hpc.state.nm.us/UNM Library/Alternative Compensation Events/No Fault Compensation for Medical Injuries.pdf [Last accessed May, 2024].
9. Chandra MS, Math SB. Progress in medicine: Compensation and medical negligence in India: Does the system need a quick fix or an overhaul? Ann Indian Acad Neurol. 2016;19(Suppl 1):S21-7.
10. Civil appeal No. 4648 OF 2022-Abhimanyu Partap Singh vs Namita Sekhon on 6 July, 2022. [Online] Available from https://indiankanoon.org/doc/186470151/ [Last accessed May, 2024].

11. Compare Your Business Costs. (n.d.). Errors and Omissions vs Professional Indemnity Policies. Compare Your Business Costs. https://compareyourbusinesscosts.co.uk/errors-and-omissions
12. Dr. Balram Prasad vs. Kunal Saha 2013(4)CPR 284(SC). [Online] Available from https://indiankanoon.org/doc/35346928/ [Last accessed May, 2024].
13. Essinger K. (2009). The Swedish Medical Injury Insurance. [Online] Available from http://www.patientforsakring.se/resurser/dokument/engelska_artiklar/Report_on_the_Swedsih_Medical_Injury_Insurance.pdf [Last accessed May, 2024].
14. Harleston J. (2003). No-fault medical liability compensation system. [Online] Available from https://www.cga.ct.gov/2003/olrdata/ins/rpt/2003-R-0386.htm [Last accessed May, 2024].
15. Panda SC. Medicine: science or art? Mens Sana Monogr. 2006;4(1):127-38.
16. Rajesh vs. Rajvir Singh2, (2013) 9 SCC 54.
17. Shaikh M. (2022). 'What to do with the money?': Families of those killed in Morbi bridge collapse. [Online] Available from https://www.indiatoday.in/india/gujarat/story/morbi-bridge-collapse-families-killed-compensation-2292482-2022-11-02 [Last accessed May, 2024].

SECTION

4

Issues Related to Different Specialties

Section Editor: Alok Gupta

Section Outline

CHAPTER 17

Medicolegal Issues in Pediatrics

Satish Tiwari

INTRODUCTION

The last few decades have seen many ups and downs in medical sciences. Some of these are positive changes such as scientific and technical advances, increasing longevity, decreasing mortality and morbidity, and overall improvement in quality of life. But there are also some negative changes such as decreasing the standard of medical education, decreasing values and morality, commercialization, and corporate culture in management of patients. In this era, where doctors are becoming specialists and super specialists, the medical faculty has evolved from a noble profession to a commercial one. The art of medicine has gradually become medical science and ultimately ended in commerce. These rapid changes in the medical field have even strained the age-old good relations between the patient and the treating physician or surgeon. Bringing the doctors under the ambit of the Consumer Protection Act (CPA) has further marginalized this relationship.

WHAT IS PEDIATRIC AGE?

There is no statutory or legal age limit of a child/adolescent. The word "Child" has not been defined precisely, neither in the Constitution nor in the General Clauses Act. This word is not identical to the word "minor." The definitions vary from act to act.

According to the Indian Majority Act of 1875, a child means 18 years old unless it falls in the category of specified exceptional case, in which it is 21 years. According to the Children Act, 1960 a child means a boy before attaining 16 years of age or a girl who is less than 18 years of age. The Indian Academy of Pediatrics recommends that a pediatrician should continue to examine and treat children up to 18 years of age. According to the American Academy of Pediatrics, adolescent means up to 10–19 years of age.

WHO IS A PEDIATRICIAN?

According to the World Health Organization (WHO), a physician is a person who, having been regularly admitted to a medical school, has successfully completed the prescribed courses of studies in medicine and has acquired the requisite qualification to be legally licensed to practice medicine using independent judgment to promote community and individual health.

A specialist is defined as one who learns more **and more** about less and less. A pediatrician or "Child Specialist" means a doctor who has specialized in managing a child. The Supreme Court in its various other judgments had made it clear that the medical practitioners should practice within the scope of one's qualifications and skills.

DEALING WITH A PATIENT

The practitioner must bring to his task a reasonable degree of skill and knowledge and must exercise a reasonable degree of care. The standard is that of a reasonable average. Pediatricians have to be more careful because while dealing with children, there may be many limitations such as the availability of reliable history, problems in investigations, and compliance/difficulties in drug administrations.

HISTORY TAKING AND EXAMINATION

The doctor should carefully listen to the history and complaints. Also, ask for significant positive or negative history. This is important to arrive at a proper diagnosis and rule out differential diagnosis. The diagnosis is never a static concept; it remains fluid and flexible. A good history may clinch the diagnosis, while a bad or misleading history may lead to wrong conclusions. In K Kumble vs. Dr Udaya Patil III (1998) CPJ 614, a patient who was being treated for fever developed skin rash and eye swelling. Medicines were stopped and a dermatologist's opinion was taken. The patient was shifted to another hospital where unfortunately he succumbed. There was no history of drug reaction in the past. The case was dismissed on the grounds that the treatment was proper and drug reactions were known to occur. In B Kaur vs. C Malhotra I (2008) CPJ 265, the skin sensitivity test done preoperatively was negative. But, on the table patient had a cardiac arrest and succumbed. The postmortem report also did not reveal any evidence of drug reaction. Negligence was not held in this case. In St Gregarious Mission Hospital vs. Raji George I (2008) CPJ 68 NC, a patient during septoplasty went into cardiorespiratory arrest, resulting in brain damage and vegetative life. The patient was known asthmatic, but details of asthma treatment were not available in the record. Critical information was withheld by doctors and surgery was started without ascertaining drug intake or prior tests.

In the present era, there is a possibility of adolescent pregnancy; if any medicines are prescribed with a fetus in utero, there is every chance of damage to this fetus. Hence, the history of the last menstrual period should be asked while examining adolescent girls. In adolescent age, there may be many sensitive issues such as sexual relationships, drug addiction, and behavioral problems; all these should be explored in history taking.

Many times, there may be allegations that a serious patient was not examined on time and was kept waiting for a long time. Similarly, there can be allegations of misbehavior with the girl child during the examination. These issues/problems can be minimized with closed-circuit audio/video recording of the events. Care should be taken with the video recording so that it should not be misused in the future by some miscreants.

A detailed *negative history* is important in arriving at the final diagnosis. We should rule out differential diagnosis and other associated diseases to prevent subsequent unexpected outcomes. If we examine the patient in a hurry, ask to come on next day.

INVESTIGATIONS

If it is not possible to diagnose the illness clinically, the help of investigations should be taken. According to the presenting symptoms and signs, the necessary investigations shall be advised. In a case, Sudhakar Gupta vs. Anugraha Nursing Home I (2008) CPJ 57 (NC), the patient was suffering from leukemia but received treatment for typhoid. Bone marrow aspiration was advised by the doctor, but complainant himself refused repeatedly. It was held that the complainant himself was negligent. If patient is not willing for any procedure or investigations, the *dissent shall also be documented.* Do not advise unnecessary investigations. In a detailed, well-reasoned, analyzed discussion Shailesh Munjal vs. AIIMS, 2004 CTJ 940 (CP) (NCDRC), the National Commission observed that the services rendered at AIIMS would be covered by the provisions of CPA as the services are not free of cost. In this case, prenatal diagnosis of thalassemia was negative, but after birth, the child was suffering from thalassemia. The prenatal diagnosis of genetic disorders is complex as the technologies are not developed and may not be free from all errors. Any scientific investigation or technology can be 100% perfect. The errors are inherent and multifactorial. No doubt, in such cases, there is thin difference between error, imperfection or fault, and negligence.

DIAGNOSIS

Sometimes, the symptoms and signs of the illness be so overlapping that it is very difficult to clinically diagnose the disease. The case Biju vs. Dr Mohammad III (1997) CPJ 316 was dismissed on the grounds that a wrong diagnosis is not a deficiency in the service. In this case, negligence was accused in investigating and treating a patient of fever. In such cases, the diagnosis may be mistaken or delayed in spite of diligence and due care by the treating doctor. In M Parimanam vs. Dr Jaganathan I (1999) CPJ 243, where the patient died due to rabies, it was alleged that there was wrong diagnosis and treatment. The defense in this case was that clinical tests were conducted and a pediatrician was called. The case was dismissed. But in J Padia vs. Dr Trivedi I (1997) CPJ 11, a child was under treatment for fever, diagnosed as measles, which did not improve. A pediatrician was called, admitted, and treated for measles for 36 hours then diagnosed with Stevens-Johnson syndrome, referred to an eye surgeon but ultimately lost vision. In this case, the pediatrician was held liable.

USE OF MEDICINES/DRUGS/INSTRUMENTS

Certain drugs should not be used in children below a particular age. There are no sufficient scientific trials/data on such drugs for their safe use in children. In special or extraordinary circumstances, such drugs may be used with special precautions or monitoring. Such emergency indications shall also be decided as per the recommendations of standard textbooks/scientific journals and not as per the leaflets provided by pharmaceutical companies.

Failure to provide proper and adequate treatment may account for a deficiency in service. This was held in Dean, Tirunelveli Medical College vs. U Subramaniyan I (2008) CPJ 188; the State Commission held that the nonproviding of intercostal drainage may not be the cause of death, but the fact remains that the treatment prescribed was not provided and this amounts to deficiency in service. In Tagore Hospital vs. Harnam Singh I (2008) CPJ 360 NC, the commission has held negligence on the following grounds. The patient with fever of 20 days, X-ray and echocardiogram (ECHO) reports could not be correlated and the patient became hypoxic, but arterial blood gas (ABG) was not done and the patient was not put on ventilator. The patient was discharged forcibly and died subsequently. It was observed that the records were fabricated and not reliable. Lame excuses regarding why ventilators from their hospital could not be spared were not acceptable and hence, deficiency was held. In Kumari Shivani Singh vs. Dr A Gokhale I (2007) CPJ 326 NC, it was alleged that due to the administration of liquid gramoneg (contraindicated <3 months), there was retinopathy of prematurity (ROP) and loss of vision. However, the commission held that there are many other causes of ROP and no evidence to exclude other causes has been produced; hence, a negligence is not held.

OUTCOME

If the complications are too remote, then it is not negligence. This defense was accepted in Sadanand Rawal vs. State of UP I (2007) CPJ 173 (NC), where a patient after a gallstone surgery died suddenly. It was held that it is a case of unfortunate and rare hazard of pulmonary embolism and every effort was made to control the same. In Administrator, Pukhraj General Hospital vs. Master M Rajput I (2009) CPJ 114 NC, it was observed that no record of nurse's chart was produced. According to the commission, this was germane to the issue at hand. In this case, the child had developed gangrene after the administration of injection. In VK Suri vs. Dr Sushma Aggarwal I (2009) CPJ 452, there was an allegation of incorrect and unwarranted treatment during pre- and postnatal care, resulting in physically and mentally handicapped child. It was informed that abortion was not possible at 34 weeks of gestation and option for the doctor to save the mother first was more important. In fact, complainant failed to follow instructions of doctors and hence, deficiency is not proved. In M Bhagat vs. Bhandari Hospital I (12) CPJ 59, sciatic nerve and right lower limb was damaged along with sensory loss with foot drop. The Medical Board findings were weakness of muscles not supplied by the sciatic nerve. According to the Board, the involvement of the right and left leg was probably due to polio. Negligence was not held.

Many illnesses are self-limiting, while many may be progressive. Some progress slowly, while some may have fulminant course in spite of adequate treatment. Hence, treating doctors should have foreseeability about common complications and diagnose and treat them adequately and at proper time. Compensation was granted to the complainant in Padma vs. Sudha Nursing Home, where a patient was treated for enteric fever and discharged but was readmitted. There was a delay in diagnosing and treating enteric perforation. Unqualified doctors gave the postoperative care. The patient was reoperated at Apollo Hospital. If a particular case is beyond skill or competence of treating doctor, the same may be referred to a higher center which is better-equipped.

IN EMERGENCY SITUATION

In practice, many times, we have to tackle the emergency situation. In such situations, the clinical features may not be very obvious to suggest a particular diagnosis. Proper history may not be available, especially if the patient is unconscious or distressed. At the same time, sufficient time may not be there to go in for investigations. In Babu Kople vs. Dr M Bhatambre III

(2000) CPJ 366, it was alleged that there was a wrong diagnosis, no investigations, and delay in blood transfusion. The doctor explained that the child was referred to him in serious condition (septicemia) after 2 days, antibiotics were started, blood culture would have taken longer time, lariago was continued as started earlier. Blood transfusion takes at least 3 hours as certain tests are to be carried out as per the government notification. The civil surgeon also certified that the treatment was proper. The doctor was not held liable.

REFERRALS

If adequate facilities are not available, patient should be referred to a properly equipped center. In Dr Rakesh Jain vs. Rakeshkumar Khare I (2003) CPJ 27, the negligence was held because in a child with rising bilirubin levels, pathological tests were not done at a proper time, proper phototherapy was not given, and referral was delayed. It was held that the treatment was not according to accepted norms and hence, it resulted in permanent disability. In T Ramarao vs. Vijay Hospital I (2008) CPJ 170 NC, a patient of mitral valve replacement suffered stroke due to clot formed from heart valve gone to brain, leading to brain damage. It was held that complications were manageable only by a neurophysician. No documents were produced in support of the contention that treatment was done in accordance with the advice of the neurophysician and hence, negligence was held. In M Vijayan vs. Vishwanathan I (2012) CPJ 43, a child with burn injuries was operated on and got infected, resulting in septicemia. According to the State Commission, third-degree burns are major problems and shall be referred to special burn centers. Not referring to a higher center is serious negligence. According to the plastic surgeon, the treatment was substandard and hence, compensation was granted.

DELEGATION OF DUTIES

A doctor can delegate his duties to a qualified and competent junior, assistant, partner, nursing staff, or laboratory assistant. Negligence was held in Birdhichand Meena vs. Dr Prabhakar Sethi I (2003) CPJ 45, where the doctor left a case of acute severe dehydration without making alternative arrangements. If the staff to whom the duty is delegated is unqualified or incompetent, then it is the liability of the doctor delegating such duty.

SOME SPECIAL SITUATIONS

Sometimes, there may be some special situations in pediatrics practice, such as immunization, injections, and blood transfusion.

Giving Injections

If there is any mishap while giving any drug or vaccine, then known complications are usual defenses. But the doctors should have taken all the precautions to manage such complications, for example, anaphylaxis after penicillin, xylocaine, and measles vaccine are known complications. A doctor must examine skin sensitivity before giving penicillin, xylocaine, etc. Oxygen, adrenaline, intravenous (IV) fluids, and steroids must be available in case a reaction occurs. It is always better to explain to the relatives that such complications can occur. A written consent is preferable before administrating injectable drugs. History of drug allergy should be recorded before prescribing any drugs which are known to cause allergic reactions.

Sometimes, if IV fluid goes at a very fast speed, various undesirable complications may occur. If the nurse is qualified and the doctor has written proper orders, the doctor may not be held negligent. But if the paramedical staff is not qualified, then doctor shall be responsible. It is always better to use pediatric bottles, microdrip sets, or chambers. At the time of starting IV line, if these are not available, extra fluid from the bottle may be discarded.

Blood Transfusion

A qualified and trained nurse or doctor should check the patient's and donor's details with their respective blood groups before starting the blood transfusion. The treating doctor shall not be responsible for wrong or mistakes by blood bank staff or in-charge (the pathologist shall be responsible for the mistakes in the blood bank). The transfusion of the blood at proper volume and proper rate is the responsibility of the treating doctor/nurse. Proper monitoring of pulse, respiratory rate, and other vital signs including early signs of mismatched blood transfusion shall be done during the transfusion. In Ms Shefali vs. Indraprastha Apollo Hospital, the patient was admitted with malaria, had a decreased platelet count, and blood/platelet transfusion was given without taking proper precautions, resulting in transmission of Hepatitis C infection. Mother's blood was not given, even though it was available. Negligence was held and compensation was awarded. In another case, J Gopal vs. Nagarjuna Blood Bank II (2003) CPJ 434, the deficiency on part of blood bank was held for issuing incorrect donor card [human immunodeficiency virus (HIV) negative]. The child became HIV positive after receiving the infected blood. Blood bank was asked to pay compensation.

SOME LEGAL ISSUES

Vicarious Liability

Vicarious liability involves the acts of staff members, partners, locum, etc. in different situations. In Rekha Gupta vs. Bombay Hospital Trust, II (2003) CPJ 160 (NC), the concept of vicarious liability was explained by the state forum. The contention of the hospital that it only provides infrastructure and the responsibility of the treatment lies with the consultant was not accepted by the forum. According to the forum, the hospital has employed the medical staff and is deducting commission while remitting the fees cannot disown the responsibility on superficial grounds. The doctors shall be liable for the acts of their staff if they are unqualified. But if the staff is qualified and make a mistake, then the doctor may not be directly responsible. For example, if doctor has prescribed some medicines or injections correctly and the nurse (qualified) makes a mistake, then in such cases, doctor is not responsible for her act. But if nurse is unqualified, then doctor shall be held responsible. In Sushma Sharma vs. Bombay Hospital II (2007) CPJ 9 (NC), it was observed that there was lack of coordination between various specialists and intensive care unit (ICU) residents. The hospital was held vicariously liable. It was observed that consultants could give orders, but actual administration is the responsibility of the parent hospital. It is up to the hospital to decide what action they want to take against the doctor/specialist.

Res Ipsa Loquitur

Res ipsa loquitur maxim means "things speak for themselves." The damages are so obvious that there is no need for any proof of negligence. Examples of such situation include giving blood transfusion to a wrong baby, operating on wrong side or wrong patient, retained sponges or forceps after surgery, etc. This principle was applied in P Ashwin vs. Manipal Hospital I (1997) CPJ 238, where a newborn child postoperatively developed burns on both legs due to hot water bags. The doctors were held negligent for the subsequent deformity. In another case, Sunil Rathi vs. Rita Dey and others I (2007) CPJ 270, negligence was held in a 10-day-old child who developed an infection at the injection site, subsequently leading to gangrene and autoamputation of the hand. The Consumer Forum agreed that the principle of *res ipsa loquitur* was applicable. In J Nathan vs. M Masane I (2008) CPJ 191 NC, a boy with epilepsy was prescribed medicines. Treatment changed without considering side effects (Stevens-Johnson syndrome after zeptol); the condition worsened and started getting more convulsions. The patient was admitted and died due to septicemia. Principle of *res ipsa loquitur* was applied and negligence was held. In B S Raj vs. M Pandharinath I (2008) CPJ 53, a patient with cough, chest pain, and blood in sputum did not respond to antibiotics. He was put on antitubercular drugs without adequate tests. No instructions were given regarding side effects of drugs. The patient deteriorated and died due to drug-induced hepatitis. The principle of *res ipsa loquitur* was applied and negligence was held. But subsequently in 2012, the National Commission in this case held that the adverse reactions were conveyed on phone and the petitioner was requested to stop the drugs. The patient did not get admitted for further treatment, had left against medical advice, and hence no negligence.

Child as a Consumer

In M/s Spring Meadows Hospital vs. Harjot Ahluwalia (AIR 1998 SC 1801), the Supreme Court has decided that both the minor child and the parents are consumers, and compensation may be awarded to both.

Limitation Period

The basic concept of the Limitation Act is that an individual must be aware of his rights and whenever these rights are infringed, one must act within a reasonable time to get back these rights. The law aids the diligent and not the indolent; one cannot sleep over the period when the rights are deprived. Thus, if a particular case of negligence is filed beyond the period of limitation (3 years according to Civil law), the defending doctor may forward this defense. In Ms Neha Kumari vs. Apollo Hospital I (2003) CPJ 145 (NC), the case was dismissed on the ground that it was time-barred. As per the provisions of the CPA, in any particular case, if the chairman of the forum feels appropriate, he may condone the limitation period after recording the reasons for the same.

Home Visits

There are some situations (including safety reasons) when a doctor can refuse or turn down a patient. In odd hours, especially if it is not an emergency, a home visit can be definitely refused. If a patient is really sick, he should attend the clinic/hospital where 24-hour emergency services are available. If the patient is not under the care of a doctor, the visit may be refused. A telephonic talk between the doctor and the patient or his relatives does not establish the relationship.

Ethical Issues

The field of pediatric healthcare is rapidly expanding. Most medical research is not complete unless experimentation on human subjects, including children, is undertaken. Children as research subjects are more vulnerable than adults. Hence, research on children should only be conducted, if the importance of the objective outweighs the inherent risks to the subjects. Now, it is widely expected that any new therapeutic, diagnostic, or preventive product that is likely to be used in children should undergo adequate safety and efficacy investigation in children. A drug trial can only be carried out after the approval of Drugs Controller General of India (DCGI). Clearance from ethics committee is required before submitting the proposal to DCGI.

Life Support Measures

Emotional feelings of adolescents may provoke them for blood donation, organ transplant, etc. Some specific, advanced, costly treatments such as ventilator therapy (including weaning from the ventilator) and euthanasia require valid consent. As per Article 21 of the Constitution of India, every individual has his own life and he can lead it as per his wishes within the framework of the law. Thus not only ethically but also legally, an individual has the right to decide whether to live or not. Probably because of this only, it is said that an individual can refuse any type of trial or treatment on his body.

Documentation

Documentation of records including history, examination, investigations, etc., should be properly maintained. A well-maintained document could be a friend of a doctor in the hours of crisis. In one case (L Meena vs. Dr S Mathur III 2001 CPJ 200), documents came to the rescue of the treating pediatrician that has been reported. In this case, a newborn with physiological jaundice who was discharged on the fifth day of life alleged deterioration and came again on the sixth day; after refusal, went to another hospital and got treated but became handicapped. In defense, doctors produced proper documents while the complainant produced fabricated documents. He took discharge against medical advice (DAMA) from the second hospital and went to the third hospital. This case was dismissed with costs in favor of the pediatrician. A doctor was held liable in HS Sharma vs. Indraprastha Apollo Hospital II (2007) CPJ 21(NC) on the ground that the complications that occurred during eye operations could have been avoided if proper care had been taken. The court also observed that according to the Indian Medical Council (MCI) Act, it is incumbent upon medical practitioners to maintain records. The discharge summary should be patient friendly and not mechanical.

Consent

Consent is routinely required in all cases of medical examinations and treatment. The adolescent may refuse treatment and demand privacy of medical records. Such consent must be taken before starting the procedure and after proper explanation of the pros and cons of the process.

Emotional feelings of adolescents may provoke them for blood donation, organ transplant, etc. A valid consent must be taken in any type of medicolegal examination. In cases of minors, parents' or guardians' consent can be taken. The consent in pediatric age may vary from situation to situation such as age of the child, place where he is residing (home, boarding school, orphanage etc.), type of illness, and availability of guardians.

Child Abuse

The term child abuse refers to any act or failure to act that violates the right of the child and endangers his or her optimal health, survival, or development. The concept of child abuse has broadened to include not only physical violence but also sexual abuse, mental and emotional maltreatment, neglect, deprivation, and lack of opportunity. Abused children, when they become parents, tend to abuse their children. The victims of suspected child abuse must be examined in detail at the earliest before signs start disappearing. The possibility of child abuse must be kept in mind, in children with multiple fractures, nonaccidental injuries, repeated admissions without significant illness, etc. The Protection of Children from Sexual Offences (POCSO) Act is discussed in detail in Chapter 40.

Effect of Media

The media should be attentive to their influence on children. This influence is related to content and total viewing time. The media has a key role to play in raising awareness about the situation of children and the challenges facing them; they should also play a more active role in informing children, parents, families, and the general public about initiatives that protect and promote the rights of children. It is recommended that the total viewing time should be restricted to 1–2 hours per day and screening of the contents of the program should also be taken care of. Children should be protected from violent or harmful websites, computer programs, and games that negatively influence the psychological development of children. There is a need for better programming, alternative leisure activities, and promoting parental involvement. We should take necessary measures, including enhanced cooperation between governments, intergovernmental organizations, and nongovernmental organizations to combat the criminal use of technologies against children and adolescents.

When to Inform Police?

A doctor has to inform the police in the following circumstances. Failure to inform the police in such cases may result in penal consequences.

Police must be informed in:
- Cases of suspected homicide
- Cases of suicidal deaths
- Unknown, unconscious patient
- Death on operation table
- Suspected unnatural death
- Sudden, unexpected, violent, unexplained death
- Instant death after treatment or reaction of medicine

It is advisable to inform the police in the following circumstances:

- Undiagnosed death occurring within 24 hours of admission or if any suspicious cause of death is there, then it is desirable to inform the police. In cases where the cause of death is obvious or can be diagnosed by the treating doctor, then there is no need to inform the police.
- Cases of poisoning
- Deaths in accidents
- Hospital deaths if:
  - Accidents unrelated to medical treatment such as falling from a staircase—though there is no legal obligation on the doctor, it is advisable to inform the police.
  - Rare or unexpected complications such as a child vomiting, aspirating the content, and may die. This is very unpredictable and it is not obligatory for the doctor to inform. But it is better if they inform because sometimes the patient's relatives may have an allegation of negligence.
  - In cases of death due to negligence, there are no specific guidelines to inform the police, but to avoid untoward incidences, it is advisable to inform. When in any case the cause of death cannot be ascertained, it is desirable to have a postmortem examination, preferably with the help of the police. It is advisable to *suggest postmortem* in the following circumstances:
    - Whenever death is sudden, unexpected, unexplained
    - Accidental deaths which may be roadside, domestic, or industrial
    - When precise cause of death is needed for insurance claim purposes, etc.
    - As a help to arrive at the final diagnosis

Information to the police shall preferably be in writing and written acknowledgment should be obtained. If the information is telephonic, one must note down the name, buckle number, and designation of the police.

Infant Milk Substitute Act

Inappropriate infant feeding practices result in feeding difficulties and malnutrition, ultimately leading to increased mortality and morbidity in children. Poor infant feeding practices and their consequences are one of the world's major problems and a serious obstacle to social and economic development. Being to a great extent, a man-made problem, it must be considered as a reproach to our science and technology and our social and economic structures, and a blot on our so-called development achievements. The World Organizations and Governments were forced to enact International Codes and National Acts [Infant Milk Substitute (IMS) Act] and regulations to restrict the unethical promotion of commercial foods. The details of the IMS Act are discussed in Chapter 41. The qualified pediatricians have moral and ethical responsibility to provide health education to the masses so as to remove misconception and food taboos from the minds of the people. In Amit Masih vs. J Iyer 574 of 2013 (decided in March 15), a lower segment cesarean section (LSCS) baby, weighing 3.1 kg, developed jaundice on the fourth day. The baby was shifted without the mother. Powder milk (Dexolac) was given with a bottle. Baby vomited and developed aspiration pneumonia, resulting in subsequent infection, septicemia, and multiorgan failure and ultimately died. The compensation was awarded.

The implementation of the Act in its true spirit will give us a chance to improve the health and well-being of our future generation by reversing the declining breastfeeding practices.

Scoring System for Risk of Medicolegal or Negligence Case

There is an overall deterioration in moral and human values. The patient's expectations are soaring and these result in frustration if something unexpected happens. The Supreme Court in CA no. 3541 of 2002, Martin F D'Souza vs. Mohd Ishfaq has observed that the medical profession is a noble profession and it should not be brought down to the level of a simple business or commerce. The law is a watchdog and not a bloodhound and as long as doctors do their duty with reasonable care, they will not be held liable even if their treatment is unsuccessful. While this Court has no sympathy for doctors who are negligent, it must also be said that frivolous complaints against doctors have increased by leaps and bounds in our country, particularly after the medical profession was placed within the purview of the CPA.

We have developed a scoring system to assess the risk of medicolegal cases **(Table 17.1)**. This scoring helps the individual practitioner in assessing the risk of negligence while caring for patient. The scoring is based on six different vital issues, criteria, or situations that one has to face daily as far as the legally safe and ethical practice of medicine is concerned.

The scoring or grading can be interpreted, analyzed, and calculated as follows:
- *High risk*: If the score is 25–30.
- *Moderate risk*: If the score is 19–24.
- *Average risk*: If the score is 13–18.
- *Minimal risk*: If the score is 7–12.
- *Negligible risk*: If the score is <7.

Table 17.1: Scoring system for risk of medicolegal or negligence case.

	Score				
Criteria	***1***	***2***	***3***	***4***	***5***
Access to medicolegal consultant (help and guidance)	All possible help	Written help/ guidance	Discussed	No guidance	No help
Behavior (communication skills)	Communication with proper skills	Communication with relatives	Communication with "so-called social worker"	With patient but not with relatives	No communi-cation
Consent	Informed	Written	Implied	Blanket	Not taken
Doctor–patient relationship	Excellent	Good	Average	Poor	Very poor
Expertise in the field	Proper qualification/ experience	No experience	No qualification	Cross pathy	Quacks
Facts/ documentation	Clear, correct, comprehensive, and chronological	Record of other colleagues	Improper	Manipulated	Not available

Limitations of this Scoring

Though care has been taken to consider various issues related to day-to-day practice, but there may be many other factors which predispose to allegations of medical negligence. The "no risk" group is not there as it is very difficult and practically impossible to learn and acquire all the skills with complete competency or perfection. The laws are interpreted and analyzed differently by different people/experts including legal experts. The scoring may change after provocation of/by the patient, relatives, or "so-called social workers."

The benefit/outcome: It is expected that those who want minimum stress or crisis in their practice should follow these parameters very meticulously/judiciously. This scoring may not give full or complete protection against medical malpractice/negligence cases but will definitely indemnify in the hours of crisis.

In Kusum Sharma vs. Batra Hospital (SC 10th Feb. 2010), the Honorable Supreme Court has agreed that a professional deserves total protection. The Indian Penal Code has taken care to ensure that people who act in good faith should not be punished. Sections 88, 92, and 370 of the Indian Penal Code give adequate protection to the professional and particularly to medical professionals. But the pediatricians and other professionals must take precautions to prevent cases of negligence against them.

CONCLUSION

The cases of negligence against doctors are increasing by leaps and bounds. Few years back, the pediatricians had less cases as compared to other specialties, but in last few years, the risk has increased. As we are moving toward the concept of small or nuclear families, the number of children in a family is decreasing, so every child is precious and parents want the best possible treatment. We have to explain to these anxious parents that we can guarantee "care" and not cure. We have to explain that in many cases, intact survival may not be possible and many times, the child may have a disability in cases of premature, low birth weight, or birth asphyxia cases. Each and every disability may not be negligence.

KEY LEARNING POINTS

- The cases of negligence in pediatrics (ROP, developmental abnormalities, fetal anomalies, etc.) are increasing.
- Give a guarded prognosis.
- Explain the abnormality by following the communication skills.
- The discharge card shall be patient friendly.
- Be more vigilant in cases of child abuse.
- Inform police if we find parental disputes or suspicious behavior.

BIBLIOGRAPHY

1. Greydanus D, Patel D, Pratt H, et al. (Eds). Indian Academy of Pediatrics—International Training Program on Adolescent Health. Adolescent Health in United States. Course Manual for Adolescent Health: Part I. New Delhi: Indian Academy of Pediatrics: 2002. pp. 1-8.
2. Gupta A, Singh CU, Jessy G. Under attack: An Indian law to protect breastfeeding. New Delhi: BPNI. DK Fine Arts Press; 1998. pp. 10-1.
3. Park K. Hospital Sociology. In: Park K (Ed). Park's Textbook of Preventive and Social Medicine, 25th edition. Jabalpur: M/s Banarsidas Bhanot; 2019. pp. 747-50.
4. Potdar RD. Consumer protection law and pediatrician. Indian Pediatr. 1997;34:283-6.
5. Sectish TC. Preventive Pediatrics. In: Behrman RE, Kliegman RM, Jenson HB (Eds). Nelson Textbook of Pediatrics, 17th edition. Philadelphia: Saunders; 2004. pp. 14-20.
6. Shah N, Paul Y. Legal safety in pediatric research. In: Baldwa M, Tiwari S, Tiwari M, et al. (Eds). Legal Problems in day-to-day Pediatrics Practice. Hyderabad: Paras Publishing; 2010. pp. 194-8.
7. Tiwari SK, Baldwa M. Doctors and Criminal Law. Indian Pediatr. 2002;39:1119-25.
8. Tiwari SK, Baldwa M. Medical negligence. Indian Pediatr. 2001;38:488-95.
9. Tiwari SK. Legal aspects in medical practice. Indian Pediatr. 2000;37:961-6.
10. Yadav B, Tiwari S. Medicolegal issues in Pediatrics. In: Tiwari S, Baldwa M, Tiwari M, et al. (Eds). Textbook on Medicolegal Issues Related to Various Medical Specialties, 2nd edition. New Delhi: Jaypee Brothers Medical Publishers (P) Ltd.; 2019. pp. 197-207.

17.1 Medicolegal Issues in Newborn Care

Kanya Mukhopadhyay

INTRODUCTION

As the neonatal survival is improving and many neonatal intensive cares are coming up in our country, several medicolegal issues are arising and there are lawsuits across the country. Major issues are related to perinatal asphyxia and its consequences, resuscitation at extremes of low gestation, decisions regarding withdrawal or withholding care for life-threatening disorders and severe illnesses which can lead to disabilities in later life. Failure to prevent blindness by adequate and appropriate intervention in preterm neonates by proper screening for retinopathy of prematurity (ROP) is a major medicolegal issue. Proper documentation, consent, and adequate counseling are key factors to prevent litigations.

The major contributory factors for neonatal death in our country are prematurity, neonatal infections followed by birth asphyxia or trauma. Along with improvements in technology, the neonatal survival is improving in all the above scenarios and parents' expectations too are also rising. In this era of more internet knowledge, people may ask more questions and can also go for lawsuits for various issues. The interventions in certain situations may lead to increase in handicapped survivors though availability of intensive care unit beds is also a major issue in resource limited settings. There is always a social pressure as well as medicolegal issues to salvage every live newborn which may not be always in the best interest of patient or family in presence of factors which may lead to a meaningless life or cause a significant burden on families, caretakers, and society. Quite often we tend to mimic western scenarios without realizing the constraints of resource limited setups. Though guidelines are available in western countries, it is lacking in our country regarding withdrawal of care in sick neonates and in life-threatening disorders where continuation of care may be futile.

Intensive care practices deal with three issues—(1) medical, (2) ethical, and (3) legal. Medical issues involve actual medical management and clinically related issues. Ethics involve to take right decisions while maintaining patients' interests in all aspects. Legal issues involve maintaining a standard care practice and providing honest and actual information to parents and care takers. Quite often neonatologists face tough decisions in neonatal intensive care unit (NICU) while providing care to a sick preterm newborn and conflicts may arise between medical care and ethics while maintaining legal aspects.

There are several situations in a neonatal unit where medicolegal issues can arise due to:
- Negligence
- Misdiagnosis
- Wrong treatment/maltreatment
- Death or permanent disability
- Lack of consent

Negligence can be an issue for preventable illnesses, e.g.—(1) inadequate treatment of neonatal hyperbilirubinemia in which delayed diagnosis or treatment of jaundice can lead to lifelong handicap due to acute bilirubin encephalopathy (ABE) which is an avoidable condition. Negligence could be (a) failure to screen and identify high risk babies, (b) failure to follow-up of babies who were discharged early, (c) failure to initiate phototherapy in time, (d) inadequate intervention in the form of intensive phototherapy and exchange transfusion. (2) Many parents may feel perinatal asphyxia and their sequelae could be due to negligence or inadequate treatment by obstetricians as well as pediatricians and may opt for legal solution. American Academy of Pediatrics (AAP) and American College of Obstetricians and Gynecologists (ACOG) have laid down strict criteria to define perinatal asphyxia which can be used in such lawsuits.

- Misdiagnosis can be a problem in cases of perinatal asphyxia where there is failure to pick up timely fetal distress and intervention, it may be failure to pick up lethal malformations in antenatal scans for which termination option was available. Death or permanent disability even can result due to this.
- Wrong treatment or maltreatment can arise in several clinical situations such as wrong medications, dosages, intravenous therapy complications, extravasation related injuries, limb gangrene resulting from arterial spasm following arterial cannulations, burns, infections, severe ROP due failure to screen timely and lack of adequate treatment, inadequate monitoring in sick children, delay in initiating treatment, retained foreign body, death, etc. Maintenance of adequate and appropriate documents is very important to safeguard these issues. Failure to maintain a document is equivalent to no documents and inadequate service.
- Death or permanent disability could arise due to the disease itself or by negligence or wrong treatment.
- Sometimes interventions are done without consent or proper explanation or documentation for the need of some investigations/treatments to the parents which can lead to medicolegal issues. All invasive procedures such as lumbar puncture, ventricular tap, etc., need a written consent from parents.

However, other than the above situations, sometimes decisions to be taken regarding continuation of critical care or end of life (EOL) decisions in NICU. There may be certain situations which are very challenging for neonatologists. Most of the time it is a complex medical, social, ethical, and moral dilemma by doctors, healthcare workers, and parents. In one hand the issue of long-term neurodevelopmental disabilities along with high cost of intensive care versus emotional and social issues regarding withdrawal of care poses a challenge to medical staffs working in NICU.

PERINATAL ASPHYXIA

When a baby suffers severe perinatal asphyxia, several issues may arise regarding antenatal management and subsequent postnatal issues.

Questions may arise regarding:

- Cause of asphyxia?
- Whether timely intervention was done?
- Was it preventable?
- Criteria of asphyxia fulfilled?
- Any supportive evidence available, e.g., cardiotocograph (CTG) tracings, partogram, scalp pH, or lactate, etc.
- Were skilled personnel available during delivery?

- Other documents such as placental examination to rule out chorioamnionitis, thrombosis, infarcts, or any evidence of metabolic diseases?
- Magnetic resonance imaging (MRI) changes and type and timing of injury

For any litigation all the above points are very relevant, however, after severe asphyxial insult if the baby develops severe encephalopathy which can lead to lifelong disabilities, questions arise regarding continuation of intensive care, ventilation, and other life sustaining care. There are guidelines how to define asphyxia and its prognosis which are required for any legal proceeding in USA.

RESUSCITATION OF EXTREMELY LOW BIRTH WEIGHT NEONATES (<1,000 g)

This is an important issue where a significant medicolegal argument can arise, regarding cut off for resuscitation in periviable births, which is defined as delivery occurring between $20^{0/7}$–$25^{6/7}$ weeks' gestation. The survival is increasing from 22 to 25 weeks' gestation (western data only, no Indian data available <24 weeks' gestation), however, long-term outcome improves with higher gestation. It should be a shared decision with parents. There are no legal guidelines of cut off gestation for limits of viability in our country, and there is a wide variation in resources in government versus private providing neonatal intensive care.

As per 2017 guidelines, ACOG and society for maternal-fetal medicine on previable birth, recommend resuscitation from $24^{0/7}$ weeks onward and consider between $22^{0/7}$ and $23^{6/7}$ weeks' gestation and not recommended <22 weeks' gestation. AAP in NRP guidelines (2010) and American Heart Association (AHA) earlier recommended noninitiation of resuscitation in confirmed cases of gestation <23 weeks and birth weight of <400 g, anencephaly, in confirmed trisomy 13 and 18 syndromes and possible 23–24 weeks' gestation if parents do not want resuscitation, however, in 2021 NRP guidelines no gestational age cut off has been provided for lower cut off for resuscitation. In India there are no laws which either say not to resuscitate or to withdraw resuscitation in such cases.

As per latest IAP-NNF textbook of NRP guidelines-2023, neonates who are after 25 weeks and >600 g, resuscitation should be initiated. For neonates born between 23 and 25 weeks, medical team should discuss with parents and decide based on local data.

One also needs to remember that gestation assignment also may be inaccurate if decided by ultrasounds done after first trimester. Parents need a detail counseling regarding short-term and long-term outcomes of an extremely low birth weight (ELBW) neonate. Local data also should be provided to parents to decide, as well as availability of expertise and infrastructure and parental support for long-term issues in these survivors.

CARE OF BABIES WITH MAJOR MALFORMATIONS/DISORDERS

Major malformation, chromosomal disorders which are either not compatible with life or associated with severe morbidities also pose a medicolegal issue whether to resuscitate these babies and to continue care or not. In such cases parents should be given a detail information regarding the clinical condition and their short-term and long-term outcomes, cost details, quality of life, extent of family care required, etc. Extended family can be involved in decision making and decision whether to resuscitate or not can be planned well before delivery and written consent should be obtained for further treatment plans. All discussion must be well documented and signed by parents, medical team, and witness. Sometimes there may be a conflict between parents and doctor's decision in continuation of care, parents wanting to continue all medical care which may not be in the best interest of child.

SERIOUS COMPLICATIONS IN PRETERM BABIES

Some extremely preterm babies or babies with significant illness can develop severe grades of intraventricular hemorrhage (IVH) or extensive periventricular leukomalacia (PVL) which can be associated with short-term as well long-term neuromorbidities. In such cases continuation of intensive care becomes a difficult decision for both the medical teams as well as parents.

As per article 21 of constitution of India, everybody has a right to live. Hence decisions should be taken at the best interest of the patient. Though there are several discussions and opinions from medical community there is no definitive court ruling regarding EOL decisions in neonates.

End-of-life Decisions in Neonates

The EOL decisions in neonates are one of the most difficult situations for both parents and medical team due to *ethical and legal* dilemmas attached to it. A very effective communication system must exist between both sides to take such a decision. The major issues regarding decisions are (1) uncertainty in diagnosis and prognosis, (2) decision making process, and (3) palliative care. Sometimes there may be a gap in the conversations between medical team and parents.

The three most common neonatal situations which may require EOL decisions are:

1. Fetuses at the lower gestational age/limit of viability
2. Neonates with life-threatening/life-limiting congenital malformations and syndromes
3. Acutely ill newborn in intensive care with very poor prognosis

Ethical Principles

While one takes the decision of EOL in any critically sick child, there are four ethical principles which must be followed:

1. Autonomy (of parents in case of neonates)
2. Beneficence
3. Nonmalfeasance
4. Distributive justice

- To have autonomy, he/she should be competent to make his/her own decisions and correct choices. In cases of children and neonates, either the parents or a legal guardian can take such decisions if own parents not available.
- *Beneficence* means action to be taken in the patient's best interest. As a doctor, he is expected to act in the best interests of the patient and his family members, and in addition to medical treatment, doctor has to provide compassionate care during the dying process. The doctor should facilitate (neither hastening nor delaying) the dying process and avoid/reduce the sufferings of the patient and his family, he should be providing also emotional support to family and family should be advised how to prevent financial losses. There are charitable

trusts, insurance schemes as well as many welfare programs by government and parents should be counseled regarding these facilities insurance schemes.

- *Nonmalfeasance* means first do no harm, and unnecessary or unacceptable burden should not be imposed upon the patient/parents.
- *Distributive justice* should be offered to parents, which means patients should be treated truthfully and fairly. Doctors should take a responsible decision and available infrastructure must be used judiciously. In developing countries financial resources and the manpower are always a constraint and hence utilization of this and human resources need to be used carefully. The doctor may decide to provide treatment and available resources to a patient who has potentially curable condition rather than a patient who has a very poor chance of recovery.

In cases of resuscitation of newborn, though the autonomy of newborn to be respected but to take decision in life-threatening emergency situations by doctors are exceptions of general rules of ethics.

Legal Dilemma in End-of-life Decisions

Certainty Regarding Prognosis

While taking a decision on EOL, one should be reasonably certain regarding outcome/prognosis of the case. In many countries there are set guidelines about when to initiate EOL decisions. In India, recently supreme court has released legal guidelines for decisions to forego life-sustaining treatment (LST) and applicable for patients—(1) who have lost decision-making capacity, and (2) who are terminally ill. If these conditions are fulfilled and if further LST would not be beneficial to the patient, a multistep approach has been legalized by supreme court.

The decision of EOL needs significant expertise and experience. Sometimes physician's opinion could be biased and depends on own attitude toward life. EOL decisions are different and difficult in pediatric and neonatal patients due to emotional attachment to parents as children are in the beginning of their life. Sometimes communication gap between doctors and parents can also lead to misinterpretation.

End-of-life Decision in Limits of Viability

In cases of EOL decisions or do not resuscitate (DNR) orders in delivery room in cases of limits of viability could pose legal issues. It is sometimes difficult to ascertain the exact gestation before delivery because the methods by which gestation is assigned are not always foolproof unless it is in vitro fertilization (IVF) pregnancy. Obstetrical dating is accurate up to $\pm$ 1 week and estimated fetal weight could vary between $\pm$ 15 and 20%. This is extremely important for preterm gestation as 1–2 weeks' gestation or 15–20% weight difference can lead to significant difference in mortality and morbidity predictions however it does not make any difference in cases of term pregnancy.

Ethical Dilemma in End-of-life Decisions

Who takes Decision if Patient is a Newborn or Minor?

As pediatric and neonatal patients cannot give consent on their own to medical treatment, they need surrogate consent from parents or local guardians. Though older children and adolescents are/can sometimes be part of decision making but neonatal patients always need surrogate decision makers. Older children and adolescent can be part of the decision making if their neurologic status, development, and level of maturity allow that.

Though it is almost universally accepted that parents decide about the treatment of newborn/minor but conflicts may arise in certain situations when parents' decisions are detrimental to the health of newborn. This situation is often faced when moral and religious beliefs of the parents prevent them taking EOL decisions. The legal options may vary from country to country. In USA usual legal options are either a court appointed legal guardian to replace parents or to take the temporary custody of the child and to involve childcare services. On the other side, a situation may arise when medical team wants to continue treatment but parents refuse to do so. In our country many times parents would ask physician to take the decision. Though the above situations can be solved to a great extent by effective communication rather than opting legal options.

The effective communication should include:
- Details of prognosis of the condition (known and unknown) both short term and long term explained to parents in local language.
- Comprehensive understanding of the existing condition by the parents.
- Explanation and providing comfort care to dying baby—providing warmth, oxygen, feeding and not ventilation, inotropes, or intravenous fluids. Parents may like to stay with the baby or can take the baby home at this point.
- Nutrition and hydration after withdrawal of care
- Discussion about mode of EOL which are:
  - Do not resuscitate
  - Withhold LST
  - Withdraw LST
- *DNR* means do not initiate any of the procedures or further resuscitation in babies who are already on ventilator in the event of clinical deterioration.
- *Withholding of LST* implies death due to the withholding of treatment which is necessary for the survival after birth which may include surgical intervention and resuscitation (it could be by hand ventilation with bag, or with endotracheal tube ventilation, or may be external cardiac massage, or administration of injection adrenaline).
- *Withdrawal of LST* implies death due to the elective discontinuation of ongoing life support. Natural death implies death occurring despite of maximal intensive care provided.

Concept of DNR came in the last quarter of twentieth century along with the promotion of patient autonomy. It has become quite familiar situation though not frequently encountered phenomenon. DNR order has to have a valid and informed consent from the patient himself or a relative in cases of comatose patients, or from parents or a legal guardian for minors such as neonates and children.

Commonly EOL decisions are taken in situation like:
- Malformations not compatible with life
- Conditions where treatment will not lead to a meaningful life.
- When there is no further treatment available and death is imminent.

The survival in these cases may lead to significant morbidities and neurodevelopmental disabilities, leading to significant burden on parents and society. Hence, the neonatal team need to make decisions to withhold or withdraw LST or to issue DNR orders in a planned manner.

Whether to Withhold or to Withdraw Life-sustaining Treatment?

There are several studies which highlight that for parents withholding LST decision may be easier than active withdrawal of treatment though ethically there is not much difference. In addition, the duration of suffering after resuscitation may be far longer for neonatal and pediatric patients than for adult patients.

Reluctance of a Do Not Resuscitate Order for Pediatric/Neonatal Patients

The ethical issues regarding EOL decisions in children are unique. These decisions are not only medical but involve the whole array of moral, social, cultural, religious, and financial issues. The last days of children and how they died are remembered by parents forever. Hence, it is a difficult decision for them and quite often they are willing to continue in spite of chances of significant morbidity associated with survival. Sometimes there is delay and hesitation from physician as both physicians and parents tend to use all available therapy options, no matter what the condition of the child though timely discussion with parents and family improves the decision of EOL in NICU. Sometimes the time given to parents to take decision is too short such as in cases of DNR at birth due to extreme prematurity or severe malformations diagnosed late in pregnancy.

Sometimes there may be a discrepancy between parents' understanding of the child's disease, its prognosis and that of treating physician. In one study, parents realized the lack of any realistic chance of cure nearly 100 days later than physicians explained it to them. This is due to delay in accepting the poor prognosis and parents may feel withdrawal may be equivalent to betraying the child. In addition, in our country the concept of "male child" or a "precious child" concept also delays significantly the decision to withdraw care.

The pediatric and neonatal patients are ethically unique due to their inability to take decisions and as a result.

- There is delay in implementing DNR order which unnecessarily prolongs their life and lead to futile investigations. This compromises their actual care of their sufferings and not taking care of their dignity (e.g., in pediatric cancer patients) and this is also very common in neonates.
- They may be subjected lot of medical interventions and tests up to the time of death.

The surrogate decision-makers should act in the best interests of the child but if the surrogate is a parent, then lot of psychological and emotional factors may make it difficult for them to act and it may not be in the in the best interests of the infant. Hence, the counseling must be adequate to avoid this and explained that prolongation of life is not in the best interests of the child.

When a newborn is affected by a life-limiting condition, a plan of preterminal care should be made along with parents. Comfort care for the newborn, pain relief, maintenance of body temperature, relief of hunger, taking care of parent's emotions, psychosocial care, and religious needs of the family are all parts of palliative care of a terminally ill newborn. This practice needs to be standardized in our country.

The practices of withdrawal, palliative care, and legal guidelines vary from country to country. Active withdrawal of treatment is common in NICUs across Europe as well as in the USA. In a multicentric survey from Europe showed that physicians from these countries have set limits to intensive interventions. Though parents take an active role in decision making but not a sole role in decision-making process. Physician should support them with clear and informed medical counseling in EOL decision making.

In a study from Portugal, a retrospective chart review data regarding withdrawing/withholding of care as well as palliative care following that during 2 time periods, 1992–1995 and 2002–2005, found withholding/withdrawal of care was significantly more in later cohort though DNR was not different. Therapeutic activities (ventilation, antibiotics, TPN, enteral nutrition) were similar in last 24 hours in both cohorts. Use of neonatal pain scale, opioids, and sedatives were significantly more in 2nd cohort. A significantly higher number of parents met neonatologist and were present at death in 2nd cohort which were more than the 1st cohort. This shows that practices are changing overtime regarding more parental involvement in decision making and accepting practices of palliative care.

In a study from Israel which collected data over 10 years (1st cohort 2000–2004 and 2nd cohort 2005–2009) showed that prematurity was the commonest cause of death and congenital malformations amongst term infants. Over the years, their maximal intensive care reduced from 65 to 46% ($p < 0.02$), whereas redirection of care (limited care or withdrawal of care) increased from 19.2 to 37.5% ($p < 0.005$) and parental role in EOL increased from 38 to 84%. These trends reflect that apart from survival, quality of life is also very important factor in decision-making process. There was a change of practice from 2006 in this unit. In all very sick babies admitted in NICU, family was approached and EOL treatment options were discussed when the situation was likely to result in a prolonged dying process or survival with severe limitations.

RETINOPATHY OF PREMATURITY

Retinopathy of prematurity is a preventable cause of blindness in children. Studies from India reported 20–30% incidence of ROP among preterm neonates and timely detection and treatment can prevent blindness. There are increasing lawsuits for not detecting ROP at right time or for delayed treatment leading to blindness.

The major risk factors are prematurity, low birth weight, high oxygen concentration and use leading to hyperoxia. Other associated factors are sepsis, acidosis, PDA, apnea, IVH, and blood transfusion. All preterm and low birth weight neonates (<34 weeks, <2 kg), higher gestation neonates (34–36 weeks) with significant neonatal illnesses, and any neonate with unstable clinical course should be screened for ROP, as per Rashtriya Bal Swasthya Karyakram-2017 (RBSK) guidelines.

CONCLUSION

In conclusion, a clear national policy is required regarding weight and gestational age cut offs for resuscitation, when to withhold care, when to withdraw care in sick neonates, how to use judiciously the limited resources, and training for palliative care in NICUs should be in place. A shared decision-making protocol along with parents/caretakers in all decisions should be followed.

The medicolegal issues in modern day neonatal care has two aspects—1st is medicolegal issues related to inadequate management or negligence leading to law suits; the 2nd aspect is EOL decisions where care seems to be futile or can lead to poor quality of life. Active parental involvement and counseling in decision-making process with honest and accurate information is important.

KEY LEARNING POINTS

- Adequate documentation of illness, treatment, prognosis, and counseling to parents must be documented.
- Decision for withholding and or withdrawal of care as well as palliative care to be discussed with parents in detail.
- Resuscitation of neonates at extremes of low gestation to be discussed with parents in advance.

BIBLIOGRAPHY

1. Million Death Study Collaborators. Changes in cause-specific neonatal and 1–59-month child mortality in India from 2000 to 2015: a national representative survey. Lancet. 2017;390:1972-80.
2. General Medical Council. Treatment and care towards the end of life: Good practice in decision making. 2010.
3. Mishra S, Mukhopadhyay K, Tiwari S, et al. End-of-life care: Consensus Statement by Indian Academy of Pediatrics. Indian Pediatr. 2017;54:851-9.
4. American College of Obstetricians and Gynecologists. Neonatal Encephalopathy and Cerebral Palsy: Defining the Pathogenesis and Pathophysiology. Washington DC: American College of Obstetrics and Gynecology, Task Force on Neonatal Encephalopathy and Cerebral Palsy, American Academy of Pediatrics; 2003.
5. Soltani Gerdfaramarzi M, Bazmi S. Neonatal end-of-life decisions and ethical perspectives. J Med Ethics Hist Med. 2020;13:19.
6. American Academy of Pediatrics Staff. Neonatal Encephalopathy and Neurologic Outcome. 2nd edition. American College of Obstetricians & Gynecologists; 2019
7. Nimbalkar SM, Bansal SC. Periviable birth – the ethical conundrum. Indian Pediatr. 2019;56:13-7.
8. Kattwinkle J, Perlman JM, Aziz K, et al. Neonatal Resuscitation: 2010 American Heart Association Guidelines for Cardiopulmonary Resuscitation and Emergency Cardiovascular Care. Circulation. 2010;122;S909-19.
9. American College of Obstetricians and Gynecologists; Society for Maternal-Fetal Medicine. Obstetric care consensus No. 6: Periviable Birth. Obstet Gynecol. 2017;130:e187-e99.
10. Limacher R, Fauchère JC, Gubler D, et al. Uncertainty and probability in neonatal end-of-life decision-making: analysing real-time conversations between healthcare professionals and families of critically ill newborns. BMC Palliat Care. 2023:22:53.
11. Gupta P, Ramji S (Eds). IAP - NNF textbook of neonatal resuscitation. 1st edition. Jaypee Brothers Medical Publishers (P) Ltd.; 2023.
12. Dettmeyer R. Extremely preterm babies—legal aspects and palliative care at the border of viability. Children. 2022;9(10):1594.
13. Mani RK, Simha S, Gursahani R. Simplified legal procedure for end-of-life decisions in India: a new dawn in the care of the dying? Indian J Crit Care Med. 2023:27(5):374-76.
14. Schouten ES, Beyer MF, Flemmer AW, et al. Conversations about end-of-life decisions in neonatology: do doctors and parents implement share decision-making? Front Pediatr. 2022;10:1-10.
15. Pant S. Ethical issues around death and withdrawal of life support in neonatal intensive care. Indian J Pediatr. 2022;89(3):274-8.
16. Mohanty N. Neonatal palliative care. NIJP. 2017;6.3:134-9.
17. Eventov-Friedman S, Kanevsky H, Bar-OZ B. Neonatal end of life care: A single centre NICU experience in Israel over a decade. Pediatrics. 2013;131:e1889-96.
18. Ministry of Health and Family Welfare, Government of India. RBSK Guidelines; 2017.

CHAPTER

Medicolegal Issues in Medicine

Anurag Verma

INTRODUCTION

It is now evident and legally accepted that the medical profession, which was regarded as an art and science has now become a commercial activity after the judgment of Supreme Court (SC) in the case of Indian Medical Association (IMA) versus VP Shanta. Now, doctors have to be treated as service providers.

Doctor–patient relationship that used to be fiduciary has now become service provider and consumer relationship where if a patient finds or alleges any negligence or deficiency in service on the part of the doctor, he/she can drag doctor to the court of law and demand for compensation where doctor may have to pay compensation in consumer cases or face punishment in criminal cases. If a complaint is filed in a medical council, the doctor may lose his license for practice.

It can be appreciated that because of the fast pace of commercialization and globalization along with the Consumer Protection Act (CPA), public has become aware of medical negligence and because of the ease of getting compensation as CPA being consumer-friendly, number of medicolegal cases against doctors has increased manifolds in recent years.

In practice of medicine specifically, a physician may face medicolegal issues related to:

- Consumer cases for compensation
- Cases of alleged criminal medical negligence
- Hospital violence
- Complaints against doctors for unethical acts and unfair trade practices

Every physician should follow principles of ethics, namely, autonomy, beneficence, nonmaleficence, justice, confidentiality, and truth-telling but should be a bit realistic as every patient may be a potential litigant. However, sweet he or she may be during counseling, may drag the doctor to the court of law.

Good rapport and communication skills are important buffers against lawsuits and violence.

A physician should be a good listener and empathic rather than reducing disease to a mechanical process.

Paramedical staff should behave humbly and should not give unqualified comments, which may lead to confusion between doctor and patient.

EXAMINATION IN OUTDOOR, PRESCRIPTION, AND MEDICAL CERTIFICATE

In outpatient department, a male physician should examine the female patient in presence of the attendant or female staff.

Proper documentation is must: On prescription paper, the correct name of the patient must be mentioned, incorrect name of the patient is treated as a gross mistake.

[Ms Samina Khatun vs. Dr SK Debnath and others, State Consumer Dispute Redressal Commission (SCDRC), West Bengal (WB)].

There should be a detailed history (past, present, family, personal, and drug-related). Clinical examination findings, investigation advised, investigation reports, provisional diagnosis, treatment plan, dietary advice, precautions, and any noncompliance must be mentioned.

The prescription must not be given without actual examination.

Writing on prescription—"Not for medicolegal purpose" has no legal validity.

A physician should write only those medical qualifications on prescription paper that are recognized by the medical council and any extraordinary achievements.

A physician should not project himself as a specialist of a branch or superspecialty of which he does not have a recognized qualification (Goyal Hospital and Research Center Pvt Ltd Jodhpur and others vs. Kishan Shukla R.P.No.4023/2011).

When issuing a medical certificate, a physician should keep in mind the following precautions:

- Identity of patient/photo ID
- Never issue a medical certificate for >15 days, reissue if needed.
- Not for the disease not treated or trained to treat
- Must address where it is to be submitted
- Never to be given in back date or fitness in advance
- Physical presence of the patient is a must.
- Medical certificate is a legal document, which is admissible in the court of law as evidence.
- A physician must not issue a false medical certificate, which is taken as a false evidence in court under Indian Penal Code (IPC) 197 for which a punishment extending up to 1 year or fine or both may be awarded.

MEDICOLEGAL ISSUES IN INDOOR TREATMENT

Medical treatment indoors is to be done only after taking proper informed consent.

A report of Nuremberg Code addresses that voluntary informed consent is required as it is the fundamental ethical principle. The participant must give their autonomy, which implies the responsibility must be given to the individual to make the decision and give consent related to their medical conditions.

In Indian context, it is to be a real and valid consent [Samira Kohli vs. Dr Prabha Manchanda and Anr 1 (2008) CPJ 56 SC].

Physician must take high-risk consent in serious cases: A legally valid consent is a must to fulfill legal requirements to refute any allegations of medical negligence without consent; it is a shared decision and has better clinical results. Knowing about limitations and probable complications, patient does not have any unrealistic expectations and so the probability of malpractice suits is less. Whatever is the result, the patient is expected to be satisfied.

Apollo Specialty Hospital, Chennai and Anr versus R Muthukrishnan, National Consumer Disputes Redressal Commission (NCDRC): Informed consent taken properly in this case saved doctors from 20 lakh rupees of compensation.

Confidential information entrusted by a patient to a physician should never be revealed unless it is required by law. However, to protect a healthy person against a communicable disease to which he/she is about to be exposed, the physician should act as he/she would wish another to act toward one of his own family in like circumstances.

The physician should not disclose secrets of the patient that have been learned in exercise of his/her profession except in the following circumstances:

- In a court of law under the order of the presiding judge
- When there is a serious and identifiable risk to a specific person or community
- In case of communicable/notifiable diseases

In case of communicable/notifiable diseases, concerned public health authorities should be informed immediately. [Mr "X" vs. hospital "Z"; (1) SCC 500: 2004].

During indoor medical treatment, some procedures can be done with oral consent, namely Foley's catheterization, Ryles tube, gastric lavage, Procto-clysis (PC) enema, oral suction, nebulization, venous or arterial blood gas (ABG) samples, and intramuscular (IM), intravenous (IV) injections.

Medical treatment indoors or for any medical treatment, which entails a risk to life, may cause sudden death or can lead to an adverse event, must be instituted after taking written consent.

A separate consent for blood transfusion must be taken. Blood that is to be transfused must be thoroughly checked for any evidence of infection, e.g., hepatitis, human immunodeficiency virus (HIV), etc. (CPL Ashish Kumar Chauhan Rtd vs. Commanding Officer and Ors Civil appeal no.7175 of 2021 SC Judgement 25th September 2023. In this, compensation of ₹1.5 crore was awarded by SC).

TREATMENT AND REFERRAL OF PATIENTS

A physician should select a case for treatment as per his competence [Dr Laxman Balkrishna Joshi vs. Dr Trimbark Babu Godbole and Anr, AIR 1969 SC 128 and AS Mittal vs. State of Uttar Pradesh (UP), AIR 1989 SC 1570].

Physician should never try to treat a case beyond their expertise, if there is a confusion regarding treatment, they should advise to take a second opinion or should refer the case to a higher center (Dr RK Sharma vs. Murtiya Devi, NCDRC Rev. Pet 1262 of 2009).

If for some reason physician in charge is not able to attend the patient, the visiting doctor should be of same specialty and competence.

In emergency, a physician must treat the patient (Clause 2.1.1 Indian Medical Council code of medical ethics), (SC Judgment, Parmanand Katara vs. Union of India, Article 21, Obligation of state to preserve life).

Any complication of the treatment should be recognized at earliest possible, and efforts should be done to correct that, and efforts should be communicated to attendants. If it is not possible to correct complications after justified efforts, patient should be referred to a higher center. A physician should never discharge such a patient to home with follow-up advice. At this point of time, it should be kept in mind that hospital should be well equipped to deal with any possible complication while admitting the patient.

If referral is on request, the same should be documented. While transferring the patient, ambulance should be well equipped and supplemented with medical officer, investigations, and treatment details of the patient (Jatinder Pal Singh vs. Escorts Heart Institute).

Physicians should know that it is the duty of the referring hospital to provide relevant records of the patient to attendants while transferring and it is the duty of the referred hospital also to ask for it when the patient reaches there. As per SC, the hospital that falls short of it is negligent.

When a patient is discharged from the hospital, advice regarding follow-up visit, if it is indicated, must be mentioned. If patient does not turn up for follow-up visit, then doctor is not at fault (Mr Mandeep Singh vs. Mata Chanan Devi hospital and Anr FA/206/2017, D.O.D. 22.09.2023).

Physicians and staff should be cautious while speaking in intensive care unit (ICU): A physician should remember that if a patient is admitted to ICU, and more so if it is a secondary or tertiary care hospital, a greater degree of care is expected from the physician, staff, and hospital.

The NCDRC held that a higher duty of care is expected from ICU staff when a patient is critical (Medical Superintendent, Mata Chanan Devi Hospital vs. Sunita Saxena).

Medical records of indoor patients should be kept in a standard format as per National Medical Council (NMC) for a period of 3 years.

Limitation period for the purpose of CPA is 2 years from the point of cause of action which is condonable as per view of the Court.

There should be no overwriting, or addition later as that is taken as tampering of evidence by the court (Indu Sharma vs. Apollo Hospital. In this case, a separate penalty was imposed by the court for tampering of records).

MEDICOLEGAL CASES

A physician always encounters medicolegal cases in practice mostly as emergencies, few facts should always be kept in mind when dealing with such cases:

- As per judgment of the SC in the case of Parmanand Katara versus Union of India, medicolegal cases including roadside accident, alleged sexual offense, acid attack, and any cognizable offense, the hospital, private or government, must provide free treatment for emergency and should not wait for any formality or police to arrive.
- In case of a brought dead patient, police is informed and if any foul play is suspected, postmortem is to be advised.
- Never certify the cause of death unless have treated the case and suspicion of foul play is there.
- Police is to be informed in cases of the death of a pregnant female or within 6 weeks of delivery, and death of female within 7 years of marriage due to burn.

Sudden Death and Hospital Violence

Another very important issue in medical practice is the sudden death of an admitted patient.

Sudden death is unexpected instantaneous death within 24 hours of onset of symptoms, with or without pre-existing conditions and there are no accidental or criminal causes.

Physicians should be very attentive and deal with this situation intelligently.

Physicians should be wise in breaking bad news to attendants who are likely to be in a volatile state from emotional trauma, and there may be emotional outburst and violence may ensue.

The following plan to deal with such a situation may be followed:

- Doctor along with the trained staff should reach the site immediately, start treatment to revive patient, and be empathic to the attendants. Bed should be cordoned off if in ward. After initial treatment, the patient should be shifted to an ICU on an AMBU bag. Documentation should be done simultaneously by a staff member.
- A senior doctor should brief the attendants about the condition of patient and the probable cause of the situation. Doctor should avoid any chance of confrontation, if there is any allegation of negligence.
- If attendants want to see patient, one or two of them should be allowed after confirming identity and relation with patient. They should be shown efforts being done to save the patient. After this, the doctor should discuss probable outcome in a separate room to prepare them mentally to accept it.
- In event of death of the patient, doctor in charge of the patient, if present, should inform the attendants. At this point, doctor should satisfy attendants in a modest way if they have any queries and should avoid any argument or provocation if they blame any staff or doctor as far as possible.
- In this way, the doctor should be able to dissipate any unwanted situation. If the situation seems to be out of control and if any violence from attendants is initiated, then doctor should take the following measures:
    - Doctor and staff members should remain calm and should not get provoked.
    - Some staff members should take photographs or audiovisuals.
    - Records should be safely taken into custody as these may be needed later.
    - A lawyer and police should be informed.
    - Colleagues, association members, and friends should be informed.
    - Someone from hospital should call media to inform its point of view.
    - Doctor should not talk to everyone in the mob, and few members from mob should be allowed to talk separately from the mob; it is very important to avoid manhandling of doctor by the mob.
    - Doctor should narrate to police whole sequence of events preferably in presence of lawyer, colleagues, and some sensible attendants.
    - In case if violence has been there, first information report (FIR) should be logged under Medicare Protection Act.
    - Do not try to "settle" the issue by paying hush money (often it is taken as admission of guilt).
    - It sends message in society that doctor was at fault and that is why money was paid. It sends the wrong message that in case of the death of a patient, by violence attendants can get compensation then and there instead of going through the tedious process of litigation.
    - Certify the cause of death only if the cause of death is identifiable.
    - Always insist on postmortem when the cause of death is not identifiable or postmortem is indicated.

LEGAL NOTICE FOR ALLEGED MEDICAL NEGLIGENCE

A physician must be aware of the fact that because of the changed scenario of medical practice, the doctor and patient relationship has been changed to a consumer and service provider relationship in which commercialization, increased cost of medical treatment, increased awareness about medical negligence, and relative ease of getting compensation, as CPA being a consumer-friendly legislation, are the factors that have played a major role. A physician should know what to do when she/he receives a legal notice either from a patient or advocate.

Not all the patients are going to file a case of medical negligence against the doctor, but a physician should treat every patient as a potential litigant as if she/he thinks it fit, can drag the doctor to court. So, a doctor should treat every patient in a professional way to be safe.

Patients likely to file a case of medical negligence:
- Uncooperative patient, always complaining during treatment
- Left Against Medical Advice (LAMA) patients, demanding medical records
- Patients who are unsatisfied with treatment bills, otherwise calm and quiet, and demand receipts and detailed summary
- Medical jousting
- Patients who are unsatisfied with treatment outcome

What a Physician Should do When He Receives a Legal Notice?

The physician should accept the legal notice as it is the right of the patient to send it if he/she feels negligence on the part of the doctor; nonacceptance serves no purpose, it is better than receiving a court summon. A physician should know about the substance of notice, replying or not can be decided later.

After receiving notice, a physician should read it carefully. Not replying to a notice is not illegal but it is not advisable.

Even if the notice appears to be on wrong assumptions and is sent by the patient himself, is not to be treated lightly and a casual reply should not be given because when the case goes to a court, it shall be read by the judge and shall leave a bad impression. On the contrary, if a sincere and justified reply is sent then the case may not go to court.

If the notice has been sent by an advocate, it means that the patient has approached him/her and intends to file a case. Here, silence on the part of the physician shall amount to acceptance and a defensive attitude on his part. If there is no reply from the physician, the court may pronounce an ex-party judgment.

The advocate should be competent in dealing with medicolegal cases, at this point of time, a medicolegal expert is of great value. It is advisable to draft a short pointwise reply only denying allegations, explaining only where necessary or of benefit. Points that need explanation if explained well even at this stage, may lead to withdrawal of the case by the patient.

CONCLUSION

In the present scenario of medical practice, a physician should be aware of the medicolegal issues of his/her specialty and should remain in touch with various medicolegal developments related thereto by attending medicolegal conferences, webinars, and various judgments of courts.

KEY LEARNING POINTS

- High-risk consent is important in serious cases.
- In emergency attend the patient, give emergency care and then refer to proper higher center.
- In your absence, have an equally competent junior or locum.
- Breaking bad news requires utmost skill.
- Advise PM examination if cause of death is not known or we suspect foul play.

BIBLIOGRAPHY

1. Mitscherlich A, Mielke F. The Nuremberg Code 1947. Doctors of infamy: The story of the Nazi medical crimes. New York: Schuman; 1949. pp. 23-5. [online] Available from xxv.http:www.cirp.org/library/ethics/nuremberg [Last accessed may, 2024].
2. Nagpal N. Incidents of violence against doctors in India: Can these be prevented? Natl Med J India. 2017;30(2):97-100.
3. The Gazette of India Part III, Section 4. (2002). Indian Medical Council (Professional Conduct, Etiquette and Ethics) Regulations, 2002. [online] Available from https://wbconsumers.gov.in/writereaddata/ACT%20&%20RULES/Relevant%20Act%20&%20Rules/Code%20of%20Medical%20Ethics%20Regulations.pdf [Last accessed May, 2024].

19

CHAPTER

Medicolegal Issues in Critical Care

Sheikh Minhaj Ahmed, Dnyanesh DK

INTRODUCTION

Pathophysiologic derangement in a patient admitted in intensive care unit (ICU) usually cuts across traditional lines of medical specialization requiring intensivist to simultaneously be both driver of care and also an integrator of diverse opinions. ICU is characterized by dynamic scenario where one keeps on monitoring the condition of patient, making interventions based on this assessment and again monitoring the effect of these interventions. The complexity and intensity of ICU care can present multiple opportunities for lapses in monitoring, assessment, judgment, or communication thus giving rise to medicolegal issues. Another peculiarity is that the typical ICU patient or caretaker is unable to participate in the decision making regarding his or her treatment. Primarily doctors especially physicians dealing with emergency and critical care have several ethical and legal obligations in performance of their duties. The doctors who are involved in critical care should know their legal obligations to avoid allegations and safeguard themselves against medical negligence.

Legal Procedure in Cases of Medical Negligence

Duty is generally not an issue in the ICU where the physician is responsible for the patient receiving medical care. In addition, a physician who holds himself out to be a specialist should have degree of learning and skill of a higher standard than that expected of a general practitioner. There are two standards utilized in determining the admissibility of scientific evidence into legal evidence. First, the Frye standard which relates to the notion of general acceptance of the scientific evidence in the relevant field; the role of the court is to prevent less than optimal science from being admitted into evidence. Another standard is Daubert standard; in this approach the court could use a broad range of criteria to establish the scientific reliability and relevance of the expert evidence. Daubert standard is increasingly being preferred and this has relevance in the ICU where new research techniques are frequently tried in innovative new therapies.

Harm forms a basis of initiating the claim. The two elements that become the subject of debate include breach and causation. It is important to point out that this standard of care represents a national standard. Causation implies that the physician's actions resulted in the alleged harm. This can have unique implications in the critical care setting where care is provided on a successive basis by multiple physicians during the course of care. Accordingly, it is generally not an acceptable defense that a physician did not cause harm if the underlying problem was precipitated by physician care provided earlier in the course of the care. Once the injured party (family) feels that thc patient has suffered an injury and obtains legal counsel, the first step relates to the concept of the statute of limitations. These are a predefined number of years established by state law during which time the medical malpractice claim can be initiated. This step typically is followed by a series of discovery during which interrogatories and depositions may be conducted and there is a thorough medical record review.

Emergency Patient Care

Medical emergency means sudden, unforeseen condition of the patient and/or where the question of life and death is there. "Doctors cannot refuse emergency treatment to a patient irrespective of his caste, creed, and ability to pay, etc., because saving human life is of paramount importance. Hospitals, nursing homes, clinics of doctors who declare that they provide emergency services are legally bound to attend all medical emergency cases, accidents, and injury cases. They cannot refuse the treatment to such cases. Honorable Supreme Court, in the case of "Paschim Bengal Khet mazdoor samity and others vs. West Bengal" has stated that Article 21 of Indian constitution imposes an obligation on the state to safeguard the right to life of every person. The government hospitals run by state and doctors employed there are duty bound to provide Medical Assistance for preserving human life. Failure to provide timely medical treatment to a person in need results in violation of his right to life guaranteed under Article 21. So it is the responsibility of state government to upgrade the hospitals at district and subdivisional level, so that serious cases can be treated there and government should make sure the all government hospitals are well-equipped and adequate staff and specialist are there. Otherwise government has to pay the compensation.

Steps to Minimize Medicolegal Liability

It is important to be up-to-date on national recommendations for various clinical conditions. It is generally not a defense that the standard of care being practiced was consistent with a local practice but inconsistent with a national standard. Ambiguity or discrepant notations in the record are usually a key focus in litigation. All contemporaneous data must agree or the discrepancy be explained. A key element of documentation, especially in ICU, is the differential diagnosis and the facts, opinions, and judgments that accompany it. Where a physician finds it necessary to deviate from an accepted guideline, protocol, or pathway, the basis for such deviations should be thoroughly and carefully documented. With the trend toward adoption of electronic health records, many of the issues related to legibility of handwriting will evaporate, but newer issues previously not addressed will emerge. It is important to have open and honest communication with families. Honesty and empathy are often appreciated and can substantiate the overall atmosphere of professionalism and caring essential to healthcare. The emerging literature from patient safety supports that full disclosure of mistakes and patient safety related adverse events to the family in a timely manner in fact reduces the likelihood of subsequent lawsuits. A confession can also eliminate triable issues off act. In the case of a lawsuit, for which there are no triable issues of fact, the plaintiff can move for summary judgment, leaving only the amount of damages to be determined by the courts or in settlement. However, the optimal policy and procedure for such disclosure remains somewhat controversial. ICU leadership and attending physicians should be aware of the applicable disclosure policy in effect at their institution and be prepared to develop it, review it, or comply with it. In addition, although hospital risk management personnel frequently oversee implementation of the disclosure policy, physicians may need to consider the personal legal ramifications of a disclosure conference and consider prior consultation with an attorney. However, in general, attorneys should probably not be present during the disclosure conference. Finally, it is important to approach the medicolegal litigation in professional manner. Typically when physicians are sued, many view this as a direct attack on their professional credibility. This is understandable. However, in order for successful resolution of the underlying lawsuit, it is important to fully cooperate with the investigation in a professional and truthful manner.

False Claims Act

The False Claims Act essentially prohibits falsification of billing to government for services provided. Besides including obvious fraudulent actions such as billing for services or procedures that were not performed. This has recently been expanded to also cover gross breaches in the quality of care provided which may be viewed as the absence of care. The potential implications for the ICU setting may be important. For example, recently in US the Centers for Medicare and Medicaid adopted policies for nonpayment of "never" events. These complications will not be reimbursed by insurance because they should never occur if the hospital care is functioning appropriately. Examples of "never" events include wrong site surgery, hospital acquired conditions such as pressure ulcers, and more recently, hospital acquired catheter associated bloodstream infections. This could create unique new problems from a billing perspective for critical care physicians and their institutions. Therefore, it is important for the critical care physician to be abreast of these new emerging rules and policies to avoid the unintentional liability that may arise because of compliance failure.

Unique Issues in the Intensive Care Unit Setting

It is important for the critical care physician to recognize the breath of legal issues that surround decision-making in the ICU setting. Several issues span underlying ethical principles, including research and policies on medical futility, end of life decisions, withdrawal of care, and determination of brain death. Medication errors are the most common type of error and account for 78% of serious medical errors in the ICU. A detailed discussion about medication errors is discussed in Chapter 10. A frequently raised bedside problem is that of triage of existing ICU resources with respect to admissions and transfers. In general, the courts seem to support the decisions made by experienced physicians, when supported by documentation. Doctors are required to behave both ethically and legally. Deferring end-of-life decision-making to courts of law should generally be viewed as a failure of bedside management. It should never be considered a "standard of care."

Vicarious Liability in Critical Care

Doctors have a duty to satisfy themselves that the persons to whom the work is delegated are qualified and have the appropriate experience to discharge the delegate task. In "Spring Meadow hospital VS. Harjot Ahluwalia" it was held that a consultant could be vicariously liable where he delegates the responsibility to his juniors with knowledge that the junior was incapable of performing his duties properly. Similarly hospital is liable for the negligence of its staff including nurses, physicians, surgeons, and anesthetists, etc. It doesnot matter whether they are permanent or temporary, full time or part time.

Telephonic Advice to a Resident in ICU

It is a dangerous practice to give medical advice on phone. In case you have examined the patient, you may give some instructions and advice on phone to the resident doctors. But ask the resident doctor to write down the instructions and to read it out what he has written to confirm. Otherwise any harm caused by telephonic advice may amount to negligence.

Research and Medicolegal Standing

Because of providing care in advance settings ICUs are also a very convenient place for medical trials of experimental therapies and research. Regarding research, Public Health Service (US) has published basic requirements that are prerequisite to Public Health Service research funding: The institutions must (1) maintain a written conflict of interest policy and enforce that policy; (2) inform research investigators of the institution's policy on conflicts of interest, the investigator's reporting responsibilities, and other applicable federal regulations; (3) designate an official to review financial disclosure statements of participating investigators; and (4) report the existence of any financial conflict of interest to the grantor agency with an assurance from the institution that the conflict has been managed, reduced, or eliminated. The Food and Drug Administration has also developed regulations that represent a combination of common rule concepts and an explicit concern for financial conflict of interest.

Informed Consent

The informed consent is an obligation of physicians to share medical decision-making authority with their patients (or caregiver in context of ICU). It has obvious ethical and legal implications. There are two broad aspects of intensive care practice for which consent is relevant. The first relates to invasive procedures and the second to participation in research. Consent to routine or everyday procedures in critically ill patients is often presumed or rather subsumed under the general consent to treatment. This is clearly not always the case. The well-being of the patient is of paramount and medical rather than legal considerations come first. No delay in medical intervention is expectable for want of consent.

In the case of Barnett vs. Bacharach, the court held that in a medical emergency in which patient lies unconscious on the operating table, the surgeon may lawfully carry out the duties of a physician in the best interest of the patient, even if these duties entail the performance of a procedure that was not originally contemplated. In Barnett vs. Bacharach, a patient who complained of abdominal pains was diagnosed with ectopic pregnancy. The patient was consented only for the removal of ectopic pregnancy. On incision, the surgeon found that the patient didnot have ectopic pregnancy but had acute appendicitis. The surgeon in the best interest of the patient, appedicectomy was performed. The patient recovered well, but refused to pay the hospital bills, saying she had not given consent for the removal of appendix. The trial court found that the surgeon acted properly because of the seriousness of the patient's condition.

Discharge Against Medical Advice (DAMA)

All patients/patient attendants have right to refuse further medical care. They can leave against medical advice to the extent that it doesnot contravene any law. They have a right to obtain details of investigations and treatment undergone. But the doctor, before sending the patient DAMA, should talk to the patient/patient attendants regarding the patient conditions and treatment given. Document the discussion in the case sheet properly and take the consent signature of patient/patient attendants.

Death Certificate in "Brought Dead" Cases

This is not an uncommon scenario in emergency rooms. Patient will be brought dead and the attendants will be forcing the doctor to give death certificate. Routinely death certificate is issued by RMP who has attended the last stages of life of the patient. So if the patient is brought dead to the hospital or dies unattended, the death certificate cannot be issued. In this situation, it is given after postmortem.

In case of unnatural (MLC) deaths, on table anesthetic and operative deaths should always be reported to the police for conducting inquest and postmortem. No consent is required for medicolegal PM as it is done as per the requirements of law.

Post Death Diagnostic Procedure

Even after death of the patient, if you want to do any procedure, you have to take the consent of parents/relatives. You have to explain to them how does this post death diagnostic test helps them. The senior doctors often encourage their junior colleagues to "practice procedure" in dead or on dying patients like endotracheal intubation. The issue may be debatable. But before doing such procedures the sensitivities of the family should be taken into consideration.

CONCLUSION

In conclusion, physicians must continue to focus their efforts on providing the best care possible to their individual patients. Nonetheless, the increasingly litigious and complex external regulatory environment will also continue to affect the practice of medicine, to enforce standards of care, and to strive to protect those most vulnerable. Physicians must increase their level of awareness of the laws relating to the delivery of healthcare so that they can best interact with patients, administrators, attorneys, and legislators.

KEY LEARNING POINTS

- Critical patient need more careful management.
- Allegations of deficiency in service or medical negligence are more common in such situation.
- Guarantee for Care and not Cure.
- Practice as per the facilities and gadgets available in your set-up.
- Don't hesitate in referring the patient if adequate facilities are not available.

BIBLIOGRAPHY

1. Camiré E, Moyen E, Stelfox HT. Medication errors in critical care: risk factors, prevention and disclosure. CMAJ. 2009;180(9):936-43.
2. Federal policy for the protection of human subjects. Final rule. Fed Regist. 1991;56(117):28003-18; codified at 45 C.F.R. §46 (2000).
3. Fisher M. Ethical issues in the intensive care unit. Curr Opin Crit Care. 2004;10(4):292-8.
4. Hamasaki T, Hagihara A. Physicians' explanatory behaviors and legal liability in decided medical malpractice litigation cases in Japan. BMC Med Ethics. 2011;12-7.
5. Hobgood C, Xie J, Weiner B, et al. Error identification, disclosure, and reporting: practice patterns of three emergency medicine provider types. Acad Emerg Med. 2004;11(2):196-9.
6. Informed consent, parental permission, and assent in pediatric. Committee on Bioetnics, American Academy of pediatrics. 1995;95(2):314-7.
7. Leape LL, Brennan TA, Laird N, et al. The nature of adverse events in hospitalized patients. Results of the Harvard Medical Practice Study II. N Engl J Med. 1991;324(6):377-84.
8. Localio AR, Lawthers AG, Brennan TA, et al. Relation between malpractice claims and adverse events due to negligence. Results of the Harvard Medical Practice Study III. N Engl J Med. 1991;325(4) 245-51.
9. Protection of human subjects; informed consent: FDA. Final rule. Fed Regist. 1996;61(192):51498-533.
10. Sachdeva RC, D'Andrea LA. Emerging medicolegal issues in the practice of pediatric sleep medicine. Child Adolesc Psychiatr Clin N Am. 2009;18:1017-25.
11. Slater A, Shann F, ANZICS Pediatric Study Group. The suitability of the Pediatric Index of Mortality (PIM), PIM2, the Pediatric Risk of Mortality (PRISM), and PRISM III for monitoring the quality of pediatric intensive care in Australia and New Zealand. Pediatr Crit Care Med. 2004;5:447-54.
12. Studdert DM, Mello MM, Sage WM, et al. Defensive medicine among high-risk specialist physicians in a volatile malpractice environment. JAMA. 2005;293(1):2609-17.
13. Szalados JE. Intensive care unit resource utilization by Medicare patients: Margin and mission meet public policy and practice economics. Crit Care Med. 2004;32:2351-2.
14. Szalados JE. Legal issues in the practice of critical care medicine: A practical approach. Crit Care Med. 2007;35(Suppl-2):S44-58.

19.1 Euthanasia and Life Support Systems

Anjan Bhattacharya, Sudhir Mishra

In medical practice, occasionally, reality brings us to the shore of ethical dilemmas. Although a doctor is bound by the ancient Hippocratic oaths to heal the infirm, **treating a person sometimes may appear more harmful** than not treating them in certain situations. In the industrialized nations of the world, academic and professional medical bodies and societies have formulated guidelines to help the doctors and the court to derive benefits of fore knowledge. In a country like India, who is at the cusp of developmental leap, a need and **demand for such guidelines is increasingly felt**. Dr Adhikary and Dr Raviraj have debated the issue few years back and brought out some salient points to ponder especially in the context of our country. The purpose of this article is to egg this discussion forward so that, using the process of peer discussion and debate, we mature to handle this difficult reality far more squarely. Let us try to have some guiding principles in place for a start.

INDICATIONS

General Medical Council of the United Kingdom has produced a guideline in 2002 **on this complex subject** for their doctors in August, 2002 named "Withholding and Withdrawing Life Prolonging Treatments: Good Practice in Decision-making". Royal College of Pediatricians and Child Health followed this up for their Pediatricians in May, 2004 with the document "Withholding and Withdrawing Life Sustaining Treatment in Children: A framework for practice". These documents have emerged with the following broad group of indications:

Brain Death

Definition: Brain death occurs when there is either (i) irreversible stoppage of circulatory or respiratory functions *or* (ii) irreversible cessation of all functions of the entire brain including the brainstem.

A determination of death must be made in accordance with accepted medical standards. Note that original definition of brain death is not applied to neonates (newborn babies) as they were thought to be affected by brain immaturity.

The "Permanent Vegetative" State

Following trauma or insult like severe hypoxia, if a person does not react or relate with the outside world and are completely reliant on others for all care, that person is considered to be in a "vegetative state".

The "No Chance" Situation

The person has such severe disease that life-sustaining treatment simply delays death without significant alleviation of suffering. Treatment to sustain life by all means is inappropriate in these circumstances.

This often arises in multiple complex congenital diseases and some terminal malignancies. For adults in such circumstances, having a "Do Not Resuscitate" (DNR) policy will mean that informed consent may be in place before the capable consenting adult drifts into phases of decreased capacity to make adult decisions-making such decisions harder to reach and consequently, prolonging the person's suffering unnecessarily. Whereas, in neonates, this example may be found in a baby who has suffered severe birth asphyxia and in whom investigations have revealed profound brain damage.

The "No Purpose" Situation

Although the patient may be able to survive with treatment, the degree of physical and/or mental impairment will be so great that it is unreasonable to expect them to bear it. For adults, this may be true in extreme situations where there is no doubt beyond reasonable limit that the prospect of his/her survival will be "impossibly poor".

In neonates, these examples are where no resuscitative measures are started as the baby is below 23 weeks of gestational age and does not respond at birth or is born anencephalic or with similar birth defect which are known to be incompatible with life.

The "Unbearable" Situation

The person or the child and/or child's family may feel that in the face of progressive and irreversible illness, further treatment is more than one can be borne. They may wish to have a particular treatment withdrawn or to refuse further treatment irrespective of the medical opinion that it may be of some benefit.

In clinical practice, scenarios arise in real life where continuation or institution of treatment or aggressive resuscitative measures seems wrong. A lack of guideline in our setting makes it difficult to make professionally sound decisions. The issues are comprehensively discussed by Dr Adhikary and Dr Raviraj. Some of the relevant ones are mentioned here along with other relevant issues:

- Written DNR policy helps doctors make professionally competent decisions. Guidelines were proposed for limiting life-prolonging interventions and providing palliative care toward the end-of-life in Indian intensive care units.
- Human rights and child's rights are important considerations in such decision-making.
- The Indian law is silent or ambiguous on most issues related to end-of-life care.
- The financial status of the patient appears to be one of the principle deciding factors. In most cases healthcare expenses are entirely borne either by the patient or by the patient's relatives. Conflict of interest may be in place when **"Proxy Consent"** is sought from family members who may be financially responsible to bear the burden of the cost of treatment.

This scenario is different in industrialized nations where the government or the insuring agency takes the responsibility. Therefore, in countries like ours, this poses a major difficulty in drawing up ethically sound guidelines which can deal with this harsh reality while respecting the human rights and child's rights at the same time. Policies should also be careful so as not to create a situation where private players are discouraged to accept terminal or potentially fatal cases.

Generally, it must be better to acknowledge the harsh realities and yet come up with agreed written policies. Surely, it is not a better option not to have any such and to keep turning a blind eye forever. We may not have perfect solutions. But we must have some bullet point guiding principles written down. The current situation of "free fall" must end sooner than later.

- Medical, Legal and Public Forums (may form "Indian DNR Forum") should come together on this very sensitive but essential subject. Government and medical societies need to spearhead the initiative and keep it apolitical.
- It is a waste of time and energy to "reinvent the wheel". The Indian DNR Forum ought to examine the current body of work and assimilate the relevant parts and raise issues that are particular to India to debate. It should also invite and examine all new suggestions made.
- Until that time, it is proposed that the following guiding principles should be followed:
  - Wherever possible, involve another competent medical practitioner in situations where DNR is considered.
  - Document, in case of dire emergencies, the reasons for not being able to do so.
  - Involve the patient/relative wherever possible in the documented decision-making process. Video evidence may not be perfect, but it is better than nothing.
  - Avoid colluding with the families. A doctor's primary responsibility is to do the best for his/her patient (who may be a minor). Consult with a colleague and document their views as much as practicable. If this is not available, write down the circumstances. As a society, we need to support wherever a sincere doctor is facing a difficult situation, analyzing it as objectively as possible.
  - DNR must indicate which of the five indications (a combination is possible, e.g., no chance in a complex life-limiting congenital heart defect, which is unbearable too from extreme shortness of breath to a degree, which no one is expected to bear) led to consideration of withholding or withdrawing life sustaining measures.
  - Do not give up on a patient just because you thought this is unbearable to the patient. Evidences have shown that an individual sufferer, even with extreme disability may still attach value to existence. Judgments on disability are bound up in people's (including doctors) fears and attitudes and can be altered by a change in the environment. It is therefore, important to be (a) objective, (b) putting efforts to find out what the individual (including a child) might be wanting and (c) cross checking with colleagues, so that your own prejudices do not discriminate the individual which your conscience may repent later (or not!).
  - In case of decisions that have to be taken in haste, document everything later. Be objective and truthful. No doctor is expected to perform at the level of the best in the subject but he/she is expected to perform which is reasonable in a professional in his/her capacity. Unless you think you are lazy and insincere, your efforts are most likely to be appreciated. So, please write down everything as truthfully as you can.

- Where there is time, any doubtful decision may be referred to appropriate authority, which may be different for each individual doctor. For example, for a hospital doctor, this may be discussed with a colleague along with medical administration and for a lone community practitioner this may be another colleague or medical association. Medical insurance advisors are often useful sources of information in legally dubious circumstances.

DNR guidelines must be drawn up. These are not easy problems. Policies may not therefore, be fullproof. This should not deter policy makers to whether for the simple reason that the situation without any is even worse. Doctors on the other hand should be reasonable in their expectations from the guidelines. There will not be the answer to every conceivable situation. Real life throws up more interesting challenges than imagination can hold! The point is that are we trying to be courageous and truthful or do we still choose to be cowardice and run away from difficult choices? Running away always makes it more difficult later. So, we better start penning down some now and start debating them straight away.

LEGAL ASPECTS OF VENTILATION IN CHILDREN

Assisted ventilation in children is now frequently used in management of children suffering from respiratory compromise due to various conditions. The availability of ventilation is gradually increasing. However, almost every unit faces a situation of lack of bed or ventilator off and on. Triaging is often required to provide optimal care to salvageable patient. Perception of a service being denied to "my child" can lead to dissatisfaction and legal problems. In such a situation, the condition of the patient should be explained to the family members and documented in case records. In. *Tagore Hospital vs. Harnam Singh I (2008) CPJ 360 NC;* the commission has held negligence on following grounds. The patient with fever for 20 days, X-ray and ECHO reports could not be correlated, patient became hypoxic but ABG was not done and patient was not put on ventilator. The patient was discharged forcibly and died subsequently. It was observed that the records were fabricated and not reliable. Lame excuses regarding why ventilators from their own hospital could not be spared were not acceptable and hence, deficiency was held. Nonavailability of the facility should be explained and documented with the signature of the parents or family members. Consequences of not providing the treatment or possible alternative treatment being provided should be explained. Possibility of shifting the patient to an alternative facility and mode of available transportation should be informed. Risk of "in transit" mishap, if any, should be explained. Consequences of not transporting the patient should also be explained and documented.

Legal issues may be involved in dealing with pediatric ventilation at various stages of treatment. These may include:

Consent for Ventilation

Ventilation is like any other intervention and requires prior active consent of patient/parents who have been given adequate information. The principles of consent were discussed by Honorable Supreme Court in Samira Kohli vs. Prabha Manchanda (discussed in Chapter 15). While taking consent for ventilation, one should inform about followings:

- Indication for ventilation
- Consequences if the child is not ventilated specially where "elective" ventilation is being proposed

- Possible alternatives, e.g., only surfactant therapy for hyaline membrane disease in newborns, especially where elective ventilation is proposed
- Complications of ventilation—both short-term and specially in neonates long-term complications
- Likely duration of ventilation based on assessment of primary disease
- Likely end point if the child does not show desired response and becomes vegetative
- Cost of treatment
- Likely outcome of the intervention especially where neurologic outcome is not certain
- The treatment being offered for primary disease and its prognosis.

Absence of Suitable Person to Provide Consent When Intervention is Urgently Needed

When a child is suffering from a disease that is life-threatening or may worsen or where ventilation may be required, e.g., in postoperative period, efforts to take an informed consent should be made at the time of admission to the intensive care unit. However, if such consent has not been taken and child is likely to die, a doctor would be right in putting the child on ventilator even without consent of parents. In this situation it would be better if another consultant's opinion is recorded in the case sheet. In similar situation if surgery is required, there is provision of administrative consent for surgery from the superintendent of the hospital. Same principle can be adopted here and administrative consent may be taken to provide ventilator support for a child at risk of dying. As and when parent(s) become available, suitable and detailed information should be provided to them. If they are not willing for continued ventilation, consequences should be explained, documented in case records and signature should be taken after which ventilation may be discontinued.

Payment for Expenses Where Treatment Prolongs beyond Expectations

This is a common problem encountered in hospitals. Initially due to emotional upsurge and social pressures, many persons would consent for ventilation. As the time passes and especially where response is not commensurate with expectations, distress sets in. Family members find themselves unable to take decisions on discontinuing life support and at the same time unable to bear the cost of treatment. There are no clear laws or guidelines to deal with such situations. However, as a general rule, treatment should not be discontinued in children who are salvageable and alternative avenues to fund the treatment, e.g., transfer to a government facility suitably equipped or support of various nongovernmental organizations should be sought.

Withdrawing Ventilator Support if Patient Cannot be Salvaged

Ventilator support cannot be withdrawn without the consent of the family members unless the evidence of brain death is absolute. Many pediatric Intensive Care Units are not suitably equipped to demonstrate this to the family members. In such a situation, appropriate counseling by more than one consultant helps family members in taking this decision. The senior most persons in the department should be involved. Sometimes involvement of administrative officers, medical social workers and support groups is also helpful. However, if family members do not give consent for withdrawing the support, it should be continued till they are convinced of the futility of treatment.

Complications of Ventilation

Ventilator support is associated with many complications which may be fatal. These may include pneumothorax, worsening of acid-base status, ventilator associated pneumonia and effect on cardiac output when high PEEP is used. Prior information to parents is always helpful. High index of suspicion toward these possibilities along with appropriate investigations ordered early will lead to prompt diagnosis and intervention to save the patient.

However, even with all such measures having been taken, parents may perceive the poor outcome as a result of negligence and seek legal help/compensation. In such a situation, it is always helpful to discuss the matter with parents. They should be informed of available alternatives and the adequacy of treatment offered/being offered. If even then parents seek legal recourse, the court should be informed of the data from your own center as well as from other centers about these complications to convince the court of inevitability of some of these complications in any given set up. Also the decisions taken after identification of these complications, involvement of specialists from other suitable subspecialties, whenever available, reference material from books or journals to demonstrate adequacy of treatment offered in the given set up helps the court in taking a favorable view. If one of the two or more possible alternatives of treatment offered are suggested in literature and there are no clear guidelines and evidence to demonstrate supremacy of one over the other, adopting one line of treatment and not the other is never held against the doctors by the court-Bolam principle. The emphasis is on early identification and prompt treatment of complications.

Death on Ventilator

Death on ventilator may be difficult to diagnose with certainty as respiratory support can prolong the functioning of heart for very long time. As stated above, video EEG is the gold standard for diagnosis of brain death in a patient on ventilator. Where ever it not available, clinical parameters like fixed and dilated pupils, absence of corneal reflexes, absence of motor response, absence of caloric response, absence of gag reflex, absence of coughing in response to tracheal suctioning, absence of sucking or rooting reflexes, lack of spontaneous respiration and absence of respiratory drive at a $pCO^2 > 60$ mm Hg and absence of motor response are used to diagnose brain death. In such a situation, it is advisable to discuss the matter with family members, counsel them and withdraw support with their consent.

Ventilator Malfunction

Ventilator malfunction is an unusual occurrence. However, in absence of a back up available, it may be life-threatening. It may lead to legal problems. There are no guidelines on this issue. Each case has to be dealt with individually and appropriate decision taken. Manual ventilation should be provided pending correction of ventilator malfunction. In case it is not possible, efforts to shift the patient to another facility should be made. In this situation, responsibility to shift the patient in good condition would lie with the treating hospital till the patient is handed over to the transporting team or the other hospital if transportation is being done by the team of treating hospital.

EUTHANASIA

The benefits of modern techniques such as cardiopulmonary resuscitation, renal dialysis, artificial ventilation, artificial nutrition and hydration are considerable. However, life has a natural end. The existence of such techniques presents doctors, patients and their families with dilemmas. In other cases, they may simply prolong the dying process and cause unnecessary distress to the patient. In these instances the question arises as to whether it is in the best interests of the patient to start or continue the treatment. Reaching a satisfactory answer may mean addressing a number of difficult ethical and legal issues.

The main questions that arise are:

- Whether the ethical principle requiring doctors to show respect for human life would mean that doctors should offer all means at their disposal to prolong a patient's life? Or would it allow for the possibility of withholding or withdrawing a life-prolonging treatment?
- Are there circumstances in which withholding or withdrawing life-prolonging treatment should be deemed unlawful?
- What are the responsibilities in the decision-making process of the patient, doctor, healthcare team, family members, and other people who are close to the patient? And what weight should be given to their views?
- These issues have caused considerable debate amongst the profession, public, and in the courts, highlighting a number of concerns within the wider community.

Recently, Supreme Court has admitted a case of Aruna Shanbaug. The issue is, "Is not keeping the women in this persistent vegetative state by force feeding violative of her right to live with dignity guaranteed by Article 21 (Right to life) of the constitution?". The Apex Court in this case has sought responses from the Union Government, Maharashtra Government, Municipal Corporation of Mumbai, Commissioner of Mumbai Police, and the KEM Hospital, Mumbai.

Doctors have an ethical obligation to show respect for human life; protect the health of their patients; and to make their patients' best interests their first concern. This means offering those treatments where the possible benefits outweigh any burdens or risks associated with the treatment, and avoiding those treatments where there is no net benefit to the patient. Benefits and burdens for the patient are not always limited to purely medical consideration and doctors should be careful particularly when dealing with patients who cannot make decisions for themselves, to take account of all the other factors relevant to the circumstances of the particular patient.

Although it may be emotionally more difficult for the healthcare team, and those close to the patient, to withdraw a treatment from a patient rather than to decide not to provide a treatment in the first place, this should not be used as a reason for failing to initiate a treatment which may be of some benefit to the patient. Where it has been decided that a treatment is not in the best interests of the patient, there is no ethical or legal obligation to provide it and therefore no need to make a distinction between not starting the treatment and withdrawing it. Decisions involving artificial nutrition or hydration may be particularly difficult and/or contentious. In part, this is because the benefits and burdens of either nutrition or hydrations may not be well known and involves difficult assessments of the patient.

In the rare circumstances where any significant disagreement about best interests cannot be resolved, legal advice should be sought on whether it is necessary to apply to the court for a ruling.

Patients who are dying should be afforded the same respect and standard of care as all other patients. Patients and their families and others close to them should be treated with understanding and compassion. Where the likely progression of a patient's condition is known, and their death is seen as an inevitable outcome, it is important to ensure that the patient's palliative care or terminal care needs are identified and met appropriately.

KEY LEARNING POINTS

- Show respect for human life.
- Consider patient's best interest.
- Consider human rights while taking DNR decisions.
- Indian laws are ambiguous on "end of life care" issues.
- Involve a team of competent consultants or board of doctors for DNR/End-of-life care decisions.
- Take proper informed high-risk consent daily in critical patients.

BIBLIOGRAPHY

1. Adhikary SD, Raviraj R. Do Not Resuscitate orders. Indian J Med Ethics. 2006;3(3).
2. Guidelines for the determination of brain death in children. Annals of Neurology. 1987;21:616-7.
3. Mahapatra D. SC admits women's plea to end her life. The Times of India. 2009;18th Dec. Nagpur page 1 (Col. 7-8).
4. Mani RK, Amin P, Chawla R, et al. Limiting life-prolonging interventions and providing palliative care towards the end-of-life in Indian intensive care units. Indian J Crit Care Med. 2005;9(2):96-107.
5. Mani RK. Limitation of life support in the ICU: ethical issues relating to end of life care. Indian J Crit Care Med. 2003;7:112-7.
6. Moolayil GF. Consent and Documentation. In: Legal Problems in Day to Day Paediatric Practice. 2nd Edition (2010). Baldwa M, Tiwari S, Tiwari M, Shah N (Eds). Official Publication of Medicolegal Group of IAP. Paras Medical Publishers, Hyderabad. pp 94-108.
7. Moore K, Persaud TVN, Torchia MG. The Developing Human. Clinically Oriented Embryology (Elsevier Saunders 2003);103.
8. Ponte J. Assisted ventilation. Indications for Mechanical Ventilation. Thorax. 1990;45(11):885-90.
9. RCPCH, UK. Withholding and Withdrawing Life Prolonging Treatments: Good Practice in Decision-making. May 2004.
10. Task force for the determination of Brain Death in Children. Pediatrics. 1987;80:298-9.
11. Tiwari SK. What is Medical Negligence? In Legal Problems in day-to-day Paediatric Practice. 2nd edition 2010. Baldwa M, Tiwari S, Tiwari M, Shah N (Eds). Official Publication of Medico-legal Group of IAP. Paras Medical Publishers, Hyderabad. pp. 14-39.
12. Wijdicks EF. The diagnosis of brain death. NEJM. 2001;344(16):1215-21.

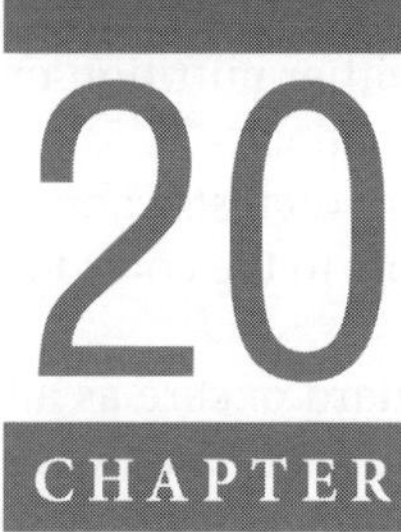

20

CHAPTER

Medicolegal Issues in Obstetrics/Gynecology

Gouri Gore

INTRODUCTION

The risk of facing a compensation suite is higher in obstetrics and gynecology. Surgeons and anesthesiologists are sued once every 4–5 years, according to a retrospective analysis. The consumer case is filed for act of omission [e.g., delay in doing lower segment cesarean section (LSCS)] or act of commission (e.g., allegation of unnecessary LSCS). A lot of sympathy factor is with the patient and newborn, considering that the specialty is supposed to deliver "wellness" rather than treating "illness." This chapter outlines various stages in surgical management of the patient, where allegations of negligence can be made. It will deal in detail about the precautions to be taken so that strong evidence can be produced in the court of law if one has to face a lawsuit.

The case references mentioned in this chapter are not limited to only obstetrics and gynecology, but the principles remain universal.

MAKING DECISION ABOUT SURGERY

A planned surgery is a teamwork for doctor and patient. Each person has a right to determine what will be done to his or her body, which includes the right to consent to or refuse any operation. This fact has to be acknowledged while advising surgery to the patient. For any procedure, major or minor, elective or emergency, patients should be informed about the following:

Nature of the Intervention and its Benefit

The outline of the procedure, in as simple terms as possible, should be communicated to the patient. The narration, if supported by visual aids such as pictures or videos, makes a positive impact on the patient. If any organ is going to be removed, the patient must fully understand the postoperative implications. It is imperative that a woman requiring hysterectomy should be made to understand that she will not get menses after the surgery and she will not be able to bear children. Highest degree of caution and care is needed in taking the decision to operate on a patient with abnormal vitals or who is unfit. If the patient is not medically fit for surgery, it is better to defer the procedure and suggest appropriate temporary conservative management options. In case the surgery cannot wait, then the doctor should have enough evidence to justify the need for surgery in critical condition in the court of law.

Performing an emergency surgery when an elective surgery can be planned later is perceived as negligence.

In cases of emergency surgery, the prime objective is to make the patient stable, for example, doing uterine packing to control postpartum hemorrhage. It is of vital importance to explain to the patient about the role, emergency surgery will have to avoid further complications in a given situation. In many of the occasions, definitive surgery cannot be offered to the patient in emergency situations. It must be emphasized in such cases that second-stage surgery may be required. For example, a patient with bowel injury during hysterectomy may need a colostomy as an emergency procedure and will require another surgery at a later date.

There is an increasing trend of surgery on demand, especially LSCS. It is the doctor's duty to decide whether a particular procedure is medically indicated or would be appropriate for that particular patient. The timing of an elective LSCS has to be determined as per the gestational age. Many times, the patients have preferred days and timing as per astrological advice. Preponing delivery before maturity or waiting for emergency LSCS due to "bad time" as per astrology cannot be a defense for doctor. A doctor is supposed to act based on scientific knowledge and current standards of treatment. If a patient refuses treatment due to "bad time," it has to be mentioned in writing and a consent for refusal of treatment has to be obtained from the patient.

Not prioritizing the surgery in case of a seriously ill patient can be considered as negligence. If there is a waiting list for any surgery, it must be communicated to the patient in writing and the patient must be given the option to avail treatment at another hospital.

SURGICAL COMPLICATION—NOT ALWAYS A NEGLIGENCE

Surgical complication is not always a negligence, if potential risks and complications are informed to the patient prior to surgery.

All major, life-threatening complications should be mentioned. It should include the risks and complications of anesthesia and procedure. Also, it is better to mention some data which can give an idea to the patient about the probability of a particular complication. It would be ideal if each center can give its own data about a particular procedure. In every procedure, certain complications are common and known to occur. Courts accept this as defense and are unlikely to hold the doctor negligent in such an event.

Many of the lawsuits are filed when an unexpected event occurs and the outcome is unfavorable. But the courts recognize that all unfavorable outcomes are not due to negligence.

Alternative Treatments

It is the patient's right to know all the available options for the ailment. If a nonsurgical treatment is also a reasonable option, the patient has to be informed about such a method. The risk of *recurrence/incomplete cure/need for surgery* after such treatment has to be explained to the patient and a specific consent must be obtained in such cases. For example, while offering medical management to a patient with unruptured ectopic pregnancy, a specific consent must be obtained about the need for emergency surgery. If more than one type of operation is possible, explain pros and cons of every possible surgery. A doctor's job is to suggest the most appropriate treatment (surgery) for the ailment under consideration. It is the patient who would decide which option to choose. However in many cases, the patient's perception and understanding of potential benefits, risks, and complications is inaccurate and misleading. It is recommended that all important facts about the surgery and its implications are noted down and patient signature is taken on the sheet at the end of consultation. If possible, it is important that the patient's family understands the risks involved because if the patient dies or becomes incapacitated, a family that is surprised by the outcome is more likely to sue.

Competence of Surgeon

In the era of superspecialties and subspecialties, it is important for any doctor to be aware of his/her limitations before venturing into any procedure. Attempting to perform any procedure without having a legally prescribed qualification for the same is definitely a negligent act. Even when a doctor has appropriate qualification for a specialty, he or she may not have adequate experience of a particular treatment or procedure. It is in the interest of the surgeon that he involves a more experienced surgeon in the case or refers the patient to another competent doctor. When a particular ailment comes in purview of different specialties, it is advisable to take the opinion of another specialty doctor before any procedure is performed.

Preoperative Evaluation

Failure to assess the patient properly and adequately prior to any surgery, particularly a planned procedure/surgery is per se negligence. Courts draw adverse inference if any standard preoperative assessment is lacking. Certain preoperative investigations are universally required for any surgery. In addition to this, there would be some tests needed in specific cases. The patient must be advised about all the required investigations before a surgery is undertaken. If a patient refuses any diagnostic procedure or investigation, it should be recorded.

In case a diagnostic surgical procedure is required such as biopsy or dilation and curettage (D&C), the patient must be made to understand that the particular procedure is not being offered as a curative surgery.

Case: A patient consulted a doctor with a breast lump who performed a biopsy. She was referred to a higher center as the biopsy suggested malignancy. The patient alleged the doctor of performing wrong surgery which did not cure her.

All possible risks and complications involved in a preoperative test should be mentioned. For example, if a patient needs to undergo a stress test as part of preoperative investigation, he/she should be made aware of the potential adverse cardiac event while undergoing stress test.

Patients should be referred to an adequately qualified doctor for fitness. Courts have held doctors negligent if fitness has been obtained from a doctor who does not have a formal superspecialty qualification. Membership of any professional body is not considered equivalent to having a formal qualification. For example, it is highly advisable to obtain fitness from a cardiologist than a general physician for a patient with an existing cardiac problem even for a minor procedure. All investigations must be duly recorded in the medical records. Failure to record any of mandatory investigations may be viewed as negligence.

It is advisable to repeat certain preoperative investigations such as hemoglobin and coagulation studies close to the scheduled surgery and record the report in the indoor papers with timing.

Preoperative Preparation

The patient has to be clearly instructed in writing about:

- Admission to the hospital
- Duration of starvation
- Preoperative procedures (enema/hair removal)
- Blood or blood products reservation
- Preprocedure medications (antihypertensive or thyroid supplement)

Any minor preoperative procedure can cause complications and the chief consultant can be held negligent even if the said procedure has been carried out by some other staff (vicarious liability).

Case: The patient was admitted for umbilical hernia repair. Proctoclysis enema was administered as part of a preoperative procedure. Subsequently, the patient was diagnosed to have rectovaginal fistula within 15 days of surgery for which she underwent repeated surgeries and required colostomy. It was alleged that the nurse was negligent in giving enema causing rectal injury. The nurse's contact could not be traced and the doctor was held negligent.

Consent

Consent provides an opportunity to establish "therapeutic alliance" between the patient and the doctor. In case of elective surgery, the process of taking informed consent starts from the first visit, as part of the process is to listen to the patient and respond to his/her queries. A detailed discussion about consent can be found in another chapter in this book.

Taking Additional Consent during Surgery

During the course of surgery, the doctor may have to perform some additional procedure or alter the nature of surgery, for which the patient has not consented. In this situation, additional consent can be obtained from the patient's relative after giving proper information about the patient's intraoperative condition. It is obvious that such a situation should be anticipated and explained to the patient during the preoperative counseling. The patient should be advised to nominate a relative who would be present during the surgery, so that an additional consent can be obtained if needed.

In grave emergency, oral consent is also valid but difficult to prove in the court of law.

Intraoperative Events

Intraoperative Complications

Law accepts that intraoperative complications cannot always be avoided, for which the surgeon cannot be held negligent. At the same, time any delay in identifying and managing the complication can be termed negligence.

Intraoperative complications due to improper functioning of equipment or nonavailability of certain backup facilities are seen as negligence. All electric gadgets used for patients (cautery/warmer) must be properly insulated and checked at regular intervals. A patient can accuse the doctor and hospital of negligence in cases such as cautery burns or burns due to warmer.

It is a must for any hospital or nursing home, however small it may be, to have all the gadgets necessary for patient resuscitation, before undertaking any operative procedure under anesthesia. Any hospital should have a ventilator and defibrillator, even if minor procedures are carried out. If the hospital does not have these gadgets, inform the patient in writing about nonavailability of these equipment. The courts perceive this as negligence on account of patient safety.

Case: A diabetic patient was taken up for hernia repair. Intraoperatively, the patient had low oxygen saturation and could not be resuscitated due to lack of ventilator. The patient was transferred to other hospital but succumbed to hypoxic brain damage eventually.

Altering Surgical Procedure/Additional Surgery

A surgeon can take on the spot decisions which can alter the course of surgery, but all such variations must be in accordance with the standard accepted medical practice and the reasons must be recorded in detail. Any deviation from preconsented surgery should be meticulously recorded in the operations notes. The reasons for doing so must also be written in detail.

Case: A patient was taken up for laparoscopic cholecystectomy but underwent partial cholecystectomy due to adherent gallbladder. The court accepted the doctor's defense and stated that doctors taking on the spot decisions which may alter the course of surgery is not a negligence per say, provided it is done in the interest of the patient.

Postsurgery Care

In many cases, the patient's condition deteriorates in the postoperative phase. Generally, the patient is monitored by a staff nurse or junior doctor in the postoperative phase. *Nonavailability of the consultant after surgery has been the prime cause of patient grievance in most of the cases.* The courts have taken cognizance of this and drew adverse inference when a particular patient is left to a junior staff. Operating surgeon must be available even in the postoperative phase till the patient is discharged or a locum arrangement must be made and informed to the patient in exceptional situations. A locum doctor should have qualifications and experience at par with the primary consultant.

If any organ/tissue is removed, it should be shown to the patient's relatives and a proper acknowledgment has to be taken and be preserved. The tissue/organ should be sent for pathological examination.

Complications in Postoperative Phase

An adverse event can occur in the immediate postoperative phase or even after the patient is discharged:

- *Sudden collapse*: If a patient has a sudden deterioration in the vital parameters in the immediate postoperative phase, it must be promptly informed to the relatives. All necessary corrective measures have to be taken in a short time. It is always better to take help from other colleagues in this catastrophic event. All the events including the time interval from diagnosis to treatment should be elaborately recorded in the indoor paper at the earliest.

If the patient needs intensive care or transfer to a higher center, the relatives should be informed promptly. The courts have ruled against the doctor for not taking a timely decision to transfer the patient to another hospital/intensive care unit (ICU).

In the event of postoperative death, a postmortem should always be asked for. The local police should be intimated about the death and all legal formalities are to be completed, even if the patient's relatives insist on avoiding the postmortem. It is more likely that the patient's relative would infer the mishap as negligence and lodge a complaint at a later date. A detailed postmortem report becomes a very solid defense for a doctor.

- *Hospital-acquired infection*: It is very common to see wound infection in most high-volume centers. All standard protocols have to be followed in the operation theater during surgery. A record has to be maintained about all asepsis measures such as fumigation, use of chemical sterilization, maintenance of laminar airflow, etc. A doctor or hospital has been sued on the allegations of improper asepsis, in cases of eye infection after cataract surgery, or failed joint replacement surgery.
- *Gossypiboma*: This is an avoidable surgical complication. The term has been coined for a forgotten mop or gauze in the patient's body, but it applies to any other foreign material as well. It has serious medicolegal repercussions. The doctrine of *res ipsa loquitur* can be applied in most of the cases. The fact should be revealed to the patient immediately and a corrective surgery must be performed.

IMPLANTS AND PROSTHESIS

Use of mesh and implants is not very common in gynecology. However, following guidelines can be followed in case gynecologists use mesh.

- In case multiple standard manufacturers are available, the patient should be given a choice to procure the mesh.
- If the patient buys the mesh from any standard company and it is to be used during surgery, the fact must be recorded.
- All the records regarding the mesh used, such as manufacturer, type, make, number, and lifespan of the implant, should be recorded in detail in the operative notes and discharge card.

CULPABLE SILENCE

It is common for a doctor to come across a patient who has been previously operated by some other surgeon. A doctor may be called for some help or opinion during the course of surgery as well. If a second surgery reveals some negligent act by the first doctor, for example, a forgotten mop or injury to any organ, it is the legal duty of the second surgeon to inform the patient about the earlier negligent act and take corrective steps. Similarly, if a surgeon is called for any intraoperative or postoperative complication which has happened due to a negligent act, it is legally binding on him/her to inform the patient about the earlier negligent act.

Case: An 11-year-old girl allegedly underwent tonsillectomy in one hospital and was shifted immediately to another hospital where another surgery was performed. It was found out later after investigations at third place that thyroidectomy had been performed on her. The court held the second surgeon guilty of not informing the patient and her relatives about the negligent act of the first surgeon.

RELAPSE OR RECURRENCE

Certain precautions need to be taken while performing a surgery where relapse or recurrence is a possibility. For example, there is a possibility of development of another fibroid after a myomectomy, a tubal recanalization surgery may not be successful or there is an increased possibility of vault prolapse after vaginal hysterectomy if the patient has bronchial asthma. While taking consent, this fact must be mentioned with appropriate statistics. Even the discharge card of the patient should have all details of surgery with a mention of specific precautions to minimize the possibility of recurrence, the telltale signs and symptoms, if the recurrence occurs and the steps to be taken by the patient if any of the symptoms are experienced. If the patient does not follow the advice or schedule of follow-up visits, it must be recorded.

ASSISTANT SURGEON

Assistance is required for lot of operative interventions. A well-trained assistant is of immense importance in a busy practice and while operating on difficult cases. However, the assistant has to have appropriate qualifications. Operation theater (OT) attendants, however experienced they may be, are unqualified assistants. In case of a lawsuit, this is perceived as grave negligence on part of the hospital and the consultant in charge.

Case: A patient underwent laparoscopy and D&C. She suffered cardiac arrest at the end of the procedure and could not be revived. In the final judgment, the court acknowledged that the treating doctor performed the surgery and managed complication as per the prevailing protocols, so there is no negligence on that count. However, the records mentioned the name of a person in the OT who assisted in the procedure, that person was not having any medical qualification; hence, it was seen as negligence and compensation was awarded.

CONCLUSION

A surgeon of any specialty is vulnerable for allegations of medical negligence.
To minimize this risk:

- A thorough presurgery assessment must be made. All required investigations should be asked for and documented properly.
- Fitness has to be obtained from an appropriately qualified specialist.
- OTs and labor rooms must be well equipped and all gadgets should be in optimum condition.
- An adverse intraoperative event must be informed to the relatives and corrective action should be taken promptly. The entire event must be recorded meticulously in the operative notes.
- Postoperative care should not be left to the junior staff solely. Operating surgeon must make appropriate arrangements in his/her absence.

KEY LEARNING POINTS

- Good communication skill and proper documentation is important.
- Take separate consent for extra investigation or additional surgery.
- Adequate and proper pre-operative work up is necessary.
- Qualified and trained assistant is good defense to prevent allegations of vicarious liability.
- Be more careful while dealing with cases of MTP, POCSO, PCPNDT, Surrogacy, etc.

20.1 Medicolegal Issues in Pregnancy and Labor

Milind Shah

INTRODUCTION

Obstetrics is a dynamic field where we deal with two lives. We all strive to reduce obstetric complications; however, it is not uncommon to land in these complications during our day-to-day practice. With doctors being pulled into court for medical negligence, it is prudent to know the medicolegal aspects of our branch so that we can give proper care to our patients without landing into litigations.

MEDICOLEGAL ASPECTS DURING PREGNANCY

First-trimester Loss—Medicolegal Aspects

- Failure to diagnose correctly may occur in this situation. A presumed completed abortion may be an ectopic pregnancy with passage of clot where the clot was thought to be tissue. Missing an ectopic pregnancy can be a life-threatening situation. Be careful. If uncertainty exists regarding whether the passed tissue is tissue or a clot, have a pathologist to evaluate it prior to sending the patient out.
- If a suction dilation and curettage (D and C) is performed, then a known complication in a small percentage of cases is Asherman syndrome or intrauterine synechiae. This situation may cause amenorrhea, infertility, or miscarriage in these patients in the future. Be gentle with the sharp curettage after the suction, and, if there is difficulty, ultrasound guidance may be helpful. Do not forget that bleeding may be occurring due to disseminated intravascular coagulation (DIC), which will not respond to a D and C but needs the missing factors replaced.
- Perforation of the uterus may occur if a suction D and C is performed. Pregnant uteri are softer than the nonpregnant state, and it is easier to perforate. Uterine perforation may occlude itself naturally because the uterus is a muscle that can undergo contraction and place its own pressure on the site until the bleeding stops. However, uncontrolled internal bleeding from a uterine perforation may require additional surgery, either a laparoscopy or laparotomy to control the bleeding. Occasionally, a hysterectomy may be the last resort to control the bleeding, which would eliminate the patient's ability to conceive in the future. Unrecognized uterine perforations may lead to significant internal bleeding that could be a life threat. Observe patients closely after a D and C and listen when patients complain of unusual symptoms (e.g., shoulder pain, unexpectedly significant abdominal pain).
- Misdiagnosis of an early intrauterine pregnancy for an ectopic pregnancy and administering methotrexate inappropriately may occur if the physician is not familiar with the laboratory and ultrasound department's discriminatory zone. Thinking about the patient's history and physical examination, differential diagnosis (including multiple gestations), the accuracy of the gestational age, the human chorionic gonadotropin (hCG) level (and pattern of hCG levels if checked every 2 days), and ultrasonographic findings are very important to make an appropriate diagnosis. This is an area of rapidly growing malpractice in obstetrics and gynecology.

- Misdiagnosis of an ectopic pregnancy as an incomplete or inevitable abortion can be a problem. In these cases, it is important to follow up on the pathology findings from the suction D and C specimen. If one is uncertain, ask the pathologist to evaluate the specimen while one is still in the operating room and proceed to laparoscopy if no chorionic villi are found in the suction D and C specimen.

Complete and Incomplete Abortions—Medicolegal Aspects

- *Ectopic pregnancy*:
  - Endometrial shedding, which clinically simulates miscarriage, may occur with an ectopic pregnancy. This misdiagnosis is the greatest potential pitfall.
  - An empty uterus on ultrasound may represent an ectopic pregnancy.
- *Retained products*:
  - Sonography for the diagnosis of retained products can yield false-positive rates, with one report of an overall false-positive rate of 34%.
  - Retained products may be more commonly found when an evacuation is performed after 15 weeks' gestation.

Threatened Abortion—Medicolegal Aspects

- *Failure to diagnose pregnancy*: Every woman of reproductive age with lower abdominal pain and/or vaginal bleeding should have a pregnancy test.
- *Failure to diagnose an ectopic pregnancy*: An ectopic pregnancy must be excluded in every pregnant woman with abdominal pain and/or vaginal bleeding. With early diagnosis, ectopic pregnancy in a patient who is stable can be treated nonsurgically.
- *Failure to provide important follow-up care*: In patients who are being monitored with serial hCG titers and sonograms, documenting a contact person with telephone number and address is prudent in the event that the patient is lost to follow-up.
- Failure to ensure patient compliance when making clinical decisions regarding definitive or expectant management.
- Failure to document discussion and patient understanding of warning symptoms and complications that require immediate medical attention.
- *Failure to prevent isoimmunization*: Unsensitized Rh-negative women should receive the appropriate dose of RhoGAM.
- *Failure to assess the true intensity of hemorrhage*: External bleeding may not accurately reflect total blood loss. Blood can be concealed in the vagina or uterus, or a hemoperitoneum may exist.

Ectopic or tubal pregnancy presents a medical emergency that requires prompt treatment in order to contain risks of maternal death and morbidity, including loss of future fertility. Medical circumstances involving individual patients and resources of the prevailing healthcare system will determine the options and means of treatment. Termination of ectopic pregnancy does not constitute or directly implicate abortion. Any practice of deliberately delaying treatment of reliably diagnosed ectopic pregnancy, on nonclinical grounds, until rupture of the fallopian tube has occurred or is imminent, in order to justify termination of the ectopic pregnancy on grounds of saving the patient's life, is unethical and illegal. Those who undertake or counsel deliberate delay of medically indicated treatment can be charged with criminal offences and civil (noncriminal) liability, and professional misconduct. On reliable diagnosis, prompt treatment to remove ectopic pregnancy is legally justified and ethically and legally required.

Septic Abortion—Medicolegal Aspects

Failure to obtain information about recent termination of pregnancy may lead to a wrong diagnosis or delayed/inappropriate treatment.

- Failure to promptly administer broad-spectrum antibiotic therapy may result in complications, including sepsis and septic shock.
- Failure to evacuate retained products of conception from the uterus leads to treatment failure and possible complications.
- Failure to diagnose uterine perforation may lead to life-threatening complications.
- Failure to diagnose bowel injury may lead to life-threatening complications.

Missed Abortion—Medicolegal Aspects

- The primary medicolegal pitfall in the diagnosis and management of missed abortion is the failure to recognize an ectopic pregnancy. Usually, findings on the sonogram confirm that the pregnancy is intrauterine. However, in rare instances, a pseudo sac consisting of retained blood clot exists and can be confused with a missed abortion. In cases in which the sonogram does not clearly show a well-developed sac, ectopic precautions should be continued until evacuated products of conception are documented by pathologic examination. In the case of pregnancy resulting from artificial reproductive technology, a coexisting ectopic pregnancy should always be a consideration.
- A second medicolegal pitfall is misdiagnosis of an early normal pregnancy as a missed abortion. This eventuality can be prevented by the use of serial ultrasonographic studies.

Abortion Complications

Postabortion complications develop as a result of three major mechanisms as follows: (1) Incomplete evacuation of the uterus and uterine atony which leads to hemorrhagic complications, (2) infection, and (3) instrumental injury.

Complications of spontaneous and therapeutic abortions include (1) complications of anesthesia, (2) postabortion triad (i.e., pain, bleeding, low-grade fever), (3) hematometra, (4) retained products of conception, (5) uterine perforation, (6) bowel and bladder injury, (7) failed abortion, (8) septic abortion, (9) cervical shock, (10) cervical laceration, and (11) DIC.

Medicolegal Aspects

Do not underestimate the amount and rate of bleeding. In the supine position, more than 500 cc of blood may collect in the vagina without severe external bleeding. Always perform a pelvic examination on a postabortion patient who is bleeding.

- Aggressively treat vaginal bleeding even if it seems minimal. Stabilize the patient with two large-bore IVs and with oxygen. Closely monitor vital signs.
- In postabortion patients with abdominal pain beyond the pelvic area, suspect perforation and evaluate with KUB (kidney, ureter, and bladder)/upright X-rays and pelvic ultrasound. Consult a gynecologist and, if suspicion is high, insist on laparoscopy.

- The chance of a missed ectopic pregnancy always exists. Do not presume intrauterine pregnancy in a patient who has just had an abortion; she may have had a missed ectopic pregnancy.
- Do not delay administration of antibiotics if a patient has signs of severe postabortion infection. Administer broad-spectrum antibiotics before completing diagnostic workup.

CONCLUSION

Early pregnancy is a very crucial period in a woman's life where there are possibilities of multiple complications. Good documentation, correct diagnosis, and proper counseling are key elements in avoiding medicolegal complications.

20.2 Medicolegal Aspects of Obstetric Bleeding

(Late) Shantanu Abhyankar

INTRODUCTION

Most obstetric litigation centers on bleeding. Of all the obstetric related medicolegal cases, 80% are following a cesarean delivery and 20% are due to mishaps following normal labor. Over half the cases in either category have an element of obstetric bleeding as a complicating factor.

Consent and Bleeding Emergencies

Every so often a doctor is faced with a bleeding patient with no possibility of legally valid consent for the necessary intervention. The law supports the doctor in such situations.

Any harm caused to a person in good faith even without the person's consent is not an offence. There may circumstances in which it is impossible for the person to sign consent and there is no lawful guardian available to do so, then the doctor may proceed with treatment in good faith. (Section 92, IPC).

Manjulaben Vinodbhai Patel vs Dr Harshida K Patel and others. CPJ 660 GUJ (1998). A patient admitted for MTP had to undergo a hysterectomy following heavy bleeding. The consent was obtained on phone, doctor not negligent as the operation was necessary to save the life of the patient.

Bleeding in the First Trimester

One is warned not to declare a woman "pregnant" on getting a positive urine pregnancy report. Even when the patient has done the test elsewhere it is prudent to caution her that a urine report tells us nothing about the viability of the embryo. An early ultrasound is a better tool to study viability.

An early ultrasound will also give us clues to other litigogenic complications such as ectopic pregnancy, heterotropic ectopic gestation, disappearing twin syndrome, gestational trophoblastic disease, early diagnosis of certain anomalies like anencephaly, and a cervical pregnancy, etc.

Patients in poor resource settings may not be willing to take the test but documentation that such a test was advised is good enough.

Of all these, cervical pregnancy happens to be most volatile situation, since it is rare and the treatment is radical. Doctors are taken by surprise and have to rush through a hysterectomy.

In some cases cervical pregnancy has been touted as defense for a hysterectomy following an MTP/abortion. Obviously having a histopathology report documenting the fact will ward off trouble most effectively.

Illegal Abortion

Bleeding and other complications following an illegal abortion are a major cause of maternal death. If one comes across a patient with history suggestive of illegal abortion it should be notified to the health authorities.

Bleeding in patients with illegal abortion can be due to trauma, infection, incomplete abortion or frank DIC.

It is mandatory to report all cases of confirmed or even suspected illegal abortion.

Consent, for an illegal act is null and void even if otherwise valid in every respect. So an abortion illegal in the eyes of the law shall remain so in spite of consent from the patient.

Late Trimester Bleeding

Major causes of late trimester bleeding are placenta previa and abruptio placenta. USG has an invaluable role in diagnosing these conditions though at times the diagnosis can be difficult or can be missed. Nevertheless the importance of a USG scan can never be overemphasized.

Equally important is the communication made to the patient and/or her relatives about the potential seriousness of the condition and need for their participation in the care of such woman. The need for complete bed rest, abstinence, need to avoid all straining at work and even stools, need for a responsible attendant with the patient at all times should be discussed and documented.

Whenever documenting any communication with the patient, put it down on the case paper with the notes. Let it be in the language that the patient can read. Enlist the names of all the persons in whose presence the counseling was done and their relation to the patient. Read out whatever you have written at the end of the visit.

Patients with Rare Blood Groups

Availability of blood is a tricky issue, especially in rural areas. Scarcity is the norm. At places where a blood bank is available autologous donation (donation by the patient for the patient) may be practiced. Medicolegally this would mean that the patient understood the risk of need for blood, and agreed to donate blood and participate in her own care.

Though obstetric hemorrhage is severe and mostly unpredictable keeping blood ready for all patients at all times is not a practicable idea. But in situations where blood loss is expected, the doctor should take reasonable care. This may mean taking informed consent, keeping blood ready, keeping alternative fluids ready, and attempting to get a rise in hemoglobin. Making enquiries about availability with a blood bank and documenting the same will also go a long way in proving reasonable care.

Urban practitioners have started the norm of keeping blood ready for all patients in labor! No textbook prescribes such practice. Since most blood so kept ready will never be used, this practice only adds to the revenue of the blood banks through 'cross-matching' charges.

In the eyes of the law it is the primary responsibility of the doctor/nursing home to make blood available as and when needed. The doctor or the hospital may be held liable in case of failure to do so.

Mismatched Transfusion

In case morbidity or mortality results from a transfusion the protocol for investigating the transfusion reaction should be meticulously followed. The transfusionist should be involved in the process. All samples from the patient, the blood bag and the transfusion set, etc., will become sources of information.

Vaginal Birth after Cesarian

Whenever a patient is being allowed a trial of labor with a scarred uterus, the operation theater should be alerted, equipment checked, and blood should be kept ready. Informed high-risk consent is in order.

Protocols for Induction and Augmentation

Protocols for induction and augmentation should be followed and their steps documented. Misoprostole is still under investigation and only 25 mg dose is accepted for induction/augmentation of labor at term.

Obstetric Hysterectomy

Torrential bleeding not amenable to any other surgical method of hemostasis will land the patient into an obstetric hysterectomy. This decision is the sole discretion of the operating surgeon. Consent from relations though desirable and valuable may not be possible in the dire situation. The obstetrician is expected to use his fair sense to decide and execute the decision in order to save the life of the pregnant woman.

Death

Maternal death leaves everyone concerned shattered. Maternal deaths have to be reported and a postmortem insisted upon.

Here is an interesting case where the affidavits of the patients in the same room were upheld and saved the doctor.

Dr Ravindra Kulkarni vs Balasaheb Gangaram Gawade CPJ 152 MAH (1999); Allegations of nonattendance after delivery which led to profuse bleeding and death were made in this case. District forum held that it was a case of PPH and not DIC and awarded compensation. State forum upheld the doctor's stand that there was no profuse bleeding but the death was due to amniotic fluid embolism. Allowed appeal and dismissed the complaint.

Affidavit of a patient admitted in the same room was relied upon. The doctor cannot be held responsible for a known complication, the bench opined.

CONCLUSION

Obstetric bleeding is a dire emergency and one wonders if one should be dealing with the patient or thinking of all the medicolegal implications. As a doctor our primary focus should of course be on the care of the patient, but the current medicosocial environment should alert us to complete and timely record keeping too.

20.3 Medicolegal Aspects in LSCS

Dilip Walke

INTRODUCTION

LSCS is one of the commonest operations in obstetric and gynecological practice. There is a growing rate at which this mode of delivery is resorted to due to several reasons:

- Women becoming mothers at late age are more likely to undergo LSCS
- Larger babies especially in mothers with diabetes or gestational diabetes are common feature of practice today
- Better monitoring leads to pick up fetal distress earlier
- Reduction in mortality and morbidity has been reported as LSCS rate raises
- Fear of litigation prompts obstetricians to take less risk and resort to LSCS earlier in high risk situations.

With this growing incidence of LSCS, there is also an increasing possibility of litigations associated with it. Most common problems which lead to litigation in cases of LSCS are associated with bleeding. One has to be vigilant about possibility of bleeding in all case of LSCS and hence, it is prudent to send blood for cross-matching for all cases of LSCS. If blood bank is situated at far away distance, at least efforts should be made to ring up the blood bank and ask for availability of blood in case of emergency.

Another situation which is prone to litigation is a case of vaginal birth after cesarean (VBAC). Documents should be able to prove that labor was meticulously monitored and OT was kept ready for emergency LSCS. 2.35 lacs compensation was awarded in DK Nayak vs. Dr Kalyani case (1997) CPJ 103 because blood was not arranged in spite of the fact that blood group was a rare (A negative) for a case of LSCS.

We need to address some medicolegal questions related to LSCS so as to become safe in our practice.

First question relates to the qualification required for performing LSCS. Ideally LSCS is expected to be performed by a gynecologist. If a general practitioner with MBBS degree or a surgeon with MS degree does it, he/she has to produce in the court proof about training in the surgery. Further there is a need to prove that gynecologist was not available for the particular surgery and that the situation was life saving and there was no time to wait for the gynecologist.

Second question relates to the place where LSCS can be performed. Infrastructure has to be reasonably well-equipped with essential equipments like oxygen cylinders, Boyle's apparatus and defibrillator. Protocol for checking the expiry dates of drugs, oxygen cylinder filling dates and annual maintenance contracts should be maintained. Standards should be followed while deciding the list of drugs, disposables, and equipments to be available in the OT.

Third question relates to the essential preoperative precautions. Preoperative questionnaire to get proper history of previous surgeries and medical problems following is ideally to be filled up by resident doctors. The minimum preoperative investigations like grouping cross-matching, hemogram, BT, CT, and urine examination should never be missed and documentary evidence of preoperative instructions to the patient like preoperative nill by mouth, medication, etc. is essential.

Documentation of proper indication for LSCS is important because common allegation related to LSCS are that doctor did unnecessary LSCS or did it too late and hence baby suffered. Courts do not usually question our opinion about the indication but it is important that our documents corroborate with indications. For example, FHR record should prove that there were problems noted in FHR if indication for LSCS is fetal distress.

Regarding Consent, the Usual Allegations in the Litigation are:

- Consent was not taken
- Consent was taken under pressure
- We were not told about the seriousness properly

In the Sameera Kohli vs. Dr Prabha Manchanda, SC Jan 2008 case, the three bench judgment has dealt with the question of consent.

1. Consent of the patient herself is most important. Others are signing as witness (unless patient is insane/minor).
2. It should be an informed consent with detailed explanation of:
   - Nature of treatment
   - Benefits
   - Possible side effects (balanced information, not to frighten her)
   - Available alternatives
   - Consequences of refusal of treatment
   - All this can be accomplished during the antenatal classes if taken.
3. Consent for LSCS does not imply consent for other associated procedures like appendicectomy or hysterectomy unless it was life, saving step.
4. With proper mention in the consent, associated procedure can be done, e.g., tubectomy or appendicectomy.
5. Consent can actually be taken by our resident doctors.

We often face a situation wherein our patient refuses to give consent for LSCS. In such a case one should do the following:

- Document informed refusal signed by the patient
- If patient refuses to sign the refusal of consent get an undertaking about the incident signed by neutral bystander
- In Mr Sakil vs. Dr P Irani 1992, doctor documented refusal of consent to LSCS as patient insisted on waiting for her father-in-law and hence negligence could not be proved in spite of hypoxic damage to the newborn
- Once consent is given one should not delay in doing LSCS. In K Murugesan vs Dr Sarladevi. I (1999) CPJ 542, doctor waited for anesthetist husband for 4 hours and did not call any other local anesthetist till then. There was IUFD and intraoperative bleeding and patient had to be shifted to Madras in ambulance. Patient died on the way and majority in the State fora held doctor liable.

There is often a dilemma regarding need for neonatologist to be present during LSCS. Legally it is enough to prove that baby was resuscitated by a person (resident doctor or staff nurse) "trained" in it. The challenge however is to prove in the court of law the extent and authenticity of training. So, a prudent practice is if available call neonatologists for all LSCS cases especially if it is for fetal indication.

LSCS is prone to complications as it is a major surgery performed under anesthesia, on several occasions performed on patients with compromised general condition. One should remember that doctors are not held liable just because there was a complication. Principles of Res Ipsa Loquitor; if, at all applied is done so with caution in cases of medical negligence. What we have to prove is:

- We acted in a manner in which any prudent and averagely qualified obstetrician would have acted in that situation
- The complication is known complication
- Supported by expert witness and textbook references.

There is a tendency to avoid doing tubectomy with LSCS, especially if it is done on a high-risk patient because of the fear associated with inquiries of tubectomy complications and deaths. One must remember that following the GOI guidelines of 2006, death or complications due to LSCS will not be considered as sterilization complication. Insurance has been started by the Government of India for doctor's indemnity and patients for any complication or death. Patients are insured for complications death and failure. We are indemnified for negligence in four cases per year. However, to avail of this insurance we have to be empanelled for it.

One of the commonest postoperative complications prone for litigation is sepsis. The documents which can save us in these cases are:

- Autoclave register
- Fumigation register
- Purchase vouchers of disposables
- Operative notes and postoperative instructions for common gynecological operations including LSCS
- Checklist of antenatal investigations
- Hospital documents
- Anesthesia-related documents.

To conclude, proper documentation, proper counseling, and sympathetic approach to any untoward complication can go a long way in averting any medicolegal problem in LSCS.

20.4 Issues in Adolescent Gynecology

Alka Kuthe

"Fear makes me tremble in my shoes,
Fear is touching stillness and makes trembling noises,
Fear makes me taste something about me,
Fear makes my ear stuff, that's not there
That is FEAR."

—Joel Fazone, Age: 10 years
(Victim of sexual abuse)

INTRODUCTION

Adolescence is a fascinating period of life that makes the transition from being a dependent child to becoming an independently functioning adult. According to Oxford's dictionary it is a period from the beginning of sexual maturity to the completion of physical growth. It is that phase of growth and development of human beings when most dramatic life transformation takes place. This is the period when aims are high and plans are plenty. It is the period of dilemma to say "Yes" or "No". It is the period dominated by split personality of stubborn but reasonable and loving but resentful. The thoughts are bundle of contradictions. The mind has wings and often leaps beyond emotions that any way is colorful. She/he wants freedom to make self-choices but hesitates to face consequences. They are generally unhappy with parent's rules and curbs; often get on each other's nerves. They look for oasis due to impending identity crisis.

Adolescents have the right to be informed, their opinions heard and above all involved in matters that affect their lives. Adults in general, world leaders, professional guards, and parents in particular need to hear their voices and see their faces. All adolescents must have best possible start to adult life. Helping adolescents begins with good health care, good nutrition, quality education, psychological support, immunization, healthy and accident-free environment, legal education, and support. In India, children <15 years constitute 42% of the whole population. Early sexual activity in this age group can pose problems of varying magnitude. The lack of attention to their health and legal issues may prove dangerous for this vulnerable class of society. Some of the important medicolegal issues involved in adolescent care are discussed.

CONSENT IN ADOLESCENTS

Ordinarily, when the adolescent is accompanied by his or her guardian while seeking the treatment, it is implied that he/she has given consent for examination and treatment. Express consent is required for any procedure beyond routine physical examination such as any invasive investigation or procedure, any operation, blood transfusion, and collection of blood, etc. It must be taken before the act. It should not be confused with the consent taken at the time of admission in the hospital.

Written consent should be taken from the guardian/parents before examining a person with the purpose to prepare a medicolegal report. Consent in these cases should be taken after informing the parents/guardian that they reserve the right to refuse the examination and that the report may go in his/her favor or against him/her.

- *Consent for sexual intercourse:* In India, definition of "child" varies from one statute to other. Protection of children from sexual offences (POCSO) Act 2012 criminalizes all sexual activities under the age of 18 years even if it was committed by consent. Bombay High Court recently has said that "balance to be struck" between protection of children against sexual abuse and age of consensual sexual intercourse. It has to be distinguished from age of marriage as sexual acts do not necessarily take place in the confines of marriage. It further said it is high time for our country and Parliament to take note of the changing scenario with respect to age of consent for adolescents to enter into a consensual sexual relationship as several countries have reduced the age of consent in the range of 14–16 years. Sexual Autonomy encompasses both, the right to engage in wanted sexual activity and right to be protected from unwanted sexual aggression. Only when both aspects of adolescent's rights are recognized, human sexual dignity can be considered to be fully respected said the High Court.

CONSENT IN RAPE CASES

As discussed before, in India, *the provisions of POCSO Act 2012, override all other laws related to child <18 years as regards sexual intercourse. Thus, even if a woman <18 years, gives consent for an intercourse, it will be considered as rape as per the present provisions of POCSO Act 2012.*

If the examiner is male the examination must be carried out in the presence of female attendant. Consent of inmates of the hostel who are >12 years is necessary for treatment. Up to 12 years, the principal or warden can give consent. If an inmate is >12 years and is suffering from disease which is likely to spread but he refuses the treatment, he can be asked to leave the hostel. However, such child can be treated even without his consent. There are few exceptions to this general rule regarding age of consent in adolescents. Consent for emergency treatment, the concept of *Loco Parentis* and other issues related to consent have been discussed in detail in Chapter 8.

When a juvenile child is arrested on charge of committing offence, e.g., smuggling and it is felt that there are reasonable grounds for believing that examination of the child will offer evidence as to the commission of the offence, the registered medical practitioner acting on the order of the court or at the request of a police officer not below the rank of sub-inspector can lawfully examine such child and use such force as reasonably necessary to ascertain the facts which may offer such evidence.

EXAMINATION OF AN ADOLESCENT CHILD

The approach to a history taking and examination of an adolescent differ from that of an adult in many respects. Consent from the guardian along with privacy and comfort are the essential things. Most teenagers will give honest answers to the questions related to sexual activity once they are assured about confidentiality. The girl child can be interviewed in the absence of her parents but in the presence of female nurse, so as to allow a rapport to be established and confidentiality to be maintained. After careful and detailed history, physical examination with appraisal of secondary sexual characters, congenital anomalies, height, and weight measurement, etc., is usually done. A gynecological examination can be performed in those who are sexually active or where history is suggestive. On completion of examination, the nature of the problem and its management options should be fully explained and discussed with the adolescent child. At the end of this, the situation is explained to the parents in presence of the adolescent. In this way the adolescent's wish can be respected and confidentiality can be maintained. There is always an inevitable conflict between the adolescent's right to confidentiality and the desire of the parents to be fully informed of all the matters relevant to their adolescent child. Patience, need of the adolescent child to be treated with respect and sincerity with some modification in the adult technique will allow proper examination of an adolescent child.

CRIMINAL RESPONSIBILITY

According to section 83 IPC, a child between 7 and 12 years is presumed to be capable of committing an offence, if the child has attained "sufficient maturity" or understanding to judge the nature and consequences of his/her conduct **(Table 20.4.1)**.

Table 20.4.1: Medicolegal importance of various adolescent ages at a glance.

Age in years	*Medicolegal importance*
7–12	A child may or may not be held responsible for his act by the court depending upon whether the child has attained sufficient maturity to understand the nature and consequence of the act
12	Nothing is an offence which is done in good faith for the benefit of the child under this age, when such act is done by his or her guardians or through their consent, even if the act ultimately causes harm to the sufferer. A child below this age cannot give a valid consent to suffer any harm which may result from an act which is done in good faith for his benefit
14	A person below this age is child and cannot be employed in factory jobs
14–15	A person can be engaged in nonhazardous factory jobs for a limited period during the day hours
15	Sexual intercourse, even with one's own wife, below this age amount to rape. A person >15 years of age can be employed in a factory like an adult, if he has a fitness certificate for the employment
16	Intercourse with a girl below this age, irrespective of whether with or without her consent amounts to rape (statutory rape)
17	Person <17 years of age shall not be allowed to work in any part of a mine which is below ground, unless a certificate of fitness is granted to him by a qualified medical practitioner
18	Below this age, an offender is a juvenile offender and is tried in a juvenile court, if convicted sent to a borstal or reformatory school. This is the age of majority except when the individual is under the guardianship of a court. It is the minimal permissible age for marriage for girls. A person above this age can give a valid consent to suffer any harm, which may result from an act, which is not intended or known to cause death or grievous hurt. A person above this age, if mentally sound, can make a valid will

JUVENILE DELINQUENCY

According to Taber's medical dictionary, delinquent means a person whose behavior is anti-social or criminal. Juvenile has been defined to mean a boy who is below the age of 16 years or a girl who is below the age of 18 years. Under the provisions of the Juvenile Act, Parliament has made provision for the establishment of the juvenile courts and the juvenile child has to be produced before the court. In its absence, the power of the juvenile court has to be exercised by the District Magistrate or the Sub-Divisional Magistrate or any Judicial Magistrate of first class, as the case may be.

In 1986, to provide care, protection, treatment, development, and rehabilitation of neglected or delinquent juveniles, the Parliament enacted the Juvenile Justice Act.

The following proposals were made namely:

- To lay down the basic principles for administration of justice to a juvenile child
- To make the juvenile justice system more appreciative of the developmental needs in comparison to criminal justice system as appreciable to adults
- To bring the juvenile law in conformity with United Nation's Convention on the rights of the child
- To prescribe a uniform age of 18 years for both boys and girls
- To ensure speedy disposal of the juvenile cases within a time limit of 4 months
- To create a special juvenile police unit with a humanitarian approach through sensitization and training of police personnel
- To minimize the stigma and in keeping with the developmental needs of the juvenile child

On 30th December, 2000, the Parliament amended the Juvenile Justice (care and promotion of children) Act to provide for effective provisions and various alternatives for rehabilitation and social reintegration.

Apprehension of juvenile in conflict with law: As soon as a juvenile in conflict with the law is apprehended by police, he shall be placed under the charge of the special juvenile police unit or the designated police officer who shall immediately report the matter to a member of the board.

- *Information to the parent guardian*: The officer-in-charge of the police station should inform the parents or guardian of the arrested juvenile child.
- *Bail of juvenile*: Detained or an arrested juvenile shall be released on bail with or without surety, but he shall not be released if that release exposes him to moral, physical or psychological danger or brings him into association with any known criminal or that release defeats the very end of the justice.
- *Release and absence of juvenile on placement*: Leave of absence can be permitted by competent authority to any juvenile, to allow him, on special occasions such as examination, death of kith and kin, accident or serious illness of parents or any emergency of similar nature to go on supervised leave for maximum 7 days, excluding the time of journey. The officer-in-charge shall maintain a roaster of the cases. Parent or guardian is given timely information regarding the exact date of release of the child, and they are invited to come to the institution to take charge of the juvenile/the child on that date. The officer-in-charge of the institution shall see that every juvenile received in the institution is searched, his or her personal effects (personal possessions) inspected. Girls shall be searched by a female staff with due respect and decency.

  When a juvenile is of unsound mind or is found to be suffering from leprosy, sexually transmitted disease (STD), hepatitis B, open case of tuberculosis, he shall be dealt with separately through various specialized reformed services or under the relevant laws. When a juvenile is found to be suffering from a disease requiring prolonged medical treatment, the competent authority may send the juvenile to any recognized place for the required treatment.

- *Death of a child*: In the event of death of a child, the death certificate should be obtained from the attending doctor, or the hospital and the details regarding the death should be recorded by the case worker. The last rites should be performed according to the known religion of the child. The name, address, school or any other particulars or any picture of any such juvenile child shall not be published by any newspaper, magazine, newssheet, or visual media.

TEENAGE SEXUALITY AND CONTRACEPTION

Adolescents account for one-fifth of world's population. In India, they constitute 22.8% of the population (Population Projections by Planning Commission), i.e., approximately 230 million Indians are adolescents. Pregnancy in adolescents is one of the main problems in the world with the prevalence rate varying from 2 to 25%. In recent years, the prevalence is increasing probably due to low puberty age, early onset of sexual activity in girls, and lack of education on contraceptive methods. It is a problem to the society contributing to high maternal and perinatal morbidity and mortality in our country. From 10 to 15% of all births in the world (about 12–18 million a year) involve teenage mothers. The demographic consequences of teenage pregnancy are important for India where about 70% of girls between 15 and 19 years of age are married. Demographers have estimated that if marriage was postponed from 16 to 20–21 years, the number of births would decrease by 20–30%. Contraceptive services and advice along with safe pregnancy termination practices should be easily accessible to this vulnerable group.

Teenage Contraception

Teenage pregnancies and incidence of STDs are increasing due to early sexual activity and lack of knowledge about contraception despite the availability of family planning methods, efforts of education department, and wide advertisement through the media. The most effective contraception method for adolescents is the oral contraceptive pill. Emergency contraception can also help in unprotected sexual act, but it cannot become routine method. Compliance, however, remains a problem, particularly in a younger patient. Barrier methods are not as effective as the sexual activity is usually not planned. Injectable contraception can be advisable but its association with amenorrhea and menstrual irregularities makes it unacceptable. The doctors looking after adolescents need to provide appropriate education and proper advice to this high-risk group.

Termination of Pregnancy

Termination of pregnancy in an adolescent girl is a serious problem not only from medical but also from social and legal angle. Abortions are usually unsafe and illegal. Out of every 20 teenagers, one is suffering from STD which may either lead to infertility and if serious; death. Pregnancies have been reported at ages as low as 10–12 years. Further, if a girl <18 years becomes pregnant, she cannot give valid consent for medical termination of pregnancy under the Medical Termination of Pregnancy (MTP) Act. Consent of legal guardian/parents is required in such cases otherwise the act of termination becomes illegal and the doctor performing such an operation is liable for punishment. Again, proper guidance to these adolescents can make a lot of difference as far as their future obstetric career and social life is concerned. Under the prevailing conditions it is essential to have medical counseling on psychological issues such as feeling of inadequacy, immorality, loss of virginity, promiscuity, premarital sex, multiple pregnancies, risk of STD, acquired immunodeficiency syndrome (AIDS), and cancer.

LIVE-IN RELATIONSHIP

Live-in relationship is not new for western countries but these days the concept is adjusting its roots in east also. The word "live in" is controversial in many terms in eastern countries. But the 2K generation is so much influenced with this concept, in the whole world. The legal definition of live-in relationship is *a living arrangement in which an unmarried couple lives together in a long-term relationship that resembles a marriage.*

India is a country, which is slowly opening its doors for western ideas and lifestyles and one of the crucial episodes amongst it, is the concept of live-in relationship. The number of unmarried partners especially adolescents living together is scaling high. At some places, policy can be shared by unmarried partners and they get legal protection as well while at other places they do not have rights, even if they have lived together for years.

Why Live-in?

It is proved by research that live-in couples who live and move in together would like to get married in future. Though they are in love, they also want to confirm their compatibility before they get married to each other instead of repenting after marriage if found incompatible, then they will have no choice other than compromising their lifestyles. Some couple remain unmarried, and some (like gay or lesbian couples) are prevented from marrying as in India as same sex marriages are not currently legal. Recently the central government has opposed legal validation of same sex marriage saying it would cause chaos in the society harming the accepted societal values and disturbing the delicate personal laws. The government submitted that despite the decriminalization of Section 377 of the Indian Penal Code, thereby decriminalized homosexuality by India's Apex Court, in 2018, the petitioners cannot claim a fundamental right for the same sex marriage to be recognized by the laws of the country.

Consequences

The unplanned pregnancy rate is high among cohabitants but its undesirable. It can prove detrimental for future of child as well as for healthy marital relationship between the couple. The unplanned, undesired pregnancy may end up in illegal abortions and whether or not it is unplanned or unwanted, if the pregnancy continues in spite of the legal status of the child whether our orthodox society would accept this child? Apart from ill effects on Indian culture, what about the impact of this lifestyle on the woman's social life? There is a possibility of increase in the cases of sexual abuse and sexual violence. In case of an adolescent, this type of behavior may have long-term effect on his/her educational career. The immature mind may not be able to cope up with the tempting moments of the cohabitation. There would be an increase in the cases of HIV and AIDS and other STDs. It is, therefore, earnestly felt that the verdict declared by Apex Court as quoted below needs rethinking. Thereby most respected Indian culture would be preserved and it would also prove that we are no more thought slaves. If at all, the modern trend has to be followed, the responsibility lies on these adolescents to protect themselves from the possible ill-effects of this modern concept of "live-in relationship" and also preserve the Indian values.

Supreme Court Judgment

A much-publicized statement of South Indian film actress Khusboo on premarital sex, virginity, and live-in relationships came for some favorable comments from the Supreme Court, which said there was nothing illegal in live-in relationships between adults. When they argued that it was virtually inducing others to commit an illegality, the bench shot back saying in that case they should also sue the Apex court, which has held live-in relationship between adults as legal. Referring to the development of law with the dynamics of social behavior, the bench also referred to the recent judgment of Delhi High Court legalizing consensual sexual relation between adults falling in the category of lesbian, gay, bi-sexual, and transgender (LGBT) group. Counsel for the actress, Mr. Anand said her client's fundamental rights of freedom of speech and expression could not be curtailed by persons with vested interest, who had systematically unleashed a series of complaints against her. In an observation that will cheer votaries of premarital sex and live-in partners, the Supreme Court opined on 22nd March, that a man and woman living together without marriage cannot be construed as an offence. "When two adult people want to live together what is the offence and under which section? The Apex Court said there was no law which prohibits live-in relationship or premarital sex. The judges repeatedly stressed that the perceived immoral activities cannot be branded as offence. The argument of the counsel was that her comments allegedly endorsing premarital sex would adversely affect the minds of young people leading to decay in moral values and country's ethos. Living together is a right to life," the Apex court said apparently referring to Article 21 which grants Right to Life and Liberty as a Fundamental Right.

CHILD LABOR

India fosters the largest number of child labor in the world. The child labor constitutes about 20% of India's Gross National Product. The child labor (Prohibition and Regulation) Act, 1986 prohibits the engagement of children in certain employments and it regulates the conditions of work of children in certain other employments. This Act also decides the hours and period of work including weekly holidays. Article 4 of the Universal Declaration of Human Rights, the International Bill of Human Rights (1948) adopted and proclaimed that "No one shall be held in slavery or servitude slavery and the slave trade shall be prohibited in all their forms." All human beings are born free and equal in rights and dignity.

Children suffer greatly when they are forced to perform as "small adults". Studies have shown that labor at such tender age can have serious effects on child's physical and mental health affecting overall development. The child's creativeness and abilities are blunted and his whole mental world is disturbed.

DRUG ABUSE

Nowadays drug abuse has become global phenomenon. Teenagers feel it as a proof of maturation and entry to "*pseudo-adulthood*". Environmental chaos or tension, economic instability or dependence, familial maladjustment, poor parental care, etc., along with complexities of today's lifestyle, and glorification by media can lead to substance abuse. It can also be a form of "*rebellion against authority*" and drug experimentation resulting in vicious cycle of drug abuse. The increasing trend of drug abuse in girls can be due to the misconception that "*modern femininity*" means behaving or adopting male lifestyle. The Cigarettes and Other Tobacco Products Act, 2003 prohibits sale of cigarette or other tobacco products to a person below the age of 18 years. Misuse or abuse of drugs may affect health and development of an adolescent child which in turn may have adverse effect on the future life.

Adolescents and Abuse

Abuse is the term commonly used to designate inappropriate and harmful treatment or exploitation of any person that affects the person either psychologically or physically or both. It encompasses a spectrum of abusive actions or acts of commission or lack of action or acts of omission that result in morbidity and mortality in the child. Adolescence abuse and domestic violence are worldwide phenomena. The exact prevalence is not known since the majority of the cases remain unreported.

Physical Abuse

It may be narrowly defined as intentional injuries to a child by care given that results in bruises, burns, fractures, lacerations, punctures, or organ damage. Short and long-term emotional consequences of the maltreatment can be more debilitating than the physical trauma. Physical neglect may affect growth, development, and learning ability. There is increased susceptibility to infection. Nutritional deprivation is the most common cause of underweight in infancy.

Sexual Abuse

Child sexual abuse is a global public health problem. It is a serious infringement of a child's rights to health and protection. The cases are seen in all socioeconomic groups. From 1970 to 1990, child sexual abuse reports are on the rising trend. The World Health Organization (WHO) estimates that globally some 40 million children aged 0–14 years suffer some form of abuse and neglect.

Figures from the USA show that one in four girls and one in six boys are sexually abused before the age of 18. Asia and Africa may have greater number. The Indian Cabinet has approved the protection of women by "*Domestic Violence Bill 2005*". It offers protection to the women from all kinds of abuse and threats—physical, sexual, verbal, emotional, and economical. Any activity with a child, before the age of legal consent, for the sexual gratification of an adult or a significantly older child is included under sexual abuse which can be oral-genital, genital-genital, genital-rectal, hand-genital, hand-rectal or hand-breast contact; exposure of sexual anatomy; forced view of sexual anatomy; and showing pornography or using a child in the production of pornography. Child sexual abuse is different from sexual play, which is defined as viewing or touching of the genitals, buttocks or chest by preadolescent children separated by not more than 4 years. No force or coercion is used in sexual play.

The role of a comprehensive forensic medicolegal examination of the victim of adolescence abuse and domestic violence, is of utmost importance in the full investigation and the building of an effective prosecution in the court. The sexually abused child should be protected from any additional emotional trauma during physical examination Medicolegal examination is one of the star evidences in the judicial proceeding. The affected children may not be able to give proper history. Therefore, a high degree of suspicion is expected from the examiner. A medical practitioner is not only morally but also legally bound to examine, document, and collect all relevant and feasible material as evidence from a victim. It is advisable to examine the victim at the earliest after the incident. The physical examination includes inspection of the whole body with special attention to the mouth, breasts, genitals, perineal region, buttocks, and anus. The next important step is the collection of biological evidence of the alleged sexual abuse that has occurred within the preceding 72 hours. Forensic experts decide cultures and serological tests according to the special circumstances of the case. Urine pregnancy test along with pelvic sonography should be performed in each case of sexually abused girl in a reproductive age if she misses her next menstrual cycle. Any medical condition (including pregnancy) traceable to sexual act done at the age <18 years of female is to be reported to police, otherwise referring doctor or any person having knowledge of it, would be punished. [Refer Protection of Children from Sexual Offences Act, 2012 (POCSO Act 2012) Section 19 and Section 21 and Supreme Court Judgement dated 11th October 2017].

Section 33(8) of the POCSO Act empowers the Special Courts to direct payment of such compensation as may be prescribed to the child, for physical or mental trauma caused or for immediate rehabilitation, in addition to punishment.

- *POCSO (Amendment) Bill, 2019:* It was introduced in Rajya Sabha by the Minister of Women and Child Development, Ms. Smriti Jubin Irani on July 18, 2019. It increases minimum punishment for offence depending upon the nature of sexual assault, the age of the victimized child, and the offender person.

Medicolegal Examination of a Sexually Abused Child

First approach: The first approach, during a medicolegal investigation of a sexually abused child is of grave importance. A forensic pathologist should spend enough time to become acquainted with the child and try to provide a simple and comprehensive overview of the process that will be followed.

The conversation should begin with the topic which is interesting and not "threatening" for the child. It should decrease the child's tension and make her relax. Vaginal and anal examination will be easier after that. Wearing a laboratory coat or other hospital and medical suit may be frightening for younger children. The history must be obtained by a highly skilled professional in an appropriate, supportive, friendly, and caring attitude without leading questions. It should be recorded in their own words.

Assessment: A full clinical inspection must be undertaken which also includes a skeletal radiological survey. It may be necessary to involve another medical professional such as genitourinary physician, psychiatrist, or family planning doctor in addition to forensic medical examiner and a pediatrician.

Medical history: History taking is story is very important. Old injuries should be recorded with extreme caution.

Examination: Each examination should include a complete physical examination with careful photographic recording of any trauma away from the genital area. Although such injuries can be serious, they can be overlooked when the examiner focuses attention only on the genital area. In some assaults, force used is severe enough to leave the marks of fingertips and bruises on the limbs or strangling marks on the neck. Quite frequently, injuries on the breast, inner thigh or other area near genital region are observed. More common in sexual assaults are bite marks. One has to measure and photograph them carefully. It helps in matching or exclusion of the teeth of the alleged assailant.

Genital examination: In the sexually abused child, it is necessary to examine the genital region along with the anal area thoroughly to note positive findings, though at times the examination findings will be normal. The reasons for absence of diagnostic findings are, firstly children are reluctant about reporting such sexual abuse incidents, so the opportunity to see and record fresh findings is lost. Secondly, children are not usually subjected to great violence. Nonabuse related conditions such as Crohn's disease, child with significant constipation, etc., should be kept in mind in the differential diagnosis of anal sexual abuse.

False sexual abuse allegation: False sexual abuse allegation is defined as the intentional reporting of a sexual abuse by the "victim" when no such activity has occurred. Obtain attention and sympathy, seek revenge, get an alibi, and protect oneself from consequences are the most common motives mainly among adolescents. In younger children, the false allegation is usually related with the dispute between parents for the child's custody. False memory syndrome includes cases in which the victims do believe that they have been sexually abused, usually in their childhood. The investigation of a sexual abuse case becomes more complicated when the findings are minor, nonspecific, or even absent.

Medical conditions frequently confused with sexual abuse: The most common dermatological condition confused with trauma for sexual abuse is lichen sclerosis. It can present in various ways. A punch biopsy may be necessary to make the diagnosis.

Evidence sampling-laboratory examination: Forensic studies, when the examination is carried within 72 hours of acute sexual assault or sexual abuse, will be of immense help to provide corroborative evidence. The swabs from mouth, anus, or vagina if taken, should be allowed to dry before they are sealed. Though the documented presence of an ejaculate is the most positive finding, its absence by no means refutes sexual abuse. Evidence should be preserved carefully, and a written record kept of every person-to-person transfer, so as to ensure that no tampering occurred during the transfer. For the identification of assailant, in addition to identification of different characteristics of scalp and pubic hair, identification tests for generic markers in the blood, saliva and serum, should be performed within 72 hours of acute sexual assault or sexual abuse. The identity of a perpetrator can be established with a high degree of certainty by deoxyribonucleic acid (DNA) finger printing. In sexually abused girls of reproductive age pregnancy test should always be performed. If the child victim has been abused under the influence of drugs, the chemical analysis of blood and urine should also be performed.

Sexual abuse is a criminal offence. Legally, it is mandatory for all physicians and care providers in all states to report all suspected cases of child abuse and neglect. The law offers protection to mandatory reporters who report in good faith. Failure to report suspected child abuse is crime and liable for punishment.

Sexually transmitted diseases: The diagnosis of STD in the child can give indirect clue of sexual abuse and will also help in treating the disease. After excluding perinatal transmission, gonorrhea or syphilis infections are diagnostic of sexual abuse. Herpes Type 2, Chlamydia, Trichomonas, and Condyloma infections are mostly due to abuse especially in children above the age of 1 year.

The responsibility of health provider is to elicit proper history, collect the best possible evidence in time, treat and above all help and support the victim. Injuries often speak for themselves. Investigation protocol should be strictly followed. Proper documentation and collection of all clinical and forensic evidences will definitely increase the value of medical evaluation of sexual offence. Empathetic attitude, prophylaxis, and proper management of pregnancy and infection along with prompt investigation and prosecution of the offender will be very much advantageous to the victim.

Adolescents and HIV infections: In 1983, the first case of AIDS in children was reported. In 1997, Global Adolescent Health Statistics shows that 5,90,000 adolescents are newly infected with HIV/AIDS. Adolescents are at the center of the worldwide AIDS pandemic. According to NACO, the majority of the newly infected people with HIV/AIDS are young people <25 years in age. According to WHO one in every 20 teenagers acquires STD each year. The disproportionately high rates of sexually transmitted infections (STIs) among adolescent girls are particularly important because the presence of STIs is known to facilitate HIV transmission. To protect the youth from this serious problem, AIDS prevention education program (APEP) was initiated in the secondary schools of Mumbai in 1993 and AIDS awareness in junior colleges (AAJ) in Mumbai was launched in the year 2000.

During recent years, although significant improvement has been made in the HIV response, children are still affected by the epidemic. Of the estimated 39.0 million people living with HIV worldwide in 2022, 2.58 million were children aged 0–19 years. Each day in 2022, approximately 740 children became infected with HIV and approximately 274 children died from AIDS-related causes mostly because of inadequate access to HIV prevention, care, and treatment (*Source:* UNICEF: July 2023).

The general bioethical principles include the right to privacy and the confidentiality of the information the adolescents provide. The additional principles and the various other ethical and legal issues related to HIV infections are discussed in the relevant chapter.

ADOLESCENCE AND RAPE

"Rape" a cognizable offence, literally means taking anything by force. The term is used to describe the criminal sexual assault on woman. A doctor is duty-bound to inform to the police about this grave offence. The number of "rape" cases has increased significantly in recent years though it exists since ancient times. The three top states in terms of rate of the crime (crime per lakh population) are Mizoram, Madhya Pradesh, and Delhi. [*Source:* Crime in India 1998, NCRB Govt. of India (1999)].

During last decade, the rape on adolescent girls <16 years of age accounts for >75% of total rape cases. In contrast to adult rape cases, the interpretation of the physical findings is comparatively easy, in adolescent rape cases (age of girls <16 years) as the plea of consensual rape is not valid in these cases. In adolescent girls presence of any feature of sexual intercourse will amount to rape.

Drug facilitated sexual assault: Date rape—in metropolitan cities especially, its increasing incidence has become the reason for deep concern. Drugs are mixed in drinks and the culprit takes the advantage of the girl's drowsy, trans-like, and confused state under the influence of drugs. The interaction of the drug with the alcohol may prove detrimental to the life of victim apart from mental injury. The characteristics of drug induced rape are:

- "Drug" is involved in about 25% of rape cases.
- Girls in the age group of 16–19 years and adult women in the age group of 20–24 years are four times more likely to be sexually assaulted than other age group women.
- Date-rape drugs are also commonly used recreationally, putting the user at risk of sexual assault. Such rapes are most common in high socioeconomic class teenagers.
- The most common drug detected in victims of drug facilitated sexual assault is alcohol. The second most common is marijuana.
- Most of these crimes either go unnoticed, unreported, unsolved, or unproven.
- Problems with the drugs are that they make the victim look like as if she is under the influence of alcohol and hence cannot be suspected, cause memory loss and are difficult to be traced in the blood of the victim as time passes by.

Adolescents need to be made alert and aware about precautions to help them to remain safe at a party, bar or just hanging out with friends. Though rape is a cognizable offence, the medical practitioner may not report it to the police in case the girl is >18 years and does not want it to be reported. But if the girl is <18 years, as per the provisions of POCSO Act 2012, it has to be strictly and legally reported to the regional police station. In general, doctors in private practice avoid reporting and admitting a case of rape because of hassles of a police and because of lack of adequate training for collection of evidence but he or she is dutybound to report if the alleged victim is <18 years.

When adolescent girls are molested, the media especially electronic media cross their limits while reporting the case. A rape case in Muzaffarnagar who was raped by her own father-in-law and gang-raped case in Gujarat are the examples. There is neither privacy nor secrecy for these women. Justice is many times delayed and even if they get justice, there is no guarantee that they will ever be able to pick up the threads of their lives once again.

Under law, rape can only be committed by man and a woman cannot commit rape although she may be guilty of an indecent assault upon him. A man cannot be raped by a man and an animal cannot be raped. These sexual acts are considered to be unnatural sexual offences.

The term "sexual intercourse" means and includes slightest penetration of vulva by penis. It is immaterial whether ejaculation takes place or not. Hence, it is quite possible that the intercourse has taken place but one finds no evidence of the same. In such situation, the accused can be convicted of indecent assault under Section 354 of Indian Penal Code. Here it is important to collect all possible corroborative evidences. Normally a female of any age would resist the unwanted intercourse.

Hence, the evidence of resistance shown by raped victim must be recorded. However, an adolescent girl, child, or an adult woman may not be able to offer resistance due to terror, feeling of helplessness or fear of risk to her life or life of others.

Age of the accused in case of rape: In India, there is no age limit under which a boy is considered as physically incapable of committing rape. The impotency is decided or excluded from the evidence in the case. The power of erection and therefore of coitus, may be present at a much earlier age than puberty. Live spermatozoa have been found in the seminal fluid of boys of 9 years of age.

The doctor in a government hospital or in private practice may come across victims of rape in various clinical situations. The doctor must know the law and its inference to give correct information to the legal authorities. The victims of rape may present to a doctor in different settings. He may be the police who brings the victim of alleged rape or she may be young unmarried girl brought for MTP. The statement of the parties may be absolutely misleading. The doctor must, therefore, stick to a systematic examination plan and report the clinical evidence to the authorities concerned.

Does Rape Victim Get Justice?

One woman is molested every 26 minutes as per the officially reported cases in 1991. If the unreported cases are taken into account, it would be matter of seconds rather than minutes. Also, the conviction rate is only 4%. It means many of the offenders get acquitted due to many factors mainly due to lack of or lacuna in evidence. Even if the girl gets justice it is too late in her life. The blame lies with shoddy investigation procedure and collection of evidence. The role of those officers who examine the rape victim, collect evidence, and send for testing to forensic laboratories is very important.

Landmark Judgments on Rape in India

In Vishakha versus State of Rajasthan and others, AIR1997 SC Justice JS Verma, Justice Sujata Manohar, and Justice BN Kirpal for the first time defined sexual harassment explicitly. It is now legally defined as an unwelcome sexual gesture or behavior whether directly or indirectly as:

- Sexually colored remarks
- Physical contact and advances
- Showing pornography
- A demand on request for sexual favors
- Any other unwelcome physical, verbal/nonverbal conduct being sexual in nature

CRIMINAL LAW AMENDMENT ACT 1983

Substantial changes in Section 375 and Section 376 of the IPC in Criminal Law Amendment Act 1983. Sections 376(A), 376(B), 376(C), and 376(D) are the newly added Sections in IPC. These new sections have been introduced with the purpose to prohibit sexual abuse of woman of any age, who is in custody, care, and control by various authorities.

CRIMINAL LAW AMENDMENT ACT 2018

By the Criminal Law Amendment Act 2018, there is change in Section 42 of the POCSO Act 2012. The Section deals with alternative punishment and Sections 376A, 376C, 376D were substituted with 376 A, 376AB, 376B, 376C, 376D, 376DA, and 376DB of Indian Penal Code.

IS LAW ENOUGH TO GET JUSTICE?

- The poor quality of investigations causes delay and denial in delivering justice. Corruption, insufficiency of the police department, and gender-biased decisions are the main reasons. The police authority has even refused to lodge FIR or lodged an incomplete FIR.
- Medical examination of the accused person and victim soon after the incidence gives good amount of corroborative evidence. The police and health department should be sensitive to use this period to deliver fair justice.
- Interpretation of the law or assessment of evidence does matter. The lower court judges often insist on evidence of physical resistance in the form of mark of injuries on the body of victim to assume that the woman has not consented, in spite of Supreme Court's decisions to the contrary. Without corroboration, woman's evidence is not considered sufficient.
- Some major impediments till the final decision are reached include the long time taken to complete rape trial, the giving of evidence of the victim before court in the presence of accused and harsh cross-examination.

GUIDELINES BY SUPREME COURT

Supreme court has given following guidelines for rape victims taking into account all above factors:

- The complaints of sexual assault cases should be provided with legal aid services which will help the victim in preparing for the case and also guide to get help from psychiatric consultation.
- Legal aid at the police station would offer guidance and support to the alleged victim.
- A list of willing lawyers should be kept and provided to the victim at police station. The police should be under a duty to inform the victim of her right to a counsel before appearing in the court.
- The advocate shall be authorized to act at the police station even before leave of court is sought or obtained.
- In all rape trials, anonymity of the victim must be maintained.
- There is need to set up Criminal Injuries Compensation Board as regard to the Directive Principles contained under Article 38(1) of the Constitution of India.

Compensation for the victims shall be awarded by the court on the conviction of offender and by the Criminal Injuries Compensation Board—whether or not a conviction has taken place. The Board will take into account pain, suffering, shock as well as loss of earnings due to pregnancy and consequent childbirth if it is the outcome of the rape. The National Commission for Women had given suggestion to frame schemes for compensation and rehabilitation to ensure justice to the rape victims.

Justice Saghir Ahmad has quoted his observation as regards to women in India as follows: *"Unfortunately, a woman in our country belongs to a class or group of society who are in a disadvantaged position on account of several social barriers and impediments and have therefore, been victims of tyranny at the hands of men with whom they, unfortunately under the constitution enjoy equal status."*

Incest

Sexual intercourse by a man within certain degree of blood relationship, i.e., between father and daughter, brother and sister, nephew and niece, and cousins, etc., is termed as incest. It is actually the betrayal of trust. It is also defined as "The imposition of sexually inappropriate acts or acts with sexual overtones by one or more persons who derive authority through ongoing emotional bonding with that child." This definition widens the traditional definition of incest to include sexual abuse by anyone who has authority or power over the child, which means immediate/extended family members, babysitters, school teachers, scout masters, or priests/ministers and others.

Incest per se is not a cognizable offence in India. It is accepted practice in some parts of the country where incestuous relations are not only allowed but are also promoted by compulsory marriages among relatives. However, any sexual relationship <18 years of age with or without consent amounts to rape even if the offender is blood relative (POCSO Act 2012). Incestuous rape is the most common form of child sexual abuse. Intra-familial sexual abuse is difficult to document and manage as in most of the cases there is coercion not to reveal or to deny the abuse while attempts are made to preserve the family unit.

Unfortunately, the evidence is lacking or scarce and sometimes extremely difficult to obtain in such situations. The police should investigate offenders and criminal prosecution should be supported. There is evidence, especially in pedophilia that incarceration may ensure access to and efficacy of simultaneous treatment of offender and victim. All juvenile and prejuvenile offenders should receive therapy to prevent recurrences.

Molestation, Indecency, and Eve-teasing

Molestation, indecency, and eve-teasing are very common incidents in society. Adolescent girls have to face these misbehaviors in their routine social life. Due to social stigma in our society, most of the cases remain unreported to the police. According to Section 294 of the Indian Penal Code 1860, whoever, to the annoyance of others does (a) any obscene act in any public place, (b) sings, recites or utters any obscene song, ballad, or words, in or near any public place shall be punished. Cases showing features of superficial injury for which a careful medicolegal examination can prove useful may be brought to medical officers for opinion. The adolescents cannot cope up with the situation due to tender age. The crime may create psychological problems in the adolescents for which they may require medical interventions.

Child Trafficking and Prostitution

Child prostitution and trafficking is the commercial sexual abuse of children. It is the sign of ultimate denial of human rights to adolescent. In spite of the number of legal provisions in India, e.g., Section 366-A IPC-Abduction, kidnapping, or seducing of minor girl, Section 372, and Section 373 IPC-selling and buying minor girls for prostitution and immoral traffic they are still beyond control. In 1998, the Government of India (GOI) formulated the National Plan of Action to combat trafficking and sexual exploitation of women and children which prescribes an exhaustive set of guidelines to the central and state governments. Other than the fact of being trafficked, the traffickers deprive the victims of their most basic human rights. Trafficking occurs not only for prostitution/commercial sexual exploitation, women, and children are trafficked for several purposes such as forced labor including bonded child labor, forced or bonded domestic work inhuman and violent conditions that include sexual abuse, forced labor in construction sites, forced employment in the entertainment industry including bars, massage parlors and similar establishments, begging, organ trade such as sale of kidneys, fraudulent or forced marriage, camel jockeying, purchase and sale of babies for adoption against the established laws and procedures for adoption.

The prohibition of "trafficking" flows out of the Constitution of India (Article 23) and not merely through legislation. Article 34 of the Convention on the Rights of the Child requires State parties to undertake the responsibility to protect the child from all forms of sexual exploitation and sexual abuse. Article 35 of the same convention requires state parties to take appropriate national bilateral and multilateral measures to prevent the abduction of the sale of or traffic in children for any purpose or in any form. Article 1(3), Article 1(4) of SAARC convention on preventing and combating trafficking of women and children for prostitution has also defined trafficking and traffickers respectively in broader sense. To substantiate the charge of child trafficking and prostitution, an adolescent may be required to be medically examined. In case of trafficking and child sexual abuse, the medical examination and its reports should be maintained in a confidential manner and must not be revealed to any unauthorized persons so as to prevent further exploitation/exposure of the victim. The medical officer, while recording the history of the case, should record only the relevant information pertinent to the case. Victims of trafficking and child sexual abuse have considerable difficulty in developing trust with any person and therefore it is necessary to conduct complete examination. It is necessary to build "trust and confidence" with the victim. Premature opinion is never to be ventured, but if feasible opinion should be given at the very earliest (within 48–72 hours of conducting the examination), since it is said that "justice delayed is justice denied." In cases where investigations and test results are awaited, the same should be mentioned in the report.

The Safe Kit

The prominent NGO "CEHAT" (Center of Enquiry into Health and Allied Themes) has come out with a unique kit called "SAFE Kit" (Sexual Assault Forensic Evidence Kit). The kit comprises manual, forms and all accessories required for the collection and preservation of forensic evidence. Use of such protocols will go long way in delivering justice to victims of both sexual assault and false allegations.

The examination of the survivors of alleged sexual offence is a very difficult task. There is a danger that the criminal may get acquitted as well as a possibility of wrong conviction. The offence itself has medical, psychological, social, and emotional attributes. It is the need of the hour that the society recognizes it as issue of human rights and health.

CONCLUSION

"We see what we look for; we look for what we know."

There is severe paucity of knowledge of law related to the medicolegal issues in adolescents. The physician must have thorough knowledge of the law and medicine both when presented with a case in adolescent. There is a great need to standardize the examination protocol, so that no piece of evidence is left out. The society also bears a moral responsibility and is duty-bound to help the adolescents, for which each one should work hard, hand in hand and shed our "SWEAT" for them, where:

S: Screening and sympathetic attitude
W: Watchful observation
E: Education
A: Awareness of the problems
T: Treatment—physical, psychological, and social

"When men are pure, laws are useless,
When men are corrupt, laws are broken."

—Benjamin Disraeli, 19th Century

It is true that law is not the only solution to each and every problem in the society. Even then knowledge about important medicolegal issues in all age groups, especially in adolescent age group is all time need. Of course law alone cannot change society, but legal protection can give confidence to fight the injustice. There should be well publicized links between adolescent friendly specialists, having knowledge about law. In this way, the adolescents would be served in a better way and not only our country but the whole world would become fit for healthy and prosperous adolescent living. Especially, free the young woman from the clutches of generation old inferiority complex and let her realize her self-worth.

KEY LEARNING POINTS

- Oxford's dictionary defines adolescence as the period from the beginning of sexual maturity to the completion of physical growth.
- Protection of Children from Sexual Offences (POCSO) Act 2012 criminalizes all sexual activities under the age of 18 years even if it was committed by consent.
- Teenage pregnancies and incidence of STDs are increasing due to early sexual activity and lack of knowledge about contraception.
- In India live-in relationship is valid while the central government has opposed legal validation of same sex marriage.
- Labor at tender age can have serious effects on child's physical and mental health affecting overall development.
- Child drug and sexual abuse are global public health problems, important reasons to cause serious infringement of a child's rights to health and protection.
- Any medical condition (including pregnancy) traceable to sexual act done at the age <18 years of female is to be reported to police else liable for punishment.
- Medicolegal examination of sexually abused child is of utmost importance from crime investigation point of view (Safe Kit).
- Pregnancy test should always be performed in sexually abused girls of reproductive age.
- The disproportionately high rates of sexually transmitted infections among adolescent girls facilitate HIV transmission.
- Drug-facilitated sexual assault is a growing menace especially in metropolitan cities.
- Commonly adolescent girls have to face incest, molestation, indecency, eve-teasing, child trafficking, and prostitution leading to psychological disturbances which often need medical interventions.

BIBLIOGRAPHY

1. Baveja R. Ethical considerations of adolescent health care needs. In: Mukherjee CG, Soonawala RP, Tank DK (Eds). Medicolegal Aspects in Obstetrics and Gynecology: A FOGSI Publication. New Delhi: Jaypee Brothers Medical Publishers (P) Ltd.; 1997. pp. 114-19.
2. Datar D. Forensic examination of rape victim. The Youth and Us: FOGSI Year of the Youth 2006: Mumbai: Sandoz Pvt. Ltd.; 2006. pp. 50-3.
3. Datar ND. Sexual abuse in adolescent. In: Bhave SY, Gandhi BA (Eds). Handbook of Adolescent Gynecology and ARSH, 1st edition. New Delhi: Jaypee Brothers Medical Publishers (P) Ltd.; 2007. pp. 176-8.
4. K Suresh. Towards a better tomorrow. In: Bhave SY, Gupta PK, Nair MKC (Eds). Course Manual for Adolescent Health. Part II: under auspices of IAP Adolescent Chapter: CII/44. New Delhi: IAP-ITPAH; 2002.
5. Mukherjee D. Adolescent scenario in India. In: Bhave SY, Gupta PK, Nair MKC (Eds). Course Manual for Adolescent Health: Part II under auspices of IAP Adolescent. Chapter: CII/44. New Delhi: IAP-ITPAH; 2002. pp. 1-5.
6. Nair MKC. Overview of adolescent problems. In: Bhave SY, Gupta PK, Nair MKC (Eds). Course Manual for Adolescent Health, Part II: under auspices of IAP Adolescent Chapter: CII/44. New Delhi: IAP-ITPAH; 2002. p. 6.
7. Sobti P, Biswas G, Sobti BS. Medicolegal issues in adolescent care. In: Bhave SY, Gupta PK, Nair MKC (Eds). Course Manual for Adolescent Health: Part II: under auspices of IAP Adolescent Chapter and IAP Task. Force On Adolescent Health: CII/44. New Delhi: IAP-ITPAH; 2002. pp. 319-31.
8. The Times of India. (2023). Age of consent under POCSO perhaps highest globally high time India takes note of-global-scenario: Bombay HC. [online] Available from https://timesofindia.indiatimes.com/india/age-of-consent-under-pocso-perhaps-highest-globally-high-time-india-takes-note-of-global-scenario-bombay-hc/articleshow/101729154.cms. [Last accessed on 1st September 2023].
9. UNICEF. Dealing with Child Victims of Trafficking and Commercial Sex Exploitation: Manual for Medical Officers. DWCD and UNICEF: 2005; pp. 1, 3, 8, 14-18, 21, 24, 25, 50.
10. Walke D. Adolescents and law. In: Bhalerao-Gandhi A, Biniwale P (Eds). Gynecological Manual on Adolescent Girls and Young Women: A FOGSI Publication, 1st edition. Jaypee Brothers Medical Publishers (P) Ltd.; 2009. 323-9.

20.5 Issues Related to the Medical Termination of Pregnancy Act

Jyoti Bindal

INTRODUCTION

The Medical Termination of Pregnancy Act, often abbreviated as the MTP Act, stands as a pivotal legal framework in the realm of healthcare and medicolegal matters. Enacted to address the complexities surrounding pregnancy termination, this legislation plays a crucial role in regulating and safeguarding the reproductive rights of individuals.

The MTP Act, which came into existence in 1971, was born out of a pressing need to provide a legal and medical framework for safe and lawful pregnancy termination. It was recognized that there are situations where pregnancy termination is not only a medical necessity but also a fundamental right, granting individuals the autonomy to make informed decisions about their reproductive health.

Documented evidence suggests a number of negative complications associated with unintended pregnancies. Unintended pregnancies have adverse effects on women's quality of life and also threaten household's economic status.

Issues delve into the various aspects of the MTP Act, ranging from its historical development to the intricate legal provisions it encompasses. It also explores the ethical considerations, challenges, and future possibilities associated with this legislation. The MTP Act plays a vital role in balancing medical ethics, legal responsibilities, and individual rights within the medicolegal landscape.

HISTORICAL CONTEXT

To appreciate the significance of this legislation, it is essential to delve into the historical context that propelled its development. Understanding this historical context helps to appreciate the transformative impact of the MTP Act on women's healthcare and the legal framework surrounding pregnancy termination in India. It represents a milestone in the journey toward ensuring reproductive health and justice for all.

- *Preindependence era*: Before India gained independence in 1947, laws pertaining to abortion were largely inherited from British colonial rule. These laws were restrictive and criminalized abortion, often accepting it only to save the life of the pregnant woman. This approach posed severe limitations on access to safe and legal abortion services.
- *Postindependence challenges*: The postindependence era brought with it a need for comprehensive healthcare reform. High maternal mortality rates and unsafe abortion practices were significant public health concerns. The restrictive legal framework led to a proliferation of unsafe and clandestine abortion procedures, endangering the lives of countless women.
- *Social and cultural changes*: As Indian society underwent transformations in terms of education, urbanization, and women's rights, there was an increasing recognition of the need

to reform abortion laws. The evolving mindset emphasized the importance of reproductive rights and women's autonomy over their bodies.

- *Landmark legal cases*: Notable legal cases emerged that challenged the existing legal framework. These cases, often involving women seeking abortions due to health risks, rape, or fetal anomalies, highlighted the need for a more compassionate and medically informed approach.
- *Medical advancements*: Advances in medical technology and techniques for safe abortion procedures added weight to the argument for reforming abortion laws. The medical community recognized the importance of providing safe and legal options for pregnancy termination.

MTP Act was initially amended because abortions had become far safer due to better, advanced medical and surgical techniques in this field. Subsequent to this, it was conceptualized to bring in the MTP Act of 1971.

This law guarantees the right of women in India to terminate an unintended pregnancy by a registered medical practitioner in a hospital established or maintained by the Government or a place approved for the purpose of this Act by the Government.

Despite gains in women's health realized by the MTP Act, the number of illegal and unsafe abortions in India continues to be very high with a large number of abortions being performed every year by untrained persons in totally unhygienic conditions. Complications of unsafe abortions remain a major factor in contributing to high rates of maternal mortality throughout the country.

This was a ground-breaking act as it would give freedom to women from the exploitation of women and society. Another main object of the Act beside elimination of illegal abortions is that women should get the right to privacy. The eight sections of this Act contain various important points and rules like when pregnancy can be terminated by medical practitioners, place where it can be terminated, and no legal proceedings will lie against any registered medical practitioner who has acted in good faith or does not have any intention of doing the act in any wrong sense.

The MTP Act of 1971 was amended by the MTP (Amendment) Act, 2002. The main objective of this amendment to the MTP Act aimed at reducing the rate of unsafe abortions by making legal abortion more widely accessible. Lack of access to MTP services at the primary healthcare level was an important reason for the high rate of unsafe and illegal abortions. The amendment aimed at decentralization of authority for approval and registration of MTP centers from the state to the district level. The existing system for approving such centers was extremely cumbersome and slow. At the same time, however, efforts at decentralization needed to be closely monitored to ensure that a speedier approval process would not compromise quality of care, and that adequate resources for both training and technology were made available. This amendment also provided an increase in punishment in violations of the Act.

Further, amendment was planned due to advances in safer methods of termination of pregnancy. The new MTP Amendment Bill 2020 and MTP (Amendment) Act 2021 expand the access to safe and legal abortion services on therapeutic, eugenic, humanitarian, and social grounds to ensure universal access to comprehensive care. The new law, will contribute toward ending preventable maternal mortality to help meet the Sustainable Development Goals (SDGs).

The changes consider the advances in medical technology, simplify requirements of providers, increase upper gestation limit for termination of pregnancy under specific conditions, and remove the gestation limit for cases that could burden the health system. The goal is to strengthen access to CAC without compromising dignity, autonomy, confidentiality, and justice for women who need safe and quality services.

Coming 50 years after the passage of the historic MTP Act of 1971, the MTP Amendment Bill 2020 is an evolutionary landmark addressing some of the challenges posed by the 15.6 million abortions we manage each year in India. As the next step, we need to work toward advocating a more rights-based approach by giving women greater autonomy and choice, operationalizing grassroots access with an expansion of provider base.

LEGAL FRAMEWORK OF THE MTP ACT

The MTP Act is a comprehensive piece of legislation that governs the termination of pregnancies in India. It sets forth a legal framework designed to ensure safe, regulated, and medically supervised procedures. Within this legal framework, several critical components shape the landscape of pregnancy termination:

- *Objectives and scope*: Objectives of the MTP Act primarily include safeguarding the health and rights of pregnant individuals while establishing lawful criteria for pregnancy termination. Scope of the Act includes the gestational limits within which termination is permitted and the conditions under which it can be carried out.
- *Categories of healthcare providers*: The Act designates two categories of healthcare providers: Registered medical practitioners (RMPs) and approved places. RMPs are qualified doctors who can perform abortions, while approved places are medical facilities where these procedures are conducted.
- *Conditions for termination*: The Act delves into the specific conditions under which pregnancy termination is legally allowed. These may include situations where the pregnancy poses a risk to the physical or mental health of the pregnant woman, cases of fetal abnormalities, or pregnancies resulting from rape or contraceptive failure.
- *Gestational limits*: The Act describes the gestational limits imposed by the Act for different conditions. For example, the Act may allow termination up to 20 weeks in cases of fetal abnormalities but restrict it to 24 weeks when the pregnancy poses a risk to the woman's life.
- *Informed consent*: The Act discusses the requirement for obtaining informed consent from the pregnant woman before proceeding with the termination.
- *Role of RMPs*: The Act outlines the responsibilities and legal obligations of RMPs, including their role in assessing the eligibility of patients for abortion, conducting the procedure, and maintaining patient confidentiality.
- *Approved places and facilities*: Medical facilities must meet to be recognized as approved places for pregnancy termination. The Act describes the role of these facilities in providing safe and regulated abortion services.
- *Reporting and documentation*: The Act highlights the requirements for maintaining accurate records, reporting cases of pregnancy termination, and the importance of confidentiality in handling patient information.
- *Legal penalties and offenses*: The Act discusses the legal consequences for violations of the MTP Act, including penalties for unauthorized providers and the consequences of conducting illegal abortions.
- Amendments and updates:
    - *Key amendments in MTP (Amendment) Act 2021*:
        - Increasing the upper gestation limit from 20 to 24 weeks for special categories of women, including survivors of rape, victims of incest, and other vulnerable women (differently abled women and minors among others).

- The opinion of one provider needed for the termination of pregnancy up to 20 weeks of gestation. Requirement of the opinion of two providers for the termination of pregnancy from 20 to 24 weeks of gestation.
- Upper gestation limit to not apply in cases of substantial fetal abnormalities diagnosed by a Medical Board.
- Confidentiality clause—the name and other particulars of a woman whose pregnancy has been terminated cannot be revealed except to a person authorized by law.
- Extended MTP services under the failure of contraceptive clause to unmarried women to provide access to safe abortion based on a woman's choice, irrespective of marital status.

CONDITIONS FOR TERMINATION UNDER THE MTP ACT

The MTP Act lays down clear and specific conditions under which the termination of pregnancy is legally permissible in India. The Act permits pregnancy termination under the following key conditions:

- The MTP Act allows for pregnancy termination if continuing the pregnancy poses a risk to the life of the pregnant woman.
- In cases where the continuation of the pregnancy would have a detrimental impact on the physical or mental health of the pregnant woman. Health risks can encompass a wide range of medical and psychological conditions.
- When medical assessments confirm significant fetal abnormalities or congenital defects. This provision acknowledges the emotional and medical complexities of such situations.
- If the pregnancy is a result of rape or sexual assault. This provision recognizes the trauma and distress associated with such circumstances.
- *Contraceptive failure*: In cases of contraceptive failure or contraceptive device malfunction leading to an unintended pregnancy.
- The Act grants flexibility by allowing healthcare providers to determine whether other medical or situational factors warrant pregnancy termination. This provision permits medical practitioners to use their judgment in exceptional cases.
    - It is important to note that the gestational age of the pregnancy can impact the availability of these conditions. The MTP Act often specifies different gestational limits for each condition. For example, the Act may permit termination up to 20 weeks in cases of fetal abnormalities but restrict it to 24 weeks when the pregnancy poses a risk to the woman's life.
    - Additionally, the Act emphasizes the importance of obtaining informed consent from the pregnant woman before proceeding with the termination, regardless of the specific condition. This ensures that individuals have a say in their reproductive choices and are fully aware of the procedure's implications.

These are the conditions which give a comprehensive understanding of the circumstances in which pregnancy termination is legally allowed under the MTP Act.

ROLE OF HEALTHCARE PROVIDERS UNDER THE MTP ACT

The MTP Act places healthcare providers, especially RMPs, at the forefront of ensuring that pregnancy termination is conducted safely, legally, and ethically. Their roles encompass a range of responsibilities and obligations, which are essential for the effective implementation of the Act:

- *Eligibility assessment*: Registered medical practitioners play a pivotal role in evaluating the eligibility of pregnant individuals for termination. They must carefully assess whether the conditions specified in the MTP Act are met.
- *Informed consent*: One of the primary responsibilities of healthcare providers is to obtain informed consent from the pregnant woman. This involves explaining the procedure, potential risks, alternatives, and ensuring that the individual fully understands and consents to the termination.
- *Medical examination and counseling*: Conducting a thorough medical examination is crucial to determine the gestational age of the pregnancy and any medical conditions that may impact the procedure. Healthcare providers should also offer counseling services to address the emotional and psychological aspects of pregnancy termination.
- *Maintaining confidentiality*: Healthcare providers must ensure that all patient information is kept confidential and not disclosed without the patient's consent, except as required by law.
- *Safe and regulated procedures*: Registered medical practitioners are responsible for performing pregnancy terminations in approved places, following medical protocols, and ensuring that the procedures are conducted safely and with appropriate medical care.
- *Documentation and reporting*: Healthcare providers must maintain detailed records of each pregnancy termination, including the medical indications, consent forms, and follow-up care. They should also report cases as mandated by the Act.
- *Ethical considerations*: Healthcare providers should approach each case with compassion and respect for the autonomy and dignity of the pregnant individual.
- *Continuing medical education*: Staying updated with the latest medical advancements and legal changes is crucial. Healthcare providers should ensure their practices align with current standards and guidelines.
- *Conscientious objection*: While the MTP Act grants the right to refuse to perform abortions on grounds of conscience, healthcare providers who choose not to provide these services should refer patients to willing providers and ensure that patients' access to care is not hindered.

By elucidating the multifaceted role of healthcare providers under the MTP Act, the responsibilities and ethical considerations that guide medical professionals in facilitating safe and lawful pregnancy terminations are specified in the Act. This understanding is fundamental to ensuring the act's effective implementation and the protection of patients' rights and well-being.

PATIENT RIGHTS AND CONSENT UNDER THE MTP ACT

Patient rights and informed consent are foundational principles in the framework of the MTP Act.

- *Right to reproductive autonomy*: It is the fundamental right of individuals to make decisions about their own bodies, including the choice to terminate a pregnancy.
- *Right to nondiscrimination*: Basic principle that all individuals seeking pregnancy termination should be treated without discrimination or bias based on factors such as age, marital status, socioeconomic status, or gender.
- *Right to information*: Patients have the right to receive clear and comprehensive information about the pregnancy termination procedure, potential risks, alternatives, and any other relevant details.

- *Informed consent*: It is critically important to obtain informed consent from the pregnant individual.

  Informed consent should be obtained after providing the necessary information and the patient should have the opportunity to ask questions and seek clarification.
- *Consent forms*: Consent forms should be used to document the patient's informed consent.
- *Confidentiality*: It is obligatory for the healthcare providers to maintain patient confidentiality.
- *Right to refuse treatment*: Patient has a right to refuse pregnancy termination even after initial consent. Consent is an ongoing process and individuals can change their decision at any stage.
- *Language and cultural sensitivity*: It is vitally important that the healthcare providers are sensitive to patients' cultural, linguistic, and religious beliefs when obtaining consent.
- *Vulnerable populations*: There are unique considerations for vulnerable populations, such as minors, those with disabilities, or individuals experiencing domestic violence.
- *Reporting violations*: Patients have the right to report any violations of their rights or unethical practices to relevant authorities or medical boards.

Elucidating patient rights and the informed consent process within the context of the MTP Act covers the ethical and legal principles that underpin the act's implementation. This knowledge is crucial for ensuring that individuals seeking pregnancy termination are empowered to make informed decisions while safeguarding their rights and well-being.

MEDICAL ETHICS IN PREGNANCY TERMINATION

Medical ethics plays a pivotal role in guiding healthcare providers when they are involved in pregnancy termination.

- *Autonomy and informed choice*: The MTP Act encompasses ethical principle of respecting the autonomy of pregnant individuals. Individuals have the right to make decisions about their reproductive health based on informed choice.
- *Beneficence and nonmaleficence*: Principles of beneficence (doing good) and nonmaleficence (doing no harm) guide healthcare providers. Pregnancy termination should be carried out with the intent of benefiting the patient's health while minimizing harm.
- *Medical indications versus personal beliefs*: Ethical dilemma arises when healthcare providers have personal beliefs or conscientious objections related to pregnancy termination. Importance of balancing these beliefs with their professional obligation to provide appropriate care or referrals to willing providers is the key feature in this.
- *Compassion and empathy*: Importance of providing compassionate and empathetic care to individuals seeking pregnancy termination cannot be overemphasized. The emotional and psychological aspects of the process and the need for healthcare providers to offer support are vital.
- *Patient-centered care*: Needs, values, and preferences of patient are central to decision-making. Healthcare providers should engage in shared decision-making processes with patients.
- *Cultural sensitivity*: It is the duty of the healthcare provider to be culturally sensitive and respectful of patients' beliefs and values.
- *Continuous education and professionalism*: Healthcare providers should engage in continuous medical education and maintain professionalism.
- *Ethical dilemmas and consultation*: Healthcare providers may encounter complex ethical dilemmas in pregnancy termination cases.

CHALLENGES AND CONTROVERSIES

The implementation of the MTP Act has not been without its share of challenges and controversies. These complexities often reflect the intersection of legal, medical, ethical, and societal factors:

- *Access to safe abortion services*: There is a definite challenge of ensuring equitable access to safe abortion services, particularly in rural or underserved areas.
- *Stigma and social attitudes*: Despite the open attitude of educated couples, there still remains the enduring societal stigma associated with abortion and the impact it has on individuals. These attitudes can deter individuals from seeking safe and legal procedures.
- *Age of consent*: There exists a debate surrounding the age of consent for pregnancy termination, especially in cases involving minors. Ethical and legal questions arise when minors seek abortions without parental consent.
- *Conscientious objection*: Controversy surrounding the conscientious objection of healthcare providers poses a challenge. While the Act allows providers to refuse to perform abortions on moral or religious grounds, it can pose challenges in terms of ensuring access for patients.
- *Late-term abortions*: A shadow surrounding late-term abortions, particularly those performed after the 24-week gestational limit lingers. Ethical dilemmas arise in cases where fetal abnormalities are detected later in pregnancy or when the health or life of the pregnant individual is at risk.
- *Sex-selective abortions*: There are serious legal concerns about sex-selective abortions. The Pre-Conception and Pre-Natal Diagnostic Techniques (PCPNDT) Act deals with legal provisions in place to prevent such practices.
- *Mental health considerations*: The inclusion of mental health considerations as a valid reason for pregnancy termination is under consideration, as it is argued that this may be open to misuse or subjective interpretation.
- *Public awareness and education*: There is ongoing need for public awareness and education programs. The lack of awareness can result in delayed or unsafe procedures.
- *Legal challenges and amendments*: There have been many legal challenges or amendments to the MTP Act that have sparked controversies or debates. These may include attempts to alter gestational limits or restrictions on certain conditions.
- *Ethical dilemmas for healthcare providers*: The ethical dilemmas faced by healthcare providers have to be addressed when balancing their personal beliefs, professional responsibilities, and the rights of patients. These dilemmas can be complex and emotionally charged.

Issues Regarding the Main Substance of MTP Act

- *Opinion regarding rights to termination*: There have been different opinions in different countries as to who should have the right to take decision about termination of pregnancy. Although some countries have given this as a right under woman's reproductive rights, other countries have reserved the rights with the state as a part to protect the life of fetus.
- *Opinion regarding time limit to termination*: Different time limits have been set regarding legality of abortion as per gestational age. In the newly amended Act in India, this time limit is 24 weeks of gestation. This period can only be extended if medical board certifies the fetus to have substantial abnormalities.

  In case of rape, if the period of gestation is more than 24 weeks, then permission has to be given only through court.

- *Opinion regarding qualification of person eligible for performing termination*: As per the amended Act, termination can only be performed by the qualified doctor—one—or two, as per the period of gestation. Due to nonavailability of qualified doctors in rural areas, in India, it leads to failure of pregnant woman to access safe abortion facilities.

By addressing these challenges and controversies, a comprehensive understanding of the complex landscape surrounding pregnancy termination under the MTP Act can be revalued.

By addressing these ethical considerations, a deeper understanding of the moral principles that guide healthcare providers in delivering pregnancy termination services under the MTP Act can be reached. This knowledge is instrumental in upholding ethical standards, ensuring patient-centered care and navigating the complexities of reproductive healthcare.

LEGAL CASES AND PRECEDENTS

XXX vs. Union of India, State of Kerala (2021)

The Superintendent, Medical College Hospital Manjeri and The Superintendent, Medical College, Kozhikode, WP(C). No. 9982 OF 2021(W) held that the pregnancy in the case of a minor girl who was raped can be terminated even after the limit of medical pregnancy as per MTP Act, 2021 has been crossed.

Facts: A minor girl aged 13 years along with her parents approached a hospital complaining of stomach pain. The doctors conducted physical examination and found that the girl was pregnant by almost 6 months. The scan report showed that the fetus was almost 24 weeks and 4 days old.

A crime was registered and during investigation, it was suspected that the minor girl was a victim of rape by her own sibling aged 14 years old. Accordingly, a report was filed before the Juvenile Justice Board.

Contention: The minor girl's father (Petitioner) contended that his daughter is a rape victim at the hands of her own brother. Accordingly, he sought direction to terminate the pregnancy. The Petitioner also contended that the victim was a premature child and due to the young age of the victim, the pregnancy may have consequences on the victim, parents, and even the unborn child.

Accordingly, the court directed the hospital (Respondent 4) at which the minor girl was admitted to constitute a medical board and report to the court as to whether medical termination of pregnancy can be performed on the victim. The observation of the Medical Board was as follows:

"As per the Medical Termination of Pregnancy Act 2021 (MTP Act), she is beyond the limit of legal medical termination (Gestational age by Ultrasound Scan is 26 weeks and 6 days). If medical termination is considered she stands certain medical risks... However, the board observed that medical termination of this pregnancy can be considered accepting the higher risks and facts mentioned above."

Law: Sections 3 and 4 of the MTP Act provide for medical termination.

1. *Section 3(2)* has been amended by the MTP (Amendment) Act 2021, which states that if the pregnancy:
   - Does not exceed 20 weeks, opinion of one medical practitioner is needed
   - Exceeds 20 weeks but does not exceed 24 weeks, opinions of at least two registered medical practitioners are needed
2. *Explanation 2* to Section 3(2) states *"Where any pregnancy is alleged by the pregnant woman to have been caused by rape, the anguish caused by such pregnancy shall be presumed to constitute a grave injury to the mental health of the pregnant woman."*

3. The Amendment Act also adds *Section 2B* which states that the provisions of Section 3(2) stated above shall not apply if such termination is necessitated by the diagnosis of any of the substantial fetal abnormalities diagnosed by a Medical Board.
4. *Section 3(3)* states that in determining whether the pregnancy poses risk of injury to the pregnant woman, account may be taken of the woman's actual and reasonable foreseeable environment.
5. *Section 4(a)* states that if the pregnant woman has not attained the age of 18 years, then written consent of the parent/guardian is required.

Analysis: The court observed in the instant case that the victim is a minor girl. The pregnancy will cause grave injury to the minor as it may possibly remind the victim of the incident of rape.

The court also stated *that "It is obviously not in the interest of the society to have this young victim to undergo the trauma of the incident of rape every day in her life."* This anguish will be shared by the parents and siblings of the victim.

The court observed that the minor victim in the instant case is also not prepared to deliver a child in the given situation. Further, the medical board suggested that medical termination can be considered if the higher risks are acceptable. Accordingly, the court took into consideration the opinion of the parents, who also wanted the pregnancy to be terminated, and it also took note of the possibility of genetic disorders in the unborn child due to the close relationship between the victim and the offender.

Decision: Therefore, taking all the above points into consideration, the court declared that the petitioner's minor daughter's pregnancy is liable to be terminated.

Voices vs. State of Kerala (2020)

This case involved a petition to the Kerala High Court challenging the mandatory two-doctor certification for pregnancy termination under the MTP Act. It questioned whether such a requirement was a violation of women's reproductive rights.

The court's decision affected the certification process and whether it eased access to safe abortion services.

A vs. Union of India (4 SCC 75) (2018)

The Hon'ble Supreme Court ordered termination of pregnancy in a case where the gestational age was 25–26 weeks.

Justice KS Puttaswamy (Retd.) vs. the Union of India and Others (2017)

Court recognized the constitutional right of women to make reproductive choices, as a part of personal liberty under Article 21 of the Indian Constitution, which despite laying a robust jurisprudence on reproductive rights and the privacy of a woman, does not translate into a fundamental shift in power from the doctor to the woman seeking an abortion.

Ms X vs. State of Kerala and Others (4) KLT 745 (2016)

Here the court ordered termination of pregnancy exceeding 20 weeks as the rape victims were not mentally prepared to deliver the child.

Ms X vs. Hospital Z (2015)

This case involved a minor girl, Ms. X, who was raped and became pregnant. Her parents sought court permission for her abortion. It highlighted the complexities of consent and confidentiality when minors are involved.

The court ruled in favor of the minor girl's right to terminate her pregnancy without parental consent, emphasizing her autonomy and the need for confidential proceedings.

Suchita Srivastava vs. Chandigarh Administration (2009)

In this case, a mentally challenged rape victim sought permission for pregnancy termination. It addressed the issue of whether mental health could be considered a valid reason for abortion under the MTP Act.

The Supreme Court of India ruled in favor of the woman, emphasizing the importance of mental health as a valid consideration for pregnancy termination and setting a precedent for a broader interpretation of the act.

Niketa Mehta vs. Union of India (2008)

This landmark case involved a pregnant woman, Niketa Mehta, who sought termination of her 25-week pregnancy due to fetal abnormalities. The case raised questions about the 20-week gestational limit under the MTP Act and the balancing of the right to life of the fetus versus the mother's right to make reproductive choices.

This case led to a review of the gestational limit in exceptional cases and how it influenced subsequent legal interpretations.

These legal cases and precedents provide concrete examples of how the MTP Act has been interpreted and applied in various situations. Implications of these cases for the act's implementation, reproductive rights, and healthcare practices in India can thus be analyzed.

AMENDMENTS AND UPDATES TO THE MTP ACT

The MTP Act has undergone several amendments and updates over the years to adapt to changing medical practices, societal needs, and evolving legal standards, which made an impact.

Amendments were made to the MTP Act in 2021, which extended the gestational limit for abortion from 20 to 24 weeks in cases where it is necessary to save the life of the pregnant woman or for substantial fetal abnormalities.

Key Amendments in MTP Act, 2021

- *Indication of contraceptive failure*: In MTP Act of 1971, this indication was limited only to the married woman, but now in the amended MTP Act of 2021, failure of contraceptive device or method is permissible as indication to unmarried woman also.
- *Opinion from number of doctors as per gestational age*: In the earlier MTP Act of 1971, opinion of one registered practitioner was needed till 12 weeks and opinion of two registered medical practitioners was required till 20 weeks. Now, in the amended MTP Act of 2021, termination of pregnancy till 20 weeks can be done with the opinion of only one registered medical practitioner. Opinion of two registered medical practitioners is needed for termination between 20 and 24 weeks.
- *Gestational age limit of fetus*: In the earlier MTP Act of 1971, gestational age limit was 20 weeks for all indications.

  Now in the amended MTP Act of 2021, termination of pregnancy till 24 weeks can be done for rape survivor, incest victim, differently abled woman, minor, etc. For substantial fetal abnormalities certified by the State Medical Board, pregnancy can be terminated beyond 24 weeks too.
- *Breach of the confidentiality of women*: In the earlier MTP Act of 1971, if confidentiality of the woman was disclosed in any way (name, personal details, identification, photograph, etc.), the fine was ₹1,000.

Now, in the amended MTP Act of 2021, if any person is responsible for breach of woman's confidentiality, he is liable to imposing fine and/or imprisonment of 1 year.

These amendments to the MTP Act were influenced by legal cases and challenges, medical advancements, changing demographics, and the evolving understanding of reproductive rights.

Legal cases

Precedent setting: Landmark legal cases can set legal precedents that challenge existing provisions of the MTP Act. For example, if a case highlights a situation where a woman's right to access safe abortion was denied due to restrictive laws, it can prompt a reevaluation of those laws.

Court decisions: Courts may interpret the MTP Act in ways that necessitate amendments. For instance, if a court rules that certain aspects of the Act are unconstitutional or in violation of human rights, lawmakers may be prompted to amend the Act to align with the court's decision.

Medical advancements

Advances in fetal diagnosis: As medical technology advances, the ability to diagnose fetal abnormalities or health risks to the mother can change. If there are developments that allow for more accurate and earlier detection of such conditions, lawmakers may consider amending the MTP Act to reflect these advancements.

Safer procedures: Improvements in medical procedures related to abortion, including medication abortion and minimally invasive surgical techniques, may prompt changes to the Act to provide safer and more accessible options for women.

Evolving understanding of reproductive rights

Changing societal norms: As societal attitudes and norms around reproductive rights evolve, there may be increased pressure on lawmakers to update the MTP Act to better align with contemporary views on women's autonomy and reproductive choices.

International human rights standards: Evolving international human rights standards and recommendations from global health organizations can influence the way a country's laws on reproductive health, including abortion, are viewed. Governments may amend their laws to align with these standards.

Overall, the process of amending the MTP Act involves a combination of legal, medical, and social factors. Legal cases often serve as catalysts for change, medical advancements provide new possibilities for healthcare, and evolving understandings of reproductive rights reflect shifting societal values. These factors together can lead to amendments aimed at ensuring that the MTP Act remains relevant, safe, and respectful of women's reproductive choices and health.

- *Expanding conditions for termination*: These amendments broadened the conditions under which pregnancy termination is permitted. This includes recognizing mental health considerations as well as expanding the range of fetal abnormalities covered.
- *Changes in certification requirements*: These amendments altered the certification requirements for pregnancy termination, which aimed to streamline the process, reduce barriers, and enhance patient privacy.
- *Telemedicine and remote consultation*: Recent amendments allowed for telemedicine and remote consultations for pregnancy termination services, thus affected access to care, especially during the coronavirus disease 2019 (COVID-19) pandemic.
- *Impact on healthcare providers*: Implications of amendments for healthcare providers were widespread, including changes in their roles, responsibilities, and obligations. New requirements have been introduced, such as mandatory training.

- *Public awareness and education*: Amendments included provisions for public awareness campaigns and education programs. These initiatives contribute to improving awareness of reproductive rights and the MTP Act.
- *Ethical and legal challenges*: Ethical or legal challenges and controversies that may have arisen as a result of the amendments continue to be debated.
- *Future directions*: It is not possible to speculate on potential future amendments or updates to the MTP Act, as changing societal norms, advances in medical technology, or legal developments may shape the trajectory of the act.

This comprehensive overview of amendments and updates to the MTP Act offers readers insight into the evolving landscape of reproductive healthcare in India and how legislative changes have influenced access to safe abortion services and the protection of patient rights.

INTERNATIONAL COMPARISONS

MTP Act versus Abortion Laws in Other Countries

The MTP Act in India is just one example of abortion laws and regulations worldwide. Comparing the Indian legislation with similar laws in other countries provides valuable insights into how different societies address pregnancy termination. Here are the key points to consider:

- *Legal framework and gestational limits*: India (MTP Act) allows abortion up to 24 weeks in certain circumstances, such as a threat to the life of the pregnant person or fetal abnormalities.

  Many European countries permit abortion on request during the first trimester and may have varying regulations for later stages of pregnancy.
- *Conditions for termination*: India (MTP Act) permits abortion based on specific conditions, including risks to the life or health of the pregnant person, fetal abnormalities, rape, or contraceptive failure.

  In the United States, abortion laws vary by state, with some states allowing abortion on request, while others have restrictions based on gestational age or reasons for termination.
- *Healthcare provider roles*: India (MTP Act) authorizes RMPs to perform abortions.

  In the United Kingdom, abortion services are primarily provided by the National Health Service (NHS) and independent clinics.
- *Informed consent and counseling*: India (MTP Act) requires informed consent and counseling for individuals seeking abortion.

  In the United States, informed consent requirements vary by state, and some states mandate counseling or waiting periods.
- *Accessibility and barriers*: India (MTP Act)—access to abortion services can be challenging in rural areas due to healthcare infrastructure disparities.

  In Canada, abortion services are widely accessible and covered by the public healthcare system.
- *Conscientious objection*: India (MTP Act) allows healthcare providers to object on conscientious grounds but requires them to refer patients to willing providers.

  In Italy, law allows conscientious objection by healthcare providers but mandates timely referrals to ensure patient access.
- *Legal penalties*: India (MTP Act) imposes penalties for unauthorized providers and illegal abortions.

In Argentina, the government legalized abortion in 2020 and decriminalized it, eliminating penalties for individuals seeking abortion.

- *Public opinion and stigma*: India (MTP Act):
  - Stigma surrounding abortion exists, particularly in certain regions, impacting individuals' willingness to seek services.
  - In Sweden: Abortion is widely accepted, and there is less societal stigma surrounding reproductive choices.
- *Recent reforms and trends*:
  - India (MTP Act): Recently extended the gestational limit for certain conditions.
  - Argentina: Legalized abortion in 2020, reflecting a global trend toward liberalizing abortion laws.
- *International human rights framework*: India is a signatory to various international human rights conventions, including those that address reproductive rights.

  International human rights organizations advocate for access to safe and legal abortion as a fundamental right.

This simplified comparison highlights that abortion laws and access to services can vary significantly worldwide. It is important to conduct more in-depth research for a comprehensive understanding of the specific laws in various countries.

By comparing the MTP Act in India with abortion laws in other countries, one gets a broader perspective on the diverse approaches to pregnancy termination and reproductive rights worldwide. This comparison can help understand how India's legal framework fits into the global context of abortion legislation.

PUBLIC AWARENESS AND EDUCATION ON THE MTP ACT

Public awareness and education are critical components of ensuring that individuals are informed about their rights and options under the MTP Act. This section focuses on the significance of awareness campaigns and educational initiatives:

- *Raising awareness*: It is vitally very important to raise public awareness about the MTP Act. Many individuals may not be aware of their rights or the legal provisions for pregnancy termination.
- *Destigmatization efforts:* There is a role of awareness campaigns in destigmatizing abortion. Any societal stigma can deter individuals from seeking safe and legal procedures. Campaigns help combat this stigma.
- *Access to information*: There is growing need for individuals to have access to accurate and comprehensive information about the MTP Act. This information should cover the conditions for termination, gestational limits, and the procedure itself.
- *Dissemination channels*: There are various channels through which awareness and educational information can be disseminated. These may include healthcare facilities, community centers, educational institutions, websites, social media, and pamphlets.
- *Role of healthcare providers*: Healthcare providers can play a crucial role in educating patients about their rights and options. It is the ethical responsibility of providers to provide information in a nonbiased and patient-centered manner.
- *Counseling services*: There needs to be a free and wide availability of counseling services for individuals considering pregnancy termination. These services can provide emotional support and help individuals make informed decisions.

- *Collaboration with nongovernmental organizations (NGOs) and advocacy groups*: Collaborative efforts between government agencies, healthcare providers, and NGOs or advocacy groups in conducting awareness campaigns and educational programs need to be built up.
- *International best practices*: Examples of successful awareness and education programs from other countries should be taken, which can serve as best practices for India.
- *Ongoing efforts*: Public awareness and education should be ongoing efforts to ensure that new generations and communities continue to be informed about their reproductive rights.

By highlighting the significance of public awareness and education, the role these initiatives play in promoting informed choices, reducing stigma, and ensuring that individuals can access safe and legal abortion services as per their rights under the MTP Act becomes available to public at large.

FUTURE DIRECTIONS FOR THE MTP ACT AND REPRODUCTIVE HEALTHCARE

While the MTP Act has come a long way in uplifting the cause of reproductive rights of women in India, there are still lacunae to be filled and need for refinement.

The recent amendment of October 2021 directs a medical board to be established by each state government for special permission for medical termination of pregnancy. However, there are yet no guidelines on how many such medical boards are to be established in each state.

- *Expanded access to services*: There is a huge potential for further expanding access to safe abortion services, particularly in underserved rural areas. Initiatives such as mobile clinics or telemedicine to bridge geographical gaps need to be considered.
- *Continued legal reforms*: There is a possibility of future legal reforms to the MTP Act. Discuss whether there is a need to revisit gestational limits, expand the list of permissible conditions or enhance legal protections for healthcare providers.
- *Comprehensive sex education*: The importance of comprehensive sex education in schools to empower young individuals with knowledge about reproductive health, contraceptive methods, and their rights under the MTP Act should be emphasized.
- *Youth-friendly services*: Development of youth-friendly healthcare services should be encouraged to ensure that young individuals feel comfortable seeking advice, counseling, and abortion services when needed.

  The Act leaves a gray zone when it comes to the issue of whose permission is most important when it comes to the issue of medical termination of pregnancy for a minor girl, whose parents/guardians are not sharing the same opinion on continuation of pregnancy as the minor.
- *Involvement of civil society*: Role of civil society organizations, NGOs, and advocacy groups in shaping the future of reproductive healthcare in India plays a vital role, including their efforts in policy advocacy and awareness campaigns.
- *International collaboration*: There are some unexplored opportunities for international collaboration and knowledge exchange on best practices in reproductive healthcare and abortion laws. These can be brought on a common platform of discussion, as per the cultural norms of the country.
- *Adapting to technological advances*: Advancements in medical technology, such as improved ultrasound techniques, can impact the detection of fetal abnormalities and the timing of pregnancy terminations.

- *Data collection and research*: Importance of ongoing research and data collection to assess the impact of the MTP Act, identify trends, and evidence-based policy decisions have to be looked into.

By addressing these future directions, a forward-looking perspective on the MTP Act and reproductive healthcare in India can serve as a starting point for discussions and actions aimed at improving access, reducing stigma, and promoting informed choices in the realm of reproductive rights.

CONCLUSION

In the heart of every legal provision and medical procedure lies a profound truth—reproductive rights are human rights. The MTP Act, with its journey of evolution and empowerment, stands as a testament to our commitment to safeguarding the autonomy and well-being of individuals. As we navigate the complexities of reproductive healthcare, let us remember that at its core, it is a journey of compassion, informed choice, and respect for the diverse paths that life may take. May we continue to strive for a society where every voice is heard, every choice is respected, and every life, including the one that chooses, is valued.

The MTP Act stands as a pivotal legal framework that navigates the intricate balance between women's reproductive rights and societal considerations. Understanding the nuances of the MTP Act is indispensable for healthcare practitioners and policymakers alike, as it not only upholds the sanctity of life but also respects a woman's autonomy over her own body and reproductive choices. As medical and legal landscapes evolve, ongoing dialogue and vigilance in upholding the principles of the MTP Act are vital to ensure that women's rights and health remain at the forefront of our society.

KEY LEARNING POINTS

- At its core, the MTP Act champions the fundamental right of reproductive autonomy.
- From its inception to present-day amendments, the MTP Act has undergone a transformative journey, adapting to societal norms, advancements in healthcare, and evolving perspectives on women's rights.
- The MTP Act is a beacon of empowerment, providing women with access to safe and legal termination of pregnancies, ensuring they are not forced into unsafe clandestine procedures that endanger their lives.
- Controversies and challenges surrounding the Act have served as catalysts for reforms and improvements, leading to a more robust legal framework that addresses emerging concerns and advocates for enhanced patient-centric care.
- Educating communities about their rights and the provisions of the Act is essential for fostering a society that respects reproductive choices and values women's health.
- Every stakeholder, from policymakers to healthcare professionals and the public, must actively engage in spreading awareness, advocating for reforms, and ensuring the effective implementation of the MTP Act.
- The MTP Act's legacy is one of progression, equality, and empowerment.

BIBLIOGRAPHY

1. Bansal JD, Bansal U. Recent Amendments to Medical Termination of Pregnancy Act in India: Boon or Bane? J Obstet Gynecol India. 2021:1-5.
2. Baru R, Bhandai P. The Role of Healthcare Providers in Ensuring Access to Safe Abortion. Health and Human Rights. 2004:102-13.
3. Dixit P, Ram F, Dwivedi LK. Determinants of unwanted pregnancies in India using matched case-control designs. BMC Pregnancy Childbirth. 2012;12(1):84.
4. Erdman JN, Cook RJ. Decriminalization of abortion—A human rights imperative. Best Pract Res Clin Obstet Gynecol. 2020;62:11-24.
5. Grover A. Reproductive Rights and Health. Indian J Med Ethics. 2014:78-82.
6. Manning V, Barot S. Access to Safe Abortion Services in India: Barriers, Challenges, and Strategies. J Health Management. 2017:577-89.
7. Messer LC, Dole N, Kaufman JS, et al. Pregnancy intendedness, maternal psychosocial factors and preterm birth. Mat Child Health J. 2005;9(4):403-12.
8. Mete A. Expanding Access to Safe Abortion in India: Key Strategies for the Future. Int J Gynecol Obstet. 2014:1-3.
9. Mishra N. Medical Termination of Pregnancy Act, 1971: A Review. New Delhi: Health and Population: Perspectives and Issues; 2004. pp. 147-56.
10. Moreland S, Talbird S. (2006). Achieving the Millennium Development Goals: the contribution of fulfilling the unmet need for family planning. [online] Available from https://pdf.usaid.gov/pdf_docs/Pnadm175.pdf [Last accessed July, 2024].
11. Nambula R, Isaac KS. Ethical and Legal Issues Surrounding Medical Termination of Pregnancy: An Overview. Indian J Med Ethics. 2013:99-103.
12. Pai SN, Chandra KS. Medical Termination of Pregnancy Act of India: Treading the Path between Practical and Ethical Reproductive Justice. Indian J Community Med. 2023;48(4):510-3.
13. Patel A. History of Abortion Laws in India: A Socio-legal Analysis. J Indian Law Inst. 2004:67-85.
14. Samant R, Khanna R. Promoting Awareness and Advocacy for Women's Reproductive Rights in India. Reprod Health Matters. 2007:193-201.
15. Shah N, Shah S. Medical Termination of Pregnancy Act and Rules: A Critical Appraisal. J Obstet Gynecol India. 2008:220-3.
16. Singh S, Sedgh G, Hussain R. Unintended pregnancy: worldwide levels, trends, and outcomes. Stud Fam Plann. 2010;41(4):241-50.
17. Sodani PR, Kothari S. Patients' Rights in the Indian Context: An Overview. Indian J Community Med. 2013: 210-3.

20.6 Issues Related to PCPNDT Act

Jyoti Bindal

INTRODUCTION

This Preconception and Prenatal Diagnostic Technique (PCPNDT) Act was brought as an important act in 1994. Its primary aim was to prevent those abortions which were done solely after sex selection. It was aimed to reduce such sex-selected abortions and improve the sex ratio. This act was brought as a measure to improve the declining sex ratio of male versus female sex ratio in our country. After the tabulation of this act, it became mandatory for genetic counseling centers to totally ban prenatal sex determination. Any kind of counseling or conducting prenatal diagnostic techniques is prohibited, which includes preimplantation genetic diagnosis in the process of in vitro fertilization (IVF) before and after conception.

Preconception and Prenatal Diagnostic Technique Act covers the act of detection of genetic or chromosomal abnormalities, metabolic or sex-linked disorders, and congenital malformations.

In historical times, when the modern technology of sex detection was not available through ultrasonography, female newborns were killed injudiciously. These female infants were denied the basic right to live. Subsequent to that, with the advent of modern techniques of sex determination during pregnancy, female feticide became more and more common in various health clinics and ill-equipped establishments. Major reason behind female fetus being killed has been dowry in all strata of society. Additionally, in the male-dominated society in India, a son is considered the only child who can carry the family name onward. This practice leads to an alarmingly disproportionate male and female ratio. In 1991, ratio was 945 girls to 1,000 boys, which went on to become 914 girls to 1,000 boys, all between 0–6 years of age ratio. Hence, it became absolute to bring in a law which will help improve this female to male ratio.

ESSENCE OF PCPNDT ACT

- Sex selection and sex determination are prohibited before or after the conception.
  - Any kind of information given to the pregnant lady or her family revealing the sex of the fetus is prohibited.
- All ultrasonography, especially for pregnant women, can only be done in registered clinics under this act and can be performed by the qualified clinicians who have also been specifically registered to work on that particular machine.
  - "Disclosure of sex of the fetus is prohibited under the law"—this has to be prominently displayed in all clinics where ultrasonography is being permitted and registered. This sign has to be written in English and also in local language of the region.
- This act permits the various diagnostic procedures, for example, ultrasonography, amniocentesis, etc., only in certain special circumstances, such as genetic, chromosomal, and congenital abnormalities.
- This act strictly prohibits advertisement in any form—printed or digital on any platform of newspaper, hoardings, flyers, or social media.

- The act includes the ultrasound machine manufacturers and agents as well and the machine cannot be sold unless the buyer medical professional and the premises is registered under this act.
- PCPNDT Act is primarily based on the concept of prevention of misuse of technological advances.

IMPORTANT DEFINITIONS

Preconception and Prenatal Diagnostic Techniques Act describes in detail the various definitions mentioned in the act, such as appropriate authority, techniques, prenatal diagnostic procedures including ultrasonography, fetoscopy, amniocentesis, tissue biopsy, etc., including analysis of any sample thus taken by a genetic laboratory for the purpose of determination of sex of the fetus.

In 2002 amendment, the detailed explanation of genetic laboratory has been explained as the laboratory with ultrasound machine, imaging machine, or scanner.

The act specifies qualified persons, including gynecologist and registered medical practitioner including their qualifications, experience, and ability to perform procedures needed in genetic laboratory.

CLEARING CERTAIN CONCEPTS PRESENT IN SOCIAL CULTURE

- *If the boys are more than girls in existence, the demand value of girls will be more and hence, their position will be elevated.*
  This myth is false, as less number of girls leads to more cases of rape, sexual violence, etc. Women folk are not commodities; they are human assets.
- *Having two daughters gives right to the parents and family for female feticide.*
  Actual fact is that many families opt for sex selection of fetus in favor of a boy even when it is the first child or if there is only one girl child before this pregnancy.
- *For sex selection to be stopped, practice of dowry has to be eliminated first.*
  Dowry system is an inherent cultural defect intricately woven in Indian society. Not having daughters will not be a solution to this. Hence, dowry system cannot be used as an excuse for sex selection. The cultural thread which brands women in lower strata of society needs to be changed.
- *Female feticide is justified as it will prevent the girls from undergoing violence.*
  Violence can be against any person, irrespective of gender. It needs to be curbed at the base, monitored by law and order agencies and violence against females is definitely not a justifiable reason for not permitting females to be born. Female feticide is the problem, not a reason.
- *Sex of the child is sole choice of the mother.*
  Any mother cannot be permitted for sex selection just because of the fact that she is going to give birth to this child. If mother is not permitted for sex selection which is prohibited under the law, it does not in any way encroach on her rights of reproduction. Due to social and cultural myths, many times a woman thinks that producing a male child will increase her status in the family and it needs to be properly counselled that sex of the child is dependent on the chromosome being genetically inherited from the father.

- *Female feticide is a just way to control the population.*
  The argument that sex selection is an effective tool for controlling population is misplaced. Population stabilization is important for improving quality of life. But for this, we cannot resort to things that damage quality of life.
- *Sex selection is only to improve the economic ratio of dependent and earner.*
  In modern scenario, this myth is totally wrong because now with advancement in social scenario about women's education, women are equal shareholders in family's economic status.
- *Sex selection is helpful in balancing the family*:
  - This is a total misconception that having equal numbers of male and female children is the rightly balanced family. There is no perfect definition of a balanced family and definitely gender of children has no bearing on it.
  - Mumbai High Court in the case of Mr and Mrs Soni vs. Union of India and CEHAT, 2005, passed the judgment, which states that "the right to life or personal liberty cannot be expanded to mean that the right to personal liberty includes the personal liberty to determine the sex of the child which may come into existence. Right to bring into existence a life in future with a choice to determine the sex of that life cannot in itself be a right."

IMPLEMENTATION CHALLENGES IN PCPNDT ACT

Inadequate Training

- *Lack of awareness*: Many healthcare professionals, especially in rural areas, might not be fully aware of the provisions of the act.
- *Continuous updates*: Medical practices evolve and the act may require periodic updates. Ensuring that all professionals are up-to-date is a challenge.

Poor Monitoring

- *Resource constraints*: Limited funding and manpower can hamper the government's ability to monitor diagnostic centers effectively.
- *Geographical barriers*: The vastness of certain regions and difficult terrains can make regular inspections and checks challenging.

Inconsistent Enforcement

- *Variation across states*: Enforcement mechanisms and priorities can vary significantly from one state to another due to differing interpretations or resource allocations.
- *Corruption*: In some instances, regulatory bodies might be susceptible to bribery or other forms of corruption, compromising enforcement efforts.

Public Awareness and Education

- *Misunderstandings*: Due to limited awareness, some communities might misinterpret the act, leading to resistance or noncompliance.

- *Cultural sensitivities*: Addressing the act within the context of deeply entrenched cultural beliefs requires nuanced communication strategies.

Technological Advancements

- *Evolving diagnostic techniques*: As new diagnostic methods emerge, the act might struggle to keep pace, leading to potential regulatory gaps.
- *Digital platforms*: With the growth of telemedicine and online healthcare services, ensuring compliance across digital platforms becomes a challenge.

Collaboration and Coordination

- *Interagency coordination*: Effective implementation requires coordination between various government departments, which can sometimes lead to bureaucratic delays or inefficiencies.
- *Stakeholder engagement*: Involving and aligning the interests of all stakeholders, including medical professionals, diagnostic centers, and civil society, is essential but challenging.

These are some of the problems and issues being faced during implementation of this act and in subsequent times to come. This, therefore, necessitates the need for a balanced and practical path to address them effectively.

SOCIOCULTURAL FACTORS CAUSING ISSUES IN THE PCPNDT ACT

Sociocultural factors play a significant role in influencing behaviors, attitudes, and practices related to gender, reproduction, and healthcare. When it comes to the PCPNDT Act, several sociocultural factors can pose challenges as follows:

Preference for Male Children

- *Deep-seated beliefs*: In many societies, especially in parts of India and some other Asian countries, male offsprings are traditionally preferred due to reasons ranging from economic considerations (inheritance) to cultural beliefs.
- *Patriarchal structures*: Societies with strong patriarchal norms might value male children more, seeing them as continuers of the family lineage.

Societal Pressures and Expectations

- *Family reputation*: In communities where family social standing is elevated with birth of a male child, there might be intense pressure on couples to ensure the birth of a son.
- *Community stigma*: Families without male heirs might face societal ostracization or face challenges in community participation, adding to the pressure for sex determination.

Misguided Notions of Balance

- *Perception of family balance*: Some families believe that having a mix of both genders ensures "balance" in the household, leading them to seek specific gender outcomes.
- *Influence of siblings*: In some instances, the gender composition of existing children can influence parents' desires regarding the gender of future offspring.

Economic Factors

- *Economic dependence*: In communities where male children are perceived as future breadwinners, families might prioritize having sons to ensure economic stability in old age.
- *Dowry system*: In societies with prevalent dowry systems, there might be a perception that raising a daughter entails more significant financial burdens, further reinforcing the preference for male children.

Cultural Rituals and Traditions

- *Lineage and ancestral worship*: In cultures where ancestral worship or continuation of family rituals is paramount, male offspring might be considered essential for performing these rites.
- *Religious interpretations*: Sometimes, religious interpretations or misinterpretations might reinforce gender biases, affecting perceptions about the desirability of male versus female offspring.

Media and Popular Culture

- *Portrayal of gender roles*: Media representations that reinforce traditional gender roles or stereotypes can perpetuate societal beliefs about the roles and values associated with male and female children.
- *Celebrity influence*: Public figures and celebrities endorsing or practicing gender selection can inadvertently or deliberately influence public perceptions and behaviors.

Addressing these sociocultural factors requires a multipronged approach involving education, awareness campaigns, community engagement, and broader societal introspection to challenge and change deep-seated beliefs and practices.

TECHNOLOGICAL LOOPHOLES IN THE PCPNDT ACT

Technological advancements can sometimes create loopholes in legislation, especially when regulations have not kept pace with emerging technologies. For the PCPNDT Act, several technological loopholes have emerged over time.

Rise of Do It Yourself Gender Prediction Kits

- *Accessibility*: Over-the-counter gender prediction kits, which can sometimes be inaccurate but claim to predict fetal gender, can be easily accessed by the public.
- *Regulatory oversight*: These kits often operate in a gray area, falling outside the direct purview of the PCPNDT Act due to their classification as nondiagnostic tools.

Online Platforms and Telemedicine

- *Virtual consultations*: With the growth of telemedicine, there is potential for sex-determination consultations to occur online, making it harder to monitor and regulate.
- *Digital forums*: Online forums and social media groups might indirectly facilitate discussions, sharing of information, or even the procurement of illegal sex determination services.

Advanced Imaging Technologies: High-resolution Ultrasound

- Technological advancements in ultrasound machines can offer clearer images, which might inadvertently facilitate more accurate fetal gender determination, bypassing the spirit of the act.
- *Portable devices*: Compact and portable ultrasound devices might make it easier for unauthorized or unregulated individuals to conduct sex determination tests discreetly.

Data Privacy Concerns

- *Unsecured data*: The digital storage and transmission of medical records, including ultrasound images, raise concerns about data privacy and potential misuse.
- *Online transactions*: If illicit services are offered online, digital payment platforms can inadvertently facilitate and such transactions may be conducted anonymously.

Cross-border Technological Access

- *Accessing services abroad*: Individuals might seek sex determination services in countries with lax regulations and then return home, circumventing the provisions of the PCPNDT Act.
- *Telemedicine across borders*: Telemedicine platforms can sometimes operate across borders, complicating regulatory oversight and enforcement.

Algorithmic Predictions

- *Predictive analytics*: Advanced algorithms can sometimes analyze a combination of factors, such as previous children's genders, maternal age, and other parameters, to predict fetal gender, though not with absolute certainty.
- *Mobile applications*: There are applications available that claim to predict baby gender based on various inputs, though their accuracy and ethical implications are questionable.

Addressing these technological loopholes requires continuous monitoring, updating of the legislation to encompass new technological developments, and international collaboration to prevent cross-border evasion of regulations.

ECONOMIC IMPLICATIONS

The Act, aimed primarily at curbing sex-selective abortions, has several economic implications.

Impact on Diagnostic Centers

- *Revenue loss*: Diagnostic centers that previously offered sex determination tests may experience a decline in revenue due to the prohibition of such services.
- *Shift in services*: To compensate for the lost revenue, some centers might focus more on other prenatal diagnostic tests or services, leading to potential overdiagnosis or overuse of certain tests.

Healthcare Expenditure

- *Increased costs*: As the act aims to prevent sex-selective abortions, families might be inclined to pursue more extensive prenatal diagnostic procedures to ensure the health of the fetus, leading to increased healthcare expenditure.
- *Accessibility issues*: Families from lower economic backgrounds might find it challenging to afford alternative diagnostic tests or travel to centers that offer them.

Economic Disparities

- *Urban–rural divide*: Urban areas with better access to a variety of healthcare services might see differential impacts compared to rural areas where diagnostic options might be limited.
- *Affordability concerns*: The act's restrictions might disproportionately affect economically disadvantaged families who might resort to unsafe or clandestine procedures due to affordability constraints.

Government Expenditure

- *Regulatory costs*: The government might incur additional costs related to monitoring, enforcement, and periodic review of the act's provisions.
- *Awareness campaigns*: Public awareness campaigns to educate communities about the act and its implications might require significant funding.

Economic Productivity

- *Gender imbalance*: Over time, persistent gender imbalances resulting from sex-selective practices can have broader societal and economic implications, such as a potential decrease in the female workforce or increased societal unrest due to skewed gender ratios.
- *Long-term social costs*: A skewed gender ratio can lead to challenges in marital markets, increased bride trafficking, or elevated dowry demands, all of which have economic repercussions.

Healthcare System Impacts

Resource allocation: The healthcare system might need to allocate resources to address the broader implications of the act, including providing support for families with female children, addressing gender-based challenges, and ensuring comprehensive prenatal care.

While the PCPNDT Act aims to address significant societal issues related to gender discrimination and skewed sex ratios, its economic implications underscore the interconnectedness of social policies with broader economic considerations.

LEGAL AND ETHICAL CONCERNS IN THE PCPNDT ACT

This Act is designed to address the critical issue of sex-selective abortions. However, like any legislation dealing with sensitive matters, there are legal and ethical concerns associated with its implementation and implications.

Legal Concerns

Ambiguities in Interpretation

- *Vague provisions*: Some sections of the act might be perceived as ambiguous, leading to inconsistent interpretations and potential legal disputes.
- *Jurisdictional differences*: Variances in interpretation or implementation across states or regions can lead to legal inconsistencies.

Enforcement Challenges

- *Resource constraints*: Limited resources might hinder effective monitoring and enforcement, potentially leading to violations going unnoticed.
- *Bureaucratic delays*: Legal processes and bureaucratic procedures might delay justice or enforcement actions.

Legal Safeguards

- *Patient rights*: Ensuring that the act respects individual rights, including privacy and informed consent, while preventing misuse is crucial.
- *Medical ethics*: Balancing medical ethics with legal requirements, especially when faced with complex medical scenarios or ethical dilemmas, can be challenging.

Ethical Concerns

Autonomy and Choice

- *Reproductive rights*: In cases where prenatal diagnosis might be crucial for medical reasons unrelated to gender, this act may prove a hinderance.
- *Parental autonomy*: The act raises questions about the extent to which the state can or should intervene in private decisions related to family planning.

Stigmatization and Discrimination

- *Stigmatizing diagnostic centers*: There is a risk of stigmatizing diagnostic centers, even those operating ethically, due to the act's stringent regulations and potential public perceptions.
- *Discrimination against female children*: While the act aims to prevent sex-selective abortions, critics argue that it might inadvertently contribute to the devaluation of female children by reinforcing negative stereotypes.

Medical Ethics and Practice

- *Professional integrity*: Ensuring that medical professionals uphold the highest ethical standards, provide unbiased counseling, and prioritize patient welfare over other considerations are essential.
- *Informed consent*: Ethical dilemmas can arise concerning informed consent, especially when patients might be compelled or coerced into undergoing or abstaining from specific diagnostic procedures.

Broader Societal Impacts

- *Gender dynamics*: The act's focus on preventing sex-selective abortions raises broader societal questions about gender equality, societal attitudes toward gender, and the underlying factors driving sex-selective practices.
- *Cultural sensitivities*: Ethical considerations also encompass respecting and understanding cultural contexts, beliefs, and practices while ensuring the act's objectives are met.

Navigating the legal and ethical landscape of the PCPNDT Act requires a balanced approach, continuous dialogue between stakeholders and periodic reviews to ensure the legislation's objectives are met without compromising individual rights and ethical principles.

IMPACT ON HEALTHCARE ACCESS IN INDIA DUE TO PCPNDT ACT

Limited Access to Essential Services

- *Reduced availability*: Many diagnostic centers, particularly in areas with strict enforcement, have stopped offering prenatal diagnostic services altogether, fearing legal repercussions. This has limited access to essential prenatal diagnostic services for genuine medical reasons.
- *Shift in focus*: Some healthcare providers have shifted their focus from comprehensive prenatal care to avoid potential legal pitfalls, leading to reduced availability of certain diagnostic procedures.

Rural–Urban Disparities

- *Urban centers*: Urban areas, with better infrastructure and resources, might still have some access to prenatal diagnostic services, albeit with increased scrutiny. However, rural areas, already facing healthcare access challenges, might experience further limited access due to reduced or no services.
- *Travel burden*: Families from rural areas might need to travel longer distances to urban centers, increasing the economic and logistical burden, to access necessary diagnostic services.

Economic Barriers

- *Increased costs*: Due to the act's restrictions, diagnostic procedures, when available, might be priced higher, given the perceived risks associated with offering such services.
- *Financial burden*: Families, especially from economically disadvantaged backgrounds, might find it challenging to afford prenatal diagnostic tests, potentially compromising maternal and fetal health outcomes.

Quality of Care Concerns

- *Overcautious practices*: To avoid legal issues, some healthcare providers might adopt overly cautious practices, such as refraining from certain diagnostic tests altogether, even when medically indicated, leading to potential gaps in prenatal care.
- *Delayed interventions*: Concerns about legal repercussions might lead to delays in necessary interventions or treatments, impacting maternal and fetal health.

Regulatory Compliance Pressures

- *Administrative burden*: Healthcare providers might face increased administrative burdens related to recordkeeping, reporting, and compliance checks, diverting resources from patient care.
- *Fear of legal action*: The stringent provisions of the act, coupled with potential legal consequences, might deter healthcare providers from offering comprehensive prenatal care services, affecting patient trust and confidence.

Deterrent for Healthcare Professionals

Professional concerns: Healthcare professionals concerned about potential legal actions or the stigma associated with offering prenatal diagnostic services, might choose to avoid or limit such services, leading to a shortage of skilled providers in this domain.

The PCPNDT Act in India underwent several amendments to address various concerns and strengthen its provisions. The 2003 amendments significantly revised the original act, which was first introduced in 1994.

KEY AMENDMENTS TO THE PCPNDT ACT IN 2003

The Amendments in the act have been implemented from December 14th, 2003.
Following are the highlights of amendments:

- The declination in the sex ratio has been contributed to a large extent by techniques of pre-conception sex selection, hence these techniques have been brought into purview of the act.
- Purchase, relocation and user identification of ultrasound machines are now under the ambit of the Act, so that any misuse of ultrasound machines for sex selection can be checked. This will be a milestone step to check female feticide.
- Central Supervisory Board has been given additional powers to ensure implementation of the Act.
- State level Supervisory Boards have been formed for decentralising the process of monitoring sex selection.
- Within the States, State Appropriate Authority has been constituted which has specific number of members to further keep checks and monitor the smooth implementation of PCPNDT Act.
- Any violation of the act now has more severe penalties and implications than earlier.

This is to send message across to ensure proper follow-up and to increase the declining sex ratio:

- Now the Authority which has been vested with power to monitor the implementation of the act has been empowered with the powers of Civil Court for search, seizure and sealing. This includes machines, equipment, premises and all the available digital and physical records.
- Use of ultrasound machine is prohibited unless a proper record is maintained of every procedure done. It specifically includes a declaration by the doctor as well as patient about not indulging in the act of sex determination.
- Further, it is now mandatory for the machine manufacturer to ensure that the machine is sold only to registered users and registered premises.

Further, following are the amended framing of the rules:

Amended Rules

- In the new rules, it has been provided that a person can appeal to the next higher authority—higher to the authority against whom the grievance is present.
- Indian Council of Medical Research (ICMR) has provided specific indications in which ultrasonography can be performed during pregnancy. These indications are twenty three in number and are vital to assess the growth and other parameters during pregnancy.
- Simpler forms have been introduced, however, filling of forms is mandatory.

Broadened Scope

In the amended rules, "prenatal diagnostic procedures" broadened to include various diagnostic procedures, e.g., ultrasonography, amniocentesis, etc., only in certain special circumstances, such as genetic, chromosomal and congenital abnormalities, etc.

Enhanced Penalties

Increased stringency: The amendments introduced more severe penalties for offenses under the act. Those found violating the provisions, including conducting or advertising sex-determination tests, faced stricter punishments, including imprisonment and significant fines.

Regulation of Genetic Counseling Centers

Inclusion: The amendments brought genetic counseling centers and genetic laboratories under the ambit of the act, requiring them to register and adhere to the prescribed guidelines.

Prohibition on Advertisements

Stricter measures: The 2003 amendments imposed a complete prohibition on advertisements, whether direct or indirect, promoting prenatal determination of sex, including online platforms, print media, or any other means.

Strengthened Monitoring and Enforcement

- *Inspections*: Local authorities are directed to form teams to inspect those clinics/institutions/hospitals which have applied for the registration, preregistered premises as well as have random inspections.
- *Seizure*: The amendments provided authorities with the power to seize records, machines, or equipment used in offenses related to sex determination.

Protection of Informers

Confidentiality: The amendments incorporated provisions to ensure the confidentiality of informers or whistleblowers who provide information about violations of the act, offering them protection from potential retaliation or harm.

These amendments in 2003 aimed to address the challenges and shortcomings observed in the original act, providing a more comprehensive framework to strengthen the regulation.

CASE LAWS

Landmark Decisions for Implementation of the Act Directions Issued by the Supreme Court and High Courts

There are a series of petitions filed either *Suo motu* or being moved by nongovernmental organizations (NGOs) in which the Supreme Court and the High Courts have issued various directions and pronounced orders to the central and the state governments for creating public awareness and for effective implementation of this Act.

- *Writ Petition (Civil) No. 301 of 2000 Decided on May 4, 2001*
- Centre for Enquiry into Health and Allied Themes (CEHAT) and Others vs. Union of India and Others

Key Issues and Legal Context

The petition raised serious concerns over lack of implementation and enforcement of the PNDT Act by the Central and State Governments—even five years after its enactment.

The writ was filed as public interest litigation (PIL) to compel the authorities to fulfill statutory duties under the Act, such as appointing appropriate authorities, establishing advisory committees, holding supervisory board meetings, and banning advertisements promoting sex determination methods.

Judgment (Order dated 4 May 2001)

The court delivered the order, issuing the following key observations and directions:

- Recognition of the grave social evil of sex-selective abortion and ongoing female infanticide, now enabled by medical advancements rather than traditional practices.
- Criticism of state inaction, noting that the PNDT Act had not been implemented effectively across the country.

Detailed directions were given:

- The Central Government must launch public awareness campaigns against sex determination and female feticide, particularly through electronic media as provided under the Act.
- CSB meetings to be held at least once every 6 months, per statutory mandate.
- CSB must collect and monitor periodic quarterly returns from State/UT authorities regarding registrations of diagnostic centers, enforcement actions, and awareness activities.
- No costs awarded, signifying the court's concern was policy-driven and public-interest focused rather than punitive.

Significance

It set a precedent for judicial activism in public health, particularly in ensuring government accountability in implementing socially critical legislation.

Writ Petition (Civil) No. 301 of 2000, Decided on September 19, 2001

CEHAT and Others vs. Union of India

The case continued through multiple further hearings, including significant orders in September 2001, December 2001, March 2003, and a major judgment on 10 September 2003.

Order Dated 19 September 2001

The Court specifically mandated that all State and Union Territory authorities must submit quarterly progress reports to the Central Supervisory Board (CSB) concerning their implementation of the PNDT Act.

This order underscores the Court's intent to monitor compliance more closely and ensure that earlier directives were being followed on the ground.

Writ Petition (Civil) No. 301 of 2000 Decided on November 7, 2001
CEHAT and Others vs. Union of India and Others

Key Order

This hearing resulted in a pivotal direction: the Supreme Court mandated the creation of a National Inspection and Monitoring Committee to oversee implementation and enforcement of the Act across all States and Union Territories.

Additionally, the Court directed States to file compliance affidavits within three weeks, reiterating its seriousness toward systematic enforcement.

Petitions Challenging Constitutional Validity of the Act

As of today, there are two decisions, both of the Bombay High Court, in which Constitutional validity of the Act was challenged but upheld. Both the decisions are landmark in the way they deal with this most sensitive and socially relevant issue.

- *In the High Court of Bombay*
  Criminal Writ Petition No. 945 of 2005 and Criminal Application No. 3647 of 2005, decided on 13/06/2005, Vinod Soni and Anr. vs. Union of India
- *In the High Court of Bombay*
  Writ Petition No. 2777 of 2007, decided on 06/09/2007

Cases Involving Procedural Issues under the Act

It has been observed that the appropriate authorities on being informed or having found any illegality usually either cancel the registration of the clinic where ultrasonography is being performed or they seal the machine or they seize the equipment. Due to nonavailability of a qualified legal counsel during this action, procedural formalities are incomplete, which makes the case of State or Appropriate Authority weak in the eyes of law. Many times, challenge is put forth by the counsellor of the professional/petitioner that his or her livelihood is hampered by this act, and thus it contradicts their constitutional right.

- *In the High Court of Bombay*
  Writ Petition No. 5295 of 2003, decided on 17/09/2004 M/s Malpani Infertility Clinic Pvt. Ltd. and Others vs. Appropriate Authority, PNDT Act and Others
- *In the High Court of Punjab and Haryana at Chandigarh*
  Civil Writ Petition No. 18365 of 2009, decided on 03/02/2010
  Dr Mrs Sudha Samir vs. State of Haryana and Others
  Civil Writ Petition No. 19740 of 2009, Dr Mrs Maninder Ahuja vs. State of Haryana and Others
  Civil Writ petition No. 19794 of 2009, Dr RD Negi vs. State of Haryana and Others

CONCLUSION

While the PCPNDT Act has made significant strides in curbing female feticide and gender-based sex selection, it is evident that challenges persist. Enforcement loopholes, inadequate awareness, and sociocultural factors continue to hinder its effectiveness. Addressing these issues requires a multifaceted approach involving robust enforcement mechanisms, comprehensive awareness campaigns, and targeted interventions to change societal attitudes toward gender. Only through concerted efforts can we hope to realize the Act's goal of ensuring the equal right to life for every child, regardless of gender.

Honorable Smt Ranjana Desai J (Vijay Sharma v. Union of India AIR 2008 Bom. 29) had stated, "That society should not want a girl child; that efforts should be made to prevent the birth of a girl child and that society should give preference to a male child is a matter of grave concern. Such tendency offends dignity of women. It violates woman's right to life. It violates Article 39(e) of the Constitution which states the principle of state policy that the health and strength of women is not to be abused. It ignores Article 51A(e) of the Constitution which states that it shall be the duty of every citizen of India to renounce practices derogatory to the dignity of women. Sex selection is therefore against the spirit of the Constitution. It insults and humiliates womanhood. This is perhaps the greatest argument in favor of total ban on sex selection."

KEY LEARNING POINTS

- Despite the act, tests pertaining to sex selection and subsequent abortions have persisted, particularly in certain regions and communities.
- One major criticism is the lack of stringent enforcement mechanisms. Many clinics and diagnostic centers violate the act without facing significant consequences.
- A clandestine market for gender determination tests exists, making it challenging to completely eradicate the practice.
- The act places the responsibility on clinics and diagnostic centers to maintain records and report to authorities.
- Deep-seated cultural preferences for male children in some communities contribute to the persistence of sex-selective practices.
- The act, has sometimes led to stigmatization of women seeking legitimate prenatal diagnostic services for other health reasons.

BIBLIOGRAPHY

1. PCPNDT Act 1994.
2. PCPNDT Act and PCPNDT Rules 2003.
3. Shalini Phansalkar Joshi; United Nations Population Fund. (1994). Compilation and Analysis of Case-laws on Pre-conception and Pre-natal Diagnostics Techniques (Prohibition of Sex Selection) Act, 1994. [online] Available from https://india.unfpa.org/sites/default/files/pub-pdf/Compilation_and_Analysis_of_Case_Laws_on_Pre_Conception.pdf [Last accessed May, 2024].

21

CHAPTER

Medicolegal Issues in Surgery

Gouri Gore

INTRODUCTION

The risk of facing a compensation suite is high in any surgical specialty. Surgeons and anesthesiologists are sued once every 4–5 years, according to a retrospective analysis. Exact statistics are not available in India, but a review of cases filed in various consumer fora from district to national level suggest that in majority of consumer cases some operative intervention, major or minor, has been done. However, it is also easier to decide the case due to the availability of clear, unambiguous evidence in most cases. This chapter outlines various stages in the surgical management of a patient where allegations of negligence can be made. It will deal in detail precautions to be taken so that strong evidence can be produced in a court of law if one has to face a lawsuit.

MAKING DECISION ABOUT SURGERY

Each person has a right to determine what will be done to his/her body, which includes the right to consent to or refuse any operation. This fact has to be acknowledged while advising surgery to the patient. For any procedure, major or minor, elective or emergency, patients should be informed about the following.

The Nature of the Intervention and Its Benefit

The outline of the procedure, in as simple terms as possible, should be communicated to the patient. The narration, if supported by visual aids like pictures or videos, makes a positive impact on the patient. If any organ is going to be removed, the patient must fully understand the postoperative implications. For example, a woman requiring hysterectomy should be made to understand that she will not get menses after the surgery and she will not be able to bear children. If a patient has to undergo amputation of a limb or removal of eye, counseling has to be done about rehabilitation after the surgery.

The highest degree of caution and care is needed in taking the decision to operate on a patient with abnormal vitals or who is unfit. The doctor should have enough evidence to justify the need for surgery in critical condition, in the court of law. In cases of emergency surgery, the prime objective is to make the patient stable, e.g., control hemorrhage after any trauma.

It is of vital importance to explain to the patient about the role, emergency surgery will have to avoid further complications in a given situation. On many occasions, definitive surgery cannot be offered to the patient in emergency situations. It must be emphasized in such cases that second stage surgery may be required. For example, a patient with bowel gangrene may need a colostomy as an emergency procedure and will require another surgery at a later date.

Performing an Emergency Surgery When an Elective Surgery is Indicated is Perceived as Negligence

Case: A patient with humerus fracture was operated upon at night during which he sustained multiorgan failure due to hypoxia (anesthesia complications) and died subsequently. The courts held the operating orthopedic surgeon negligent as he could not produce evidence to justify surgery at night, as emergency.

There is an increasing trend of surgery on demand, especially for cosmetic purposes. It is the doctor's duty to decide whether a particular procedure is medically indicated or would be appropriate for that particular patient. It is imperative for any doctor to explain to the patient **WHY** he/she needs a particular procedure.

The Patient's Consent Cannot be Presumed as Permission to Perform an Inappropriate Surgery

Case: An orthopedic surgeon performed one surgery of a multistage procedure for limb lengthening, on a man with height of 5' 10". Subsequently, the patient refused to go ahead with the remaining procedure, so a reversal was done. The patient experienced some walking disability thereafter. The courts did not accept the defense that it was on the patient's demand that such a procedure was undertaken. In fact, it stressed upon that the doctor should have explained the patient inappropriateness of the said surgery for him and refused to operate.

Surgical Complication is Not Always a Negligence

All major and life-threatening complications should be mentioned. It should include the risks and complications of anesthesia and procedure. Also, it is better to mention some data which can give an idea to the patient about the probability of a particular complication. It would be ideal if each center can give its own data about a particular procedure. In every procedure certain complications are common, known to occur. Courts accept this as defense and are unlikely to hold the doctor negligent in such an event.

Case: Common bile duct was injured during laparoscopic cholecystectomy. The injury was detected and repaired by open surgery. The courts upheld that it is a well-known risk during cholecystectomy and cannot be correlated as the act of negligence or carelessness on the part of the operating surgeon. Hence, the judgment was in favor of the doctor.

Many of the lawsuits are filed when an unexpected event occurs, and the outcome is unfavorable. But the courts recognize that all unfavorable outcomes are not due to negligence.

Alternative Treatments

It is the patient's right to know all the available options for the ailment. If a non-surgical treatment is also a reasonable option, the patient has to be informed about such a method. The risk of recurrence/incomplete cure/need for surgery after such treatment has to be explained to the patient and a specific consent must be obtained in such cases. For example, while offering medical management to a patient with unruptured ectopic pregnancy a specific consent must be obtained about the need for emergency surgery. If more than one type of operation is possible, explain pros and cons of every possible surgery. A doctor's job is to suggest the most appropriate treatment (surgery) for the ailment under consideration. It is the patient, who would decide which option to choose. However in many cases, the patient's perception and understanding of potential benefits, risks, and complications is inaccurate and misleading. It is recommended that all important facts about the surgery and its implications are noted down and patient signature is taken on the sheet, at the end of consultation. If possible, it is important that the patient's family understand the risks involved, because if the patient dies or becomes incapacitated, a family that is surprised by the outcome is more likely to sue.

Scheduling Surgery

Not prioritizing the surgery in case of a seriously ill patient can be considered as negligence. If there is a waiting list for any surgery, it must be communicated to the patient in writing, and the patient must be given the option to avail treatment at another hospital.

Case: A patient was advised to undergo bypass surgery and was on the waitlist. The patient died due to a cardiac event before undergoing the procedure.

Postponing a surgery for astrological reasons, particularly in an emergency, cannot be a doctor's defense. In India, it is very common for patients to demand surgery on a specific day or time. A doctor has to record his/her advice and schedule surgery as per medical conditions.

Competence of Surgeon

In the era of super specialties and subspecialties, it is important for any doctor to be aware of his/her limitations before venturing into any procedure. Attempting to perform any procedure without having a legally prescribed qualification for the same is definitely a negligent act. Even when a doctor has appropriate qualifications for a specialty, he/she may not have adequate experience of a particular treatment or procedure. It is in the interest of the surgeon that he involves a more experienced surgeon in the case or refers the patient to another competent doctor. When a particular ailment comes in purview of different specialties, it is advisable to take the opinion of another specialty doctor before any procedure is performed.

Case: A patient underwent a spine surgery from an orthopedic surgeon for leg pain. The pain persisted even after the surgery, so the patient consulted a neurosurgeon who performed another surgery. The court after perusing all medical records observed that the patient's problem was concerning the nerves, and the orthopedic surgeon should have consulted a neurologist before surgery.

Preoperative Evaluation

Failure to assess the patient properly and adequately prior to any surgery, particularly a planned procedure/surgery is per se negligence. Courts draw adverse inference if any standard preoperative assessment is lacking. Certain preoperative investigations are universally required for any surgery. In addition to this, there would be some tests needed in specific cases. The patient must be advised about all the required investigations before surgery is undertaken. If a patient refuses any diagnostic procedure or investigation, it should be recorded.

In case a diagnostic surgical procedure is required like Biopsy or D&C, the patient must be made to understand that the particular procedure is not being offered as a curative surgery.

Case 1: A patient consulted a doctor with a breast lump who performed a biopsy. She was referred to a higher center as the biopsy suggested malignancy. The patient alleged the doctor of performing wrong surgery which did not cure her.

All possible risks and complications involved in a preoperative test should be mentioned. For example, if a patient needs to undergo a Stress test as part of preoperative investigation, he/she should be made aware of the potential adverse cardiac event while undergoing stress test.

Patients should be referred to an adequately qualified doctor for fitness. Courts have held doctors negligent if fitness has been obtained from a doctor who does not have a formal super-speciality qualification. Membership of any professional body is not considered equivalent to having a formal qualification. For example, it is highly advisable to obtain fitness from a Cardiologist than a General Physician, for a patient with an existing cardiac problem, even for a minor procedure.

All investigations must be duly recorded in the medical records. Failure to record any of mandatory investigations may be viewed as negligence.

Case 2: Intraocular test prior to cataract surgery was said to be done, but was not recorded in indoor papers. Hence, the doctor could not produce any evidence in the court, for doing a mandatory preoperative investigation.

It is advisable to repeat certain preoperative investigations close to the scheduled surgery and record the report in the indoor papers with timing.

Case 3: A patient underwent a cardiac surgery and died within a few days of the operation. The hemoglobin test done 3 days prior to surgery showed a normal level, but hemoglobin done on the day of surgery was very low. The complainant argued that the hemoglobin test was done before the surgery and without waiting for the report the surgeon proceeded with the operation. The doctor's defense, that the hemoglobin test was done after the procedure and necessary action of blood transfusion was taken in accordance with the report, was not granted.

Preoperative Preparation

The patient has to be clearly instructed in writing about:

- Admission to the hospital
- Duration of Starvation
- Preoperative procedures (enema/hair removal)
- Blood or blood products reservation
- Preprocedure medications (antihypertensive or thyroid supplement)

Any minor preoperative procedure can cause complications, and the chief consultant can be held negligent even if the said procedure has been carried out by some other staff (vicarious liability).

Case: The patient was admitted for umbilical hernia repair. A proctoclysis enema was administered as part of the preoperative procedure. Subsequently, the patient was diagnosed to have rectovaginal fistula within 15 days of the surgery, for which she underwent repeated surgeries and required a colostomy. It was alleged that the nurse was negligent in giving enema causing rectal injury. The nurse's contact could not be traced, the doctor was held negligent.

CONSENT

Consent provides an opportunity to establish "Therapeutic Alliance" between the patient and the doctor. In the case of elective surgery, the process of taking informed consent starts from the first visit, as part of the process is to listen to the patient and respond to his/her queries. A detailed discussion about consent can be found in another chapter in this book.

Taking Additional Consent during Surgery

During the course of surgery, the doctor may have to perform some additional procedure or alter the nature of surgery, for which the patient has not consented. In this situation, additional consent can be obtained from the patient's relative after giving proper information about the patient's intraoperative condition. It is obvious that such a situation should be anticipated and explained to the patient during the preoperative counseling. The patient should be advised to nominate a relative who would be present during the surgery, so that the additional consent can be obtained if needed.

In grave emergency, oral consent is also valid but difficult to prove in the court of law.

INTRAOPERATIVE EVENTS

Intraoperative Complications

Law accepts that intraoperative complications cannot always be avoided, for which the surgeon cannot be held negligent. At the same time any delay in identifying and managing the complication can be termed as negligence.

Case 1: A patient underwent phacoemulsification for cataract, during which the nucleus was dropped in the vitreous cavity. It was removed 25 days after surgery after repeated attempts of vitrectomy. The multiple vitrectomy attempts were due to malfunctioning of the vitrectomy machine. The court held the doctor negligent NOT because the nucleus was dropped, as it is a known accident during phacoemulsification, but due to the DELAY in corrective surgery and improper functioning of the equipment.

Intraoperative complications due to improper functioning of equipment or non-availability of certain back up facilities are seen as negligence. All electric gadgets used for patients (cautery/warmer) must be properly insulated and checked at regular intervals. A patient can accuse the doctor and hospital of negligence in cases like cautery burns or burns due to warmer.

It is a must for any hospital or nursing home, however small it may be, to have all the gadgets necessary for patient resuscitation, before undertaking any operative procedure under anesthesia. Any hospital should have a ventilator and defibrillator, even if minor procedures are carried out. If the hospital does not have these gadgets, inform the patient in writing about non-availability of these equipment. The courts perceive this as negligence on account of patient safety.

Case 2: A diabetic patient was taken up for hernia repair. Intraoperatively, the patient had low oxygen saturation and could not be resuscitated due to lack of ventilator. The patient was transferred to another hospital but succumbed to hypoxic brain damage eventually.

ALTERING SURGICAL PROCEDURE/ADDITIONAL SURGERY

A surgeon can take on the spot decisions which can alter the course of surgery, but all such variations must be in accordance with the standard accepted medical practice and the reasons must be recorded in detail. Any deviation from pre consented surgery should be meticulously recorded in the operations notes. The reasons for doing so also must be written in detail.

Case: A patient was taken up for laparoscopic cholecystectomy but underwent partial cholecystectomy due to adherent gallbladder. The court accepted the doctor's defense and stated that doctors taking on the spot decisions which may alter the course of surgery is not a negligence per say, provided it is done in the interest of the patient.

Post-surgery Care

In many cases, the patient's condition deteriorates in the postoperative phase. Generally, the patient is monitored by a staff nurse or junior doctor in the postoperative phase. Non-availability of the consultant after surgery has been the prime cause of patient grievance in most of the cases. The courts have taken cognizance of this and drew adverse inference when a particular patient is left to a junior staff. The operating surgeon must be available even in the postoperative phase till the patient is discharged or a locum arrangement must be made and informed to the patient in exceptional situations. A locum doctor should have qualifications and experience comparable to the primary consultant.

If any organ/tissue is removed, it should be shown to the patient's relatives, and a proper acknowledgement has to be taken and preserved. The tissue/organ should be sent for pathological examination.

Complications in Postoperative Phase

An adverse event can occur in the immediate postoperative phase or even after the patient is discharged.

- *Sudden collapse*: If a patient has a sudden deterioration in the vital parameters in the immediate postoperative phase, it must be promptly informed to the relatives. All necessary corrective measures have to be taken in a short time. It is always better to take help from other colleagues in this catastrophic event. All the events including the time interval from diagnosis to treatment should be elaborately recorded in the indoor paper at the earliest.
- If the patient needs intensive care or transfer to a higher center, the relatives should be informed promptly. The courts have ruled against the doctor for not taking a timely decision to transfer the patient to another hospital/ICU.
- In the event of postoperative death, a postmortem should always be asked for. The local police should be intimated about the death, and all legal formalities are to be completed, even if the patient's relatives insist on avoiding the postmortem. It is more likely that the

patient's relative would infer the mishap as negligence and lodge a complaint at a later date. A detailed postmortem report becomes a very solid defense for a doctor.

- *Hospital acquired infection*: It is very common to see wound infections in most high-volume centers. All standard protocols have to be followed in the operation theater during surgery. A record has to be maintained about all asepsis measures like fumigation, use of chemical sterilization, maintenance of laminar airflow, etc. A doctor or hospital has been sued on the allegations of improper asepsis, in cases of eye infection after cataract surgery or failed joint replacement surgery.
- *Gossypiboma*: This is an avoidable surgical complication. The term has been coined for a forgotten mop or gauze in the patient's body, but it applies to any other foreign material as well. It has serious medico-legal repercussions. The doctrine of *res ipsa Loquitur* can be applied in most of the cases. The fact should be revealed to the patient immediately and a corrective surgery must be performed.

Implants and Prosthesis

Many specialties use implants for various surgeries. It is almost universal to use an artificial lens after cataract surgery. Orthopedic surgeons use implants at various sites. General surgeons use Mesh for the majority of hernia repairs.

A few guidelines must be followed when an implant of any nature is used:

1. The patient should be informed about the need to use the implant and its nature.
2. In case multiple standard manufacturers are available, the patient should be given a choice to procure the implant.
3. If the patient buys the implant from any standard company and it is to be used during surgery, the fact must be recorded.
4. In case the patient is unable to procure the implant or refuses to procure the implant, a declaration must be taken from the patient permitting the hospital or doctor to procure the implant and use it for the patient.
5. All the records regarding the implant used like manufacturer, type, make, number, lifespan of the implant etc. should be recorded in detail in the operative notes and discharge card.
6. In case the implant is found to be defective/nonfunctioning/broken and has to be removed, it has to be informed to the patient, and the removed implant should be handed over to the patient. A proper acknowledgment has to be taken from the patient of receipt of the defective implant. Ideally, the manufacturer also should be informed about the defective implant. However, this may not always be possible as the patient may approach different doctors in different parts of the country for primary surgery and implant removal.

Case 1: A hip replacement surgery was done for femur fracture. After 2 years, the patient approached another hospital with complaints of pain and inability to walk. Another surgery was performed in which the implant was found to be broken, hence it was removed and replaced. The allegation was made against the first hospital that the initial implant used was of substandard quality. The judgment was in favor of the doctor as the evidence was produced that the implant used was of international quality.

Case 2: A patient underwent a phaco surgery and the lens was implanted. A month later the same eye had to be removed. The judgment was in favor of the patient as no record could be produced of the lens asserting the quality.

Culpable Silence

It is common for a doctor to come across a patient who has been previously operated by some other surgeon. A doctor may be called for some help or opinion during the course of surgery as well. If a second surgery reveals some negligent act by the first doctor, e.g., a forgotten mop or injury to any organ, it is a legal duty of the second surgeon to inform the patient about the earlier negligent act and take corrective steps. Similarly, if a surgeon is called for any intraoperative or postoperative complication which has happened due to a negligent act, it is legally binding on him/her to inform the patient about the earlier negligent act.

Case: A 11-year-old girl allegedly underwent tonsillectomy in one hospital and was shifted immediately to another hospital where another surgery was performed. It was found out later after investigations at third place that thyroidectomy had been performed on her. The court held the second surgeon guilty of not informing the patient and her relatives about the negligent act of the first surgeon.

Relapse or Recurrence

Certain precautions need to be taken while performing a surgery where relapse or recurrence is a possibility, e.g., hernia repair or myomectomy has a definite risk of recurrence. Any joint replacement surgery may need a revision surgery after a certain period. While taking consent this fact must be mentioned with appropriate statistics. Even the discharge card of the patient should have all details of surgery with a mention of specific precautions to minimize the possibility of recurrence. The telltale signs and symptoms, if the recurrence occurs and the steps to be taken by the patient if any of the symptoms are experienced. If the patient does not follow the advice or schedule of follow up visits, it must be recorded.

The above protocol must be observed even in cases where a multistage procedure (correction of deformity/Limb lengthening operation/Dental procedures/cosmetic surgery, etc.) is planned. It is very useful to give an information sheet to the patient about how the entire procedure will be carried out. It should include the number of surgeries, hospital stay, precautions to be taken during the entire period of treatment. Non-compliance to any advice or follow-up schedule must be recorded.

KEY LEARNING POINTS

- A thorough pre surgery assessment must be made. All required investigations should be asked for and documented properly.
- Fitness has to be obtained from an appropriately qualified specialist.
- Operation theaters must be well equipped, and all gadgets should be in optimum condition.
- An adverse intraoperative event must be informed of the relatives and corrective action should be taken promptly. The entire event must be recorded meticulously in the operative notes.
- Postoperative care should not be left to the junior staff solely. The operating surgeon must make appropriate arrangements in his/her absence.

BIBLIOGRAPHY

1. B.H. Parmar v Dodiya Manharbai alias Manubai. National Consumer Disputes Redressal Commission, New Delhi. 2011;6.
2. Budetti PP, Waters TM. Medical malpractice law in the United States. Menlo Park (CA): Kaiser Family Foundation; 2005.
3. CHL Apollo Hospital, Indore & Ors v Ashish Sanyal & Ors.
4. Dr. A. Ramesh Reddy v R. Venkata Krishna Murthy & Ors. Andhra Pradesh State Consumer Disputes Redressal Commission, Hyderabad.
5. Dr. Ch. Raghuram v Kasuladev Anusha & Ors. Andhra Pradesh State Consumer Disputes Redressal Commission, Hyderabad.
6. Dr. Gopinath Menon v N.K. Dayanandan & Ors. Kerala State Consumer Disputes Redressal Commission, Thiruvananthapuram; OP No. 984/03.
7. Dr. Joydeb Kundu v Rabindranath Pal & Ors. Med Law Cases Doctors. 2010;3(3).
8. Dr. Mahendra Borana v Fateh Singh Sishodiya. Rajasthan State Consumer Disputes Redressal Commission.
9. Dr. R.K. Sharma & Ors v Vinit Mehta. National Consumer Disputes Redressal Commission.
10. Dr. S.G. Nagral v Janglisab M. Balannavar. Rajasthan State Consumer Disputes Redressal Commission.
11. Janab Fazai v Dr. Hamza Thayyil. Kerala State Consumer Disputes Redressal Commission, Thiruvananthapuram.
12. M/s Bone & Joint Clinic & Ors v Anusuya. Tamil Nadu State Consumer Disputes Redressal Commission, Chennai.
13. Mahendra Singh v Sanjeev Agarwal & Anr. Uttarakhand State Consumer Disputes Redressal Forum, Dehradun.
14. Medical Law Cases for Doctors. 2011;4(12):185-6.
15. N. Duraiswamy v Prof. Dr. M. Ramdoss & Ors. Tamil Nadu State Consumer Disputes Redressal Commission.
16. N. Ramakrishnan & Ors v Isabel Hospital. Tamil Nadu State Consumer Disputes Redressal Commission, Chennai.
17. Postgraduate Institute of Medical Education and Research, Chandigarh v Bimla Devi.
18. Satyanarayan Agarwala & Ors v Dr. (Mrs.) Alaka Goswami & Ors. Assam State Consumer Disputes Redressal Commission, Guwahati.
19. Smt. Syamala v Dr. D. Vijay Devi & Ors. Kerala State Consumer Disputes Redressal Commission, Thiruvananthapuram.
20. Smt. Tilat Chaudhry & Anr v All India Institute of Medical Sciences & Anr. National Consumer Disputes Redressal Commission.
21. Somraj Sen & Anr v [Respondent]. Consumer Case No. 428 of 2015.
22. Vimal Kumar Mundra & Anr v Pardaya Memorial Hospital & Ors.
23. Vinod Kumar Rawat v Dr. Suresh Gupta & Ors. Rajasthan State Consumer Disputes Redressal Commission, Jaipur; Case No. 671/2005.

22

CHAPTER

Medicolegal Issues in Orthopedics

Vijay Kuthe, Alka Kuthe

INTRODUCTION

Orthopedics is a specialized surgical branch concerned mainly with muscles, bones, and joints. A patient consults orthopedic surgeon for disorders or injuries affecting any of them. The seemingly endless horizons of orthopedics have many known complications, the skillful management of which requires knowledge, experience, and a standard treatment protocol. Deficiency or negligence in above cases can lead to deformities and subsequent litigations. It is easy to measure orthopedic outcome irrespective of the surgeon's performance unlike other specialties. There were no controlled clinical studies and there was inadequacy of research. To examine the completely healed acute fracture of patella or to assess the proper functioning of a leg was much easier for the court as these are the concepts that even common people can understand. There is still a lack of unanimity in specialties over the definition of *"standard practice"*. However, intraoperative or follow-up X-rays are very much helpful in orthopedic surgery. They can provide photographs of a surgeon's skill and work. The failure to return to a desired function can give a fair measure of dissatisfaction. The specialty has played an important role in developing many of the key doctrines which are discussed in this chapter and used often in medical malpractice law.

EXPERT TESTIMONY

Slater versus Baker and Stapleton is one of the first cases dealing with medical malpractice law that was tried in England in 1767. It marked the beginning of the concept of a professional standard, that is, whether physicians and surgeons have committed right or wrong is to be judged by "the usage and law of surgeons... the rule of the profession as testified to by surgeons themselves." A patient in this case consulted two doctors to change the bandages on a partially healed fracture. The doctor decided to refracture the leg to improve alignment and placed the leg in an unorthodox apparatus to get proper alignment. The aggrieved patient filed a case against that doctor, and before court, he produced similarly trained other physician expert who opined that the treatment used was contrary to standard medical practice. Since this historical case, the concept of expert opinion to support a claim against a professional is included in modern law.

PROFESSIONAL STANDARD

A patient can be blindsided by a poorly executed surgery, especially when they expect their surgeon to perform the procedure with the utmost care. As with any other invasive procedure, orthopedic surgery presents inherent risks. In many instances, these risks can be avoided so long as the orthopedic surgeon can avoid these inherent risks by always following the standard of care. In *Pike versus Honsinger (1898),* the patient got his patella fractured. The plaster and bandages came off before the duration of treatment and the patient joined work in his farm. The result was poor in terms of fracture healing, knee stiffness, and torn ligaments. It was alleged that it was due to delayed diagnosis of ruptured ligaments, inadequate treatment, and the improper follow-up instructions given to the patient. The decision was in favor of defending doctor in trial court but on appeal, a higher court reversed in favor of the patient based on expert opinion. Pike established immunity from liability for "an honest error in judgment". These case laws have proved the important role that orthopedic cases have played in the evolution of the "American law of medical malpractice."

CORPORATE LIABILITY

In *Darling versus Charleston Memorial Hospital (1965)* case, a high school athlete had to undergo amputation due to complications related to compartment syndrome and gangrene. It was after cast treatment of a lower extremity fracture. Prior to Darling, there was no special obligation on the hospital to assure the quality of the care rendered by independent medical staff. The concept of hospital corporate liability was generated from this Darling case. The court held that a hospital could not limit its liability as a charitable corporation. The hospital board of trustees should be sure about the competency, qualifications, and proficiency of individual staff in the hospital. Other landmark cases related to orthopedic injuries that broadened the Darling precedent include *Johnston versus Misericordia Hospital* and *Elam versus College Park Hospital.*

INFORMED CONSENT

The doctrine of informed consent was developed by the landmark orthopedic case, *Canterbury versus Spence*. The patient underwent a lumbar laminectomy for a herniated disc. Before operation, the surgeon told the family that the operation is relatively simple. Contrary to the assurance, the operation landed in complication resulting in incontinent and paralyzed patient. The court delivered its decision by observing that *"the record we review tells a depressing tale".* There was incomplete information about the risks of surgery. In this case, the court held: "The average patient has little or no understanding of the medical arts, and ordinarily has only his physician to whom he can look for enlightenment to reach an intelligent decision. From these almost axiomatic considerations springs the need, and in turn the requirement, of a reasonable divulgence by a physician to make such a decision possible". *Canterbury versus Spence* was decided in 1972 and it marked the beginning of the present era of informed consent. Thus, orthopedic specialty has played a major role in establishing legal precedent than any other medical specialty. Why the specialty of orthopedic surgery has been so influential in shaping judicial decision-making? Following hypotheses perhaps can explain this phenomenon:

- *Outcome*: It is easy to know the result in orthopedic surgeries irrespective of the surgeon's skill.

- *Personality*: The facts in Darling case showed that the orthopedic surgeon was elderly and uninsured. Although the hospital was held liable, the surgeon should have known his limitations. This continues to be a major liability issue. Many surgeons may not be aware of new technologies that they were never taught during their residency.
- *Communication*: Poor communication skills can be the reason for lawsuits in orthopedic cases. This is the specialty where there is a need for enhanced communication and dialogue. The patients expect a full and complete recovery. Therefore, one must develop good communication skills, which is mandatory to prevent the ill effects.

WHAT IS ORTHOPEDIC SURGEON'S MALPRACTICE?

Orthopedic surgery involves invasive procedures, which require the utmost care and attention. A deviation from this duty resulting in injuries may leave an injured or aggrieved patient with the right to legal recourse. As with other types of surgeries, orthopedic surgery carries the same risks such as anesthesia issues and nursing staff errors; however, the following may indicate negligence on the part of the orthopedic surgeon:

- Failure to diagnose fractures
- Harmful delay in diagnosis of a health problem
- Improper treatment of fractures
- Improper placement of orthopedic hardware when repairing fractures
- Failure to diagnose nerve impingement
- Misinterpretation of *X-rays, computed tomography (CT) scans,* or *magnetic resonance imaging (MRI) scans*
- Improperly setting a broken bone
- Improper placement of a replacement bone
- Operating on the wrong part of the body
- Leaving surgical instruments, sponges, or towels in the patient
- Failure to recognize postsurgical problems
- Applying a cast too tightly, which can lead to compartment syndrome

Negligence by an orthopedic surgeon could lead to fatal blood clots, nerve damage, spine damage, hip or other joint problems, blood vessel damage, infection or sepsis, motor function loss in hands and other extremities, and decreased mobility. Failed or incorrect surgeries could compromise future revisions.

Common causes of litigation in orthopedics include femur fracture and complications, meniscal injuries, spinal stenosis surgery, knee arthroplasty, operating on wrong site, and lack of communication.

Apart from these specific issues, the following are a few common issues that are important for each branch of medicine. As the numbers of litigation are more in orthopedics they need special mention from orthopedic point of view.

The issues are patient–physician communication, documentation, and informed consent.

Patient–Physician Communication

When surveyed, patients and colleagues describe orthopedic surgeons as *"high tech but low touch".* In the United States of America (USA) and other advanced countries, there is more of a trend for Internet-based communication with orthopedic surgeons. It also helps to improve patient satisfaction and also allows the provider to demonstrate empathy, concern, and humanism. That gives them a sense of security and peace of mind. But the tendency of patients to come to the surgeon with a preconceived treatment choice poses many vexing legal issues. Overall, orthopedic surgeons are described as having poor communication skills and empathy for their patients. As communication issues are the number one cause of medical litigation, this is an area where orthopedic surgeons need to improve.

Learning communication skills allows the orthopedicians to build trust, promote healing, and ultimately improve outcomes. Interestingly, not only do successful encounters improve patient outcomes they have also been shown to improve professional satisfaction. It also leads to professional respect among the physician's peers. Finally, interviews with patients who have filed malpractice suits against their physicians often cite poor communication and lack of empathy as a factor in pursuing legal action.

The American Academy of Orthopedic Surgeons (AAOS) urges orthopedic surgeons to use patient-focused communication skills during their direct patient encounters. These include:

- Sitting down during patient encounters
- Developing an understanding of the patient as an individual, not as a disease or a musculoskeletal condition
- Showing empathy and respect
- Listening attentively and creating a partnership
- Eliciting concerns and calming fears
- Answering questions honestly
- Informing and educating patients about treatment options and the course of care
- Involving patients in decisions concerning their medical care
- Demonstrating sensitivity to patients' cultural and ethnic diversity

When time counts, it is the quality, and not necessarily the quantity of physician–patient communication, that is vital. The patient often measures quality by how well the specialist listens, validates his or her musculoskeletal complaint, and acknowledges concerns. Quality is also measured by the skill by which he/she explains the diagnosis and treatment options, and how well the physician involves the patient in decisions concerning his or her care. These factors play an important part in the way patients perceive, recall, and evaluate their visits with the physician.

In order to prevent litigation, the orthopedic surgeon should avoid:

- Using terms such as "cure" if no cure truly exists
- Using terms such as "painless" or "bloodless" to describe surgery
- Overstating credentials such as "board certified in joint replacement", if no such qualification exists
- Using terms such as "world-renowned"

The AAOS believes that orthopedic surgeons must place an emphasis on good communication with patients and the quality of the interaction, especially when time is limited.

Documentation

Documentation of the consent process is critically important in Orthopedic specialty. Institutional consent forms are made available to allow patients to verify with their witnessed signature that they have been fully informed and agree to the proposed treatment procedure. The surgeon should document the complete informed consent process with a comprehensive note in the patient's medical record. Finally, the note should report that the patient (guardian) wishes to proceed with the recommended treatment.

The World Health Organization (WHO) and the AAOS recommend that the surgeon verify the correct surgical site with the patient. This site should be "signed" (usually with the surgeon's initials) and witnessed by the patient prior to the patient being brought into the operating room. The surgeon should be familiar with national and institutional regulations requiring permission for observers in the operating room. Surgeons should also obtain specific consent for intraoperative medical photography for the purpose of documenting the patient's condition.

Informed Consent

Orthopedic surgeons routinely obtain informed consent prior to surgery. Nowadays, online sources provide patients with nearly unlimited access to information about treatment choices. Many patients consult the internet about their symptoms. This results in a preconceived idea of which treatment choices are most beneficial prior to consulting with a surgeon. While there is merit in informed decision-making, the internet has eliminated some of the "magical mysteries" of medicine that may have a positive impact on patient outcomes.

Some implants have inherent problems with their design leading to an increased failure rate, metallosis, infection, dislocation, immobility, and an increased cancer risk. Some implant recipients who experienced pain, swelling, nerve, muscle and bone damage, or blood poisoning can sue claiming the product design was defective. All these things should be discussed at length beforehand in order to make them aware about the forthcoming complications, if any. In order to minimize these, the orthopedic surgeon should adopt the practice of proper patient selection and use standard quality of implants.

Any adult patient who is capable to make a decision has the legal right to refuse care, even if this refusal may ultimately result in the loss of a limb or death. Surgeons may be able to decrease the risk of a malpractice claim by obtaining informed consent in their offices, rather than in the preoperative holding area, and by documenting the informed consent discussion within their dictated office or operative notes.

Minors

Minors are not legally permitted to consent to surgery. Despite this, it is well recognized that children should actively participate in the discussions related to their healthcare. The degree of involvement will depend on the age of the child and his or her individual capacity to understand the discussion. In 1994, the American Academy of Pediatrics, Committee on Bioethics released a position statement entitled "Informed Consent, Parental Permission and Assent in Pediatric Practice". A 16-year-old with normal capacity scheduled for surgery for idiopathic scoliosis should actively participate in the discussion and assent to the procedure. Many physicians actually have the adolescent child and the guardian both sign the informed consent.

One of the additional protections provided by the law to minors is their right to receive limb- or life-saving treatment even when this treatment is refused by the guardian. Thus, the surgeon may provide, e.g., a blood transfusion to the child of parents who refuse this treatment, if he or she believes that the child's life is at risk without the transfusion. The surgeon should be familiar with the institutional and legal processes to be followed when providing limb- or life-saving treatment to a child against the wishes of the child's parent. Because the conditions for which minors are emancipated vary from state to state, orthopedic surgeons should familiarize themselves with the specific requirements of the states and institutions in which they practice.

The AAOS urges orthopedic surgeons to provide information and education to their patients about treatment alternatives and the course of care, especially expectations for surgical outcomes. Discussing the risks of surgery and possible complications in a kind and compassionate manner, can create realistic expectations on the part of the patient, increase patient satisfaction, and minimize the risk of malpractice claims.

PHYSICIAN ERRORS

Unlike other branches of medicine, orthopedics is more likely to have communication errors leading to wrong-site surgeries, medication errors, diagnostic delays, or loss of follow-up. Wrong-site surgery can be very well prevented by involving the patient in identifying the correct site, following fixed protocol for the patient's preoperative preparation, verifying the correct procedure, and accepting self responsibility, but not blame. Any surgical intervention is a team work and the surgeon is the most important team member in reducing complications when using a surgical checklist and "time-out".

In addition to these common issues, orthopedic surgeons may get caught in the clutches of law due to some specific specialty-related issues as follows:

Issues Related to Fracture and Spine

Fractured Femur

Sanjay Verma versus Janpriya Accident and Fracture Hospital, 2001 (3) CPR 2

In this case, the complainant had suffered a fracture in the neck of the femur and was operated. Even after operation, he had persistent pain and fever for which he consulted another doctor who performed a second operation to remove Richard Plate fixed by the first, and the neck of the femur bone was removed. The complainant claimed compensation on account of shortening of leg by 3.5 "due to the negligence of the doctor. It was observed that in spite of taking all preoperative and postoperative precautions by the first doctor, the patient developed an infection in the wound." The only difference that the complainant's witnesses/doctors stated was that some strong antibiotic must have been given. The doctor was not held negligent by the court as a mere difference of opinion about treatment by doctors may not amount to negligence.

Fractured Elbow

Ashok Kumar versus Ms Agadi Nursing Home, 1995 (1) CPR 517

An 8-year-old boy suffered a fracture of the hand. The respondent fixed the fracture and plastered the hand. It was alleged that the pain continued and there was no improvement. On the contrary, he developed a deformity. The medical testimony proved that the fracture was corrected properly and then the plaster was put. The exact cause for deformity can not be definitely said. Admittedly the boy had taken physiotherapy treatment elsewhere. It was held that the deformity, if any, in the left elbow of the minor boy was due to the negligence of the minor in tampering with the plaster and giving movement to the fractured elbow without waiting for the full removal of the plaster.

Fracture Fixing

Sachin Aggarwal versus Dr Ashok Arora, (1993) 1 CPJ 113

In this case, the doctor fixed the femur fracture of a student with "INOR" quality of dynamic compression plating. Subsequently, the boy suffered another fracture due to a fall. It was alleged that the doctor was negligent. But it was established that the doctor followed the procedure correctly, and as the children in this age group keep on growing, the plate had been fixed on the nongrowing part of the bone. It was also established that the plate would not break itself and could merely loosen. The court held that though consumer agencies should protect patients from malpractices, complaints of careless and unscrupulous patients cannot be entertained. The patient was held negligent and the complaint was dismissed.

MB Gajinkar versus St Martha's Hospital, 1994 (1) CPR 490

The patient had a fall and suffered fracture on his right elbow along with dislocation. It was alleged that due to the negligence of doctors, he could not fully recover from the injury. It was a case of type IV fracture, a serious injury. X-rays revealed subluxated elbow joint. Therefore, under general anesthesia, gentle manipulation of elbow joint was conducted followed by physiotherapy after discharge. Radial head was broken into fragments. So, two fragments were removed during the operation. Expert evidence proved that restricted movement of the elbow was due to: (a) subluxation of the elbow, (b) myositis ossificans, which are the consequences of fracture dislocation of elbow on account of injuries sustained by the complainant. The complaint was dismissed.

Arthroscopy of Knee

SA Qureshi versus Padode Memorial Hospital and Research Centre, 2002 CCJ 98

The patient got his knee joint operated and suffered permanent disability for which the district Medical Board had issued a certificate stating post-traumatic ankylosis—permanent physical impairment to left lower limb is 50%. The doctor's defense was that the arthroscopy method of surgery was fully explained to the patient for which he willingly agreed and also that recovery was out of question. It was contended that the knee was totally unstable prior to the operation and the patient was not able to walk. It was also pleaded that the patient could not prove how the repair of anterior cruciate ligament was necessarily to be done before the repair of posterior cruciate ligament. Disagreeing with this contention, it was observed that a duty is also cast upon the opposite party to prove that there was no negligence on its part. As stated by the Medical Board, post-traumatic ankylosis may not be ruled out to be a postoperative complication. The medical specialties should have at least explained the probable cause for the deformity as quoted in the disability certificate and similarly the doctor could have explained that the disability was not due to any kind of negligence in the performance of operation by him by quoting medical literature. The burden lay on the doctor. The respondent stated that the record of case sheets and operation theatre notes of surgery had been destroyed after 3 years. Admittedly, the surgery took place on 5 February 1995 and complaint was filed on 17 October 1996 while the reply was filed on 8 May 1997. It was the duty of the doctor to preserve the record till the final decision of the court, since he alone knew the facts of operation and the burden of proof lay on him to show that he was not in breach of any duty. Compensation of ₹50,000 was granted.

Slip Disc

Akhil Bhartiya Grahak Panchayat versus Dr Jog Hospital, III (1993) CPJ 1447

In this case, the complainant was a working woman and was suffering from pain in her left leg and waist. She got done her myelography after about a week's treatment by the respondent doctor. Thereafter, she was operated upon for decompression of prolapsed disc in the lumber region. It was alleged that due to the negligence of the surgeon in performing the operation, she could not live a normal life and suffered defect in her leg and pain and claimed compensation to the sum of ₹4 lakh. The allegations were rebutted by the doctor. Finally, it was held that the complainant failed to prove the allegations of negligence on the part of the doctor, and hence the complaint was dismissed. The Maharashtra State Commission observed that the complaint was founded on the ignorance of the complainant about her ailment and was filed on account of mental distress and extreme physical discomfort with a view to find some solace to her sufferings.

Issues Related to Use of Implants

There are many issues related to the use of implants such as:

- The inherent problems associated with metal-on-metal hip systems is with their design, leading to an increased failure rate, metallosis, infection, dislocation, immobility, and an increased cancer risk.
- Serious complications associated with metal-on-metal hip implants include:
  - The implanted device does not stay attached to the bone in the correct position.
  - The bone around the implant breaks.
  - Dislocation of the two parts of the implant
  - Metallosis (metal poisoning)
  - Eroding of the ball and socket components

These complications lead to a second surgery in a large number of patients. To prevent these, firstly, one must have acquired the requisite skill to perform these surgeries. Secondly, before using implants always ensure that they are from standard companies, having requisite certificates/licenses and are procured through official channels/distributors. In case of legal proceedings wherein the quality of the implant is challenged, requesting the manufacturers/distributors for attested copies of the requisite certificates/licenses and producing the same in the court of law is beneficial. In *Vijaya Menon versus BK Thampi*, the patient challenged the quality of implants alleging that the implant used by orthopedic surgeon was of inferior quality. The hospital produced the attested copies of ISO certificate, and the license for manufacturing the orthopedic implants, proving that the implants were nationally and internationally approved. The allegation was obviously rejected by the court. The court has observed that "no liability can be cast upon the hospital who used the certified orthopedic implant for the surgical procedures".

Complications Associated with Hip Replacement Surgeries

Like any other surgery, this surgery also has its share of complications but occur very rarely. Less than 2% cases report problems such as blood clot, infection, or loosening/wearing of joints. Although uncommon, one should discuss the ways to reduce the risks with the patient before the surgery. All these are taken care of by orthopedic surgeon by continuous monitoring, medications, and precautionary measures.

DO'S AND DON'TS FOR AN ORTHOPEDIC SURGEON

The orthopedics is a vulnerable branch from a legal point of view. In order to prevent and defend litigations, there are certain do's and don'ts an orthopedic surgeon needs to follow such as:

Contemplate before Refusing to Refer the Patient to Another Facility

Refusing to refer the patient to another facility must be done with great care and contemplation. The patient/*relatives* may draw adverse inferences from the same. In *Dr SK Gupta versus RR Dobhal (7MLCD a129;j336-September 2014)*, the patient's husband specifically alleged that he had requested the orthopedic surgeon to refer the patient to a higher medical center for total knee replacement but the same was refused.

Discharge Card Should be Patient-Friendly

Like in other branches of medicine, the discharge card should contain all the details about the investigations and treatment given, operative notes in short, and postoperative follow-up advice. Specific postdischarge advice should be clearly explained and mentioned on the discharge card. Whenever a patient is found acting contrary to medical advice, the same must be specifically recorded in the patient's records. In *Rohini Morghade versus Dr AV Sapre (7MLCD a 118;j313-August 2014)*, postsurgery, the orthopedic surgeon had instructed the patient to bed rest with minimum movement, but contrary to this medical advice, found the patient walking with the help of walker when he visited her house. The orthopedic surgeon did specifically raise this aspect in defense. In *Rachel Sumitrarao Salunke versus Bombay Hospital (7MLCD a124;j324-August 2014)*, the patient admittedly did not follow the postsurgery advice given by the orthopedic surgeon to keep the aeroplane splint for 12 weeks and got it removed within 3 weeks on the advice of another doctor. The complaint and allegations of the patient were rejected. Thus, failure or refusal of the patient to follow medical advice is a valuable defense and one should not make a mistake to forget to record the aforesaid.

Before Performing an Operative Intervention, Always Assess the Patient First

Before taking a decision to perform a major elective nonemergency surgery, the surgeon must take into consideration the physical and mental status of the patient and the same must be duly recorded. The necessary preoperative investigations must be done. If required, opinion from relevant specialists must also be obtained. All this should be duly recorded. In *Sheuli Das versus Dr Kanchan Bhattacharya (7MLCD a13;j26-January 2014)*, the patient had obtained an opinion of another doctor, who had opined that the time chosen by orthopedic surgeon for performing total hip replacement surgery was not ideal after taking into account the patient's condition. The orthopedic surgeon was successful in rebutting this allegation as the necessary presurgery investigations were done and the opinion of the relevant specialist was obtained, and only after getting fitness from all the surgery was performed.

Incomplete Diagnosis, Misdiagnosis or Missed Diagnosis

Defending in a court that at least a part of the diagnosis was correct will not rectify the wrong. In *Mrs Savita Suneja versus Dr RS Oberoi (7MLCD a30;j66-February 2014)*, the patient had suffered a *"Monteggia fracture"* (fractured ulna, and dislocation and fracture of the radial head), but the orthopedic surgeon had diagnosed it as comminuted fracture of the ulna. In the court, the misdiagnosis was requested to be justified pointing out that a *Monteggia fracture* variant also includes comminuted fracture of the ulna. The court rejected this defense as an illogical claim, thinking that how even with an incomplete diagnosis, the treatment given to the patient could be complete. The court also observed that there was no explanation for how dislocation of the elbow could have been treated if it was not even diagnosed.

Medical negligence does not depend on the outcome of the treatment/intervention. The only factor that law takes into consideration is whether the medical decisions and actions were appropriate or not. In *Rohini Morghade versus Dr AV Sapre (7MLCD a118;j313-August 2014), the* orthopedic surgeon had performed two unsuccessful surgeries and the third surgery performed by another orthopedic surgeon was successful. The patient put this as proof of negligence, but court rejected this. Law accepts that the treatment, course of action, or the decision to intervene may change with doctors/hospitals.

Law accepts all such variations provided each one of them should be as per the accepted medical practice. In the above case, patient alleged that suprapatellar (SP) nailing technique was obsolete. The court rejected this observing that "the best method of treatment.... shall vary from one hospital to another". Medical negligence could be broadly divided into two parts: An improper decision/diagnosis/course of action and/or improper implementation of an otherwise proper decision/diagnosis/course of action. The court's decision in *Dr G Swaminathan versus G Rajendran (7MLCd a145;j385-October 2014)* very well explains this. The court held that "the choice of the line of treatment of the orthopedic surgeons can not be faulted for choosing the plate and screw method and not external fixation method. But having chosen the line of treatment, they failed to do it properly".

Proceeding by a Wrong Method/Preference

Courts generally do not interfere with the medical decisions unless the same is palpably wrong or done for some dishonest purpose. The court asks doctors to issue a discharge card to every hospitalized patient. The discharge card must have a brief summary of treatment, precautions to be taken, and instructions for follow-up. If a patient insists on discharge or transfer to another hospital contrary to medical advice, a proper "discharge against medical advice declaration" must be taken from the patient clearly explaining the risks of such a step. Refusal of the patient to perform or follow medical advice should be specifically noted in the medical records. Indian courts follow the English law which is proprofessional. That means in all cases of medical negligence, the patient has to prove in the court of law that the doctor was negligent. The patient has to make reports to collect medical records from the doctor/hospital. The doctor/hospitals were not bound to produce medical records in court or give copies thereof to the patient on their own. If a hospitalized patient wants to seek a second opinion, then doctor/hospital should cooperate in getting that. The court delivers its judgments on the basis of accepted medical practice, which includes knowledge of medical practice and the procedure available at the time of the operation and not on the date of trial. The following case will explain all these issues.

Dr Prakash M Bhandari versus Venkati Narhari Watamwar 8MLCD (j19): In this case, the patient met an accident and sustained a fracture of the right tibia/fibula and was admitted to the hospital where he underwent X-ray. A closed reduction under C-arm was performed with a plaster cast applied under general anesthesia. A senior orthopedic surgeon and a plastic surgeon were consulted during hospitalization. About 3 weeks later, the patient was transferred to another hospital in an ambulance, about 400 km away, where the patient's right leg was amputated. The patient's allegations of negligence were as follows:

- The doctor should not have applied plaster in the first place as there was swelling and the next day after the plaster was slit opened, fasciotomy, which was indicated, ought to have been performed.
- The orthopedic surgeon failed to put a round plaster during transfer so as to prevent infection in transit which led to complications. The orthopedic surgeon gave only the discharge card and not the complete medical records.

Doctor's Defense

- It was pointed out that the orthopedic surgeon had advised an anti-inflammatory drug for reduction and avoidance of swelling. But on postoperative day when he observed that the swelling continued, the plaster cast was immediately slit open which improved the circulation to distal limb.
- It was stated that the patient and his relatives forced the doctor to discharge and refer the patient to a hospital about 400 km away.
- It was also pointed out that as per the wish of the patient, a senior orthopedic surgeon from another city was called, who examined the patient, approved the line of treatment, and in addition advised skeleton traction which was given.
- A senior plastic surgeon from another city was called on the patient's request, who advised and was even ready to perform *"a cross-leg flap"*, but the patient refused and decided to shift to the other hospital.

Findings of the Court

The court held that the fasciotomy was not needed as the pulsation was regained as soon as the plaster cast was slit open by the orthopedic surgeon. The doctor can not be held negligent even if he preferred the wrong method of treatment by applying plaster cast instead of fasciotomy. It also can not be inferred that his conduct fell below the standards of a reasonably competent practitioner. The court also held that it is for the patient to make efforts to collect medical records and produce them in the court, which he failed to do. The patient's allegation regarding medical records was meritless as a "discharge card giving brief of summary of treatment was issued".

The court drew adverse inference against the patient for not following the advice given by the plastic surgeon and insistence for discharge and transfer. Hence, the orthopedic surgeon was not held negligent.

The general principles of safe medical practice as in other *specialties* also hold true in orthopedic practice.

The following cases will explain what one must do and not do to maintain standards of orthopedic practice:

- In *Satyapal Jain versus Mohan [I (2008) CPJ 176]*, a case of fractured hand, orthopedic surgeon applied plaster and pain persisted even after that. For that matter, another operation was done. It was alleged that there was monetary burden along with physical suffering. The court awarded compensation for the said deficiency of not advising X-ray before replastering.

- In another *Ms Soni Kumari versus Dr N Narain [I (03) CPJ 196]*, it was alleged that there was a loss of sensation due to tight plaster along with infection, which resulted in the amputation of the limb. The defense was that the complainant left after first aid and the plaster was not applied. The burden of proof was on the patient, which she could not prove. No negligence was held.
- In *Parminder Singh versus General Hospital [II (05) CPJ 205]*, the court delivered the judgment in favor of doctor accepting that the management skills may differ from one doctor to another and there can be more than one treatment modality. In this case, the expert who managed subsequently stated that a reasonable degree of skill was used by the former orthopedic surgeon who died during pendency of the case. Once again onus of proving negligence was totally on a person who set up the case. After the death of the doctor, the General hospital was only remaining party. The complainant failed to prove negligence, so the complaint was rightly dismissed.
- In *KS Sridhar versus Rajkumar [I (07) CPJ 362]*, a 40-year-old patient with a *fractured* hip joint was advised to undergo joint replacement surgery. Usually, replacement is advised in age group between 50 and 55 years and such a procedure may further lead to complications. Therefore, deficiency and negligence were proved.
- In *United India Ins versus Ghisaram [I (10) CPJ 612]*, a case of *fractured* hand, it was alleged that plate/bolt were fixed improperly and steel rod not inserted leading to malunion. The patient then changed the doctor. The court came to the conclusion that the decision of fixing the plates was not wrong and the doctor was qualified and experienced having deep knowledge of the subject. No doctor can undertake a guarantee of cure. The doctor cannot be held liable simply for not exercising better method. Only ₹25,000 were awarded on humanitarian grounds.
- In *Dr S Mohan versus S Singh [I (2008) CPJ 458 NC]*, an alleged case of *fracture* united with angulation and leg shortening, it was contended that the fracture united properly but got bent subsequently and that the petitioner adopted for traction as surgery was refused by patient. But the documents *"advised surgery but refused"* were not genuine. The court also found that the petitioner tried to conceal the fact of leg shortening. This act of petitioner is a violation of professional ethics, and therefore order was upheld.
- In *Jagbir Singh versus S Sabharwal [I (10) CPJ 375]*, a case of postfracture shortening of leg, the allegation was that the shortening was due to a wrong medicine. It was defended that it was not due to a wrong medicine but the result of nature of fracture. The complainant was not present for follow-up and removal of plaster as was advised and failed to produce an expert witness. No negligence was held.
- In *VM Rao versus Miot Hospital [I (08) CPJ 179 (NC)]*, a hip replacement case, there was an allegation regarding the use of longer screws and that the cup was fixed vertically instead of 45°. The defense was that the surgery was performed 10 years back and the screw did not damage any organ till the hearing of case. The court observed that snapping of wire is an accepted complication and fixing in a vertical direction is the surgeon's decision. No expert evidence was brought by the complainant. No negligence was held.
- In *R Sahu versus Akhilesh Dubey (I (10) CPJ 3)* case, a rod was implanted. The bone being loose, no proper union could take place and the pain persisted. A second surgery was performed by another doctor. There was a possibility of infection at the fracture site, which

was deliberately concealed by the patient. The court observed that before 6 months nonunion cannot be commented. Therefore, no negligence was proved.

- In *Shaqeel Quireshi versus Dr AK Dubey [I (10) CPJ 600]* case, it was alleged that the defect persisted due to a delay in operating upon the fracture in neck femur and because of not doing a *second* operation. The defense was that fracture in neck femur sometimes takes months and there is no necessity for *second* operation. The court observed that the orthopedic surgeon failed to diagnose fractured neck properly and he is also negligent in not doing a *second* operation.
- In *BN Gurudev versus N Ramanna [I (2008) CPJ 84 (NC)]* case, leg got fractured in an accident. There was delay in admission. X-ray was taken followed by arteriogram. The orthopedic surgeon found no possibility of reviving leg gangrene. A team of doctors unanimously decided on amputation. It was alleged that the surgery was done without consent. Denial by patient not accepted as consent was given by wife. The defense was that the operation of amputation was done as an emergency procedure to save the life of the patient. The complainant was given a prosthetic leg. No negligence was held.
- In *Dr PS Grewal versus CS Chawla [I (2007) CPJ 125 (NC)]*, a patient underwent surgery for shoulder dislocation. Pain still persisted. The orthopedic surgeon had followed standard operative procedure. However, it did not work due to axillary nerve damage. Various experts opined that it is due to accident and not due to surgery. Thus, negligence was not proved. But the court observed that the records were not meticulously maintained. The court also guided the medical fraternity to make the records available to the patients as a matter of right and in this case awarded ₹10,000 costs for the said deficiency.
- In *Jangeer Singh versus Kochar Hospital [II (05) CPJ 223]*, a case of accident, after treatment, the medical certificate was denied. The court opined that the patient cannot be deprived from getting a certificate and failure to issue a certificate is taken as a deficiency in service.
- In *Ashthana versus Sh Ramsingh Hospital [I (09) CPJ 132]*, a patient requested for bedpan but the attendant refused. Patient slipped due to slippery entrance and got tibia/fibula fracture. The administrative deficiency was proved and compensation was awarded. The patient was awarded additional compensation as the fractured bone not plastered properly. The patient needed compensation for future treatment.
- In *Sarangpani versus Bones/Joint Clinic [I (2008) CPJ 488 NC]*, a patient had fracture in neck femur which did not improve even after surgery. Deficiency allowed by district forum. State commission said there can be different causes of nonunion. Affidavit in support was filed by an MBBS and not by an orthopedic surgeon. No expert opinion was available to counter the treating doctor. No negligence was held.

CONCLUSION

All these judgments highlight the importance of having knowledge about the ethics and legalities governing the specialty, which in turn allow the specialist to practice safely to lessen the pain and suffering. This also leads to building up the bond of trust, which ultimately helps to improve doctor–patient relationship.

KEY LEARNING POINTS

- Skillful management of orthopedic problems requires knowledge, experience, and a standard treatment protocol; deficiency or negligence in which can lead to deformities and subsequent litigations.
- In a charitable corporation, the hospital board of trustees is duty-bound to assure the competency, qualifications, and proficiency of each and every staff in the hospital.
- Orthopedic specialty has played a major role in developing the doctrine of informed consent.
- Communication skills can help to prevent litigation in case of residual deformity.
- Proper documentation, unlike other specialties, can be assured to win defense in the orthopedic field.
- Proper patient selection and use of standard-quality implants can protect a orthopedic surgeon from malpractice claims.
- Surgical checklist should be strictly followed and physician errors should be avoided by following standard practice protocol.
- Refusal to surgery should be properly documented.

BIBLIOGRAPHY

1. Bajpai M, Srinivasan B (Eds). Medicolegal year book 2015. Institute of Medicine and Law publication. Mumbai: Wolters Kluwer Health/Medknow; 2015. pp. 15-16, 133, 162-3, 259-65.
2. Bal BS, Lawrence H, Brenner JD. Healio. (2008). Malpractice law evolved via orthopedics. [online] Available from https://www.healio.com/news/orthopedics/20120325/malpractice-law-evolved-via-orthopedics [Last accessed May 2024].
3. Bhattacharyya T, Yeon H, Harris MB. The medical-legal aspects of informed consent in Orthopedic surgery. J Bone Joint Surg Am. 2005;87(11):2395-400.
4. Drugwatch. (2024). Hip Replacement. [Online] Available from https://www.drugwatch.com/depuy-hip/replacement.php [Last accessed May, 2024].
5. Gurunanak Institute of Professional Studies. Proceeding by a wrong method/preference is not necessarily negligence in medical law cases for doctors. Institute of Medicine and Law Publication. 2015;(8):1-16.
6. Informed consent, parental permision, and assent in pediatric practice. Committee on Bioethics, American Academy, of Pediatrics. Pediatrics. 1995;95(2):314-7.
7. Kaushal AK. In: Arora M (Ed). Medical Negligence and Legal Remedies, 3rd edition. New Delhi: Universal Law Publishing; 2004. pp. 127-201.
8. Levinson W, Roter DL, Mullooly JP, Dull VT, Frankel RM. Physician-patient communication. The relationship with malpractice claims among primary care physicians and surgeons. JAMA. 1997:277(7);553-9.
9. Moore DW. (2022). Orthobullets. Legal Considerations in Orthopaedic Practice. [online] Available from http://www.orthobullets.com/basic-science/9074/legaland-ethics [Last accessed May, 2024].
10. Morgan and Morgan. (2024). Orthopedic Malpractice. [online] Available from http://www.forthepeople.com/medical-malpracticeattorney/orthopedic-injury/. [Last accessed May, 2024].
11. Schattner A. The silent dimension: Expressing humanism in each medical encounter. Arch Intern Med. 2009;169:(12)1095-99.
12. Tongue J, Epps HR, Forese L. Communication skills for patient-centered care; research-based, easily learned techniques for medical interviews that benefit Orthopedic surgeons and their patients. J Bone and Joint Surg Am. 2005;87:652-8.

23

CHAPTER

Medicolegal Issues in Anesthesia

Shivakumar F Kumbar

INTRODUCTION

Anesthesiology is a specialized branch of medical speciality wherein anesthesiologists plays very vital role in surgical interventions and smooth recovery of patient. He also acts as acute physician, pain specialist, intensivist, active role in operation theater, labor analgesia, CPR training, emergency medicine, etc. Over the last two decades, this profession is recognized as most wanted speciality with advent of sophisticated monitoring gadgets and specialized skill of anesthesiologists. He is dedicated to deliver his services just like pilot. With the advancement of the technology, Nowadays, it has become safer for all surgical procedures.

ETHICAL ISSUES

Anesthesiologists are confronted with many ethical, medical, legal, social issues in their day-to-day practice. Anesthesiologists are highly regulated by ethical standards, legal rules and regulations in order to achieve ethical practice. The Indian Society of Anesthesiologists (ISA) and the American Society of Anesthesiologists (ASA) have come up with guidelines for ethical practice. The basic principles are:

Basic Principles of Medical Ethics

- *Nonmalfeasance*: This is the doctrine of—"do no harm" to their patients
- *Autonomy*: The patient can make fully informed decisions about his own health care
- *Justice*: Anesthesiologists should be fare when providing their service to surgical patients.
- *Beneficence*: This requires anesthesiologists to—"do good" for the patient in every situation.

Ethical Issues

Anesthesiologists invariably use sophisticated machines and gadgets in many procedures which may result dehumanisation of the patient care which may result ethical dilemma.

Preoperative Issues

Effective communication is necessary to establish good rapport with the patient. And also, he should know what is to be explained to the patient in order to get—informed real consent from the patient. Surgeon may not agree with the anesthesiologists who explain all the risks related to the anesthesia and surgery as patient would refuse for surgery. In such cases, anesthesiologists shall be under dilemma what to put forth to the surgeon or patient. Balancing the ethical issues with truthfulness toward the patient and maintaining harmony with the surgeon plays a vital role. Here skilful interaction should be made without having a direct conflict with the surgeon, not compromising the safety of the patient.

Intraoperative Issues

Anesthesiologists should be very diplomatic, assertive and avoid domination by other professionals during patient care.

POSTOPERATIVE PERIOD

Anesthesiologists has greater responsibilities in the postoperative care. He should not rely on the surgeon for the postoperative care and should not delegate to the juniors. If any complications occur, he shall be liable for delegating the postoperative care to the juniors.

Role of Consent

In view of the CPA 2019 and IMC guidelines (NMC), informed written consent must be obtained before performing any anesthetic procedure and it should be a separate consent. It includes proper discussions, risks involved, alternative procedures which shall be brought to the notice of the patient wherein he can take independent decision regarding anesthesia and the procedures. The consent should be comprehensive, should be in the vernacular language, understandable to the patient. Patient should not be influenced by undue pressure or influence, coercion while giving the consent. Patient should not be under the influence of drug, alcohol, and should be above 18 years as per the Indian Evidence Act to give the valid informed consent.

Blanket Consent

Here the patient has been asked to sign a printed format in which consent is taken in a mechanical fashion to say that—Consent is given for any type of procedure, without specifying any treatment and also under any type of anesthesia. This is legally invalid and should be avoided.

Withdrawal Consent

Here the patient can withdraw his/her consent at any time. It is unlawful to continue treatment once he withdraws the consent and it must be recorded with date and time, so that, anesthesiologist is not held responsible for any deterioration in the patient condition due to delay in treatment for want of consent.

High-risk Consent (Practical Point of View)

Surgical patient where the probable mortality is more than 5% or twice the risk of population undergoing the same procedure. Surgical patients for whom the probable mortality is greater than 20%, should be considered as—extremely high-risk patients.

IMPORTANCE OF RECORD

The Indian Society of Anesthesiologists guidelines in India provide guidelines on how to maintain good anesthesia records which can play a vital role in defending the medico legal cases. Anesthesiologist should follow the following points while record keeping:

- Anesthesia - regional/block—name of the block, concentration, volume, etc.
- General anesthesia—premedication, induction agent, relaxation, etc.
- Airway management device
- Maintenance of anesthesia
- Ventilation technique
- Hemodynamic parameters settings
- Postoperative orders

DEATH IN THE OPERATION THEATER

Anesthesiologists are likely to come across such situations many times, which is very stressful and cause for burn out syndrome. If anesthesiologist knows the cause of death, he can always declare and certify the cause of death. If the cause of death is not known or death is unexpected following steps can be taken:

- If the cause of death is sure, death certificate can be given.
- Complete documentation
- Do not clear the OT, preserve all ampoules used during the procedure
- Death should be communicated to their relatives in a sympathetic and sensitive manner.
- If the cause of death is not known—inform the Police.

JUDICIAL BINDINGS ON ANESTHESIOLOGISTS

Anesthesiologists shall come under purview of CPA 2019, criminal procedures, respective medical councils, administrative authorities, human rights commission, and Anesthesiologists need to be very vigilant in their professional works.

CONSUMER PROTECTION ACT—2019 (CPA 2019)

The doctor-patient relationship, which forms the corner stone of healthcare, has swung from the idealization of doctors to their devaluation. Whatever said and done—medical professionals come under the purview of CPA 2019. The relationship between doctor and patient is contact for service. There is no relationship of master and servant between the doctor and patient. This is very well said by S/C in VP Shanta v/s IMA.

Pecuniary Jurisdiction

It would depend on the consideration paid by the patient to the doctor or toward the hospital and not compensation claimed. It refers to the amount of money paid by the patient to obtain the services provided by the doctor. Here district commission—consideration paid up to Rs. 50 lakh, State commission—consideration paid from ₹50 lakhs to 2 crore, national commission—consideration paid >2 crore.

Place

Patient can file the complaint either at a place where cause of action has taken place (treatment), either at a place where the patient resides or works for gain.

Mediation Cell

It is an ADR mechanism. Patients and anesthesiologists settled their dispute through the mediation cell, which operates at district, state, national commission levels. Once the settlement is mutually agreed upon, no appeal is allowed. Medical negligence that results in grievous hurt or death is excluded from the scope of mediation.

Appeal

If the anesthesiologist wants to appeal to the higher commission, he should deposit 50% of the awarded compensation at the lower court.

Compensation

There is no provision in the Act, for the capping of the compensation. It means, complainant can claim any amount of compensation, depending upon the consideration paid at the respective jurisdiction.

PREANESTHETIC EVALUATION AND FITNESS FOR SURGERY

The preanesthetic evaluation (PAE) is very important for anesthesiologist. In the following case, it has been explained by the State commission. Fitness for surgery is actually misnomer. Anesthesiologist takes the opinion of the physicians or cardiologists depending upon the pre-existing diseases of the patient and ask for the optimization of the conditions wherein patient can withstand anesthetic and surgical procedures.

Case

Aruna ben Kotari v/s Navadeep clinic and ors. - SCDRC - 1993 Gujarat. Here patient was seen by the cardiologist for the fitness for the surgery and he gave opinion that patient is fit for the proposed surgery, even though BP was 150/100 mm Hg and ECG was showing ST - T changes in AL leads. Anesthesiologist induced the patient for the orthopedic procedure and intraoperatively patient had cardiac arrest and died. Cardiologist certified cause of death without subjecting for PM. The court held that—why was PM not done? It is no excuse that patient's relatives refused for the PM and signed for the same. Why cardiologist certified death certificate, who himself was not present in the OT? Why did the anesthesiologist rely on the cardiologist's opinion and since it was elective case, why was the patient not investigated further. Anesthesiologist should have seen for the availability of defibrillator before starting the procedure and a compensation of ₹4.15 lakh was awarded which was to be shared by anesthesiologist - 60%, surgeon - 30%, cardiologist - 10%.

New BNS Act 2024 (Bharatiya Nyaya Sanhita)

Whoever causes death of any person by doing any rash or negligent act not amounting to culpable homicide shall be punished with imprisonment of either description for a term which may extent to 5 years and shall also be liable to a fine. And if such act is done by RMP (registered medical practitioner) who is registered under the NMC and respective state medical councils, while performing medical performance shall be imprisoned for a term which may extent to 2 years and shall also be liable to a fine. Under the current law—both the imprisonment and fine are mandatory. BNS section - 117 and 124—there is ambiguous language which can be misinterpreted and misused by the Police. Any act which causes permanent damage, deformity, or vegetative state is punishable with rigorous imprisonment for 10 years, which may extent to life imprisonment. A permanent vegetative state may occur at any time after the patient is revived following the cardiac arrest in the OT or ICU or perioperative period. This is draconian for the anesthesiologist.

Transfer of the patient to the higher or tertiary care center. Many times anesthesiologists are requested to assist in the transfer of the patient to a higher center for various reasons reasons. There are legal hurdles if the proper care is not taken by the anesthesiologist during the transferring.

■ Case: (Mr Shakil Mohammad Vailkhan vs Miss Dr Perin Irani – SCDRC – MS 1999)

In this case, a patient underwent cesarean section and intraoperatively patient had desaturation which was warned by the surgeon to the anesthesiologist. Ultimately, patient was to be shifted to a tertiary care hospital in an ambulance. Anesthesiologist did not accompany the patient in the ambulance, but instead followed the ambulance in his own car. By the time patient reached the hospital, they had developed hypoxic encephalopathy and remained in a vegetative state. The court held that it was the responsibility of the anesthesiologist to accompany the patient in the ambulance—professionally, ethically, and legally. The anesthesiologist was held negligent and asked to pay ₹4.1 lakh as compensation.

Intraoperative Issues

Anesthesiologist are to be very careful in monitoring throughout the surgical procedure and should be very vigilant. In Texas - Court said - Treat, but do not tweet—A 60-year-old lady who underwent low risk cardiac procedure died intra-operatively. Here anesthesiologist did not notice fall in the SPO_2 for 15-20 minutes and ultimately patient had de-saturation and died. It was held that anesthesiologist was on his iPod throughout the procedure and surgeon testified that anesthesiologist did not notice dangerous fall in the SPO_2 which led to the death of the patient.

Medication Errors in Anesthesia

This is very common and may lead to morbidity and mortality. So, anesthesiologist needs to be very vigilant and should use standardized color coding labelling, standardized drug preparations, familiar with the bar code scanner and double checking shall prevent the ongoing mishaps.

Medical Indemnity

Anesthesiologist should not practice without the medical indemnity cover. He should be indemnified at least ₹1 crore. in the ratio of AOA:AOY (any one accident:any one year).

Case: (Master PM Ashwin vs Manipal Hospital, Bangalore)

A 65-day-old child underwent a hernia operation and developed hypothermia during the procedure. A warm water bag, duly wrapped in sterile towel, was kept under the child legs. Severe burns occurred on both the legs. It was held that surgeon and the anesthesiologist were held negligent, applying - Doctrine of *res ipsa loquitur*, and they were awarded compensation of ₹5 lakhs to be paid by the surgeon, anesthesiologist and hospital jointly and severally.

BIBLIOGRAPHY

1. Parakh SC. Legal aspects of anaesthesia practice. Indian J Anaesth. 2008.
2. Shenoy GN, Shenoy GG. Anaesthesiology and Law of Medical Negligence, Bombay Ritanjan Publications; 2002. pp. 22-4.
3. Singh J. Medical negligence and compensation. Jaipur; Bharat Law Publications; 2007. p. 105.
4. Thomas J. Medical records and issues in negligence. Indian J Urol. 2009.

24

CHAPTER

Medicolegal Issues in Ophthalmology

Purendra Bhasin, Priyamvada Bhasin

INTRODUCTION

No branch of the allopathic system of therapy has remained untouched by the scientific and technical developments in the recent years and ophthalmology is no exception to it. The ophthalmic diseases that were earlier considered incurable have now become curable with the induction of sophisticated types of equipment such as laser, phacoemulsification, angiography, optical coherence tomography (OCT), etc. These equipment help the ophthalmologists to diagnose the disease and provide better and effective treatment. Since the pretreatment diagnosis (involving various tests and examinations) and the treatment thereafter involve a lot of money, the patients expect better results with improved visual outcomes within a short time and without any physical harm. Since the treatment outcome depends on the quality of the treatment and the biological response of the patient, the results vary from patient to patient.

Among all ophthalmic surgeries, cataract surgeries have a major share of about 70%. These surgeries with intraocular lens (IOL) implantation have been successful and have given excellent visual recovery to cataract patients. These surgeries are performed in private and government hospitals and eye camps organized by various charitable hospitals on a mass scale. The patients have other surgical and medical options too for their vitreoretinal (VR) conditions, which require the latest types of equipment and surgical skills. Sometimes, the patients do not realize the fact that their other medical problems besides cataracts, namely diabetic retinopathy, maculopathy, age-related macular degeneration (ARMD), retinal detachments, vitreous hemorrhages, glaucoma, etc., can adversely affect the surgical outcome.

The poor results arising out of incomplete preoperative workup and/or negligence in the postoperative care or showing the cold shoulder to the genuine grievances of the patients may sometimes result in unwanted and undesirable litigations.

The Courts of Law have, by and large, termed medical services the noblest of all services and the profession as being life-saving but risky, requiring high degree of intellectual and manual skill; thus, there is a need to protect the medical professionals from being prosecuted in frivolous and unjust litigations filed against them for medical negligence. The Honorable Supreme Court has, therefore, rightly held that a surgeon, plagued by the fear of legal repercussions, is unable to carry out a successful operation with trembling hands and a hesitant physician, fearing criminal prosecution, may struggle to administer the appropriate medication dosage to a patient.

With the winds of globalization, every profession has become commercialized and the medical profession, to some extent, has no longer been an exception to it. It is true that some doctors are going astray for their selfish ends and making money by adopting unfair and unethical ways, forgetting the solemn oath they had taken at the time of entering this noble profession. The Consumer Protection Act of 1986 was enacted with the objective of giving speedy justice. The erring and negligent medical professionals practicing allopathy, homeopathy, and naturopathy are liable to be prosecuted under this Act.

NEW LEGISLATIONS

Governing Body for Medical Practice

The medical profession is now regulated by the National Medical Commission (NMC), the new regulatory body replacing the Medical Council of India (MCI) through the National Commission Act, 2019 (Act 30 of 2019). Medical ethics, registration, and grievance redressal now come under the purview of NMC.

Eye Donation and Retrieval

Earlier, the Transplantation of Human Organs Act of 1994 mandated that corneal tissue retrieval was to be done by a registered medical practitioner (RMP) only. An amendment passed in 2014 stated that the cornea is to be considered as a tissue and not as an organ, which in turn authorized trained technicians to harvest it during enucleation. Also, consent for eye donation has now been extended to include more relatives as legal next of kin.

NEGLIGENCE

Malpractice and Criminal Negligence

Professional negligence by act or omission by a health care provider is called medical malpractice in which the care provided deviates from accepted standards of practice prevalent in the medical community, resulting in harm to the patient. On the other hand, criminal negligence involves a doctor being subject to legal action under criminal law for failing to perform an action that no competent and ordinarily sensible medical professional would carry out or fail to do.

Standard of Care

The term "standard of care" is linked to medical negligence and therefore, it is imperative to understand its meaning. It means an ordinary competent person exercising ordinary skills in that profession. Hospitals are held to the same standard of care as individual physicians, but there is a distinction in the liability framework. While individual physicians bear personal liability, hospitals face corporate liability, being accountable and responsible for any negligence on the part of their staff.

The same standard of care applies to hospitals as to individual physicians with the difference that the liability of hospitals is the corporate liability and the hospital is accountable and responsible for any act of negligence of its staff.

Whether Error of Judgment Amounts to Negligence

To err is human and in several cases, the courts have also held that no human being is perfect. Even the most eminent specialist is likely to be at fault in diagnosing the disease and therefore, error in the judgment in this profession is a common phenomenon. As such, an error of judgment does not and should not amount to an act of negligence. Whether any medical practitioner is guilty of negligence depends on the nature of the error coupled with his duties toward a patient.

Duties to be Discharged by the Doctor

The Honorable Apex Court in a case *AS Mittal and Ors vs. State of UP* laid down primary duties to be discharged by a medical practitioner as under:
- A duty of care in deciding whether to undertake the case
- A duty of care in deciding what treatment to give
- A duty of care in the administration of that treatment

If a medical professional commits a breach of duty, the immunity they benefit from can become the ground for judicial interference, ultimately granting the patient a right of action to pursue negligence.

Analytical Overview of Clinical Negligence in Ophthalmology

In England, an overview of the clinical negligence claims in ophthalmology was presented in the National Health Service (NHS) from 1995 to 2006. All the claims on NHS Litigation Authority were analyzed and categorized by ophthalmic subspecialty. Out of 848 claims, 651 claims were closed. 46% of closed claims resulted in payment of damages. Cataract made up the largest share of claims of 31%, pediatric ophthalmology had the highest mean damages, and 64% of claims related to glaucoma were most likely to result in payment of damages.

Clinical negligence claims in ophthalmology in England are infrequent, but most ophthalmologists will face at least one in their career. Ophthalmic subspecialties show marked differences concerning their litigation profiles. The ophthalmic subspecialties are ranked by the number of claims. Cataract accounts for nearly a third of claim numbers, with retinal specialties (VR and medical retina) comprising the next largest group.

Even in our country, it is noteworthy that cataracts and VR surgery form a major part of the claims filed before various forums. In several cases, it is observed that the patient knocks on the door of the court after the surgery when he gets a very poor/nil visual outcome. The grievances raised before the court arising out of cataract surgeries are more than glaucoma, VR, and other subspecialties.

Negligence: Legal Aspect

It is to be remembered that no law aims at punishing all acts that cause harm or injury to the patient. A medical practitioner is punished only when he is found guilty of carrying out his duties enumerated earlier. It is crucial to emphasize that mere difference of opinion, error of judgment, patient not getting cured despite correct treatment, operation not being successful without any negligence on the part of the surgeon, etc., do not constitute grounds for holding doctors liable. It is an acknowledged fact that no human being is infallible and even distinguished specialists may make mistakes in detecting or diagnosing the disease.

PROTECTIVE FACTORS

The adage "A stitch in time saves nine" will definitely help prevent litigation in respect of medical negligence against a medical practitioner.

Factors that can aid medical professionals in safeguarding themselves from unnecessary lawsuits are enumerated further:

- Establishing an atmosphere that engenders trust.
- Doctors have a valid insight regarding their abilities and limitations.
- Doctors and their staff listen, hear, and treat their patients respectfully.
- Doctors and their staff sincerely care for patients.
- Ensuring clear and sufficient communication among patients, staff, and doctors involves the following:
    - Maintaining comprehensive medical records
    - Encouraging patients to manage their medical records
    - Advising patients to bring written lists of their concerns, medications, and topics for discussion
    - Providing patients with written instructions regarding recommended medications
    - Sending letters to patients that outline the outcomes of their visits, along with copies of letters being sent to consultants.

The actions, especially by doctors and their staff, which create an environment in which patients feel cared for, heard, and respected are essential. At the very top of the list is engendering trust—trust in the doctors, trust in their staff, and trust in their recommendations.

Many years ago, Francis Peabody said that "the secret of the care of the patient is caring for the patient." This simple commentary encapsulates most of what is trying to be pointed out in this chapter. Doctors who genuinely care for their patients will avoid inappropriate treatments and will avoid going beyond their capabilities to prevent any harm. Their genuine concern extends to providing appropriate information, ensuring realistic patient expectations and maintaining clear communication channels.

PRACTICES AND/OR PRECAUTIONS

There is no smoke without fire. Contrary to his expectations, when the patient gets dissatisfied with services and treatment prescribed by the medical professional that causes him agony, harm, or loss, be it of any kind, then the patient prefers to knock on the door of the Court of Law. What is important here is that the causes that lead to litigation should be looked into and efforts be made not to let any cause arise by giving proper treatment and sticking to the standard of care that would keep the patient from approaching the court. The patient approaches the court when he gets the "cause." Following practices or precautions will avoid litigation and even if the litigant approaches the court, he may not get any relief from the court, as mere judgment of error cannot be said to be negligence.

- A proper and complete workup of a patient going for cataract surgery should be done by recording vision, tension, type, and grade of cataract along with any associated pathology of adnexa, anterior and posterior segment, etc.

- The duration of treatment for which medicine has to be used or consumed should be clearly mentioned and explained. For example, in cases of vernal catarrh, consequences of corticosteroid use such as cataract/glaucoma development as a side effect must be noted and informed.
- Cases of suspected retinopathy of prematurity (ROP) should be timely referred to a retina specialist for screening.
- Invasive procedures such as surgical capsulotomy or surgical iridectomy should be avoided in view of risk of endophthalmitis. Noninvasive procedures such as yttrium-aluminum-garnet (YAG) laser capsulotomy and iridectomy should be suggested and informed to the patient and then only performed.
- Lacrimal sac evaluation should be done before all invasive intraocular procedures to avoid the risk of endophthalmitis.
- Any complaint either with the spectacle power or improper spectacle making should be looked into or rectified accordingly to the fullest satisfaction of the patient.
- For any medicine which has to be used for a long time, the tapering regimen along with the duration should be particularly explained and recorded in the prescription.
- It must be clearly mentioned in the prescription as to which medicine is to be used in both eyes and which one in a single eye (especially in right or left eye) with frequency and duration.
- In case of any surgical complications during cataract surgery or any other ocular surgery, the surgeon must try his best to manage the complications sticking to minimum basic guidelines.
- Explain additional precautions to be taken in simple and easy words.
- Inform side effects along with cure.
- Clearly explain any deviations from standard care and indicate whether the prognosis has been thoroughly discussed with the patient as well as the attender.
- Always mention "diagnosis under review" or "under evaluation" until a final diagnosis is determined.
- If the patient or attendants deviate from recommended actions (such as providing unreliable history, refusing investigations, or declining admission), document these instances or obtain written refusals, preferably in the local language and with a proper witness.
- Record the patient's history of drug allergies, clearly specifying the drug names and outlining the method and interval of administration.
- It is advisable to make a note if either the patient or the attendant is under the influence of alcohol or drugs at the time of examination.
- Regularly update your knowledge and skills, as well as those of your staff.
- Ensure that facilities and equipment are consistently being updated to meet the prevailing standards in your area.
- It is imperative that we obtain legally valid consent only from the patient duly witnessed or from his relatives when the patient is serious and/or unable to sign it due to any reason, before undertaking a surgical/diagnostic procedure.
- In case of an intraoperative posterior capsule rent and nucleus drop, inform and refer the patient to a VR surgeon for further management. Take the patient and his attendant into confidence and with your personalized self and humanitarian attitude, you can win the patient and avoid grievances even in poor outcome cases.
- A surgeon's responsibility extends beyond the surgery itself to encompass postoperative care and it is imperative for the surgeon to ensure the proper care of the patient during this period.

- In the unfortunate event of a patient's death, it is crucial to promptly inform the police or hospital authorities to facilitate autopsy and other necessary formalities.
- When a hospital or clinic asserts the provision of 24-hour emergency services, it is mandatory that all essential equipment is readily available in good working condition and competent staff is on hand to deliver the required services.

CONSENT

Before obtaining a valid consent, the patient and/or his relatives must be apprised of the nature of the patient's condition, the treatment options available, pros and cons of the possibilities, associated complications, and material risk with each modality of treatment. This will help the patient decide for the modality of treatment he wants his doctor to adopt. Consent of guarded/poor visual prognosis due to specific causes such as corneal opacity or corneal decompensation, glaucoma, macular degeneration, retinal pathology, amblyopia, and optic atrophy must be obtained.

Honorable High Court of Kerala in a case of TT Thomas vs. Elisa has observed that "Consent from the patient is evidently not for the safety of the patient but for the protection of the physician or the surgeon as the case may be."

The following legal case substantiates the importance of obtaining consent:
A boarder while in hostel of an institution was hit in his right eye by a firecracker during his stay in hostel and the official in the school immediately took the boy to an eye hospital. After detailed examination, it was observed that the right eye had been shattered to pieces and totally damaged. The parents were residing far away from the hostel. Left with no option, the school authorities, without further delay and waiting for the arrival of his parents gave consent for evisceration to save the boarder. The father filed a complaint stating that it was a case of evisceration and major surgery was done without obtaining consent from the parents.

The Tamil Nadu State Commission held that there was no deficiency of service on the part of the doctor and dismissed the complaint. In this case, the consent was given by the school authorities who were having lawful charge over the child at the time of injury to his eye and the consent was given for evisceration to avoid sympathetic ophthalmitis.

It is very important to note that it does not give total immunity from being held negligent just because the patient has given consent for an operation. This has been held by the Maharashtra State Commission in a case Nirmala R Parab vs. Dr Kalpana Desai that "Merely signing the consent form does not exclude doctors' responsibility if he is negligent, in carrying his duty." In another complaint, the complainant alleged that his eye was operated but vision was lost. The contention regarding lack of hygiene in hospital was falsified, as no postoperative infection had developed in the patient—no deficiency in service on part of treating doctor proved—no relief entitled on this ground.

However, the doctor did not obtain consent of the patient himself, but it was obtained from his grandson when the patient was conscious, mentally alert, and in a position to give it. The forum held that no one else can give consent on his behalf unless any proof is produced to show the rationale behind this for performing surgery and that attendant's risk is involved and is communicated to patient prior to operation. The Forum held deficiency in service in not obtaining consent from the patient and awarded compensation.

PRACTICES THAT SHOULD BE AVOIDED

- Do not advise the patient to abruptly stop the medicines having been used by him/her with any prejudice, especially antiglaucoma medicines. Explain him properly with reasons if there is a need to change the treatment.
- Do not perform refractive surgery procedures on a teenager below 18 years of age or who has unstable myopia.
- Do not operate on both eyes simultaneously unless there is a real, documented emergency.
- Prescriptions should only be issued after you have examined the patient and one should not assume always true of the statement by the patient/attendant.
- It is the patient's right to leave against medical advice (LAMA) and this choice should not be refused.
- Patients have the right to be informed about their diagnosis and treatment.
- One should provide first aid and medical care promptly in accident and emergency cases, even if it is a medicolegal case.
- Avoid smoking while examining the patient.
- Refrain from examining patients when you are unwell, exhausted, or under the influence of alcohol or any other intoxicating substance.
- Exercise extra caution in elective surgeries involving both eyes simultaneously; ensure a comprehensive preoperative workup of both eyes and document it.
- When uncertain about the course of action, consult with your senior, colleagues, or a specialist.
- Avoid speaking negatively about your colleagues, even in the face of professional competition. Criticism of fellow professionals, especially in front of patients and/or their attendants, should be avoided.
- In the case of injured persons seeking medical treatment, provide immediate medical aid and allow procedural criminal law to follow; there is no legal impediment to doctors attending to such cases promptly.

CASES IN WHICH NO SUIT AGAINST THE DOCTORS

- A 20-year-old patient was advised to have a femtosecond-assisted laser-assisted in situ keratomileusis (LASIK) for recruitment purposes in the Merchant Navy, as he was having a refractive error. The complainant claimed that his vision started deteriorating post-LASIK due to which he could not join the Merchant Navy. The patient was eventually diagnosed with post-LASIK ectasia (PLE) and was advised cross-linking procedure. The patient and his father filed a case of medical negligence against the treating ophthalmologist. PLE is a rare but well-known postoperative complication of LASIK, which may occur even in otherwise normal corneas. It was concluded by the jury that the concerned doctor exercised his skills with reasonable competence and knowledge during the preoperative workup as well as during surgery. Hence, the court passed judgment in favor of the doctor and found him not guilty. The case was dismissed as being devoid of merits.
- A keratoconus patient who underwent collagen cross-linking, unfortunately developed infection postprocedure and was eventually advised corneal transplant. The complainant then approached the State Consumer Disputes Redressal Commission, filing charges of

utter medical negligence against the concerned ophthalmologist, but negligence could not be established by the prosecution on two grounds:

i. The infection with which the complainant suffered was a known and well-documented complication.
ii. The doctor was treating the patient's complication with due diligence and did not fail to exercise his duties toward the patient in any way.

It may be helpful to enumerate the following cases in which a cause for legal action was there, but in fact, no suit was brought. It cannot be known with certainty why no suit was initiated in these situations, but it seems likely that the patients had realistic expectations about what could happen, and therefore, were not surprised at a particular outcome and that the patients felt that they had been treated respectfully and competently.

An elderly man lost his only eye due to an expulsive choroidal hemorrhage that occurred intraoperatively during an intracapsular cataract extraction combined with a trabeculectomy. An elderly woman's visual acuity deteriorated from 20/200 to finger counting following a peripheral iridectomy for angle closure glaucoma, complicated by malignant glaucoma, necessitating a cataract extraction. Postoperative acuity was poor due to cystoid macular edema. An elderly woman was first seen with far-advanced glaucomatous ocular nerve damage in both eyes and visual acuity is reduced to 20/60 in both eyes due to the severe glaucoma damage which already involved fixation. Intraocular pressure was in the 40s and did not respond to medical therapy. A trabeculectomy was performed in each eye and both procedures appeared to be uncomplicated. The postoperative visual acuity was finger counting in each eye.

PRACTICES THAT WILL HELP

No matter how competently one practices and no matter how sincerely one cares for patients, there is a reasonable chance of a doctor being sued sometime during his/her career. It is prudent to be prepared for such a situation and to act in a way that will lessen the likelihood of being held liable or culpable. Many articles advise wisely in this regard, most originating with attorneys who defend doctors.

Important tips to prevent oneself from being held liable if a suit is brought:

- Documentary records should be kept meticulously:
  - Records must be maintained thoroughly, appropriately, and legibly.
  - If not following standard procedure, make sure that this has been discussed with the patient and note in the chart that the patient has agreed and ideally have the patient sign the note.
  - Be sure that communications are clear and accurate and if errors are made, they are corrected promptly and the date of the correction is indicated.
  - Make sure that notes are placed in the chart regarding the dates, subject matter, and recommendations that relate to telephone calls or other oral communications.
- Make sure that copies of all authorizations, including suggested diagnostic procedures and treatments are noted accurately and legibly in the chart:
  - Indicate in the record when a patient does not keep an appointment and document that the patient was informed of the missed appointment and that an attempt was made to schedule a new appointment.

- When a patient initiates a contact through a letter, e-mail, or telephone call, make sure the record indicates who responded, when the response was made, and the outcome of the response. If the patient cannot be reached, clearly indicate the efforts that were made in order to try to reach the patient.
- In ordinary course, the medical record of the patient must be maintained for 3 years from the date of commencement of treatment.
- Obtain truly informed consent customized for the individual patient. Make sure that these are designed to be carried out in a way that is clear to the patient that the intent is to help the patient make a decision and that the obtaining of the informed consent is not primarily to protect the doctors.
- Do not make comments that would be easily misinterpreted or worse, properly interpreted as indicating disrespect for the patient. This applies to whether or not the patient is apparently able or unable to appreciate the comment.

CASES SETTLED OUT OF COURT

Cases Resulting in Judgment for the Plaintiff

The parents of a child with a rare metabolic disease alleged that they told the pediatrician that their 1-year-old child had excessive tearing and was extremely light sensitive. The pediatrician reassured the parents by telling them that tearing and light sensitivity were a routine occurrence in children. A doctor friend of the parents advised getting a second opinion with an ophthalmologist who informed the parents that the child had advanced congenital glaucoma.

A business executive was told he could expect to have 20/20 vision without glasses following cataract extraction, without correction was 20/40, and with correction 20/20.

An elderly man developed endophthalmitis following an otherwise uncomplicated cataract extraction; the operating surgeon had not ordered antibiotics preoperatively and had not used intraoperative antibiotics.

Cases Settled

- A severely diabetic patient was referred from another hospital to the ophthalmologist's hospital because of the onset of severe neovascular glaucoma associated with severe pain. The patient's wife was unhappy because the nurses did not appear to pay attention to her husband's complaint of back pain. The patient had cyclocryotherapy which resulted in lowering intraocular pressure to a satisfactory range and relief of the eye pain. The ophthalmologist, learning of the back pain, ordered a medical consultation. The medical consultant immediately requested an X-ray examination of the back, which was negative. The patient was returned to the hospital from which he had come and the back pain increased. The diagnosis of an epidural abscess was made and surgery was performed, resulting in paraplegia. The plaintiff sued the ophthalmologist and the hospital where the cyclocryotherapy was performed and a settlement was reached.
- A psychologist with bilateral cataracts and early glaucoma had a cataract extraction performed, during which a rupture occurred in the posterior capsule. An anterior chamber lens was placed. Postoperative visual acuity was 20/20, but the eye remained mildly inflamed. The operating surgeon assured the patient and turned the patient over to an

associate while he went on vacation. On return from vacation, the eye was more inflamed than before. Gonioscopy showed the haptic of the IOL to be in the proper position, but the end of one of the feet was broken and the sharp edge irritating the eye. A lens exchange was performed, following which acuity was 20/20 and the eye quiet.

It is likely that one of the reasons why the parents of the child with congenital glaucoma initiated the suit was because the ophthalmologist who first examined the infant commented to the parents that the pediatrician should have recognized that the child had glaucoma. Had the ophthalmologist indicated that many healthy infants do have tearing and light sensitivity and the distinction between those common symptoms and the rare situation of glaucoma was not easy to make, it is likely that parents would not have brought legal action. Understandably, a person who has a serious illness would want to find somebody to blame.

NEGLIGENCE IN DECIDING TREATMENT

Once it is decided to treat the patient, the next important duty is the duty of care in deciding what treatment to be administered. The decision to be made is whether the patient requires a surgical or medical line of therapy. If the surgical line of therapy is decided upon, then the type of surgery to be done and whether the patient is fit for surgery or not—should be given careful consideration. If medical therapy is advised, contraindications (if any) should be ruled out first and precautions to be taken before the use of certain drugs should be borne in mind before starting the treatment.

The following case laws will illustrate this point:

In one particular case, the allegation against the opposite party doctor was that he was negligent in performing filtration surgery followed by radial keratotomy (RK) operation of the left eye of the complainant's son aged 14 years, resulting in total loss of sight in his left eye.

To decide the complaint, the Madhya Pradesh State Commission referred to various textbooks on the subjects of RK. The textbook authored by Dr George Warring categorically stated that "Patients younger than 21 years of age are not fit for keratotomy because their refraction may not be stable and an increase in myopia in teenagers might affect the surgery."

Another textbook by Dr KR Mehta also reiterated the same instructions with respect to RK.

"Age: Keratorefractive surgeons all over the world use 18 years as the minimum age for exposing a cornea to radial keratotomy procedures. There are many reasons for this age selection. The promise offered by the RK procedure is a decrease in myopic power and in addition, safety and minimal optical problems. In young people, the myopia is not stable and the power tends to increase again, thus vitiating the advantage of the procedure." The book further mentions as under.

"Finally, and most important of all, the patient must be given time to think, evaluate the details, and make up his mind prior to surgery. Overpromotion of radial keratotomy or an attempt at a fast shall only result in a large percentage of dissatisfied patients whose expectations have not and could realistically have been met."

Another textbook produced before the State Commission (by Dr Sanders) fortified the view that to be considered a candidate for RK, the patient must be at least 18 years of age and demonstrate a stable myopic refraction.

From the above case, the State Commission held that the opposite party ophthalmologist had committed a breach of duty by performing an operation on a teenager which he, as a reasonable and prudent surgeon, should not have performed. A compensation of ₹1 lakh with interest was awarded to the complainant in this case.

CASES WHERE NEGLIGENCE WAS PROVED

- The consumer filed a case of medical negligence against the doctor alleging that complications developed after a cataract operation. The patient was referred to the hospital and a fungal infection was found; hence, eyeball was removed. The doctor was found guilty of suppression of fact and in administering follow-up treatment, and the court observed deficiency in service and awarded compensation. The appeal filed was also dismissed.
- In this case, the eye was operated but the aperture of the operated eye was deformed due to shortcomings/imperfections in operation which was later on rectified by the removal of the thick layer from the operated eye with the help of a laser. As a result, the vision became low and the eye could not be opened fully. The complainant had a feeling of swollen eyeball. The Forum found the doctor guilty of medical negligence and awarded compensation for expenses and mental agony.
- Medical negligence was observed in cataract surgery as necessary postoperative care was not taken. Patient was admitted for simple cataract surgery, with no high-risk factors, but he lost his vision. Requirement of three repeated surgeries after operation was not explained and opposite parties failed to follow normal medical practices as per standards of medical parlance. They were liable to pay compensation toward medical expenses and cost.
- Usual and normal practice of conducting minimum tests before zeroing on diagnosis was not followed and the step was taken to abruptly decide on diagnosis and commence the treatment held—it was a case of negligence, deficiency in service, and not maintaining proper record. The complainant alleged that mandatory preoperative laboratory investigations were not conducted; thus, negligence and deficiency in service on part of the concerned doctor proved. The patient died due to operative septicemia leading to renal failure. The hospital failed to maintain day-to-day treatment record of the patient. District Forum held that the cause of death cannot be ascertained in the absence of a postmortem report and dismissed the complaint. In appeal, the order of the District Forum was set aside, holding the negligence, deficiency in service, and nonmaintained hospital records proved and granted compensation.
- The patient had cataract and glaucoma. Prior to the operation, intraocular pressure was not measured. After surgery, the patient lost his vision. The court held it as a case of negligence and awarded compensation. The court directed the doctor to pay to the complainant a sum of ₹456,000 as compensation for loss of eyesight on various heads inclusive of costs.
- In this case, the patient had cataract operation in her right eye but lost eyesight completely after surgery. The doctor advised him to undergo an operation within the next 2–3 days, but the patient came after about 3 weeks and the operation could not bring the desired result. The commission held District Forum concluding that it was not a case fit for operation at all; the doctor should not have conducted the same and awarded compensation of ₹50,000. The State Commission also upheld that it was fully established from the admission of the doctor himself that it was not a case fit for operation, but he conducted it after asking the complainant herself, who was an illiterate woman from a village. If it was not a case fit for surgery, the doctor should not have conducted the same and should have advised accordingly. The State Commission found no reason to interfere with the judgment of the District Forum.

Retinal Detachment—Negligence

The complainant alleged that he was not able to see anything when the bandage was removed 3 days after the operation performed by the doctor on his right eye. He was referred to Dr Ahuja who told him that his eyesight was lost as a result of the operation. The State Commission observed that the opposite party should have carefully examined him during the removal of the bandage after 3 days, should have recorded the findings, and advised him of treatment. He must have carefully watched for glaucoma. Vitreous hemorrhage should have caused some anxiety to the opposite party and he should have advised the complainant for proper treatment and should have watched him at short intervals. Chances of proliferative vitreoretinopathy (PVR) are increased in such cases for which no instructions appear to have been given to the complainant. The State Commission held the opposite party negligent and allowed the complainant a sum of ₹180,000 on account of loss of wages and ₹10,000 on account of travel, lodging consultation fee, and purchase of medicines to be paid by the opposite party.

Retinopathy of Prematurity—Negligence

Retinopathy of prematurity unfortunately is the leading cause of preventable infant blindness in the world. With the widespread expansion of neonatal intensive care unit (NICU) services and increased survival rate of premature neonates, there is a need for greater emphasis on the ROP screening programs in our country. The challenge is the large cohort of babies waiting for screening and relatively few ROP specialists to manage. The problem in our country gets compounded by the survival of infants in rural settings where there are no or very few ROP specialists to screen the infant as compared to the urban population. As new cases are coming to light every day, the medicolegal aspects about it have also gained attention.

The emerging medicolegal concerns revolve around ensuring timely screening and treatment of ROP, as well as addressing potential negligence or malpractice cases, and thus, there is an emerging need for addressing the important paradigms regarding patient safety, ethical practice, and accountability.

Hereby, we have highlighted some of the ROP-related landmark judgments passed by the Court of Law. These judgments will help us improve our working by reducing the number of ROP cases and developing early diagnosis and management strategies.

1. A neonate having a birth weight (BW) of 1,280 g and gestational age (GA) of 28 weeks was incidentally diagnosed with stage 5 ROP at 7 months of age by a relative who happened to be an ophthalmologist. A case was filed by the parents against the treating pediatrician regarding the inability to inform the parents about timely ROP screening. Despite the pediatrician's claim that he had verbally informed the parents about a retina specialist consultation, the parents filed an affidavit denying this fact. The pediatrician was not able to defend himself as he could not produce any evidence to support his claim. Also, the pediatrician's records showing the eye findings as "Eyes-WNL" (within normal limits) further weakened the case. At the time of conclusion of the case, a judgment was passed in favor of the complainant and the pediatrician had to pay a compensation of ₹5 lakh.

Take-home messages:
- All verbal communications to the parents or guardian must be documented in the medical records.
- Standard and very commonly used medical abbreviations such as WNL are not adequate enough in such cases. All details must be meticulously recorded.

2. An infant having BW of 1,250 g and GA of 29 weeks was born in a tertiary care government hospital. Eventually, stage 5 ROP was accidentally detected during a routine vaccination visit at 4.5 months of age. The Supreme Court fined the treating pediatrician with a hefty compensation of ₹1.8 crore on the grounds of failure to advise the parents regarding ROP screening. The total value assessment was based on the principle of "Restitutio in integrum" which cumulatively accounted for all past and future medical expenses, psychological trauma, lifelong dependence, and care, along with annual interest and RBI's future inflation rates.
3. A newborn having BW 1,340 g and GA 31 weeks was found to have stage 5 ROP 4 months later. A lawsuit was filed against the concerned doctors claiming that ROP screening was not advised during the patient's hospital stay of 30 days in the NICU. The treating pediatrician actually had requested a cross consultation, wherein an eye specialist had examined the baby at 8 days of age and found that there was "no ROP." The jurisprudence was based on the fact that neither the eye specialist nor the pediatrician could produce any documented evidence of such cross-reference and examination. Also, it was alleged that parents were not asked for any further follow-ups. The doctors were held guilty of medical negligence on account of "gross deficiency" in service and were made to offer compensation of ₹7.5 lakh to the parents.
4. A lawsuit was filed against the pediatrician by the parents of premature twin babies, alleging too much use of oxygen and improper care on the part of the doctor. The babies were diagnosed with stage 5 ROP at 3 months of age. The case was taken up by the parents to the High Court, since they felt that the compensation amount offered by the district court was too low. The pediatrician was accused of medical negligence on account of the fact that he or she did not refer the twins for ROP screening during their 40 days of NICU stay under his care and secondly did not document the quantity of supplemental oxygen that was given to the infants. Final judgment was passed in favor of the complainant and a quantum of compensation amounting to ₹1.2 crore was decided upon by the jury, which also included 6% per annum interest for 23 years.

Take-home messages:
- A proper referral to a concerned eye specialist must be done and should be in accordance with the current national guidelines.
- Details of the supplemental oxygen therapy must also be documented.

5. Stage 5 ROP was diagnosed in an infant at 8 months of age. Both the pediatrician and ophthalmologist were alleged to be medically negligent stating that the ROP screening of the premature infant under their care was "casual" and "improper" and consequently were made to pay a compensation of 64 lakh to the parents. Despite a proper ROP screening being done by a senior ophthalmologist, the deficiencies as highlighted by the Court of Law were that the examination details such as the name of the doctor along with

the drugs and anesthesia used, pupillary dilation, indirect ophthalmoscopy findings, and other intraocular/extraocular findings were not documented.

Take-home message: Documentation of ROP findings must be detailed and meticulous, stating the name of the doctor and the method used (indirect ophthalmoscopy/imaging/ telemedicine) and details of the pupillary dilatation along with the anterior and posterior segment findings.

Following are some good clinical practices along with general recommendations from an ophthalmologist's perspective in order to mitigate undesirable litigations:

- Detailed and meticulous record maintenance by the treating ophthalmologist is imperative.
- The importance of timely referral for ROP screening on the part of the pediatrician/ neonatologist cannot be overemphasized.
- Parents' counseling regarding the nature of the disease and regular follow-ups should be given equal importance.
- Ophthalmologists should be well informed and should keep themselves updated regarding the current published national guidelines pertaining to ROP management.
- The treating specialist must have good professional indemnity insurance.
- A well-informed and detailed consent form should be filled at every screening and/or treatment session, duly signed by the parent(s) or guardian.
- The history and examination findings should be descriptively mentioned in the "ROP card" along with the next follow-up date and this should be well communicated to the parents as well.
- In case the screening mode is via telemedicine, then that shall also be documented in the consent form.

CASES DISMISSED FOR WANT OF DOCUMENTARY EVIDENCE

- Vision was affected after a cataract operation. No expert evidence was produced in support. Even the oral evidence of the complainant was not supported by any medical evidence. The Forum held that the burden of proof lies on the complainant, which was not discharged, hence, dismissed the complaint. The order of the Forum was upheld in appeal.
- The complainant was operated on for a cataract in the right eye and IOL was implanted. Till December 14, 1992, he was recovering normally. On December 15, 1992, he got severe inflammation and burning in the same eye. He consulted an eye surgeon and he was under close observation of the doctor. There was a slight improvement in vision over the next 2–3 months, but again due to repeated infection, his vision deteriorated, probably due to the carelessness of the doctor. He consulted an eye surgeon and again consulted the opposite party and had to undergo an emergency vitrectomy, but his vision deteriorated. He took treatment from several other doctors and hospitals and was still under treatment. The complainant did not file any affidavit of experts nor adduced any evidence. The State Commission in the absence of proof dismissed the complaint, but looking into the seriousness of the allegations and the voluminous evidence that would be required for the intricate issues therein, observed that the complainant was at liberty to approach the Civil Court.

CASES WHERE NEGLIGENCE NOT PROVED

- It was alleged that the left eye was operated on instead of the right eye. The operation was unsuccessful. Eye was removed later on to save her life. Complaint was allowed by the Forum, but the order of the forum was set aside in appeal. In revision, it was held that no expert evidence was produced in support of allegations—negligence on the part of a doctor was not proved; hence, the complainant is not entitled to any relief. Moreover, the eye was operated in a government medical college by paying a token amount of registration only. No amount was paid for the surgery. It was held that the complainant is not a consumer and is not entitled to any relief.
- The patient had cataract in both eyes and after surgery for cataract and IOL implantation, he developed headache and severe pain in the operated eye on the very next day and he was reoperated. IOL was removed and a vitrectomy was done. But the patient developed an infection in the eye and the eyesight was lost due to negligence and lack of aseptic precautions. In the other eye, which was operated on in Belgium a year later, he regained vision with no complications. The complainant had disfigurement of the face with loss of business. The State Commission observed that the certificate given by the surgeon who performed the operation on the other eye did not show that there was negligence on the part of the surgeon who performed the operation on the first eye. The commission also observed that as the doctor performed the operation only after looking into the urine and blood reports, it cannot be said to be an act of negligence in finding out the state of diabetes of the patients. Regarding the allegation that the very fact that the complainant lost his vision in his right eye shows negligence, the Commission held that in spite of taking the best care, a patient may die, but that does not itself establish negligence on the part of the doctor. The complaint was dismissed.
- The complainant was operated on for a cataract in her right eye and IOL was implanted by the doctor, but the vision in the eye did not return to normal in 6 months. The doctor guaranteed that on reimplantation of the lens in the eye, her vision would certainly return to normal. He did the reimplantation of the lens, yet she did not regain her vision. She ultimately consulted a doctor in another hospital and the lens was removed. The State Commission observed that there is nothing to show that the complainant felt any pain or trouble for about 5 months after the operation or that she took any postoperative treatment during the period. Had there been any negligence, she would not have got the second operation done by the same surgeon. The commission held that the complainant herself was neglectful in the follow-up treatment and hence, the complaint was dismissed.
- There was no restoration of vision after extraction of cataract and IOL implantation apprised of all surgical options and advantages and risks of the operations; the patient gave his consent of his own free will and accepted responsibility of all its benefits and ill effects. The doctor had taken all due care, but there is always a chance that the human body may reject the implant which is a foreign body; any allergies that may develop following implantation can be countered by drugs. While the complainant was responding to such a course of drugs, the patient voluntarily discontinued the treatment and did not come for reevaluation, thus contributing to the damage to the eye. The State Commission held that the complainant had failed to discharge the burden of establishing negligence of the opposite party and ordered him to pay a cost of ₹1,000 to the doctor. However, the National Commission set aside the cost and upheld the dismissal of the complaint.

EYE CAMPS

Often, eye camps are organized by nongovernmental organizations with the laudable thought of providing either free service or services on a concession or subsidized rate to the underprivileged. Sometimes, in such eye camps, patients develop postoperative infection or other such complications, defeating the very purpose of conducting such eye camps, i.e., to restore vision.

The Lions Club of Khurja in Uttar Pradesh had conducted an eye camp, as a part of a social service program. The Club invited an ophthalmologist and his team of doctors from Jaipur. In this camp, a total of 108 patients were operated on, out of which 88 patients were operated on for cataract. Out of those operated, at least 84 persons suffered permanent damage to the operated eye owing to a postoperative infection noticed on the very day of the operation. In addition, around 15 similar cases were reported where 380 patients were operated in Moradabad. Inquiries showed that this happened due to a common contaminating source and in all the cases, probably the source of the infection was *Escherichia coli* (*E. coli*) in the saline, which was used to irrigate the eyes during the surgery to maintain turgidity of the operational surface.

In the instant case, the doctor has himself brought all the medicines and surgical instruments for use at the camp. The Lion's Club was granted permission to conduct the eye camp on the basis of certain norms and guidelines for the conduct of eye camps contained in a circular issued by the Ministry of Health and Family Welfare, Government of India.

Two social activists filed a writ petition (public interest litigation) before the Supreme Court under Article 32 of the Constitution requesting for the following:

- Rehabilitation of the affected patients
- Compensation for the affected patients
- Inquiry into the cause of a mishap of such magnitude
- Evolving guidelines and norms to prevent such mishaps in the future

After the writ petition was instituted, a committee was set up by the central government to update and revise the earlier guidelines. The MCI also submitted recommendations in regard to the conduct and management of eye camps. The Supreme Court lamented the standards of cleaning and hygiene in public hospitals. It observed that:

"The necessity of maintenance of the highest standards of aseptic and sterile conditions at places where ophthalmic surgery or any surgery is being conducted cannot be overemphasized. It is not merely on the formulation of the theoretical standards but really on the professional commitment with which the prescriptions are implemented that the ultimate result rests. Government, States, and Unions incur enormous expenditure of public money on health care. But the standards of cleanliness and hygiene in public hospitals, unfortunately, leave a lot to be desired. The maintenance of sterile septic conditions in hospitals to prevent cross-infections should be ordinary, routine, and minimal incidents of maintenance of hospitals. Purity of the drugs and medicines intended for man use would have to be ensured by prior tests and inspection."

"The remedy lies in a ruthless adherence to the virtue of method and laying down practical procedures in the minutes of detail and by exacting not merely expecting strict adherence to these procedures." The Supreme Court directed that the following points be considered to be incorporated in the revised guidelines:

"Staff—the operations in the camp should only be performed by qualified, experienced ophthalmic surgeons registered with the Medical Council of India or any State Medical Council.

The camp should not be used as a training ground for postgraduate students and postoperative work should not be entrusted to postgraduate students."

"There should be a pathologist to examine urine, blood sugar, etc. It is preferable to have a dentist to check the teeth for sepsis and a physician for general medical checkups."

"Medication—all medicines to be used should be of standard quality, verified by the doctor in charge of the camp."

In view of the limited scope of the writ petition, the Supreme Court did not decide on the issue of medical negligence on the part of the doctor. This issue was pending before the criminal court and hence was left for the trial court to decide on the issue of medical negligence. The Supreme Court on humanitarian consideration directed the State Government to pay a sum of ₹12,500 to each of the victims in addition to the sum of ₹5,000 already paid to the victims.

MEDICOLEGAL ASPECTS OF TELEMEDICINE PRACTICE IN OPHTHALMOLOGY

Since the advent of telemedicine, it has gained tremendous popularity [especially after the coronavirus disease 2019 (COVID-19) pandemic] and has now been incorporated into the mainstream of all medical specialties. Ophthalmology, per se being a tech-savvy branch, has its own limitations in terms of affordability and accessibility. On that front, telemedicine has broadened the horizons of eye care services by providing high-quality community service to remote areas. But it also comes with this huge responsibility of catering to its medicolegal aspects in order to safeguard ourselves from undesirable lawsuits.

Legalities

Currently, there is a lack of defined ethical standards and regulatory laws pertaining to telemedicine practice in India. However, various committees and boards have laid down certain guidelines to streamline it.

Qualification

Any RMP can practice telemedicine anywhere in India. He/she is expected to exercise the same professional, ethical norms and standards as one would follow during a conventional physical consultation practice. An RMP would be required to take a mandatory online course within 3 years of its notification, conducted by the Board of Governors in supersession of the MCI.

Identity

During teleconsultation, both the doctor's and patient's identity should be known to each other. Identification of the patient has to be done accurately by means of documenting the patient's name, age, address, phone number, and registered ID proof. Also, the doctor's credentials, qualifications, and registration number should be displayed for the patient's information. It is the responsibility of the RMP to carry out their due diligence in maintaining the patient's privacy by all means.

Consent

Patient consent is necessary even for any kind of telemedicine consultation, which can be in the form of implied consent or explicit consent. Consent is said to be implied if the patient has initiated the teleconsultation, whereas if an RMP or healthcare worker initiates it from his end, then it is explicit.

Mode

The mode of consultation can be decided by the RMP based on his/her judgment as per the patient's complaints (textual, audio, or video interaction). It is up to the discretion of the RMP to recommend an in-person examination to the patient if it is warranted.

Emergency Care

Teleconsultation can be provided for emergency cases also with the motive of providing first aid depending upon the seriousness, urgency, and stage where an in-person consultation is not possible. The concerned doctor can then refer the patient for a detailed in-person examination thereafter if required.

As far as the examination of the patient is concerned, there are certain obvious limitations with telemedicine as a medium of consultation. So wherever required, depending upon the treating doctor's professional judgment, it is advisable that he/she should do a video consultation or an in-person examination.

Medicine Prescription

The patient has to be provided with a proper prescription. A RMP has the option of providing a photograph or giving a scanned or digital copy of a physical prescription. An electronic prescription via email or other online portals can also be issued. Additionally, a RMP is bound to furnish a receipt or invoice to the patient.

The consensus is that cycloplegics and steroid medications should be avoided in telemedicine practice, owing to the limitation of a proper eye examination. Schedule-X drugs which have a high potential for abuse cannot be prescribed with telemedicine as a means of consultation.

Documentation

It is imperative for the RMP to have a detailed and meticulous record maintenance as one would expect in a traditional in-person hospital consultation.

PROFESSIONAL INDEMNITY INSURANCE

All medical practitioners must have professional indemnity insurance coverage from any recognized insurance company to meet the claim of compensation awarded under the Consumer Protection Act. From a medical protection perspective, the indemnity premiums should be tailored according to the subspecialty areas an ophthalmologist is involved in.

In the simplest terms, documenting that care is competent, respectful, and thorough is the best way to build a record that will protect the doctors if sued.

Published literature highlights cases reviewed by the National Consumer Disputes Redressal Commission (NCDRC) for nearly 942 cases pertaining to ophthalmology from 2002 to 2018, in which about 73.3% of the judgments proved the doctor to be guilty and compensation for the cases ranged between ₹200,000 and ₹10 million.

An online survey aimed at assessing the knowledge, attitude, and practice patterns (KAPP) of the medicolegal aspects and awareness regarding professional indemnity insurance among Indian ophthalmologists revealed that 19.4% of the respondents were totally unaware of the entity. Of the 81.6% of respondents who were aware of the entity, only 54% had taken indemnity insurance.

Given the current scenario of rising litigations against ophthalmologists, it is the need of the hour that there should be a sincere attempt in this direction to generate more awareness which can be achieved by means of webinars, physical conferences, and discussions in open forums or meetings. Every practicing ophthalmologist should have good professional indemnity insurance (preferably ₹1 crore or more).

CONCLUSION

Doctors are members of a privileged community. Most are relatively wealthy and live interesting lives. Understandably, members of the Forum and the jury will not give the benefit of the doubt to doctors who appear arrogant, cocksure, uninterested in the well-being of their patients, or frankly dishonest. A doctor must come across as willing to speak the truth and to be held accountable for what happened. Suggestions that a doctor has misinterpreted the facts or has altered the medical records understandably destroy defendants' lawyers' attempts to create an environment in which the jury is likely to look favorably on the doctor. In summary, doctors are quick to blame others for the "malpractice crisis." But doctors themselves bear a heavy responsibility for legal actions being initiated or being indefensible.

KEY LEARNING POINTS

- Bad outcomes by themselves do not trigger lawsuits, but unhappy patients, families, and staff are likely to sue if their issues are not addressed properly.
- Thorough, honest, legible, appropriate documentation helps doctors to protect themselves from being held responsible.
- Creating a trustworthy environment, ensuring patient satisfaction, being aware of limitations, clear communication, providing descriptively written instructions, and an ethical practice can prevent medical negligence litigations.
- Truly caring for the patient, truly respecting the patient, and practicing competently are the best ways to avoid becoming a defendant or being held liable for malpractice.
- "Loose-cannon" comments about others, especially from doctors, can trigger a suit. Unity and respect within our own medical fraternity breed a culture of collaboration, ensuring the best care for our patients and the advancement of healthcare as a whole.
- While it is important to consult legal professionals who specialize in healthcare laws to navigate the complexities of the legal system effectively, it is equally vital for doctors to defend themselves in a malpractice lawsuit if they believe they are innocent.

ACKNOWLEDGMENTS

This chapter is based on my experience of ophthalmology practice over the years. I am grateful to Dr Satish Tiwari, Dr Mukul Tiwari, Dr Priyamvada Bhasin, and colleagues who have encouraged me to write a chapter on this topic. I want to thank Dr Savitri Kumari Deval for her contribution in shaping the content of this edition and enriching its impact and also would like to thank Mr Vikas Savita for his support in the technical aspect of this chapter. A heartfelt thanks to everyone on the publishing team as well.

BIBLIOGRAPHY

1. A.S. Mittal and Ors. Vs. State of U.P. and Ors., In the Supreme Court of India, Writ Petition No. 1247 of 1986 & Decided On: 12.05.1989, Equivalent/Neutral Citation: AIR1989SC1570, 1989 INSC 188, JT1989(2)SC419, 1989(1)SCALE1535, (1989)3SCC223, [1989]3SCR241,1989(2)UJ276.
2. Agrawal D, Heda A, Ghosh S, et al. Knowledge, attitude, and practice patterns of Indian ophthalmologists regarding medicolegal issues. Indian J Ophthalmol. 2023;71:3690-5.
3. Air Commodore Satyanarayana Vs. L.V. Prasad Eye Institute and Ors. Andhra Pradesh State Consumer Dispute Redressal Commission, Hyderabad, C.D. No. 30 of 1990 & Decided On: 26.08.1997, Equivalent/Neutral Citation: I(1998)CPJ110(AP).
4. Akash Mayur Shridharani vs Dr Sharmila Mallya And Others on 2 February, 2012, State Consumer Disputes Redressal Commission, Mumbai, Maharashtra, Complaint Case No. CC/09/104 (http://indiankanoon.org/doc/60366700/).
5. Ariga M, Sinnasamy M, Fredrick NT, et al. Medicolegal aspects in ophthalmology in India. TNOA J Ophthalmic Sci Res. 2023;61:290-6.
6. B.P. Sharma and Ors. Vs. N.L. Shrivastava, Chhattisgarh State Consumer Disputes Redressal Commission, Raipur, Appeal No. 464 of 2006, Decided On: 14.06.2007, Equivalent/Neutral Citation: III(2008)CPJ376(Chhat.).
7. Board of Governors in Supersession of the Medical Council of India. (2020). Telemedicine Practice Guidelines: Enabling Registered Medical Practitioners to Provide Healthcare Using Telemedicine. [online] Available from https://esanjeevani.mohfw.gov.in/assets/guidelines/Telemedicine_Practice_Guidelines.pdf [Last accessed July, 2024].
8. D. Rama Krishna Vs. K. Sree Kumar Reddy and Ors, Andhra Pradesh State Consumer Disputes Redressal Commission, Hyderabad, C.D. No. 131 of 2001, Decided On: 11.07.2007, Equivalent/Neutral Citation: I(2008) CPJ126(AP).
9. Dmc vs Sanjiv Bhasin on 16 April, 2012, Punjab State Consumer Disputes Redressal Commission, Chandigarh, First Appeal No.175 of 2009, Date of institution: 16.02.2009, Date of decision: 16.04.2012, Indian Kanoon (http://indiankanoon.org/doc/40136277/).
10. Dr.T.T. Thomas vs Smt. Elisa And Ors. on 11 August, 1986, Equivalent citations: I(1987)ACC445, AIR1987KER52, AIR 1987 KERALA 52,(1987) 2 TAC 50, (1987) 1 ACC 445, (1986) KER LT 1026, (1987) ACJ 192, (http://indiankanoon.org/doc/600254/).
11. Gurdip Singh Sidhu Vs. Dr. Daljit Singh Eye Hospital Pvt. Ltd., Punjab State Consumer Disputes Redressal Commission, Chandigarh, Original Complainant No. 81 of 1993, Decided on: 15.03.1994, Equivalent/Neutral Citation: 1995(2)C.P.C.267, 1994 (2) CPR 706, 1994 (2) CPR 293.
12. Jallella Venkata Subbamma vs DM Anjaneyulu, (2008) 09 NCDRC CK 0001, National Consumer Disputes Redressal Commission, Date of decision: 30-09-2008, Citation : 2008 4 CPJ 305 (www.courtkutchehry.com).
13. K.N. Lal Vs. R.K. Akhaury, Bihar State Consumer Dispute Redressal Commission, Complaint Case No. 5 of 1994, Decided On: 27.08.1997, Equivalent/Neutral Citation: 1998(1)C.P.C.27, III(1997)CPJ112(SE), 1997 (3) CPR 398.
14. Kailash Kumar Sharma Vs. Hari Charan Mathur, National Consumer Disputes Redressal Commission New Delhi, First Appeal No. 117 of 1994, Decided on: 29.05.1997, Equivalent/Neutral Citation: 1997(2)C.P.C.345, III(1997)CPJ41(NC), 1997 (2) CPR 126.
15. Kamla Bai Pandey Vs. P. C. Dwivedi and Ors., National Consumer Disputes Redressal Commission, New Delhi, Revision Petition No. 233 of 2004 and Appeal No. 1331 of 2001, Decided on: 03.12.2008, Equivalent/Neutral Citation: 2009(1)C.P.C.588, I(2009)CPJ263(NC), 2009 (1) CPR 200.

16. Kapil Bajaj vs Ahuja Child Eye Clinic And Ors. on 1 April, 2022, Complaint Case No.-37/2010, In The Delhi State Consumer Disputes Redressal CommissionCC/37/2010 D.O.D: 01.04.2022, Indian Kanoon - http://indiankanoon.org/doc/177375107/.
17. Laxmibai and Ors. Vs. B.R. Kappalguddi and Ors., Karnataka State Consumer Disputes Redressal Commission, Bangalore, Appeal No. 1316 of 2006, Decided on: 17.08.2007, Equivalent/Neutral Citation: 2008(3)C.P.C.123, II(2008)CPJ562(SP), 2009 (1) CPR 173.
18. Maharaja Agrasen Hospital and Ors. Vs. Rishabh Sharma and Ors., Supreme Court Of India, Civil Appeal No. 6619 of 2016 and Civil Appeal No. 9461 of 2019, Decided on: 16.12.2019.
19. Ministry of Law and Justice. Government of India. (2019). National Medical Commission, NMC. [online] Available from https://www.nmc.org.in/nmc-act [Last accessed July, 2024].
20. Ram Babu vs Dr Anjani Kishore Prasad, Bihar State Consumer Disputes Redressal Commission reported in II (1998) CPJ 684 (Bihar SCDRC). Complaint Case No. 64 of 1994, Decided on 27 April 1998 (https://lawyerservices.in/Ram-Babu-Versus-Dr-Anjani-Kishore-Prasad-1998-04-27).
21. Ram Gopal Varshney vs Laser Sight India Pvt Ltd I (2009) CPJ 23 NC, LAWS(NCD)-2008-9-48 NCDRC, Decided on September 29,2008, https://supremetoday.ai/doc/judgement/01200024982.
22. Rohini Devi v. Dr. H:S. Chudawat & Anr.on 9 october 2001, 1995 (I) CPI 334: 1994 (3) CPR 621 (Raj. SCDRC). (https://indiankanoon.org/doc/25511/).
23. S.B. Jain Vs. Munni Devi and Ors., Haryana State Consumer Dispute Redressal Commission, Chandigarh, First Appeal Nos. 124 and 99 of 1997, Decided on: 20.03.1998, Equivalent/Neutral Citation: 1998(2)C.P.C.100, II(1998)CPJ239(Har.).
24. Shikhar Chand Jain vs Ku Dimple; http://www.scconline.com/DocumentLink/1wC77c8y.
25. Shubham Bansal vs Kapil Eye Hospital on 20 July, 2017, State Consumer Disputes Redressal Commission Haryana, Panchkula, Complaint No : 180 of 2015. Date of Institution: 08.10.2015, Date of Decision : 20.07.2017 (http://indiankanoon.org/doc/117938980/).
26. SS Vats vs Avtar Singh Gill (Dr) IV (2008) CPJ, In The State Commission Delhi, Date of decision: 01-04-2008, Complaint Case No. C-24/2000 (http://indiankanoon.org/doc/26421158/).
27. Tandon R, Singh A, Gupta N, et al. Upgradation and modernization of eye banking services: Integrating tradition with innovative policies and current best practices. Indian J Ophthalmol. 2017;65:109-15.
28. V Krishnakumar vs State of Tamil Nadu &Ors., Supreme Court Of India, Civil Appellate Jurisdiction on 1 July, 2015, Civil Appeal No. 8065 OF 2009 (http://indiankanoon.org/doc/86607695/).
29. Vidya Devi vs R Mehindru (Dr) II (2008) CPJ (NC)., National Consumer Disputes Redressal Commission, New Delhi, Revision Petition No. 2348 OF 2003 (Against the order dated 14/02/2003in Appeal/ Complaint No. 198/1999 of the State Commission, Haryana) (http://indiankanoon.org/doc/183845094/).

25

CHAPTER

Legal Issues in ENT

Rupali Patil Jain

INTRODUCTION

Otorhinolaryngology (ENT) practice is continuously evolving. Only one study showing statistics for litigation cases in otolaryngology is available in India. Although there are a number of cases filed against ENT surgeons in various courts and cases are pending. ENT surgeons mainly deal with airways and also their surgeries have outcomes on the senses of smell, hearing, taste, and speech. ENT surgeons have a broad scope of practice and treat conditions ranging from tympanoplasties, mastoidectomies, tonsillectomies, septal corrections, dacryocystorhinostomies (DCRs) to rhinoplasties, functional endoscopic sinus surgeries (FESS), anterior skull base surgeries, lateral skull base surgeries, cochlear implant surgeries, ossiculoplasties, auriculoplasties, thyroid surgeries, voice surgeries, allergies, neuro equilibrium, cancer surgeries, obstructive sleep apnea (OSA) surgeries, etc.

New procedures, techniques, technologies, and research have reshaped the entire healthcare system. But with newer technologies comes more challenges, more risks, and also more expectations from patients. As expectations increase, so do litigations.

In a study published in the Indian Journal of Medical Ethics in 2023 following data from the National Consumer Disputes Redressal Commission has been presented of the last 5 years. The highest compensation claimed in the ENT specialty was ₹ 19,600,000. Compensation has been awarded to four patients and highest compensation awarded was ₹ 1,000,000. In ENT, the nature of the error was a lack of skill/care in two patients, deficient medical records in three patients, and failure to take a specialist opinion in one patient.

Once a case is filed in the court of law against an institution, hospital, or healthcare professional, he has to go through a series of legal events. These events then affect the accused's personal, social, and professional life. Only a strong defence in the form of proper informed consent, documentation, etc., can save the surgeon from legal injuries. So, the best way is to prevent these events.

The major issues which can affect the ENT surgeon are:

INFORMED CONSENT

"Consent is not merely a piece of paper on which patient and his relative should sign but consent should be considered as a document of proof of communication and counseling done to the patient and his relative."

Taking informed consent is a mandatory process. Whatever is going to be done has to be communicated to the patient and relative. It is a contract between the physician and the patient which helps in strengthening the confidence between doctor and patient. The procedure of consent has been delivered in a landmark judgment Samira Kohli vs. Dr Prabha Manchanda. There are certain principles as to how consent should be taken.

- The physician has to seek consent before commencing any procedure.
- Consent should be real and valid with "adequate information" containing.
  - *Purpose of the treatment*: Diagnosis of the patient
  - *Nature and procedure of the treatment*: The routes, e.g., in ear surgeries whether endoscopic with a minimal scar or post aural/endaural incision will be given; the organs going to be removed, e.g., tonsils along with adenoids, hemi or total thyroid gland removal; and the steps of the procedure in brief.
  - *Benefits and effects of the procedure*: The outcome of the procedure, e.g., hearing improvement, voice change, relief from nasal blockage, relief from pain, etc., should be mentioned.
  - *Alternative treatments*: Medical or surgical alternative treatment, e.g., hearing aids in patients suffering from otosclerosis, nasal decongestants in case of deviated nasal septum, etc., have to be included in the consent form.
  - *Outline of substantial risks*: Risks that are remote or distant need not be mentioned in the consent form which might confuse or frighten the patient from undergoing the necessary surgery, similarly, remote or distant risks of not undergoing surgery which might persuade the patient from undergoing the unnecessary or fanciful surgery, need not be mentioned. A balance should be achieved. Risks that are less than 1% need not be told to the patient. It is also important to remember that certain patients may place high importance on certain risks. For example, a chef or sommelier may find the risk of anosmia following endoscopic skull base surgery to be unacceptably high.
  - *Adverse consequences of refusing treatment*: The consequences the patient might face if he fails to undergo the particular surgery must be mentioned. For example, risks of intracranial complications in cases of cholesteatoma or cerebrospinal fluid (CSF) rhinorrhea, chances of SN loss if surgery for otosclerosis is delayed must be conveyed to the patient.
- If consent has been taken for the diagnostic procedure, you cannot do a therapeutic procedure. For example, If consent has been taken only for direct laryngoscopy you cannot perform any further procedure like taking a biopsy. Or while doing bronchoscopy, you cannot do any further therapeutic procedure like Balloon dilatation for stenosis. The fact that the unauthorized additional surgery is beneficial to the patient, or that it would save considerable time and expense to the patient, or would relieve the patient from pain and suffering in future, are not grounds for defence in an action in tort for negligence or assault and battery.
- There can be a common consent for a diagnostic and therapeutic procedure where they are contemplated. For example, If you suspect a growth in the larynx and you might need to take a biopsy you should take informed consent for both procedures. Similarly, while doing nasal endoscopy on a child, if you suspect a foreign body, the patient's legal guardians should be told the facts.
- There can be a common consent for a particular surgical procedure and an additional or further procedure that may become necessary during the course of surgery. For example, If the surgeon suspects the need for the removal of adenoids too while taking the patient

for Tonsillectomy surgery, he can take common consent for both surgeries. Similarly, while doing surgery for septal correction, polyps are detected in the nasal cavity when a patient is under the effect of anesthesia, one cannot perform the additional surgery if consent has been taken only for one particular surgery. However, in certain cases "Principle of necessity" can be applied where a doctor is permitted to perform further or additional procedures, the delaying of which would be unreasonable because of the imminent danger to the life or health of the patient. For example, If the need for emergency tracheostomy arises to save the life of the patient, during any surgical procedure it will be accepted in a court of law.

- Consent can be taken by an assistant doctor, provided he/she is able to explain the adequate information to the patient. It can be the Residents or Junior ENT surgeons working in your hospital.

A consent form is a contract according to section 13 of the Indian Contract Act 1872, between a doctor and a patient, so it should be signed by the patient, his attendant, and the physician. If a neurosurgeon, maxillofacial surgeon, or any other surgeon is a part of the surgery, then their signature is also mandatory. Consent should be taken in a language that the patient understands. Consent should be patient and procedure specific. There is no consensus about the timing of the consent but try to take the consent of the patient as soon as they get admitted to your hospital so that they have sufficient time to decide whether they want to undergo the surgery or not. Video consent is not mandatory but it can definitely be useful in high-risk cases. If you are video recording or taking images of the patient, he/she should be informed, and consent should be taken. There should be a different consent form for admission, surgery, anesthesia, and blood transfusion.

MEDICAL DOCUMENTATION

"If it was not documented, it was not done."

Good documentation is a good defence in court and poor documentation is a poor defence. Apart from its benefits as important evidence in medicolegal cases, medical records play an important role in clinical research and audit and help in patient assessment, management, and progress.

Medical records range from outdoor patient department (OPD) prescription letters to indoor patient department (IPD), operation theater (OT), surgical, anesthesia, nursing notes, implant notes, discharge cards, transfer/referral letters, medical certificates, and postmortem reports and are equally important. The first point of contact with your patient is the OPD prescription letter. Symptoms, histories (allergy, medication, any major illness, last menstrual period), examination findings, probable diagnosis, and investigations advised should be written on the prescription letter itself along with the name of the patient, date and time of examination, and signature/designation of the physician. There is a practice seen among physicians who write "This is not valid for medico-legal purposes" on their prescription letters or X-ray/ultra sonography (USG)/computed tomography (CT) scan reports. It holds no value. Whatever the physician has signed and documented holds in the court of law.

All documents should be legible, comprehensive, and confidential. Never use medical abbreviations. Do not overwrite or overcorrect. It is an offense under section 192, 204 IPC. Records should always be kept in a safe and secure place and if stolen, police should be notified. Always keep copies of all documents with you. If documents are asked by the patient or any legal authorities, xerox copies have to be given within 72 hours. Original copies have to be submitted only in courts.

OPERATION THEATER ISSUES

The majority of an ENT surgeon's time is spent in the OT and this is the place where surgical as well as medical errors can happen. Errors can create legal issues. The causes of such issues can range from drug allergies, non-working of OT machines, intraoperative bleeding, and injury to vital structures; to leaving behind sponges or instruments in the patient's body. As ENT surgeons work within the domain of airways, anesthesia-related adverse issues remain a rare but real possibility. This could make the concerned ENT surgeon partially liable along with the Anesthetists. Anesthesia issues could be displaced endotracheal tube or loose endotracheal tube which can cause aspiration as was seen in the case of Dr Suresh Gupta vs. Government of National Capital Territory (NCT) of Delhi.

The WHO has prepared a surgical safety checklist which should be followed by every surgeon. These checklists should be a part of the protocol in every hospital.

A day prior to OT, anesthesia machines, oxygen cylinders, monitors, drills, suction machines, microscopes, and emergency drugs should be checked. If dealing with high-risk cases, appropriate machines for that particular surgery, nerve monitors, navigation systems, and defibrillators should be in the operation theater.

1. *Before induction of anesthesia (with nurse and anesthetist)*:
   - The patient's name, procedure, and site should be identified. Operating on the wrong ear is considered negligence. Chances of errors are more in cases of bilateral chronic symptoms with similar audiometry and imaging findings on both sides. Tuning fork test and study of images can be done again in OT to confirm the ear findings.
   - An anesthesia machine, pulse oximeter, medication check, and xylocaine sensitivity check should be completed.
   - Known medication allergies should be identified.
   - Difficult airway, aspiration risk, and assistance available should be confirmed especially in cases of laryngeal and OSA surgeries.
   - If there is a risk of more than 500 mL blood loss, especially in pediatric patients, e.g., juvenile nasopharyngeal angiofibroma, there should be the availability of two IV lines/ central access. IV fluids should be planned according to weight and blood loss expected.
2. *Before skin incision (with nurse, surgeon, anesthetist)*:
   - All team members should introduce themselves by name and their role.
   - Patient's name, procedure, and site of the incision should be confirmed.
   - Antibiotic prophylaxis should have been given within the last 60 minutes of the procedure accordingly.
   - Surgeon should anticipate the critical or non-routine steps, especially in skull base cases, how much time the case will take, and how much blood loss is expected.
   - Anesthetists should anticipate any patient-specific concerns.
   - Nursing team should confirm the sterility and equipment issues.
   - Essential imaging should have been displayed.
3. *Before a patient leaves the operating room (with nurse, anesthetist, and surgeon)*:
   - The nurse should verbally confirm the name of the procedure.
   - Completion of instrument, sponge, and needle counts should be done.
   - The specimen should be properly labelled along with the part and name of the patient.
   - The equipment problems should be addressed.

POSTOPERATIVE COMPLICATIONS

Complications can occur with any surgery, and it is the duty of the surgeon to identify, address and notify the complications to patient and their relatives. The patient should not be discharged until his complications are taken care of. If any surgeon is planning to travel immediately after the surgery, they should hand over the responsibility of the patient to another equally competent ENT surgeon who can handle the complication efficiently. The surgeon who has operated on the patient is liable for any injury the patient may face if it is not addressed. Postoperative bleeding, nerve palsies, neuropathies, headaches, vertigo, and vision deterioration should be identified and addressed immediately. If the ENT surgeon who has performed the surgery is unable to handle the complication, the patient must be referred to another competent surgeon. Not identifying or not addressing the complication after its identification, considers a surgeon negligent by a court of law. ENT surgeons have been held liable for not distinguishing between unilateral and bilateral nerve injury in several cases, especially when bilateral nerve injury necessitated airway intervention. In OSA surgery, 8% of claims arise from lack of CPAP utilization after surgery and due to postoperative management of patients arising due to securing of the airway in already compromised airway. Informed consent for tracheostomy should always be taken in such patients before surgery. 20% of litigation cases in OSA surgery were due to medical management. In pediatric otolaryngology most common lawsuits were stemming from adenotonsillectomy (bleeding and burn injuries from cautery). Residual tissue, medication-related, misdiagnosis leading to meningitis, injury secondary to otitis media management and thyroidectomy, airway related, mainly tracheostomy.

Delay in Diagnosis or Missed Diagnosis

Delayed diagnosis, missed diagnosis and misdiagnosis can make an ENT surgeon liable in court. However, in delayed diagnosis , the patient will have to prove that the delay has directly harmed their clinical outcome. A missed or delayed cancer diagnosis is frequently cited as the grounds for a non-surgical malpractice claim in head and neck surgery. Many of these patients required more extensive intervention including laryngectomy as a result of delayed treatment. A delay in diagnosis of > 1 month often contributes to the diagnosis of later-stage disease in oral and oropharyngeal squamous cell carcinoma and subsequent poorer prognosis. Patients with early-stage disease can be managed with single modality treatment, with fewer recurrences in follow-up and better overall survival compared with advanced-stage disease. Just a laryngeal mirror examination cannot do justice in cases of laryngeal complaints, there are chances of growths being missed. Misdiagnosis or wrong diagnosis can change the treatment, investigations advised and can lead to harmful effects of the treatment. For example, base tongue tumors, unilateral hearing loss due to acoustic neuromas, unable to differentiate between peripheral and central vertigo, missing CSF otorrhea or rhinorrhea, not doing a direct laryngoscopy in uncooperative patients

Contributory Negligence

If the patient due to their lack of reasonable care has contributed to the damage caused by the doctor, it is termed as contributory negligence. In the case of Dr Sunny Varghese vs Satyprabha Sujathan and Anr the patient had hidden the history of known bleeding disorder. He died due to heavy blood loss after tonsillectomy was performed on him.

Negative history, history of any known major illnesses, and advices given to the patient postoperatively should always be documented.

Sudden Death

Sudden death can occur in any OT or ward. It can be preoperative because of anesthesia issues even before giving the incision, intraoperative due to bleeding, anaphylactic shock, embolism, cardiac arrest or postoperative because of any complications. There can be a lot of commotion or agitation post-death of a patient. Patients are unable to accept the fact that their conscious, otherwise healthy patient has suffered mortality. Whatever efforts the doctor and their team have put up go unnoticed. Relatives can create a ruckus in your hospital as seen previously in many incidents in recent years. To reduce the intensity of such kind of situations one must:

- Always keep emergency drugs and resuscitative measures ready.
- Politely ask only close relatives to stay in the ward or your cabin. Explain them the whole situation in a sympathetic way.
- Always inform the police in case of sudden or unexpected death. Postmortem of such cases is mandatory how much ever relatives disagree for that. It will reduce your chances of future legal complications.
- Remove all the tubing, tracheostomy tubes, catheters, IV cannulas, and instruments from the patient's body before sending it for postmortem or handing it to the police.
- Complete all the documents like operation theater notes, nursing notes, and anesthesia notes. All notes should be contemporaneous.

Medical Negligence

Medical negligence is defined as an act of commission which a reasonably competent medical practitioner guided by such medical knowledge and practice and guided by such other considerations which ordinarily regulate the conduct of a reasonably competent doctor would not do (e.g., doing laryngectomy without taking a biopsy, doing stapedectomy on a patient who has known sensorineural hearing loss, leaving behind sponges in the body during surgery, giving drug to a patient who has known allergies to that drug); or omission to do something which a reasonably guided and prudent doctor would do (e.g., performing surgery without doing basic investigations, not arranging for blood during surgery where major blood loss is expected, giving local ansthesia without doing xylocaine sensitivity).

For example: An ENT surgeon has advised and performed a tonsillectomy on his patient, so the duty of care has been established. Postoperatively after few hours, that operated patient starts bleeding. The ENT surgeon is called to attend to the patient. Due to some reasons, there is a delay by the ENT surgeon in reaching the hospital, so there is a breach of duty. The patient suffers an injury, goes into hemorrhagic shock due to excessive bleeding, and succumbs to death, so there is damage caused by the breach of duty. These damages can also be in the form of aggravation of the pre-existing condition, complications or side effects of treatment, pain, and suffering, prolonging the illness, disability, reduction in expectation of life, expenses incurred by the patient in form of hospital charges, travel, medicine, specialist consultation, etc., and loss of earning due to absence of work. Here the ENT surgeon will be considered negligent as he has not given the reasonable standard degree of care to the patient. In Halsbury Laws of England, the degree of skill and care required by a medical practitioner is stated as follows: "the practitioner must bring to his task a reasonable degree of skill and knowledge, and must exercise a reasonable degree of care. Deviation from normal practice is not necessarily evidence of negligence. To establish liability on that basis it must be shown (1) that there is a usual and normal practice; (2) that the defendant has not adopted it; and (3) that the course in fact adopted is one no professional man of ordinary skill would have taken had he been acting with ordinary care."

For example: A patient comes with epistaxis which needs immediate control of bleeding. Normal practice is to either do anterior or posterior nasal packing or electro cauterization of the blood vessel to control the hemorrhage. If the ENT surgeon has just prescribed medication and the patient has suffered any damages, the ENT surgeon will be held liable.

The complainant (patient in case of civil negligence and police in case of criminal negligence) needs to prove the negligence. Only in OT and intensive care unit (ICU) where the patient does not have an access, the onus lies on the defendant (doctor) to prove they are not negligent.

SOME IMPORTANT ENT-RELATED CASES

- Dr Ravishankar vs. Jery K Thomas and Anr—Mr Jery K Thomas underwent septoplasty. After surgery patient had pain and breathing problems for which he was given antibiotics but no relief. The patient went to St John's hospital where a CT scan and endoscopy were done and a ribbon gauze piece was removed from one nostril. ENT surgeon who had performed septoplasty was held negligent.
- Dr G Vivekananda Verma vs. Chinta Bharamaramba and Ors-Tonsillectomy was performed after giving local anesthesia by the ENT surgeon himself in the absence of the anesthetist. Anoxic encephalopathy occurred and the patient suffered diffuse brain damage which the ENT surgeon could not manage himself. The patient had probably laryngeal or broncho spasm which led to cardiac arrest. The patient died after 11 days. Doctrine of Res Ipsa loquitor was applied and the ENT surgeon was held responsible.
- Siddiqi Shah Nawaz Ahmed vs. Managing Director of Bombay Hospital: The patient came to ENT surgeon for deafness. Stapedectomy was performed. Hearing loss did not improve for which the patient filed the case in the state consumer disputes redressal commission, Maharashtra. ENT surgeon was held negligent as proper informed consent was not taken and postoperative instructions were not given.
- Dr Gagandeep Tathgur vs. Veerpal Kaur & Anr 27 Jan 2021—Patient was given injection triamcinolone intralesionally in a keloid over the dorsum of the nose after she lost her eyesight partially in one eye and totally in another eye. ENT surgeon had to pay compensation as the patient was not informed of the risks of triamcinolone injection given in and around the eye.
- Prem Kumar Batra vs. Dr OM Parmar: Tonsillectomy was performed on a 13-year-old child. After surgery, he was shifted in the ward. After some time he vomited blood and died in some time. Autopsy reports revealed that the child had died due to suffocation because of aspiration of blood and blood clots which directly resulted from the site of operation which was sufficient to cause death in the ordinary course. ENT surgeon was held negligent as he had left the hospital before the child came out from the effect of anesthesia as bleeding and aspiration were foreseen and expected complications which could have been avoided if the ENT surgeon had taken due care.

CONCLUSION

There is a complex relationship between law and ethics. Medical ethics determine what should and should not be done while medical law deals with various aspects of healthcare; including the practices of caregivers and the rights of the patients. Violation of the laws creates civil or criminal liabilities. Medical errors can occur despite the utmost care in day-to-day practice. Such errors can create legal issues. All measures should be taken to prevent these errors by ensuring that everyone follows all the protocols of the hospital, documenting all clinical information, maintaining a good relationship with patients, and following all the ethics of medicine.

KEY LEARNING POINTS

- Effective, transparent, and simple communication by the doctor with the patient/his-her immediate kin is as critical to the patient's well-being. Allow them the opportunity to ask questions, keep your language simple, be accessible, and convey the feeling of being approachable even during non-verbal communication.
- Giving disease/procedure-specific booklets to patients helps in familiarizing them with the procedure and avoids too high expectations, especially in high-risk or complicated cases.
- Consent should be taken even for minor procedures like wax removal and skin prick tests as they can cause vasovagal syncope and anaphylaxis respectively. Try to review the consent on the day of the surgery.
- Documentation of things such as missed appointments, investigations not done, medications not taken, and instructions not followed (e.g., avoiding swimming, voice rest, avoiding forceful blowing of the nose, and postoperative speech therapy, especially in CI patients) should be done.
- It is important to be judicious with steroids and obtain informed consent with communication of risks posed by steroids, particularly in high-risk patients, those with long-term requirements, advanced age, alcohol abuse, and those with significant co-morbidities.
- Always document flexible/rigid laryngoscopy, nasal endoscopy, and otomicroscopy/endoscopy findings during every patient visit.
- Complications should be responded with accepted medical practice and at the earliest.
- Hoarseness and neck masses should be evaluated properly.
- ENT surgeons performing skull base surgeries should be well trained before handling such cases single-handedly. They should have good coordination with rhinologists, neurosurgeons, maxillofacial surgeons, head and neck cancer surgeons, neuro-otologists, and radiologists.
- Small acoustic neuromas may be missed even with appropriate imaging studies and can lead to delayed diagnosis. In such cases, the patient's first visit complaints, tuning fork test, audiometry reports, and imaging findings must be properly documented with date and timing.
- Patient positioning, and protecting pressure points which can lead to neuropathies, especially during long procedures is important.
- Insufficient irrigation during skull base surgeries can cause cranial neuropathy because of thermal injury and can make you liable.
- Dietary advice, advice pertaining to the disease, and precautionary postoperative advice should always be mentioned on the prescription letter or discharge card.

BIBLIOGRAPHY

1. Allisson P, Locker D. Role of diagnostic delays in prognosis of oral cancers: a review of the literature. Oral Oncol. 1998;34(3):161-70.
2. Gartland RM, Bloom JP, Parangi S, et al. A Long, Unnerving Road: Malpractice Claims Involving the Surgical Management of Thyroid and Parathyroid disease. World J Surg. 2019;43(11):2850-5.
3. Lydiatt DD. Medical malpractice and cancer of the larynx. Laryngoscope. 2002;112(3):445-8.
4. Nash JJ, Nash AG, Leach ME, Poetker DM. Medical malpractice and corticosteroid use. Otolaryngol Head Neck Surg. 2011;144:10-5.
5. Simonsen AR, Duncavage JA, Becker SS. A review of malpractice cases after tonsillectomy and adenoidectomy. Int J Pediatr Otorhinolaryngol. 2010;74(9):977-9.
6. Sukumar S. Medical negligence in cases decided by the national consumer dispute redressal commission: A five-year retrospective study. Indian J Med Ethics. 2023;8(4):273-8.
7. Svider PF, Pashkova AA, Folbe AJ, et al. Obstructive sleep apnea: strategies for minimizing liability and enhancing patient safety. Otolaryngol Head Neck Surg. 2013;149(6):947-53.

26

CHAPTER

Medicolegal Issues in Dentistry

Shivali Vaid

INTRODUCTION

In the current era of consumer satisfaction, dentists are increasingly facing legal challenges from dissatisfied patients. With this changing scenario, dental surgeons have to be more careful and may sometimes have to face legal problems, which are intangible and disturbing. Thus it is important that all dentists should be aware of the medicolegal aspects of the field and also the important role they play in forensic cases. Most of these issues in dentistry are due to negligence of either doctor/staff or sometimes patient himself.

Like any other medical practitioner, it is the duty of dentist to practice dentistry with certain standard of care. A breach of this duty that results in injury to the patient is called negligence. Dental practitioners must be aware of the legal elements, as there are greater possibilities of the dentist encountering such cases, particularly in the context of patient empowerment and increased desire for improved personal appearance.

A FEW DENTAL NEGLIGENT ACTS

- Any doctor can take up an emergency. A patient cannot be refused treatment on the ground that it is a medicolegal case and therefore to be seen in a government or approved hospital. Failure to attend an emergency is negligence
- Prevention of infection should not be restricted to only the health provider. It is the dentist's responsibility to prevent cross infection between patients. Endangering the health or lives of other patients (even without injury) can invite criminal negligence (as under Sec 336 IPC)
- Another cause of negligence usually involves general dentist's attempt to treat beyond their level of competence and failure to refer cases to the appropriate specialist. For example, in periodontal cases when there is any question as to the degree of difficulty or outcome, case should be referred to a periodontist to avoid legal pitfalls or in case of impactions/fracture the patients should be referred to oral surgeons
- Lack of informed consent is a cause of malpractice action, and without it, battery (unlawful touching) can be alleged. In practical terms, this means physically or emotionally harming the patient. If there is a procedure, which has complications or undesirable consequences, which a prudent patient does not anticipate, it is necessary to get an informed consent

- Dentist must engage in acceptable practice that is usually the product of evidence-based dentistry as opposed to customary practice, which is usually anecdotal. For instance, arsenic has been traditionally used to devitalize the pulp in endodontic. However, current endodontic practice unequivocally disapproves the use of arsenic due to potential complication, it may therefore be said that, while the use of arsenic was customary it is not an accepted practice today. A complication produced by arsenic, may therefore be said to be negligence
- Failure to give advice clearly results in complication. Dentist must give clear instructions regarding diet and postoperative care
- If prescriptions are not clear and if they do not have proper instructions, the dentist is deemed to have been negligent
- Failure of dentist to advice a crown for root canal filled tooth with significant loss of tooth substance can result in fracture of tooth. Dentist will be held liable. Similarly, making defective dentures is a negligent act
- Accidental ingestion of crowns, dental instrument, teeth, etc. can also be considered as negligence
- Patient was given local anesthesia without test dose and developed anaphylaxis and died. Dentist will be held liable
- Under Public Liability Insurance Act, a dentist can be held liable for harm caused to the public by inadvertent exposure of harmful substances like mercury, arsenic or for that matter even radiations.

NON-NEGLIGENT ACTS

- Patient's dissatisfaction with the progress of treatment cannot be called negligence
- Not getting desired relief is not negligence
- Charging, what the patient thinks exorbitant is not negligence
- When patient does not follow advice of the doctor and does not get satisfactory results, dentist cannot be held negligent.

HOW IS DENTIST LIABLE FOR NEGLIGENCE?

Dentists are liable under four headings:

1. Tortuous liability
2. Contractual liability
3. Criminal liability
4. Statutory liability.

Liability means an obligation that legally binds an individual to settle a debt, i.e., the state of being legally responsible for something. Usually liabilities are settled over time through the transfer of economic benefits including money, goods or services.

Tortuous Liability (Civil Liability)

Two types:

1. Primary liability
2. Vicarious liability

Primary Tortuous Liability

When a dentist is directly liable for an act of negligence in his clinic or hospital it is called primary liability. Most dental negligence's come under this category. The remedy for breach of tortuous liability is un-liquidated damages (damages that are unascertained) as awarded by the judge; it is usually in the form of compensation by cash.

Vicarious Liability

Dentist who is employed by a hospital or institution is often not primarily responsible for negligence. They may be said to have vicarious liability through the hospital. The hospital has the liability for the negligence of an employee. However, if the patient is admitted by a dentist in his personal capacity, then the dentist will be personally liable.

Contractual Liability

In a doctor-patient relationship, an implied contract is established when a dentist accepts a patient for treatment. A breach of any aspect of this implied contract, where the dentist is under duty to treat with care as well as continue to treat and not terminate until patient is cured or till patient discontinues treatment, may be considered a contractual liability. However, in most instances if there is no written contract, their liability will essentially lie within the realm of tortuous liability.

Criminal Liability

Criminal liability normally lies with an identifiable individual or groups of individuals. However, recent trends indicate that hospitals also may be held vicariously liable just as in civil liabilities. The important offences inviting criminal liability with regard to negligence are:

- *Section 304A Indian Penal Code (Sec 304A IPC)*: Negligent homicide. A rash or negligent act resulting in death, e.g., death on the dental chair
- *Sec 336 (IPC)*: An act endangering the life of a person (even if there is no injury), e.g., extracting a tooth for a patient with valvular heart disease without antibiotic prophylaxis against endocarditis (even if he does not develop endocarditis)
- *Sec 337 (IPC)*: A rash or negligent act causing simple injury, e.g., pain and swelling after extraction due to negligent extraction
- *Sec 338 (IPC)*: A rash or negligent act resulting in grievous injury, e.g., fracture of jaw during extraction due to excessive or improper force
- *Sec 339 (IPC)*: A rash or burn or negligent act resulting due to chemical used in various dental procedures, e.g., Eugenol burn during root canal treatment or dental filling or due to over-heating of dental instruments.

Statutory Liability

A dentist is liable if there is any infringement of statutes. They then become accountable to a statutory body. The liability depends on the kind of infringement and the provisions in the statute to deal with it. There are many statutes dealing with practice of doctors and dentists, as well as hospitals.

Who is Liable?

- Dentists with independent practice rendering only free services
- Private hospitals charging all
- All hospitals having free as well as paying patients; they are liable to both
- Doctors and hospitals paid by an insurance firm for treatment of their client or by an employer for the treatment of an employee.

Who is Not Liable?

- Dentists in hospitals who do not charge for any kind of treatment from their patients
- Hospitals offering free services to all patients.

A FEW LEGAL TERMINOLOGIES

Cognizable offence: An offence where a police officer can be based on his investigation, arrest a person without a judicial warrant.

Non-cognizable: An offence, where an arrest can only be made by a judicial warrant.

Bailable: The arresting officer can give a bail. Bail is a matter of right and has to be given unless the officer apprehends that the accused may abscond or tamper with evidence.

Non-bailable: Bail can be secured only from a judge. Heinous and violent crimes fall in this category, e.g., if there is a significant risk that the offender may commit further crime, abscond or tamper with evidence.

Compoundable: A crime in which a compromise between the suspected offender and the victim or his representatives can be worked out is said to be compoundable.

Non-compoundable: If the crime is against society and is of a serious nature, no compromise can be made between the accused and the victim. These cases are said to be noncompoundable.

Sec 304A is cognizable, bailable and non-compoundable. It can be punished with imprisonment of either description for a term of two years or fine or both.

Sec 337 and 338 are cognizable, bailable, and compoundable.

What should a Dentist do in the Event of a Medical Mishap?

When some mishap happens following a diagnostic or therapeutic procedure, or when a patient or relative makes a complaint, the dentist must take appropriate steps, some of which may be:

- Complete the patient's record and recheck the written notes
- Be frank enough and inform clearly of the mishap. Show that you were genuinely concerned about the unfortunate mishap. Answer all the queries of patient/relative and do not mind their repeated questioning, harsh attitude and at times even abusive language. Keep in mind the mental state of the close relatives/friends. Be compassionate, try to remain on the scene as long as possible, try to engage less excited attendants into discussion on the mishap and indirectly try to bring into focus the circumstances under which the

mishap occurred. Doctors who are open-minded and communicative are much less likely to be complained against as patients/attendants are extremely forgiving of errors made by a friendly and concerned medical attendant. A high proportion of complaints are precipitated or escalated into legal action by a progressive breakdown of the doctor-patient communication
- After initial responses, the dentist should contact some other doctor/protection organization to seek advice. The Dental Associations can form groups/cells to advise and assist in such situations.

LEGAL PROCESS

Dental negligence falls under Section 2(0) of the Consumer Protection Act (CPA) because Indian Dentist Act (IDA) had no provision to:
- Entertain any complaint from the patient
- Take action against dentist in case of negligence
- Award compensation.

Procedure

Complaint means any allegation in writing by the complainant that he has suffered loss or damage due to deficient services. It can be related to deficiency causing discomfort, loss of activity, loss of money, loss of workdays and quality of life, etc.
- As per section 13 of CPA, first a copy of complaint has to be sent to dentist directing him to give his version within a period of thirty days, which may be extended up to 45 days. After 45 days, if no reply is provided, then the court orders contempt proceedings against the dentist.
- *During reply, dentist may deny the allegation of the complaint:*
  - The machinery is required to decide the cases speedily, i.e., within a period of three months. If, after the proceedings, the District Forum is satisfied that any of the allegations contained in the complaint about the services are proved, it shall issue an order to the opposite party directing him to do one or more of the following things:
    - To return to the complainant the charges paid
    - Pay such amount as may be awarded by it as compensation to the consumer for any loss or injury suffered by the consumer due to the negligence of the opposite party.
- Where a complaint instituted before the District Forum, the State Commission or the National Commission, as the case may be, is found to be frivolous or vexatious, it shall, for reasons to be recorded in writing, dismiss the complaint and make an order that the complainant shall pay to the dentist such cost, not exceeding 10,000 rupees, as may be specified in the order.

Some Interesting Dental Cases in India

- Parmley vs Parmley (1945) 4DLR81. Dentist was held liable for extracting few more teeth in upper arch without patient's consent though they were advanced by the periodontitis

- Garner vs Marrell (1953) Times 31 Oct. CA. Dentist held liable for the death of the patient as a piece of gauze slipped into his throat during extraction causing asphyxia
- Ishwardas vs VK Gupta (1992) CPJ118NC. Soreness and ulcers caused due to ill-fitting denture, dentist was held liable.

DENTAL NEGLIGENCE CASE STUDIES IN UK

Detached Reamer

In this claim the client was elderly and of nervous disposition. She visited her dentist to undergo a root canal treatment on her lower left wisdom tooth. During the course of that treatment a reamer being used by the defendant became detached and fell onto the back of her tongue. Unfortunately the client involuntarily swallowed it. The client was taken to hospital and an X-ray was undertaken confirming that the instrument/implement had lodged in her intestine. Surgical intervention was not attempted and a month later X-ray examination confirmed that the reamer had been passed. The client suffered shock and anxiety as a result of this incident. The client received £2,000 in full and final settlement of her claim.

Fractured Dental Instrument

A piece of fractured dental instrument was left in a patient's tooth which subsequently required extraction due to infection. Damages were awarded in the sum of £1,000.

Failure to Recognise Decay

The client consulted her dentist for treatment for tooth pain. The dentist failed to recognise decay in a tooth which demanded prompt treatment. The failure to treat led to pain and extraction of the tooth, which needed replacing with an implant retained crown. The defendant dentist also unnecessarily extracted a wisdom tooth and removed and replaced a filling. The client received £3,000 for damages for pain and suffering, which included an element of future inconvenience as the crown would have to be replaced every 7 years.

Failure to Exercise Due Care and Skill

The client consulted a dentist to replace a removable double denture to the lower left jaw and of one crowned tooth. The client underwent extensive treatment involving the placing of fixed bridges in the lower left and lower right jaw. Four teeth were crowned and one of those crowns had to be replaced 5 times. The client had several operations on her teeth, which permanently affected her inability to eat hard foods or to drink hot or cold liquids. The client received £10,000 in damages for pain and suffering and £7,090 for future treatment.

Negligently Fitted Bridge

The client underwent dental work. Five crowns which were intended to carry a bridge were negligently fitted. They fell out leaving the sides of some teeth exposed. The client received

£3,250 for damages for pain and suffering and £3,462 for damages for the cost of restorative treatment.

Inadequate Fitting of Bridge

The client received £15,000 in respect of the dentist's failings in the bridge provision. The client returned to the dentist complaining of pain on biting and the temporary bridge was eased. The client then returned again and the temporary bridge was then removed and the client was advised of the need for root canal treatment. The client suffered pain and suffering as a result of repeated infections and could have avoided root canal treatment. The client would need to undergo future implants.

Wrongful Extraction

Wrongful extraction of baby or deciduous teeth, damages were awarded of £1,850.

Poor Canal Root Treatment

The client received £2,500 in respect of poor root canal treatment and failure to diagnose and treat an infection of another tooth.

Failure to Warn of Nerve Paresthesia

Nerve paresthesia on surgical extraction of lower wisdom tooth is common and the patient must be informed prior. The dentist failed to give adequate warnings of the risks associated with extraction of wisdom teeth. The client had slurred speech and also had numbness on her tongue. The client brought an action against the defendant alleging that he failed to advise her of the proximity of the inferior dental nerve and the dentist failed to obtain the client's consent to extract the tooth or adequately advise her of the risks of parasthesia. Damages were awarded of £12,000.

Substandard Placement of Titanium Dental Implants

The client received £4,000 for substandard placement of her titanium dental implant. The defendant dentist purported to be an expert in dental implants and extracted the claimant's teeth to place the titanium dental implant. The dentist poorly positioned the implant. The client suffered pain and social embarrassment due to the poor placement of the implant.

Failure to Diagnose and Treat Periodontal Disease

The client attended the dental practice from 1993 to 2007. During this period, the client had veneers fitted, underwent deep scale polishing, a replacement veneer was fitted, had a crown fitted and various root canal treatments. In 2007, the client attended an alternative dental practice complaining of immense pain. It was noted that the client was suffering from advanced adult periodontitis and had several mobile teeth. By 2007 the prognosis for various teeth was extremely poor and was advised that those teeth may require extraction. It was alleged that the dentist failed to diagnose the client's periodontal disease and failed to appropriately interpret the radiographic evidence. The dentist failed to investigate the client's deteriorating periodontal condition and failed to advise her of the disease and the treatment required. The dentist also failed to monitor the client's disease and failed to refer her to a periodontal specialist. The client received £7,500 damages in respect of the dentist's failure to diagnose and treat the client's periodontal disease.

Failure to Diagnose and Treat Periodontal Disease

The client was a 61-year-old woman who received £25,000 in respect of the dentist's failure to diagnose, monitor and treat periodontal disease, resulting in the loss of several teeth and likely future loss of further teeth. The client had root canal treatment and crowns fitted and prolonged gum treatment in 1988. She further had prolonged gum treatment again in 1989. The client regularly attended between1990 and 2006. During this period, regular radiographs were taken. Radiographs were taken in September 2005 which confirmed significant bone loss due to advanced periodontal disease. The client brought her case, arguing that the dentist failed to use reasonable care and skill in the provision of root canal treatment and in the provision of periodontal treatment from 1987–2005. The client also argued that the dentist failed to use reasonable care and skill and monitoring of the progression of the periodontal condition and failed to use reasonable care and skill in recording periodontal indices.

THE ROLE OF FORENSIC ODONTOLOGY IN LEGAL MATTERS

Forensic odontology helps the law in the administration of justice. Though in developed countries this branch of dentistry is playing a useful role but as far as India is concerned its role is definitely being recognized now-a-days. An overview of the basic and recent trends of this emerging branch of dentistry is presented to make the concerned professionals aware of their role in medicolegal matters. Forensic odontology deals with proper handling, examination and evaluation of dental evidence which are presented in the interest of justice. The information, so obtained is concerned primarily with:

- Establishment of identity
- Investigation of criminal cases
- Research purposes.

But dentists are responsible for the following main areas of practice:

- Identification of human fragmentary measures
- Identification in mass disasters
- Assessment of bite marks, injuries
- Assessment of abuse, i.e., child, spousal and elder
- Civil cases involving malpractice
- Age estimation
- Criminal liability.

Identification can be further studied under two categories:

1. General or reconstructive identity, i.e., to classify unknown persons by age, sex, race, occupation, and habits, etc.

2. *Comparative methods*: A person's identification is indicated or excluded when the postmortem dental record is compared with the antemortem dental record.

Dental evidences represent one of the most scientifically reliable methods of identification. On exposure to physical injury and putrefactive changes the human dentition preserves itself, but the enamel which is the hardest part of the body, lasts much longer than the other tissues. The preservation of teeth in ancient human relics buried for centuries attests to this fact. The adult dentition is comprised of 32 teeth, each tooth has five surfaces. The innumerable combinations of missing teeth, filling materials, carious lesions, restorative work, and prosthesis involving these 160 surfaces form the basis of dental identification. Considering additional identifying features incorporated within the root canal, periapical, and surrounding bone and soft tissue, it may be realised how specific the oral structures can be in terms of identification. The concept that no two dentitions are alike is the basic premise of dental identification.

Three organizations are dedicated to the field of forensic odontology. These organizations include:

1. The Bureau of Legal Dentistry (BOLD)
2. The American Board of Forensic Odontology (ABFO) and
3. The International Organization for Forensic Odontostomatology (IOFOS).

In 1996, BOLD was created at the University of British Columbia to develop new technology and techniques in forensic odontology. The University of British Colombia Program is the only one in North America that provides graduate training in forensic odontology. The Bureau of Legal Dentistry encourages the use of multiple dental impressions to create a "dental line-up", similar to a suspect line-up used to identify/alleged perpetrators of crime. Currently, dental impressions collected as evidence are compared only to these collected from a given suspect, which may bias the resulting outcome. Using multiple dental impressions in a lineup may enable forensic odontologists to significantly decrease the current bias in matching bite marks to the teeth of a suspect. The organization BOLD also support the creation of a database of dental records, which could help in verifying dental uniqueness. This database could be created using criminal records or possibly all dental patients.

In 1984, the ABFO began making an attempt to diminish the discrepancies and increase the validity of bite mark analysis by creating bite mark methodology guidelines. The guidelines attempt to establish standard terminology in describing bite marks and that reduces the risk of biased results. The ABFO also provides advice on how to effectively collect and preserve evidence. For example they recommend that the collection of DNA evidence and detailed photography of bites be taken together at the crime scene. The guidelines also outline how and what a forensic odontologist should record such as the location, contours, shape, and size of a bite mark. They also provide a system of scoring to assess the degree to which a suspect's dental profile and bite mark match, i.e.:

- *Positive identification*: The antemortem and postmortem data match in sufficient detail, with no unexplainable discrepancies, to establish that they are from the same individual.
- *Possible identification*: The antemortem and postmortem data have consistent features but, because of the quality of either the postmortem remains or the antemortem evidence, it is not possible to establish identity positively.
- *Insufficient evidence*: The available information is insufficient to form the basis for a conclusion.
- *Exclusion*: The antemortem and postmortem data are clearly inconsistent.

According to the ABFO, the guidelines are not a mandate of methods to be used, but a list of generally accepted methods. The guidelines are intended to prevent potentially useful evidence from being thrown out simply because the forensic odontologist's collection methods were not standardized. Kouble and Craig used a simplified version of the ABFO scoring guidelines in order to return accuracy with a large sample of comparison. A numerical score was assigned to represent the degree of similarity between the bite mark and model/overlay. The higher the score, the greater is the similarity. In order to simplify the model, some features that were individually scored in the ABFO guidelines such as arch size and shape were assessed together while certain distinctive features such as spacing between teeth were treated as a separate variable.

In an attempt to improve guidelines used to collect dental evidence IOFOS developed one of the most recognized systems for collection of forensic dental evidence. Antemortem loss or fracture of tooth in assault cases is a criminal act U/S 320 of Indian Penal Code (IPC) clause 7. If such cases are to be examined medicolegally, then determination of nature and age of injury (loss or fracture of tooth) is very important to corelate the history with the occurrence of crime from medical and dental facts. It is not only the examination of injured tooth which is important, but associated injuries to the surrounding structures and on the face should be recorded along with the examination of the stump/root or empty socket. The X-ray examination of the jaw is equally important to find associated fracture of the thin bony plate surrounding the alveolus which is usually seen in local trauma thereby ruling out natural fall of diseased tooth. The role of teeth in providing age estimation, sex determination, race, and misidentification is undisputedly well documented. Recently cheiloscopy and rugoscopy have established their unique role in identification just like superimposition technique.

India is far behind both in the theoretical as well as practical aspect of forensic dentistry. Practically, there is no laboratory which may do the work of forensic dentistry except Forensic Science Laboratories of Centre and States where only superimposition technique is done for identification. The routine medicolegal cases/forensic autopsy cases where examination of teeth/bite marks is required are handled by forensic physician, forensic pathologist or dentist by routine conventional methods. But no specialized procedure in relation to forensic dentistry is adopted except routine dental X-rays and clinical examination of teeth and related structures.

So, it is high time, that the dental fraternity should realize their role in the criminal investigation system. They should take the forensic dentistry to such heights in the society that it may be become a very useful tool for the investigating agencies in solving the disputed cases and the courts should not hesitate to base their verdict on the undisputed dental evidence tendered by forensic dentist in the court of law.

CONCLUSION

It is the duty of dentist to practice dentistry with certain standard of care. Dentists are increasingly facing legal challenges from dis-satisfied patients. Dentist must engage in acceptable practice that is usually the product of evidence-based dentistry as opposed to customary practice, which is usually anecdotal. Be frank enough and inform clearly of the mishap. Show that you were genuinely concerned about the unfortunate mishap. Forensic odontology helps the law in the administration of justice as it deals with proper handling, examination and evaluation of dental evidence. The Dental Associations can form groups/cells to advise and assist in such situations.

KEY LEARNING POINTS

- Dentist must engage in acceptable evidence-based dentistry as opposed to customary practice, which is usually anecdotal.
- Making defective dentures is a negligent act. Accidental ingestion of crowns, dental instrument, teeth, etc., can also be considered as negligence.
- The principles of Informed consent, civil, criminal or statutory liability are same as in other fields of medical establishments.
- The role of forensic odontology is increasing in the present circumstances.
- The bite marks, shape of the teeth, artificial/implanted teeth can give clue in cases of criminal offences or legal matters.

BIBLIOGRAPHY

1. Ishwardas vs VK Gupta (1992) CPJ118NC. https://www.google.com/search?q=Ishwardas+vs+VK+Gupta+(1992)&oq=Ishwardas+vs+VK+Gupta+(1992)&aqs=chrome..69i57j0i512i546l4j0i751.13755j0j9&sourceid=chrome&ie=UTF-8
2. Parmley vs Parmley (1945) 4DLR81 https://www.google.com/search?q=Parmley+vs+Parmley+(1945)&oq=Parmley+vs+Parmley+(1945)&aqs=chrome..69i57j33i10i160l2.19616j0j9&sourceid=chrome&ie=UTF-8
3. Garner vs Marrell (1953) https://www.google.com/search?q=Garner+vs+Marrell+(1953)&oq=Garner+vs+Marrell+(1953)&aqs=chrome..69i57j33i10i160l2.3607j0j7&sourceid=chrome&ie=UTF-8.

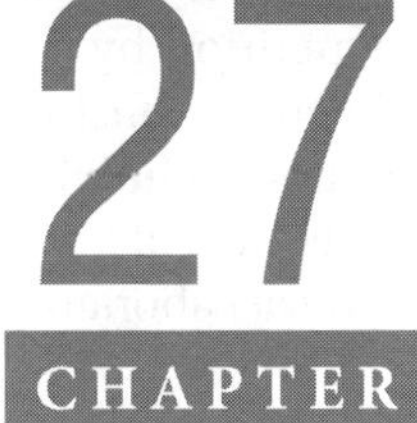

27

CHAPTER

Medicolegal Issues in Pathology and Microbiology

Varsha Baldwa, Mahesh Baldwa, Namita Padvi, Sushila Baldwa

"Pathology and medical laboratory practice has revolutionized medical treatment always."

INTRODUCTION

The role of pathologists in patient care is undergoing a transformation, with pathologists now playing a more active role in patient management. Modern society's expectations regarding laboratory medicine are leading to increased scrutiny regarding the accuracy of laboratory data, the timely execution of laboratory tests, and the communication of results. Healthcare professionals in medical laboratories must grasp the fundamental medicolegal principles applicable to laboratory medicine to navigate the complex intersection of law and medicine effectively. They must adhere to established standards for laboratory medicine in their practice. However, it is crucial to note that pathologists also have a responsibility to patients and can be held accountable for medical negligence, even when delegating tasks to non-pathologists and support staff, which is essential for the efficiency of laboratory medicine. Common challenges often revolve around errors in diagnosis and documentation. Nonetheless, a significant distinction between pathologists and clinicians is that pathologists typically have minimal direct interaction with patients.

REGISTRATION AND LICENSING OF A PATHOLOGIST

In the case of Rajni Shukla versus Rajendra Kumar Agrawal Madhya Pradesh S.C.D.R.C. 1 (2003) CPJ: 551.

The pathology laboratory lacked both registration and a license. The court ruled that government laboratories are exempt from registration and licensing requirements. This exemption applies when government doctors are employed or providing services on a part-time basis. However, all private pathologists and laboratories in Madhya Pradesh are required to obtain registration and licensing from the local authority.

SHORTAGE OF PATHOLOGISTS AND MICROBIOLOGISTS

As of September 25, 2023, there are a total of 24,842 pathologists in India, with only 4,500 members belonging to the pathology association. India, with its vast population of 1.4 billion, also hosts approximately 100,000 diagnostic laboratories.

In light of the Supreme Court's judgment on July 10, 2018, in the case of "*North Gujarat Unit of Association versus North Gujarat Pathologists,*" where the review petition by the Gujarat-based Association of Laboratory Technicians was rejected, it has been established that laboratory reports can only be countersigned by registered medical practitioners holding a postgraduate qualification in pathology. This decision significantly impacts the role and responsibilities of individuals with qualifications such as BSc and Diploma in Medical Laboratory Technology (DMLT) cannot sign reports.

SHOULD HOSPITALS PROVIDE 24-HOURS SERVICES?

In the case of Shahul Hameed versus Apollo Hospital Enterprises Tamil Nadu S.C.D.R.C. II (2002) CPJ, 395.

Hospitals, expected to operate round the clock, cannot claim to have fixed working hours when it comes to handling laboratory samples from the public. When a patient provides a sample, it is essential that the necessary tests are carried out within a specified time frame. Failing to do so constitutes a failure to act within the required time frame, which can prevent the treating doctor from taking corrective actions for the patient.

In a specific case, the complainant was suffering from fever and was referred to Apollo Hospital for certain tests. The hospital collected the required sample, but the tests were not conducted on the same day the sample was received. The hospital's explanation that its microbiology department ceased operations after 5 PM was not acceptable to the court. The court ruled that the laboratory associated with the hospital should operate 24 hours a day. Therefore, the failure to conduct tests on the same day as the sample collection amounted to a service deficiency, and the complainant was entitled to compensation.

VARIATION OF PLATELET COUNT—NO NEGLIGENCE

In the case of Vikram versus Jagdamba Medical Centre (HSCDRC)(Panchkula), First Appeal No. 963 of 2014. D/d. 17.11.2014.

There was no evidence demonstrating any discrepancies in platelet count reports, leading to a deficiency in service. As a result, the initial complaint was dismissed. An appeal was subsequently filed, but no evidence was presented in the record suggesting that incorrect reports were deliberately generated for financial gain. It was established that platelet levels can fluctuate during treatment, and minor variations do not necessarily imply negligence or malicious intent on the part of the opposing party. Therefore, the appeal was dismissed as it lacked merit.

PATHOLOGIST CANNOT BE HELD RESPONSIBLE FOR NEGLIGENCE OF PEDIATRICIAN

In the case of Shyam Sunder Tantia (Dr.) versus Deepika, Rajasthan S.C.D.R. I (2002) CPJ, 411.

The pathologist doctor performed the required pathological tests based on the pediatrician's recommendation and charged a professional fee. However, the pathologist doctor did not prescribe any medication. Therefore, the pathologist doctor cannot be held accountable for negligence. The infant was under the care of a consulting pediatrician who recommended the use of Gardenal tablets without conducting tests, which led to the child's condition deteriorating. Consequently, the pathologist is not responsible for providing compensation. The negligence in delivering professional services was solely attributed to the pediatrician, and therefore, the pediatrician is liable to compensate the patient party.

NON-DIAGNOSIS OF BLOOD CANCER

In the case of Wahid Khan versus Dr. Mohd. Abdul, 1999 (3) CPJ 304 (UP SCDRC).

The complainant's son was suffering from blood cancer, and the opposite party (OP) was unable to treat the condition within a 40-day period. Eventually, the patient was taken to a medical college where the diagnosis of blood cancer was confirmed. According to the appellant's counsel, the family doctor who was treating the complainant's son should have arranged for a blood cancer examination with the assistance of a pathology report. However, this blood report has not been presented to the District Forum, nor has a copy of it been provided to the Commission.

The State Commission determined that in the absence of this report, it cannot be asserted that there was any clear indication that the complainant's son was suffering from blood cancer. Consequently, it is not possible to conclude that the doctor who was treating the complainant's son acted negligently or provided deficient service.

ANTENATAL EXAMINATION—VENEREAL DISEASE RESEARCH LABORATORY—FALSE POSITIVE

In the case of Chandrasagar D. Rajput versus Dr. Dinesh J. Shah, 1999 (1) CPJ 434 (Maharashtra SCDRC).

The complainant's wife underwent antenatal examinations, including a VDRL (venereal disease research laboratory) test. The certificate issued by the doctor indicated a "positive" result with a "titer of 1:8," implying that one of the spouses might have a venereal disease. However, this certificate did not mention that it was preliminary and subject to confirmatory tests.

Subsequent tests from another doctor's laboratory revealed that the complainant tested "negative" for VDRL, while his wife's result was nonspecific and a biological false positive. The initial certificate had a damaging impact on the complainant's reputation within society. While corrective certificates were later issued, the stigma associated with the initial result persisted.

The lack of clarity in the initial certificate caused significant social distress and suspicion between the husband and wife. This resulted in social turmoil and damage to their reputation. To compensate for this social trauma, an award of ₹50,000 in cumulative damages is appropriate, signaling to society that neither spouse is afflicted with VDRL disease. This award serves the interests of justice, considering the status of the husband and wife.

WRONGLY REPORTED AS CANCER: PAN-HYSTERECTOMY—NEGLIGENCE

In the case of Dr. Sanjay J. Batra versus Jagrut Nagrik, (NCDRC), Revision Petition No. 567 of 2015 (Against the Order dated 24/12/2014 in Appeal No. 2997 of 2012 of the State Commission Gujarat). D/d. 12.4.2016.

A misdiagnosis occurred in the case of dilatation and curettage (D and C) and the biopsy specimen, leading to an incorrect cancer report from Tata Cancer Hospital. On November 6, 1999, Dr JJ Vyas performed a pan-hysterectomy (removal of the uterus). The histopathology report initially indicated "no cancer." Subsequently, the District Forum ruled in favor of the complainant and directed the hospital to pay a lump sum compensation of ₹1 lakh with 9% interest.

Diagnostic errors represent a significant and costly portion of medical errors. An erroneous diagnosis by a clinical pathologist can result in delayed or inappropriate treatment and potential legal action from the patient who suffered harm. Such errors are considered acts of omission and do not align with the standard of practice. The goal is to establish a clear distinction between reasonable and unacceptable pathology practices without relying on hindsight.

The misdiagnosis caused unnecessary mental distress and suffering to the patient and their family; therefore, the hospital is liable to a certain extent. The compensation amount has been adjusted to ₹50,000, and the petition has been resolved accordingly.

ANTENATAL WRONG DIAGNOSIS OF SICKLE CELL ON DEOXYRIBONUCLEIC ACID TEST

In the case of Ravindra Dnyaneshwar Patil versus Dr. Vinay Tule, (NCDRC), First Appeal No. 1291 of 2017, (Against the Order dated 03/05/2017 in Complaint No. 13/2015 of the State Commission Maharashtra). D/d. 17.7.2017.

The complaint was initially dismissed by the State Commission, and an appeal was filed against this decision. In cases involving alleged medical negligence in treatment or diagnosis, the burden of proof lies with the person making the allegation of negligence. In this specific case, it was the responsibility of the complainants/appellants to demonstrate that the medical service provider (OP) had been negligent in conducting the testing or recording the results.

The complainant couple had a history of Sickle Cell disease, a blood disorder, and sought medical advice due to concerns about the possibility of their unborn child inheriting the disease. Dr Bharati Taori, an Obstetrician and Gynecologist, recommended a prenatal deoxyribonucleic acid (DNA) test to assess the risk to the fetus. A sample was collected and sent to the OP's laboratory for examination. The initial report from the OP indicated that the fetus was a carrier of the sickle cell trait, not the sickle cell SS pattern, so the pregnancy continued.

However, after the child's birth, a different specialist conducted a similar test and issued a report that contradicted the OP's earlier findings, indicating that the child had the "SS Pattern Sickle cell trait." Subsequent examinations confirmed that the child was affected by sickle cell anemia.

Despite these discrepancies, the complainants did not present any medical experts to comment on whether the OP's testing procedure was negligent. Consequently, they failed to establish negligence on the part of the OP. The State Commission's decision was deemed appropriate, and the appeal was dismissed.

CANCER STAGE IV MISSED

In the case of Raj Kumar versus Dr Ajay Gupta, 2001 (I) CPJ 495 (UP SCDRC).

The pathological examination conducted by the second party (OP No. 2) consisted of a report based on the examination, and they did not provide any advice for the treatment of the complainant's wife. None of the parties involved (OP Nos. 1, 2, and 3) indicated that the complainant's wife was suffering from cancer or any other illness. They merely submitted their reports, leaving it to the surgeon who performed the operation to determine if cancer was present in the complainant's wife's body. OP Nos. 1, 2, and 3 were not responsible for this part of the diagnosis.

Furthermore, ultrasound examinations cannot detect cancer if the tumor is <2 cm in size. Therefore, OP Nos. 1, 2, and 3 cannot be held responsible for the death of the complainant's wife because they were not involved in diagnosing the case. Consequently, no case has been established against OP Nos. 1, 2, and 3.

PATHOLOGICAL LABORATORIES—DIFFERENT READINGS OF BILIRUBIN

In the case of Smt. Supriti Modak versus Dr. Gokul Ch. Modak, 2001 (2) CPJ 219 (WB SCDRC).

During the hearing, it became evident that the baby had been delivered through a cesarean section, and there were significant allegations of negligence against the attending physician and pathological laboratories regarding the baby's treatment. It is acknowledged that the baby's blood was tested three times at different pathological laboratories, resulting in varying bilirubin readings. Eventually, the baby was transferred to NRS Hospital in Kolkata, where the illness was accurately diagnosed, and the baby was successfully treated.

The Forum recognized that substantiating the claims of negligence against the opposing parties would require the testimony of several witnesses, including medical, gynecological, and pathological experts. Citing the precedent set by the Honorable Supreme Court in the case of *Indian Medical Association versus V.P. Shantha (reported in AIR 1996 SC 550)*, the Forum chose not to adjudicate the dispute. The State Commission upheld the Forum's decision, deeming it entirely reasonable.

LITIGATION EVEN AFTER REFUNDING BLOOD EXAMINATION CHARGES

In the case of Madhyamgram Consumers Welfare Society versus Dr. Kalyan Kumar Chatterjee and others, 2002 (2) CPJ 381 (WB SCDRC).

The Forum, however, did not grant any compensation to the petitioner. Their reasoning was based on the petitioner's failure to provide evidence of any harm or injury resulting from the incorrect reports issued by the Opposite Parties (OPs). The time gap between the two reports was only 9 days. The first report from the OPs indicated a subnormal reading, while the second report from another laboratory showed a higher reading within the normal range. Although a third report was not obtained to determine the accuracy of either report, the Forum found insufficient evidence to support the petitioner's claim for compensation.

It should be noted that the OPs refunded ₹250 to the petitioner, and they also covered the cost of the litigation, which the petitioner accepted. There is essentially no evidence to suggest that the petitioner suffered any harm due to the first report. The consulting physician did not rely on the initial report and instead recommended obtaining a second report. Additionally, no treatment was initiated based on the first report. Given these circumstances, the Forum's decision not to award compensation and to refrain from awarding a higher amount for litigation costs was entirely justified.

WRONG PATHOLOGY REPORT OF BREAST CANCER—NEGLIGENCE

In the case of Smt. Yashoda Goyal versus Dr. Ahuja's Pathology and Imaging Centre, (USCDRC) (Dehradun), Consumer Complaint No. 4 of 2006. D/d. 13.03.2018.

The patient received an incorrect pathology report from OP Nos. 1 and 2, erroneously indicating that she had breast cancer (carcinoma breast). Subsequently, OP No. 3, relying on this erroneous report without conducting any additional laboratory tests, performed an unnecessary surgery on the patient's left breast, which resulted in its removal.

The patient presented a histopathology report dated 11.12.2003 from Dr. Lal Path Laboratories Pvt. Ltd. to support her case. The surgery was performed based on the biopsy report provided by the patient herself. Given these circumstances, OP No. 3 cannot be considered negligent as they acted upon the report issued by OP Nos. 1 and 2. Therefore, there is no medical negligence on the part of OP No. 3.

In light of the above, the consumer complaint has been upheld, and OP Nos. 1 and 2 are directed to pay compensation of ₹10,00,000.

NO REAL CONSENT FOR BLOOD TRANSFUSION

In the case of Sulochana Lad versus Dr. Mohan Gerra, (NCDRC) (New Delhi), First Appeal No. 138 of 2008 (against Order dated 12.4.2007 in Consumer Complaint No. 237 of 1997 of Maharashtra SCDRC, Mumbai). D/d. 29.3.2016.

A blood transfusion was administered, but the blood was infected with human immunodeficiency virus (HIV) virus, leading to both the mother and newborn child being diagnosed as HIV positive. It was alleged that the necessary tests were not conducted before the transfusion, and the risks and alternatives were not properly communicated, depriving the patient of the right to self-determination. The State Commission dismissed the complaint, but on appeal, it was found that the treating doctor failed to obtain valid consent for the blood transfusion, making it an unauthorized act akin to assault and battery.

Although there was no clear evidence linking the contaminated blood transfusion to the complainant contracting HIV, the deficiency lay in the treating doctor's failure to secure valid consent, not in the procedure itself. The complainant's life expectancy depends on strict medication and a healthy diet. She has already endured considerable suffering and will continue to face HIV-related stigma, discrimination, and negative community reactions fueled by misconceptions about HIV transmission routes. As a result, a compensation of ₹5,00,000 has been awarded.

SPINAL SURGERY—FOOT DROP—STEM CELL THERAPY—PATIENT WORSENED—NEGLIGENCE

In the case of Vikas Yadav versus ReeLabs Pvt. Ltd., (HSCDRC)(Panchkula), Complaint No.301 of 2016. D/d. 23.10.2018.

In 1997, the complainant underwent spine surgery, resulting in a condition of foot drop, requiring the use of a walker. Stem cell therapy was administered through a spinal route, with the complainant paying ₹4 lakh to Dr. Narender Rohilla (OP No. 2). Unfortunately, Dr. Narender

Rohilla's treatment did not yield positive results, and the complainant's condition worsened after the second dose administered by Dr. Mohit Lathar (OP No. 3) and Vikas Gupta. This situation warrants serious attention, and Dr. Narender Rohilla (OP No. 2) and Dr. Mohit Lathar (OP No. 3) are held responsible for their negligence.

Dr. Narender Rohilla (OP No. 2) is obligated to refund the medical expenses of ₹4 lakh paid by the complainant, and Dr. Mohit Lathar (OP No. 3) is required to indemnify ₹5 lakh to OP No. 4, who serves as the insurer for OP No. 3. Additionally, ₹2,00,000 is to be awarded to the complainant for physical and mental distress.

MISSED ABORTION URINE TEST FOR PREGNANCY MAY SHOW NEGATIVE

In the case of Rajani Shukla versus Rajendra Kumar Agrawal, 2003 (1) CLD 347: 2003 (1) CPJ 551: 2003 (2) CPR 238 (MP SCDRC).

Opposite Party Nos. 1 and 2 operate an unregistered pathology laboratory staffed by qualified personnel, including a doctor with MBBS and MD in pathology overseeing operations. The complainant was admitted to a Maternity Home for a Missed Abortion case. The doctor requested a urine pregnancy test, which was conducted around 11.00 a.m. by the complainant's husband. However, due to the nature of a Missed Abortion, the urine test returned a negative result, which is typical after a missed pregnancy.

The complainant was admitted on the night of March 13, 1994, and diagnosed with Missed Abortion, defined as the retention of a deceased fetus inside the uterus for >4 weeks. Therefore, the allegation that the wrong report led to a change in medication resulting in abortion is baseless. The missed abortion was already established, and a Dilation and Curettage (D and C) procedure may have been necessary to remove remaining fetal tissue. The pathology laboratory, Mani Pathology Laboratory, cannot be held negligent for providing a negative pregnancy report. The District Forum's finding that the wrong report led to medication changes and subsequent abortion lacks merit, as there was no negligence on the part of the OP. Consequently, the complainants are not entitled to any relief.

WRONG REPORT CARCINOMA OF UTERUS

In the case of Santosh Kaur Sodhi versus Dr. Vijay Mujoo, 2003 (2) CLD 751: 2003 (2) CPJ 344 (Chd.-UTCDRC).

The OP pathologist issued a report diagnosing the complainant with uterine carcinoma. Relying on this report, the complainant was taken to the renowned Tata Memorial Hospital in Mumbai, where her uterus was removed. However, post-surgery histopathological tests revealed the absence of cancer in the uterus. The hospital should have conducted further tests before resorting to a major surgery like uterine removal solely based on the pathological report.

No negligence can be attributed to the OP, as doctors may offer opinions and treatments based on established medical practices, which may differ from those of more experienced doctors. The District Forum correctly emphasized that a reputable hospital such as Tata Memorial Hospital in Mumbai would not have solely relied on the respondent's report and would have conducted tests in Mumbai before deciding on a major surgery such as uterine removal. Furthermore, the histopathology report after the uterine removal was not substantiated by credible evidence.

The respondent cannot be deemed careless or negligent in conducting the tests and providing the report. It is a well-established legal principle that differences in medical opinions can arise, and merely having a different opinion does not warrant holding the respondent liable for negligence or carelessness, especially given the complexity of diagnosing diseases such as cancer.

WRONG BLOOD GROUP

In the case of Bharat Pathology Laboratory versus Mangi Lal Vyas, 2003 (3) CPJ 94 (NCDRC).

Two separate blood group tests were conducted, resulting in different blood group recordings, raising concerns about the possibility of blood transfusion errors. Both the District Forum and the State Commission concurred in their findings that providing incorrect reports amounted to negligence, and they awarded compensation of ₹5,000. The National Commission did not overturn this determination.

Both forums determined the case to be a matter of medical negligence and ordered compensation of ₹5,000. However, during the admission stage, it was brought to our attention that the parties had settled the matter in accordance with the District Forum's order dated March 20, 2002. Consequently, the case is dismissed as withdrawn.

DENGUE NEITHER SUSPECTED NOR DIAGNOSED–CAUSED DELAY–DEATH

In the case of Umakant Rajaram Chauhan versus Dr. Anil M. Gupta, (GSCDRC) (Ahmedabad), Complaint No. 42 of 2011. D/d. 06.11.2020.

Patient was not diagnosed with dengue and seems to have been treated for sepsis, anemia, chronic obstructive pulmonary disease (COPD), but not for dengue, which he doubted only on 29th. He doubted it from very fever, tachycardia, anemia not responding to standard treatment as answered by him. The root cause of sepsis, pleural effusion, abdominal distension was not tried to be found out vide WHO guidelines under clause 2.1.2 critical phase for dengue nor treated the dengue that way at least before it was detected on 29.10.2010 by seeing laboratory report of reduced platelets and dengue immunoglobulin G (IgG) which was carried out at Divine Micropath Laboratory on 29th and it was found that she was positive. She was shifted Nidhi Hospital, there she was diagnosed of dengue fever, brain white matter edema, paralytic ileus on 01.11.2010; was found with remote possibility of encephalopathy, on discharge on 09.11.2010, she was diagnosed of dengue fever with white matter edema with acute respiratory distress syndrome (ARDS) with acute renal failure (ARF) with obstructive sleep apnea + paralytic ileus. All these clearly prove negligence of Dr Gupta. The underlying causes of sepsis, pleural effusion, and abdominal distension were not thoroughly investigated, as per WHO guidelines (clause 2.1.2, critical phase for dengue). Additionally, dengue was not treated appropriately until it was detected on October 29, 2010, based on laboratory reports showing reduced platelet levels and a positive dengue IgG test conducted at Divine Micropath Laboratory on that day.

Failure to employ the necessary diagnostic skills resulting in incorrect treatment can be considered negligence. Upon discharge on November 9, 2010, she was diagnosed with dengue fever, white matter edema, ARDS, ARF, obstructive sleep apnea, and paralytic ileus. These conditions highlight the patient's deteriorating health due to the failure to diagnose and treat dengue promptly. All these factors collectively indicate negligence on the part of Dr Gupta, for which compensation of ₹14,14,000 awarded. No negligence of laboratory.

WRONG REPORT OF SMALL CELL CARCINOMA OF LUNG

In the case of Leena Bhattarcharjee versus Nightangle Diagnostic and Eye Care Research Centre (P) Ltd., 2003 (6) CLD 706: 2004 (1) CPR 130 (WB SCDRC).

Chief pathologist initially indicated the presence of small cell carcinoma of the lung. Subsequently, the patient was admitted to another hospital and underwent a surgery, during which the left upper lobe of the lung was removed. However, further pathological tests revealed no signs of cancer. Allegations of negligence were made against the chief pathologist.

These allegations of negligence are unsustainable because the chief pathologist had not provided a final report, and it was the responsibility of the surgeon who performed the operation to make the final decision before proceeding with the surgery. Therefore, there is no evidence of negligence on the part of the chief pathologist.

HEMOPHILIA—HEPATITIS C VIRUS POSITIVE—NO NEGLIGENCE

In the case of Sandeep Kumar versus Post Graduate Institute of Medical Education & Research, (NCDRC) (New Delhi) 2016(4), First Appeal No. 407 of 2012; (Against the Order dated 01/06/2012 in Complaint No. 12 of 2011 of the State Commission Chandigarh). D/d. 13.12.2016.

The complainant, a patient with Hemophilia-A, received treatment from OP-1 through FFP transfusion. It was alleged that the complainant contracted hepatitis C virus (HCV) following the fresh frozen plasma (FFP) transfusion, with the infection being detected from a blood sample 3 weeks after admission to OP-1 Hospital.

In cases of negligence, it is necessary to establish a breach of duty and the omission of required actions. However, there is no evidence to prove negligence on the part of the treating doctors or the hospital. A letter from PGI dated 07.06.2011 indicates that the incidence of transfusion-associated HCV infection is estimated to be between 0.01 and 0.001% per unit transfused, indicating that the chances of contracting the infection are negligible. Therefore, negligence cannot be attributed to the treating doctors at OP-1 Hospital. As a result, the revision petition has been dismissed.

HIV INFECTION CAUSED BY NEGLIGENCE NOT PROVED

In the case of Gulshan Kumar versus Dr. Rajan and Others III (2012) CPJ 415 (NC).

In this case, it has been determined that the burden of proof lies with the complainant to demonstrate that the HIV infection was a result of carelessness or negligence on the part of the hospital. However, the complainant has failed to establish negligence.

REMOVED SPLEEN AND GALLBLADDER–BLEEDING FROM GASTRIC ARTERY—NO CRIMINAL NEGLIGENCE

In the case of Dr. Ashok Ladha versus State of Madhya Pradesh, (Indore Bench), Miscellaneous Criminal Case No. 2662 of 2017. D/d. 16.04.2018.

On 3.7.2012, Kamal Parmar was admitted to Vishesh Hospital as an emergency case due to severe sickle cell anemia. Dr Manish Neema, a Consultant Hematologist, requested the petitioner, a Gastroenterology Surgeon, to perform surgery to remove both the enlarged spleen and gall bladder. The surgery was conducted on 7.7.2012, and a wide bore abdominal tube drain was placed to monitor for postoperative bleeding, which did not occur. However, on the same day around 7.30 PM, Kamal Parmar became unconscious and was transferred to the ICU, where he subsequently passed away on 8.7.2012.

A postmortem revealed a cut and open short gastric artery, with the cause of death determined as shock and hemorrhage from the operated short gastric artery. A medical board was formed to assess whether the petitioner's surgery involved negligence, and their report dated 23.10.2013 concluded that Kamal Parmar's death resulted from the petitioner's negligence. While the petitioner's actions may be considered negligent, the review committee did not find gross negligence on the part of the doctor. Consequently, the case was dismissed.

BLOOD TRANSFUSION—HIV INFECTION—RES IPSA LOQUITUR

In the case of Care Hospital M/s. Quality Care India versus Vemuganti Venu Gopal (NCDRC), Revision Petition No. 4236 of 2014 from order dated 22.9.2014 in Appeal No. 488/2013 of Andhra Pradesh State Consumer Disputes Redressal Commission Hyderabad with IA/8352/2014. D/d. 9.12.2014.

Misdiagnosis of any disease or condition can be fatal as it can result in untreated or incorrectly treated conditions. In cases of false-negative HIV diagnoses, the consequences can be catastrophic. Patients not only miss out on essential treatments but may unknowingly transmit the virus to others.

The case involves a blood transfusion leading to an HIV infection due to alleged medical negligence. The District Forum partially accepted the complaint, while the State Commission dismissed the appeal. A revision petition was filed before the National Commission. It questions whether the hospital and laboratory's carelessness and wrong diagnosis of HIV were acceptable standards, especially for a superspecialty hospital.

Upon reviewing medical records, it appears that the patient's HIV status was indeed positive post-blood transfusion during an aortic valve replacement (AVR) operation. There is a possibility that the blood donor was in the window period for HIV detection, as HIV tests after 3 months are highly accurate but not infallible. The principle of *res ipsa loquitur* applies, signifying negligence through the actions and inaction of the hospital and laboratory.

Therefore, the revision petition is dismissed, and the awarded compensation of ₹5 lakh is upheld.

HUMAN IMMUNODEFICIENCY VIRUS NEGATIVE GIVEN POSITIVE REPORT

In the case of P Bhopal Reddy versus Alekya Diagnostic Centre, Andhra Pradesh State Consumer Disputes Redressal Commission, Hyderabad.

Exhibit A1 clearly indicates that the HIV-1 and HIV-2 tests returned a positive result. However, there is no accompanying note or information explaining that a positive result does not necessarily mean the presence of acquired immunodeficiency syndrome (AIDS). It is unreasonable for the respondent to argue that the appellant hastily sought another opinion from a superspecialty hospital. When a report states that HIV-1 and HIV-2 tests are positive, a patient typically seeks confirmation or a second opinion from another diagnostic center. The absence of such explanatory notes in Exhibit A1, issued by the respondent, implies that an incorrect report was provided, and the mental distress experienced by the appellant should not be underestimated.

RETENTION AND OWNERSHIP OF SPECIMENS AND REPORTS

It is important to note that the statute of limitations is 3 years. It is reasonable to retain wet, formalin-fixed tissue specimens for a duration that allows the consulting clinician to review the report thoroughly and for the pathologist to collect additional samples if needed after consulting with the clinician. If the clinician has indicated to the pathologist that the case might have legal implications, it would be prudent to preserve the specimen for a longer period. There is a recommendation to retain histopathological slides for at least 3 years. Ideally, these slides should be handed over to the patient or their representative if a second opinion and continued patient reviews are required, with acknowledgment.

LIABILITY OF LABORATORY STAFF

Within any laboratory, specific responsibilities are assigned to technical and supporting staff members. Errors made by these staff members can have significant consequences for patients and may even lead to negligence claims, such as specimen mislabeling or incorrect patient name or reference number typing. The crucial question is—Who should be accountable for these errors? In hospitals, the general principle that "*the employer is liable for the actions of their employees*" typically applies. This means that all staff members, from attendants to consultants, share a level of responsibility.

However, the pathologist, as the leader of the laboratory team, carries additional responsibilities and may be held accountable for mistakes made by the general laboratory staff. It is important to recognize that the pathologist is generally responsible for professional matters as the individual in charge of the laboratory.

TEST THE TEST BEFORE ADVISING

Advancing technology and easy availability of investigatory modalities including imaging, genetic and immunological tests have made many doctors depend on them for diagnosis of diseases, avoiding detailed history and physical examination. Test results must be correlated with clinical impression and hence are not meant to diagnose diseases but only to confirm, support or rule out the provisional clinical diagnosis. Test results are not always right and dependable. A positive test may be seen without an active disease and a negative test may not rule out the disease. Without a provisional diagnosis, test results could add to confusion besides wasting time and money. There is nothing like "routine tests." Doctors must know what they expect out of a test rather than treat what they see in the test results. Rationality demands minimum and appropriate tests based on provisional clinical diagnosis.

In evidence-based modern medicine, ideally, clinical bedside diagnosis should be confirmed by relevant laboratory tests. However, it may not be necessary for every patient and it may not be possible for various reasons. Rational practice demands provisional clinical diagnosis before ordering relevant laboratory tests. Tests are not meant to search the diagnosis but just to confirm, support or rule out clinical bedside provisional diagnosis. Test results must be correlated with clinical profile and not considered in isolation. Test results are at times confusing and there may be a disparity between test results and clinical judgment that must be cautiously addressed. Hence, a test must be tested for its worth in a given situation.

Clinical bedside diagnosis of any disease consists of four components—anatomy (site of disease), pathology (type of disease), etiology (cause of disease), and functional status of an affected organ (normal, compensated, or de-compensated function). The tests should be planned accordingly to confirm either or all the components of the diagnosis as per the need.

CONCEPT OF SENSITIVITY AND SPECIFICITY

Assessing the reliability of a diagnostic test is crucial to determine its accuracy in predicting a suspected disease. The "gold standard" test is considered 100% reliable, serving as the benchmark against which all other tests are compared. For example, the detection of a malarial parasite in a blood smear is the "gold standard" for diagnosing malaria, and the reliability of other tests is measured against this standard.

Sensitivity measures a positive test's ability to accurately predict the presence of a disease, while specificity gauges a negative test's accuracy in predicting the absence of a disease. In practical terms, a test with 80% sensitivity can accurately diagnose the disease in 80% of cases but may miss it in 20% of cases. Similarly, a test with 80% specificity can correctly rule out the disease in 80% of cases, but 20% of cases may yield false negatives. Ideally, a test would have 100% sensitivity and 100% specificity, but such perfect accuracy is rare. Therefore, physicians should always consider the possibility of false positive or false negative results and correlate test findings with the patient's clinical presentation.

In summary, modern medicine relies on diagnostic advances to support evidence-based practices, emphasizing the need for a confirmed diagnosis to guide treatment. However, there are inherent limitations in diagnostic modalities. Laboratory tests should serve the purpose of confirming, supporting, or ruling out a provisional diagnosis made at the bedside and should not be used as the primary means of diagnosing a condition.

Regrettably, there is a growing trend of overreliance on tests at the expense of traditional clinical bedside medicine, which is diminishing in importance.

ALWAYS PLEAD GAUSSIAN DISTRIBUTION AND REFERENCE RANGE FOR NORMAL READINGS

The Gaussian distribution, also known as the normal distribution, presents as a bell-shaped curve, and it is assumed that measurements will adhere to this distribution, with an equal number of measurements falling above and below the mean value. To comprehend the normal distribution fully, it is essential to understand the definitions of the "mean," "median," and "mode." The "mean" represents the calculated average of all values; the "median" corresponds to the value at the midpoint of the distribution, while the "mode" denotes the value observed most frequently during the measurement process. If a distribution is normal, the values of the mean, median, and mode are identical. However, in the case of a skewed distribution (non-Gaussian), the mean, median, and mode values may differ.

CONCLUSION

Various methods employed in reporting surgical pathology and laboratory medicine can introduce error rates. Differentiating between errors, diagnostic variations, test sensitivity, and specificity can sometimes be challenging. Nevertheless, it is evident that the most common issue leading to pathologists being involved in medical malpractice litigation is misdiagnosis. Beyond the legal considerations, it is beneficial to pragmatically assess which tests, specimens, or diseases traditionally pose the greatest risk for pathologists in terms of potential errors that may result in medical negligence lawsuits.

It is essential to bear in mind not to assume that you possess superior knowledge compared to patient party lawyers. While facing a lawsuit is one thing, presuming expertise in malpractice law is another. Regardless of your medical expertise, it is crucial to acknowledge that legal matters require a distinct set of skills and knowledge.

KEY LEARNING POINTS

- Avoid inaccurately recording the patient's name.
- Ensure the patient's age is accurately documented.
- Verify that the patient's gender is correctly indicated.
- Refrain from placing the report in an envelope intended for a different patient.
- Do not mix up or interchange samples.
- Avoid copying and pasting content or formatting without proper modification, as this can lead to errors.
- Double-check readings that appear excessively low or high.
- Verify the results of serological tests, such as Widal, Australia antigen, HIV, HCV, RA, VDRL, for both false positives and false negatives.

BIBLIOGRAPHY

1. Amdekar YK. What Doctors Must Learn: Testing a Test. Volume 3. Clever Pen Publishing Llp; 2022.
2. Baldwa M, Baldwa V, Padvi N, et al. Legal Issues in Medical Practice. 2nd edition. New Delhi: CBS Publishers and Distributors Pvt. Ltd.; 2023.
3. Baldwa M, Baldwa V, Padvi N, et al. Legal Issues in Critical Care. New Delhi: CBS Publishers and Distributors Pvt. Ltd.; 2022.
4. Care Hospital M/s. Quality Care India versus Vemuganti Venu Gopal (NCDRC), Revision Petition No. 4236 of 2014 from order dated 22.9.2014 in Appeal No. 488/2013 of Andhra Pradesh State Consumer Disputes Redressal Commission Hyderabad with IA/8352/2014. D/d. 9.12.2014.
5. Chandrasagar D. Rajput versus Dr. Dinesh J. Shah, 1999 (1) CPJ 434 (Maharashtra SCDRC).
6. Dr. Ashok Ladha versus State of Madhya Pradesh, (Madhya Pradesh) (Indore Bench), Miscellaneous Criminal Case No. 2662 of 2017. D/d. 16.04.2018.
7. Dr. Sanjay J. Batra versus Jagrut Nagrik, (NCDRC), Revision Petition No. 567 of 2015 (Against the Order dated 24/12/2014 in Appeal No. 2997 of 2012 of the State Commission Gujarat). D/d. 12.4.2016.
8. Gulshan Kumar versus Dr. Rajan & Others III (2012) CPJ 415 (NC).
9. In Bharat Pathology Laboratory versus Mangi Lal Vyas, 2003 (3) CPJ 94 (NCDRC).
10. In Santosh Kaur Sodhi versus Dr. Vijay Mujoo, 2003 (2) CLD 751: 2003 (2) CPJ 344 (Chd.-UTCDRC),
11. Leena Bhattarcharjee versus Nightangle Diagnostic and Eye Care Research Centre (P) Ltd., 2003 (6) CLD 706: 2004 (1) CPR 130 (WB SCDRC).

12. Madhyamgram Consumers Welfare Society versus Dr. Kalyan Kumar Chatterjee and others, 2002 (2) CPJ 381 (WB SCDRC).
13. P Bhopal Reddy versus Alekya Diagnostic Centre, Andhra Pradesh State Consumer Disputes Redressal Commission, Hyderabad.
14. Raj Kumar versus Dr. Ajay Gupta, 2001 (I) CPJ 495 (UP SCDRC).
15. Rajni Shukla versus Rajendra Kumar Agrawal Madhya Pradesh S.C.D.R.C. 1(2003) CPJ:551.
16. Ravindra Dnyaneshwar Patil versus Dr. Vinay Tule, (NCDRC), First Appeal No. 1291 of 2017, (Against the Order dated 03/05/2017 in Complaint No. 13/2015 of the State Commission Maharashtra). D/d. 17.7.2017.
17. Sandeep Kumar versus Post Graduate Institute of Medical Education and Research, (NCDRC) (New Delhi) 2016(4) C.P.R. 639: 2017(1) CLT 259: 2017(2) C.P.J. 157: 2017 NCJ 631, First Appeal No. 407 of 2012; (Against the Order dated 01/06/2012 in Complaint No. 12 of 2011 of the State Commission Chandigarh). D/d. 13.12.2016.
18. Shahul Hameed versus Apollo Hospital Enterprises Tamil Nadu S.C.D.R.C. II (2002) CPJ, 395.
19. Shyam Sunder Tantia (Dr.) versus Deepika, Rajasthan S.C.D.R. I (2002) CPJ, 411.
20. Smt. Supriti Modak versus Dr. Gokul Ch. Modak, 2001 (2) CPJ 219 (WE SCDRC)
21. Smt. Yashoda Goyal versus Dr. Ahuja's Pathology and Imaging Centre, (USCDRC) (Dehradun), Consumer Complaint No. 4 of 2006. D/d. 13.03.2018.
22. Sulochana Lad versus Dr. Mohan Gerra, (NCDRC) (New Delhi), First Appeal No. 138 of 2008 (against Order dated 12.4.2007 in Consumer Complaint No. 237 of 1997 of Maharashtra State Consumer Disputes Redressal Commission, Mumbai). D/d. 29.3.2016.
23. Umakant Rajaram Chauhan versus Dr. Anil M. Gupta, (GSCDRC) (Ahmedabad), Complaint No. 42 of 2011. D/d. 06.11.2020.
24. Vikas Yadav versus ReeLabs Pvt. Ltd., (HSCDRC) (Panchkula), Complaint No. 301 of 2016. D/d. 23.10.2018.
25. Vikram versus Jagdamba Medical Centre (HSCDRC) (Panchkula), First Appeal No. 963 of 2014. D/d. 17.11.2014.
26. Wahid Khan versus Dr. Mohd. Abdul, 1999 (3) CPJ 304 (UP SCDRC).

CHAPTER 28

Medicolegal Issues in Organ Transplant

Suchismita Mallick, Sumanta Ghosh Maulik

INTRODUCTION: THE ETHICS AND LEGALITY

The main ethical question regarding organ transplantation revolves around the commodification of human beings, right to bodily autonomy and the right to life. In developing countries like India where there is a possibility of misuse and exploitation of human resource and unrelated donors with the commercial angle, the basic human rights are guarded by legislations and judicial pronouncements. The Transplantation of Human Organ Act (THOA) was enacted in 1994 stating the laws pertaining to organ transplantation. Certain facets of the act were to establish brain death as a form of death, to legalize cadaveric organ transplantation, to stamp monetary transactions a punishable offence, and to promote living related donation program. The main arms of the statute are the authorities responsible for its actual execution and they are given the responsibility to maintain strict norms and follow the statute meticulously. However, the proper implementation of the THOA depends much on its interpretation and implementation by these authorities and there lies the margin of error. With regenerative medicine such as stem cells transplants, cloning, and tissue re-engineering, the organ transplantation law comes more into focus and relevance, obviating the need for Transplantation of Human Organs and Tissues Act (THOTA) and the execution of the statutes under the control of the authorization committees (ACs).

The present situation in India is that it has >500 transplant centers undertaking over 10,000 organ transplants annually, coming in third position in the global rank after USA and China. Most of these are living donor transplants, most common being renal transplants. However, the demand for organs are in lakhs and the demand supply gap needs active organ donations and laws relating to it. The cadaveric donation program from brain dead patients will not only cater to the patient population needing kidney transplants but also liver, heart, pancreas, and lung transplants. The huge number of road traffic accident cases with head injury and other patients with neurologic injury and subsequent brain death can be source of cadaveric donation and it would eliminate the crisis for organs and therefore reduce the unlawful and exploitative activities associated with living healthy donations. The cadaveric donation and brain death declaration has ethical dimensions. These are addressed in the current legal recommendations and the organ transplantation program and the strict cognizance of commercial dealings in organ trade are probably the hallmarks of the newly amended transplantation act.

TYPES OF TRANSPLANTATION

- Live organ donation or transplantation from genetically matched individual to another individual
- *Cadaveric donation*: In case of brainstem death, where the heart is beating but there is apnea or no respiration, or no signs of brainstem activity
- Cadaveric donation after cardiac death

TRANSPLANTATION OF HUMAN ORGANS AND TISSUES ACT

The THOA, passed in the year 1994 to legally regularize organ transplantation and formulate guidelines, was subsequently amended in 2011, further under section 24 of THOA and the new rules of the act were passed in 2014. The 1994 Act laid the rules for removal, storage, and transplantation for therapeutic purpose.

The (Amendment) Act 2011

The (Amendment) Act 2011 introduced certain amendments:

- Inclusion of "tissues"
- "Near relative" now includes grandchildren and grandparents. Swap donation and altruistic donation possible with permission of authorizing committee.
- Cautious dealings with minors and foreign nationals and mentally challenged persons were prohibited from organ donation.
- Mandatory inquiry about potential donors from the intensive care unit (ICU) and counseling for organ donation and mandatory "Transplant Coordinator" in hospitals registered with the Act.
- *Brain death certification*: In absence of a neurophysician, an anesthesiologist or an intensive care physician can be a member of board, provided that he does not belong to the transplant team.
- Strict punitive actions for commercial dealings
- National Organ and Tissue Transplant Organization (NOTTO) and National Level Registry for better coordination
- Registration under THOTA of retrieval centers and tissue banks
- Advisory committee to aid Appropriate Authority (AA)
- Technician aided enucleation of corneas.

Rules Pertaining to Alive and Cadaveric Donation

Section 2 in the 2011 Act added the donation of organs for therapeutic purpose. Before this, under section 297 of IPC 1860, causing any indignity to the corpse was considered criminal cognizable and a nonbailable offence. Section 2(o) states the rules of live and cadaveric organ donation mainly to relatives and also to strangers.

Near Relatives Definition Expanded

Section 9(1) states that in case of Indian nationals and near relatives, permission of the third party or AC is a mere formality. The 2011 amendment added four types of relations as near relatives to spouse, son, daughter, father, mother, brother, and sister, and, i.e., grandfather, grandmother, granddaughter, and grandson. Therefore, for live donation, donation without any legal formalities is possible in such cases. The first relatives are supposed to produce documents as proof of their relationship by genetic testing or by legal documents. As per section 2(i) of the 2011 amendments, the mentally ill or challenged persons were not allowed to donate their organs.

In Nonrelated Cases

The case of a nonrelative organ donation requires further proof of their emotional closeness and need to give their vocational proof or salary in the preceding 3 years in the Form 3 of 2014 rules. The AC is guided by rule 6F when dealing with such cases of nonrelatives. They can demand for additional proof of relationship such as photographs, residence, and disparity of financial status and are advised to interview the donor personally and record the minutes of the proceedings. The form 11 is another form, which needs to be submitted to the AC by such patients and donors. Human leukocyte antigen (HLA) and tissue matching of the organs is a problem and to overcome the problem subsection 3A of clause 7 of 2011 amendment act was introduced. Two donors and their near relative two recipients can swap places for the tissue matched organ. They can do so under a single agreement with the permission of the AC.

The THOA has 13 different forms for various procedures.

Cadaver Organ Donation

Organ donation for therapeutic purpose can be done by donors before their death in Forms 1(A), 1(B), and 1(C) as legally valid authorization. The above forms need corroborative documents such as identity proof and address proof attested by a public notary. Prior to removal of an organ from the donor, a physician should ensure that the respective authorization forms as in Form 1(A) for a close relative, Form 1(B) in case of a spouse and Form 1(C) for other relatives are in order. He should also confirm the fitness for organ donation (Form 2) and the relation with recipient (Form 3). A registered medical practitioner before removing a human organ from the body of a person after his death should confirm that the donor had, in the presence of two or more witnesses (at least one close relative of the recipient), provided for the authorization in Form 5 before his death. As per section 3(3), near relatives can deny the permission to donate, and therefore, after brain death has been certified, the medical practitioner needs to communicate with a near relative and record the said consent in Form 8. In case of brainstem death, confirmation is needed in Form 8 with signatures of medical experts constituting the board and Form 9 signed by either of the parents in case of a minor are required. Brain death confirmation is required at an interval of 6 hours by at least two medical practitioners chosen by the AC. It is to be given in form 10 under rule 5(4c) of 2014 THOA. The board should consist of a registered medical practitioner of the hospital where brain death occurred, a registered medical practitioner treating the person, an independent medical practitioner, and a nominated neurologist or neurosurgeon, the last two names to be decided by the practitioner in whose hospital the brain death occurred.

In Case of Unclaimed Bodies

Person in-charge of hospital or prison may grant permission for organ donation in Form 9, but only after being sure that there is no relative.

Body due for Medicolegal Autopsy or Entrusted for Cremation

Under section 6, organ donation of such bodies is not legal. Failure to seek permission of legal authorities is punishable under section 18(1) with a fine of 20 lakh rupees and imprisonment of 10 years.

Punishment for Commercial Dealing

This act also ensured strict laws against commercialization of organ transplantation. Section 19A of the act dealt with the unauthorized dealings in transplantation penalizing the offenders for a minimum period of 5 years of imprisonment and 20 lakh rupees fine. As of the 2011 amendments of the THOA, the court can no longer reduce the punishment with proper reasons and the punishments were made more strict and severe.

Authorization Committee and Appropriate Authority

These are two important bodies responsible for the execution of the rules under the statute. The AC is a regulatory body for authorization of approval or rejection of transplants from donors other than first relatives. The AC is set up by the central government for the union territories and by the state government for the states under section 9(4). Under section 13(2) of the THOA, the AA is also set up by the central government for the union territories and by the state government for the states. The AA are not offices but appointed officials. The AA regulates the hospitals performing removal, storage, and transplantation of human organs. The AA provides permission to hospitals to perform specific transplant procedures with licensed from the authority. The eye removal can be done from a donor after death at other places without licensing formalities. Under section 13(3) of the THOA, the AA can carry out investigations and not the police. The court directs the investigations from the police or court to the AA. A court can take cognizance of the case only when the AA approaches the court under section 22. An AA can proceed suo moto to the court or after receiving a notice of 60 days. The AA are in charge of granting registration to hospitals, tissue banks, to ensure their proper functioning by periodic inspection and to investigate complaints. In case of a nonrelated donor and recipient transplant applications in Forms 1, 2, 3, and 11, the AC is supposed to carry out further inquiries. It grants permission under section 9(5). If refusal is there, then it is done under section 9(6) only after a thorough inquiry and explanation given by the AC.

Psychiatrist's clearance is required for the assessment of the donor's mental state, psychiatric conditions, and the capacity to consent. The necessary forms should be filled up and duly signed and completed as procedural work and video recording should be kept for the interviews. Final decision needs to be taken by the AC within 24 hours of the meeting for permitting or rejecting a transplant. Transplant hospitals need to have their own website and the decision needs to be displayed on the website of the hospital or notified in the institution within 24 hours. When the hospital or transplant applicant has a grievance against the AC with an order under section 15(2) or section 9(6) by the AC, there is scope of an appeal to the state or central government under section 17. A person aggrieved with the decision of the AC can appeal to the state government by 30 days of passing of the order.

Recognized Qualification

Medical practitioners possessing recognized medical qualification vide section 2(h) of the Medical Council of India act 1956 in the three schedules were allowed to do the organ transplantation.

National Organ Transplantation Program

The central government formulated certain rules and guidelines on kidney transplantation and the NOTTO has put them up on their web portal. The guidelines are on the method of organ availability and who gets the organ first. It is the recipient living in the same city who gets the first preference followed by a person living within the state, then cross state. There is also a scoring system that guides the preference to the person with the highest score. Each parameter is assigned a number, either positive or negative, for example, a previous recipient, a critical person receiving dialysis for the past 3 months are positive scorers, whereas patients with hepatitis positive condition, high risk for general anesthesia, and significant atherosclerosis will get negative points. The highest scorer and the longer waiting patient will get the priority for transplantation. The AC should consider other factors as well such as location and age of the donor and stage of dialysis. The priority list should be reviewed by the state transplant advisory committee at 3 months interval and update the status of patients.

JUDICIAL PRONOUNCEMENTS

The role of AC has been scrutinized in a number of cases and their role in granting permission or refusal in unrelated donors need to be substantiated with proper reasoning and unnecessary harassment has been criticized by the courts. In BL Nagaraj and others versus Kantha and others case, a writ petition was filed before the High Court of Karnataka against the order of the AC that rejected the application for organ donation by the sister-in-law of the recipient on the grounds that close relatives were not appropriate donors. The High Court order reflected that there is no prohibition in near relatives and held the AC order as wrong or misdirected.

As was also observed in the cases of Samson versus AC, the AC only added one sentence and refused the transplant application, and the court redirected them the case for reconsideration. Also observed in cases of Ganesan versus state IP and Fortis hospitals limited versus state of Karnataka, the role of AC and AA was reinforced as per the THOA guidelines. Even though the strict legalities were introduced to prevent foul play, the hospitals on the contrary did not have the right to refuse patients just to avoid legalities. As was observed in the case of Smt. Vandana Dixit versus visitor SGPGI and others, 2010 in Allahabad with Fortis hospital and SGPGI.

In a case between N Ratnakumari versus State of Odisha 2014, a hospital director was arrested for committing cognizable offence under sections 120, 468, 471, and 342 of section 34 IPC and under section 19 of THOA. His wife filed a writ petition of habeas corpus. The petitioner in her husband's defense put forward that section 19 of THOA was inapplicable in the case as in Andhra Pradesh THOA of 1995 was the relevant statute wherein the maximum term of imprisonment was 5 years. Thereby, the arrest by the police without a warrant was illegal as police can only arrest without warrant under section 41(1) when the cognizable offence is punishable by imprisonment for 7 years. The court ruled that the arrest was illegal. The jurisdiction of Orissa police was not applicable and under section 13(3) of the central act, the jurisdiction remained with the AC. The court ruled it was their responsibility to investigate the case and the aggrieved party was supposed to serve a notice of 90 days to the AC about the grievances. Under section 22 of the THOA, the court did not have the power to take up the issue. The court ruled that the arrest was illegal but the transplantation was done in an illegal manner violating the rules of section 9(4b) of the 1994 act, without an appropriate AC recommendation. The rule states that the AC should belong to the state in which the donee and donor are from. In this case, both donee and donor needed to fill up Form 11 and seek permission of the AC of the state they are from, that is Orissa. Finally, the court ruled that although Andhra Pradesh, where the transplant hospital was, was outside the jurisdiction of the central act, as both the donor and donee were from Orissa, which was under the jurisdiction of the THOA, therefore the transplantation was illegal.

FALLACIES IN THE ACT

The THOT Act was introduced to curb the illegal financial dealings in organ donation and commoditization of the unrelated donor in a developing country like India. However, due to the inherent weakness of its main instrument that is the AC, the legislation has not been able to attain its final goal. Subsection 3 of the THOT Act dealing with nonrelated donors need the AC and their approval for the organ donation. However, the interpretation of closeness of relations by the medical professionals and the AC or the failure to ascertain the lack of it has created certain weaknesses in the system.

In the recent times, globalization has opened up medical tourism for patients and commercialization of the transplants. As observed in the organ bazaar by Raj Chengappa, there are certain villages where people live off the money from illegal transactions, for example, Pandoli near Ahmedabad and "Kidneyvalkam" near Chennai. And the infamous kidney rackets as observed by Faizan Haider. This kind of live donor exploitation can only be tackled with increasing cadaver donation.

As rightly pointed out by Dr MK Mani, a leading Nephrologist, he noted the fallacy of the Act and the law. The failure of section 9 of the Act, the unacceptability of middlemen, and more stringent methods to be assumed by the AC were all noted in his article.

Among other important observations made, "the Bellagio Task Force from the Department of Anthropology, University of California, Berkeley" with the Open Society Institute (from the Soros Foundation) made important observations from their ethnographic research in Brazil, India, and South Africa. They noted that inequalities of societies and injustices prevalent led to the illegal harvesting of organs along with the noncompliance of laws, moral degradations of society, etc. As Mr Soros noted the opening up of the global market in presence of marked inequalities in social structure is one of the leading factors. Similar findings were also noted in a report given by the United State Congress in 2001 to the international operations and human rights. The increase in the medical tourism along with vast economic differences of the developing and the developed countries have resulted in increased exploitation and increase of this illegal practice further, as was noted by them.

The question of individual autonomy and the fundamental right of a person was debated by Francis Delmonico in the New England Journal of Medicine. He stated that although the commoditization of the human body was for the preservation of life in another, the monetary angle conflicted with the basic values and our fundamental rights.

Although lesser in number, yet, some purely altruistic organ donation not just from the relatives alone, but also from some unrelated donors do occur still today. Allowing a market with professionalism and commercial intent in such noble conjectures of human values will erode the possibility of such altruistic donations in future days. It is the duty of both the *executive* and *judiciary* to prevent such erosions and formulate such means either in terms of law or proclamation of policies so that such objectives are not overlooked in the zeal of increasing the availability of the organs in the market ready for transplantations. The difference between demand and supply of the organs and tissues for transplantation has progressively widened so much so as to promote international travelling to avail such organs. Countries such as Brazil, China, Pakistan, Ukraine, Russia, and India have been victims of such human organ trade because of their weak regulatory mechanisms. The World Health Organization categorically proclaims that there is violation of Universal Declaration of Human Rights if the human body part is used for commercial transaction and prohibits the physicians from performing such transplants "if they have reason to believe that the organs concerned have been the subject of commercial transactions." In a meeting of the world transplant committee held in Istanbul, it was proclaimed that organ transplantation despite being a lifesaving procedure cannot conflict with the basic rights of a financially weaker section and lead to their exploitation.

CONCLUSION

So, to sum it up, the financial dealings in organ donation were against the fundamental rights of human beings and the commoditization of human body cannot be accepted by moral and ethical standards. With this in mind, the legislations were introduced. But even with the best of intentions, the corrupted practitioners and middlemen of this trade are continuing with their illegal practices, giving it a legal face. This is obviously due to the weakness of the system. The lack of uniformity of the legislation across the whole country, certain clauses of the legislation that are grossly misused, the weakness of the AC in identifying such cases, and the increased medical tourism along with lack of stringent international laws have resulted in the failure of the statute in part. Another extremely important factor being the growing population along with increased longevity of the people and the ever increasing demand for organs. In this respect, the importance of cadaveric organ donation comes into the picture. That would reduce the load and demand for live organ donation and reduce the financial angle to the situation. But obviously the question of declaration of brainstem death will with itself bring about further legal implications and complications, which would then be needed to be addressed. Therefore, a more stringent and uniform legislation with more severe punishments in case of lapses to increase its legal binding, negative feedback checks for the working of the AC, the effort of the government to increase social awareness along with the media, and increase in cadaveric transplantation can all help to tackle the problem in a multimodal approach.

KEY LEARNING POINTS

- There is a possibility of misuse and exploitation of human resource.
- The THOA, passed in the year 1994 to legally regularize organ transplantation.
- AC is a regulatory body for authorization of approval or rejection of transplants.
- The AA regulates the hospitals performing removal, storage, and transplantation of human organs.
- The difference between demand and supply of the organs and tissues for transplantation has progressively widened.
- Organ transplantation despite being a lifesaving procedure cannot conflict with the basic rights of a financially weaker section and lead to their exploitation.
- The commoditization of human body cannot be accepted by moral and ethical standards.

BIBLIOGRAPHY

1. BL Nagaraj and Others vs Dr. Kantha and Others on 12 July, 1995. [online] Available from https://indiankanoon.org/doc/537327/ [Last accessed May, 2024].
2. Chengappa R. (2006). The organ bazar. [Online] Available from http://indiatoday.intoday.in/story/india-has-largest-number-of-kidney-transplants/1/180170.html [Last accessed May, 2024].
3. Delmonico FL, Arnold R, Scheper-Hughes N, et al. Ethical incentives—not payment—for organ donation. N Engl J Med. 2002;346(25):2002-5.
4. Ganesan vs. State, Represented by the Inspector of Police and others crl.O.P.No.17336 o 2013 and MP no. 1 of 2013. [Online] Available from https://indiankanoon.org/doc/117140644/?type=print [Last accessed May, 2024].
5. Haider F. (2016). Kidney racket rampant across India as crackdown proves difficult. [Online] Available from https://www.hindustantimes.com/india-news/kidney-rackets-rampant-across-india-as-crackdown-proves-difficult/story-R6M3s4HVxOq7BGErOQJ26L.html [Last accessed May, 2024].
6. M/s. Fortis Hospitals Limited vs. State of Karnataka Writ Appeal No. 8767/2012 (gm-res), 17 September 2013. [Online] Available from https://indiankanoon.org/doc/122216077/ [Last accessed May, 2024].
7. Mani MK. Making an ass of the law. Natl Med J India. 1997;10(5):242-3.
8. Ministry of Health and Family Welfare. (2014). Transplantation of Human Organs and Tissue Rules. [Online] Available from https://main.mohfw.gov.in/sites/default/files/THOA-Rules-2014%20%281%29.pdf [Last accessed May, 2024].
9. National Medical Commission. First Schedule of Medical Council of India Act. [Online] Available from https://www.nmc.org.in/acts-amendments/the-first-schedule-of-imc-act/ [Last accessed May, 2024].
10. NOTTO. Allocation criteria or deceased donor kidney transplant (draft guidelines). [Online] Available from https://notto.mohfw.gov.in/WriteReadData/Portal/News/807_1_807_1_UpdatedKidneyAllocationPolicy-Publish__1__edited.pdf [Last accessed May, 2024].
11. Ratnakumari vs. State of Odisha 2014 W.P (crl) no 266 of 2014. [Online] Available from https://indiankanoon.org/doc/156479333/ [Last accessed May, 2024].
12. Rothman DJ, Rose E, Awaya T, et al. The Bellagio Task Force report on transplantation, bodily integrity, and the International Traffic in Organs. Transplant Proc. 1997;29(6):2739-45.
13. S. Samson vs. Authorization committee of human organ transplantation W.P.no.3584 of 2008 and M.P.no.s1 and 2 of 2008. [Online] Available from https://indiankanoon.org/doc/928791/ [Last accessed May, 2024].
14. Smt. Vandana Dixit vs. Visitor SGPGI and Others Writ Petition No. 4310 (MB) of 2010. [Online] Available from https://indiankanoon.org/doc/124839/ [Last accessed May, 2024].

CHAPTER

Forensic Issues in Clinical Practice

Padmakumar K

INTRODUCTION

Forensic medicine is a branch of medicine which deals with application of medical knowledge for the administration of law and justice. A medical practitioner must have a fair knowledge in all branches of medical sciences to aid legal system and elucidation of various problems of medicolegal interest. This will help the practitioner in medicolegal examinations and drawing up various medicolegal reports. In addition to various medicolegal examinations and reporting, legal responsibilities of registered medical practitioners are police intimation, documentation, evidence preservation, intimation of death, and recording of dying declaration. Various medicolegal examinations and reporting are:

- Wound certification
- Drunkenness certification
- Female victim of sexual assault
- Male accused in sexual offence
- Certification of a victim alleged to have been drugged
- Recent delivery
- Postmortem examination

POLICE INTIMATION

Registered medical practitioners are legally bound to report the legal authority all medicolegal cases which comes for examination and treatment. A medicolegal case is a case of injury or ailment when investigation by law enforcing authority is essential to fix the responsibility regarding the causation of injury or ailment. This intimation is prepared in duplicate on a structured pro forma, the original must be issued to police and an acknowledgment must be received from the police for future reference. Prompt reporting is must in all medicolegal cases. While attending to a patient, saving life must be given priority. If intimation cannot be given immediately, a telephonic intimation must be given, and this must be documented. This must be recorded while transmitting the written intimation later.

INTIMATION OF DEATH

Intimate all deaths to registration authority as per death and birth registration act. Intimate all cases of unnatural deaths and brought dead cases to police. When a registered medical practitioner is not able to differentiate between natural and unnatural deaths, inform such cases also to police. Whenever a death is informed to police, transfer the body to mortuary. Reporting to registration authority is not required if death is intimated to police.

RECORDING OF DYING DECLARATION

Dying declaration is a statement made by a dying person about the cause and/or circumstances leading to his/her impending death. It is accepted as legal evidence in a court of law after the death of the person. Ideal officer to record dying declaration is judicial magistrate.

Legal responsibility of medical practitioner is examining the person and issuing a certificate as to the fitness of patient's condition to make a declaration.

If the condition of the dying person is so serious that there is a chance of unconsciousness or death occurs before the arrival of magistrate, medical practitioner should record the declaration. It should be recorded in own sentence of declarant. Presence of two disinterested witnesses is a must, whose signatures should be there after the declaration is signed by the medical practitioner. The dying declaration so recorded should be forwarded to the judicial magistrate in a sealed cover.

A dying declaration is valid even if the declarant dies some days after making the declaration, but if the person survives declaration ceases its legal value.

ACCIDENT REGISTER CUM WOUND CERTIFICATE

Whenever a registered medical practitioner attends an injured person, while examining, record all injuries in the accident cum wound certificate. Record alleged cause of injury and history in patient's own words in the columns specified for it. Note who brought the case. In case brought by the police, details such as name, number, and name of the police station must be documented. If brought by others, enter their name, address, and contact number. If patient is brought unconscious, history must be recorded as per the version of accompanying person.

- *Injuries*: Record injuries with reference to type of injury, dimension, direction, site, and exact position from anatomical landmarks. Even a trivial injury needs adequate description. Complaints of pain also must be documented, investigated, and kept under observation. General description about the person, general condition, and investigations with results must also be noted. Registered medical practitioner must record all findings in his own handwriting.
- *Transfer of patient*: When a patient is transferred to another center, the registered medical practitioner first attending the patient is bound to document the accident cum wound certificate. Record the condition of the patient and mention if documentation of injuries could not be made. This must be informed to the other center along with reference letter, ideally a copy of the certificate.
- *Consent*: Consent from the injured person or from those who brought the injured person is not required to prepare an accident cum wound certificate. Consent from parents or local guardian is also not required if the injured person is a minor.

- *Treatment/discharge certificate*: Treatment and/or discharge certificate following wound certification must be given by the registered medical practitioner who treated the patient or by the doctor under whom the injured person was being treated.

DRUNKENNESS CERTIFICATION

Drunkenness is a condition resulting from intake of alcohol and the person is under its influence such that (1) person loses control over mental faculties, (2) person is not able to perform duties which are engaged by that person at that particular time, and (3) the person is a source of danger.

Drunkenness is not a crime where drinking of alcoholic beverages is not prohibited but becomes a crime when accompanied by an act of commission or omission. Registered medical practitioner can examine an accused person at the request of the police even without consent and by using reasonable force if necessary. Important clinical signs of drunkenness are:

- Alcohol smell in breath
- General demeanor
- Loss of self-control
- Clothing—disorderly/disarranged
- Dilated pupil, sluggish reaction
- Alcoholic gaze nystagmus (fine lateral)
- Slurring of speech
- Gait, which is unsteady, staggering on sudden turning
- Impaired coordination
- Confusion or impaired memory especially for recent events

Alcohol Smell in Breath

Do not ask the subject to blow. Persistent smell during the course of examination must be present. Do not smell nose or mouth. Identify the smell during the normal course of conversation or breathing while examining the subject. Conditions to be ruled out during examination of a case of drunkenness are:

- Head injury
- *Metabolic disorders*: Insulin induced hypoglycemia, hyperthyroidism, and uremia
- *Central nervous system (CNS) disorders*: Epilepsy, Parkinson's disease, intracranial tumor, and disseminated sclerosis
- *Drugs*: Insulin, antihistamines, morphine, and barbiturates
- Carbon monoxide poisoning

Sample Collection

- *Blood*: Collect 5 mL of blood by venipuncture using a fresh disposable syringe and needle. Spirit should not be used as a disinfectant. Instead, soap and water can be used.
- It is ideal to collect urine sample also. Ask the patient to void urine prior to examination. Collect the sample of urine voided at the end of examination.
- *Preservation and transmission*: Collect 5 mL blood and 5 mL urine in separate containers which should be stoppered tightly to avoid evaporation of alcohol. Label the container with name, age, reference number, date and time of collection along with signature of registered

medical practitioner. Handover the sealed containers to police for onward transmission to chemical examiner's laboratory or forensic science laboratory. Samples should be refrigerated if they cannot be transmitted immediately.

Opinion

Opinion can be given as person has consumed alcohol if there is persistent smell of alcohol in breath. Along with persistent smell of alcohol in breath, if there is muscular incoordination and impaired higher functions, the opinion can be given as person has consumed alcohol and is under its influence. Preservation of alcohol is mandatory in drunken driving and it is ideal to preserve samples in all cases of act of commission or omission with drunkenness and also to prove nonconsumption of alcoholic beverage.

EXAMINATION AND CERTIFICATION OF FEMALE VICTIM OF SEXUAL ASSAULT

Examination of a victim of rape or attempted rape soon after the alleged incident will give valuable information, while any delay will result in loss of such evidences. As per rule, the examination must be conducted by a registered medical practitioner employed in a hospital run by state government or local authority. In absence of such facility any registered medical practitioner can examine the woman. Details discussed in Chapter 20.4.

Opinion

Based on the examination and chemical analysis findings, opinion can be furnished as:
- There is evidence of general bodily injuries or there is no evidence of general bodily injuries.
- There is evidence of genital injuries/penetration or there is no evidence of genital injuries/penetration.
- There is evidence of recent sexual act/there is no evidence of recent sexual act.

Reason for each opinion must be explained. To conclude there is evidence of recent sexual act, human spermatozoa or semen must be detected in the vaginal swab or smear.

It is ideal to prepare the certificate in triplicate. Issue the original certificate to the investigating authority. Third copy can be preserved as official one. When the victim comes directly to the registered medical practitioner, she is entitled to receive the duplicate of the certificate.

EXAMINATION AND CERTIFICATION OF MALE ACCUSED IN SEXUAL OFFENCE

A male accused and arrested on a charge of committing the offence of rape or attempt to rape may be brought for examination to get evidence for proof of offence. Examination must be conducted by a registered medical practitioner (irrespective of the gender) employed in a hospital run by state government or local authority. In absence of such facility within a radius of 16 kilometers from the place of occurrence, any other registered medical practitioner can be requested to conduct examination. Consent is not required if the person is arrested and reasonable force can be applied for the purpose of examination. The role of doctor is to search for any signs that corroborate with allegation.

- *Record*: (1) Name and address of the accused person (2) age of the person, (3) name and details of the person who brought the accused. Date and time of commencement and completion of examination must be recorded.
- *Examine*:
  - Clothes—for tear, any stains such as blood, semen, mud, etc.
  - Foreign hairs—scalp or pubic hair of the victim
  - Injuries, bite marks, and nail marks. Document injures in detail—type, dimension, site, and location with reference to anatomical landmarks.
  - Genital injuries, if any
  - *Absence of smegma*: Indicates recent sexual intercourse if not washed
  - *Evidence of sexual act*: Presence of vaginal epithelial cells in glans penis.

    Apply cotton swab wet with saline or distilled water on glans penis. Prepare a smear with this swab, *or* wash glans with distilled water. Collect the wash and centrifuge. Prepare a smear with the centrifuge deposit. Stain the smear with iodine. Vaginal epithelia cells if present will stain blue.

  Dry the clothes in shade, pack, seal, and send for analysis if stains are present.

  Examination and certification of potency is required if the accused person pleads impotency.
- *Opinion*:
  - There is evidence of general bodily injuries or there is no evidence of general bodily injuries.
  - There is evidence of genital injuries or there is no evidence of genital injuries.
  - There is evidence of recent vaginal intercourse/there is no evidence of recent vaginal intercourse. Reason for each opinion must be explained.

RECENT DELIVERY—EXAMINATION OF FEMALE

Delivery is the expulsion of products of conception from the uterus at term. Circumstances under which question of delivery of a woman may come before law are (1) abortion or infanticide—When there is an allegation against the woman that she has aborted or delivered a child and then killed the child, (2) concealment of birth after delivery, (3) *Feigned delivery*: Pretend pregnancy and delivery, (4) producing a supposititious child.

For examination and certification of a female for signs of delivery consent of the female is mandatory. The examination should be undertaken by a gynecologist. If a gynecologist is not available, examination should be undertaken preferably by or under supervision of a lady medical officer.

Detailed history must be recorded, especially gestational period, place of delivery, attempt to abortion, etc. Record injuries if present in the body or external genitalia in detail. Signs of recent delivery in the living are: (1) general appearance, (2) features of breast, (3) abdominal features, and (4) features of external genitalia.

- *General appearance of indisposition*: Woman look pale, exhausted, and ill. Pulse will be feeble and rapid. Body temperature is slightly raised. Intermittent painful contractions of uterus will be present for a period of 4–5 days after delivery.
- *Features of breast*: Breast will be full, firm, and tense with prominent surface veins. Striae are seen on the breast. Areola is darkened with prominent Montgomery tubercles. Colostrum can be squeezed out of the breast for few days after delivery which is replaced by milk later.

- *Abdominal features*: Pendulous and wrinkled, stretch marks called striae gravidarum (pink), striae albicantes (silvery white), Linea nigra (brownish or black) will be present.
- *Features of external genitalia*:
  - Vulva—bruised and with gaping
  - Labia—tender, swollen, bruised, or lacerated
  - Vagina—smooth walled, relaxed, and capacious, rugae will reappear only after few weeks.
  - Cervix—soft and dilated, internal os closes in 24 hours after delivery, edges torn and lacerated transversely.
  - Uterus—enlarged and contracted, reaches normal size only in 6 weeks after delivery.
  - Lochia—a vaginal discharge seen after delivery and is a part of healing process of uterus after delivery. Initial discharge is blood stained and red in color and persists for 4–5 days and is called lochia rubra. For the next 4 days discharge becomes pale and serous and is called lochia serosa. Lochia alba is the next stage and is greenish initially and later becomes white. Discharge gradually loses its color and disappears in 14–15 days after delivery.

EXAMINATION AND CERTIFICATION OF VICTIM OF DRUG ADDICTION

Use and possession of narcotic drugs and psychotropic substance is punishable. If a police officer brings a victim alleged to have been drugged, doctor must examine such patients for certification. Examine the victim after taking the consent. Police intimation must be given if the victim has directly approached the medical practitioner. Record the history in victim's own words. Note the mode of administration. Examine the oral cavity, circumoral region, and whole body for any injuries. Look for any injection marks and tattoos which mask the injection marks. Describe the injuries in detail—type, site, dimension, and location in relation to anatomical landmarks and age.

Common features of drug addiction are: (1) Drowsy or sleepy appearance of the person, (2) emotional outbursts and loss of temper, (3) dress and appearance, (4) poor hygiene, (5) staggering or stumbling gait, and (6) miosis if narcotics are used and mydriasis in case of use of stimulant drugs.

Preservation of material objects for analysis is mandatory. Various material objects that can be collected are: (1) nasal swabs (2) vomitus (3) blood (4) urine (5) clothing, and (6) any other material when found necessary. Preservation of material objects for chemical analysis may not be useful if the victim is brought for examination 7 days after alleged drug intake.

Based on the physical findings and result of chemical analysis, an opinion can be furnished.

POSTMORTEM EXAMINATION

Postmortem examination or medicolegal autopsy is a type of scientific examination of dead body under the laws of the state. Authorization for medicolegal autopsy is given by the police or magistrate. Postmortem examinations can be conducted only in institutions authorized to undertake medicolegal work and with a mortuary facility. The authority who conducted the inquest can order any registered medical practitioner to carry out medicolegal autopsy. However, a doctor employed in state government, health services from the primary health center level to Forensic department of a government medical college is permitted to do autopsy unless specified by the state government to authorize a registered medical practitioner.

The objectives of medicolegal autopsy are:

- To determine the cause of death
- To determine the time since death
- To give clue regarding manner of death (accident, suicide, or homicide)
- To determine identity in case of unidentified corpse
- *Skeletal remains*: To find out whether it is human or not. If human—age, sex, stature, probable cause of death, and approximate time since death.
- *Fetal autopsy*: To determine whether live-born or dead-born, age of fetus.

Clinical autopsy is done by a pathologist if requested by the treating doctor to determine the diagnosis. It is not done under any legal obligation and hence authorization from police or magistrate is not required. But consent of relative is must to perform clinical autopsy.

CONCLUSION

It is an important obligation of the doctor to register medicolegal cases and inform the police. Consent of family is not required for registration of a case as medicolegal case. In addition to basic medicolegal duties such as police intimation and death intimation a registered medical practitioner may be approached by the legal authority for various medicolegal examinations and reporting. Such reporting is must for determining the link between the offence and the harm suffered. A proper reporting and opinion will help the legal system for fair administration of justice.

KEY LEARNING POINTS

- Registered medical practitioners are legally bound to report all medicolegal cases to the legal authority.
- Intimate all cases of unnatural deaths and brought dead cases to police.
- While recording dying declaration, it is the legal responsibility of medical practitioner to examine the declarant and certify whether he/she is mentally fit to give declaration.
- Whenever a registered medical practitioner attends an injured person, while examining, record all injuries in the accident cum wound certificate.
- Examination of a victim of sexual assault must be conducted by a registered medical practitioner employed in a hospital run by state government or local authority. In absence of such facility any registered medical practitioner can examine the woman.
- For examination and certification of a female for signs of delivery, consent of the female is mandatory.
- Postmortem examination or medicolegal autopsy is a type of scientific examination of dead body under the laws of the state.

BIBLIOGRAPHY

1. Aggrawal A. Medicolegal autopsy. In: Aggrawal A (Ed). Forensic Medicine and Toxicology for MBBS, 1st edition. New Delhi: Avichal Publishing Company; 2016. p. 93.
2. Bakshish singh vs State of Punjab AIR 1957 SC 904.
3. Bharatiya Sakshya Adhiniyam, 2023. Government of India.
4. Bharatiya Nagarik Suraksha Sanhita, 2023. Government of India.
5. Parikh CK. Inebriant Poisons. In: Parikh CK (Ed). Parikh's Textbook of Medical Jurisprudence and Toxicology, 6th edition. New Delhi: CBS Publishers and Distributors; 2007. pp. 10.21-25.

6. Parikh CK. Injuries-Medicolegal aspects. In: Parikh CK (Ed). Parikh's Textbook of Medical Jurisprudence and Toxicology, 6th edition. New Delhi: CBS publishers and distributors; 2007. pp. 4.56-60.
7. Parikh CK. Virginity pregnancy delivery. In: Parikh CK (Ed). Parikh's Textbook of Medical Jurisprudence and Toxicology, 6th edition. New Delhi: CBS publishers and distributors; 2007. p. 5.23.
8. Samira Kohli vs Dr. Prabha Manchanda and another SC 1949 of 2004.
9. Umadethan B. Principles and Practice of Forensic Medicine, 1st edition. Kochi: Swami Law House; 2008.
10. Vij K. Abortion and Delivery. In: Vij K (Ed). Textbook of Forensic Medicine and Toxicology, 5th edition. Gurugram: Elsevier; 2011. pp. 389-90.

29.1 Issues Related to PM Examination of Fetus

Gautam Biswas, Rajinder Gulati

INTRODUCTION

Fetal autopsy encompasses a varied spectrum of cases—from aborted fetuses, discarded fetuses/infants, birth-related deaths, natural deaths, to traumatic deaths, including deaths from accidental and homicidal trauma. Various questions are required to be answered by an autopsy surgeon while handling such cases. These include establishing the identity of the mother (who is the mother?), estimating the gestational age of an infant (was the fetus "viable"?), determining whether there are indications of live-born, stillborn, or deadborn (was the baby born alive or died during the process of delivery or died in utero?), examining the existence of life-threatening underlying organic conditions, recording both deadly and nondeadly injuries, and establishing the potential cause, process, and mode of demise, when feasible.

MEDICOLEGAL ISSUES

The autopsy surgeon has to deal with the practical issues of abortion and infanticide as they exist today. The fetus may be brought for the examination so as to settle some of the matters cited further:

- *Inquiries related to artificial or deliberate abortion* (intentional ending of pregnancy prior to viability):
  - Is the abortion legal or justified? Abortion is considered legal and justified when carried out in good faith to safeguard the woman's life and conducted in accordance with the lawful stipulations outlined in the Medical Termination of Pregnancy Act (MTP Act). Under MTP (Amendment) Act 2021, pregnancy cannot be terminated beyond 20 weeks' pregnancy except under special categories of pregnant women and in case of substantial fetal abnormality. Opinion of only one provider will be required up to 20 weeks' gestation and of two providers for termination of pregnancy of 20–24 weeks' gestation. Upper gestation limit not to apply in cases of substantial fetal abnormalities diagnosed by Medical Board. The pregnancy can be terminated to save the life of the woman at any gestational age. In such cases, decision can be taken by a single doctor.
  - Whether this is a case of criminal abortion? Criminal abortion is induced destruction and expulsion of fetus from womb unlawfully which is outside the ambit of MTP Act. At times, when the female is sure of her unwanted pregnancy and has crossed the duration prescribed under the MTP Act or when the fetus is of female sex, she may approach for such abortions.

Issues regarding feticide, criminal abortion, concealment of birth and abandonment, and infanticide are dealt under various sections of the Indian Penal Code (IPC) **(Box 29.1.1)**.

- *Question on negligence*: Charges could be formulated and a legal action for a wrongful or negligent act might be initiated against the healthcare provider if such action leads to a miscarriage or stillbirth of the fetus. The medical practitioner may be held accountable for compensation if the harm endured arises from their wrongful behavior.

  Allegations of not monitoring the fetus during labor and providing a cesarean section when the stress is discovered or overstimulating contractions during augmentation of

Box 29.1.1: Criminal liability in fetal/infant deaths.

- *Section 103 BNS*: Infanticide is charged under Section 103 BNS which is punishable by death or imprisonment for life and also fine. In infanticide, the maturity is not legally material as it is the deliberate killing of any baby that has attained a separate existence, and this does not depend directly upon the gestational age. Infanticide does not include the death of fetus during labor, when it is destroyed by craniotomy or decapitation
- *Section 88 BNS*: Whoever voluntarily causes criminal abortion with the consent of the patient is liable for imprisonment up to 3 years and/or fine, and if the woman is quick with child, imprisonment may extend up to 7 years
- *Section 89 BNS*: If miscarriage is caused without the consent, imprisonment up to 10 years and fine
- *Section 91 BNS*: Any act done with intent to prevent the child being born alive or cause its death before birth is punished with imprisonment up to 10 years and/or fine
- *Section 92 BNS*: Any act which cause death of quick unborn child amounts to culpable homicide and imprisonment up to 10 years and fine
- Section 93 BNS deals with abandoning by the father or mother of the child under the age of 12 years with imprisonment up to 7 years and with/without fine
- Section 94 BNS deals with concealment of birth by secret disposal of dead body. In a case where infanticide (murder) is not proved, the person is usually charged under this section. Whoever, by secretly burying or otherwise disposing of the death body of a child whether such child die before or after or during its birth, intentionally conceals or endeavors to conceal the birth of such child is punished with imprisonment of for a term which may extend to two years, or with fine, or with both. It does not matter whether the child died before or after or during its birth, there must be a secret disposal of the body. Leaving the dead body of a neonate in the compound of a house or in public place where it can be easily seen does not constitute an offence under this section

(BNS: Bharatiya Nyaya Sanhita)

labor or not managing seizures of eclampsia or not maintaining blood pressure in case of hemorrhage, which resulted in stillbirth, may be levied against the doctor. The death may occur mainly due to asphyxia. Many a time, termination of pregnancy is not always based on a correct antenatal diagnosis. In one study, discrepancies between ultrasound and autopsy findings were observed in about 40% of the pregnancies.

- *Question on trauma resulting in abortion or fetal death*: Accusations could be made against an individual suggesting that the alleged assault caused the pregnant woman to experience an abortion. This scenario might involve a situation where a mother becomes a target of an assault, leading to preterm labor and the birth of an extremely premature infant who manages to survive for a brief period, but subsequently succumbs due to the severity of prematurity. In such an instance, there is potential for treating the case as a homicide, possibly resulting in the pursuit of criminal charges. In similar cases where the fetus dies in utero as a result of alleged trauma, criminal charges are framed under various sections of IPC/BNS. Postmortem changes take place between traumatic event, delivery, and subsequent examination of the fetus. Fetal autopsy findings may help in estimation of time of intrauterine fetal demise, particularly in context of maternal trauma.

  It is important to highlight that, excluding cases of trauma, traveling does not raise the likelihood of abortion. Infrequently, trauma might lead to an abortion, provided it does not result in substantial harm or danger to the mother's life.

- *Question on false reporting*: The medical practitioner may falsify the ultrasonographic report of fetal age and viability so as to bring it within the ambit of the MTP (Amendment) Act 2021. They may underestimate the gestational age of pregnancies and/or determine that viable pregnancies were nonviable in order to avoid having to obtain the concurring opinion from a second physician that is the mandatory requirement for the late abortion (after 20 weeks) under the MTP (Amendment) Act.

Identification of the Mother

The identification of the mother is difficult since in most cases, there is delay in discovery or the fetus/infant is removed from anything that could link the newborn with the mother and then discarded. A thorough investigation might result in finding the possible mother. The material used to wrap the infant with the body, such as bags, blankets, supermarket bags, and newspapers may help the police to identify or locate the maternal residence. Deoxyribonucleic acid (DNA) testing can provide a conclusive answer to the identification question, but only if a presumptive mother can be identified and DNA sample is collected from her.

Viability of Fetus/Infant

As of now, there exists no legally established threshold for intrauterine development, age, or weight that definitively designates a baby as viable. Irrespective of gestation period, any newly born infant can be subject to infanticide if they are born alive. When a child is identified as premature, there is a significant assumption that their chances of survival greatly diminish outside of medical care during and after birth. In instances where an infant is extremely premature from a rural setting within a developing nation, the likelihood of survival is notably low. Therefore, viability in one place means something quite different from viability in another.

The point of viability differs across nations, often falling between 24 and 28 weeks as the recognized thresholds for potential survival. In India, the age of viability is considered to be 28 weeks' gestation. In the context of English law, the legal age of viability is set at 24 weeks, a reflection of advancements in neonatal medicine and obstetric practices.

Autopsy

A complete autopsy includes a head-to-toe examination along with internal organ dissection and examination (including the brain). It may include retrieving and preserving organs for later study (formalin fixed). A partial autopsy can also be done in case of pathological autopsy. In this scenario, the family determines which body cavities can be investigated. They might choose not to have the head examined internally, instead granting permission only for an external assessment. With this knowledge, some families become more open to the idea of an autopsy.

The postmortem examination could coincide with radiological procedures such as X-rays, magnetic resonance imaging (MRI), computed tomography (CT) scans, or advanced ultrasounds. These tests aim to reveal any worrisome intracavitary abnormalities. If such issues are identified, needle biopsies can be employed to investigate the presence of infections, tumors, or malignancies. X-rays can be taken in case of suspected skeletal anomalies such as osteogenesis imperfecta or dwarfism.

Conducting an autopsy can offer significant insights in cases where multiple anomalies are detected but do not align with a specific syndrome **(Fig. 29.1.1)**. Additionally, it proves beneficial in examining renal irregularities and investigating potential causes of nonimmune hydrops, especially in instances without a cystic hygroma present **(Fig. 29.1.2)**. Capturing photographs of identified abnormalities is crucial, as they can be shared with other healthcare professionals. This collaborative approach aids in determining the cause of stillbirth and provides guidance for future pregnancy management.

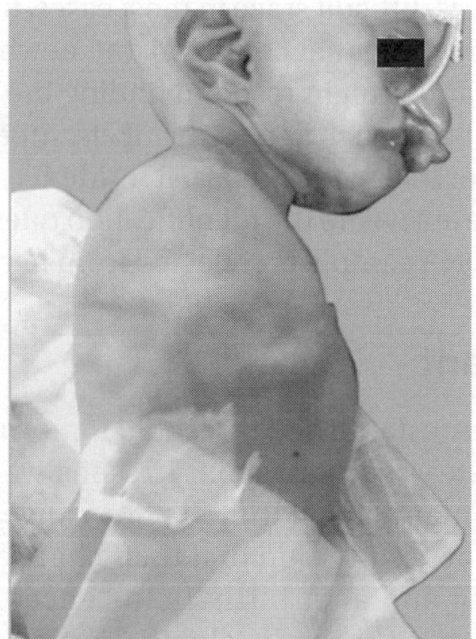

Fig. 29.1.1: Newborn with cleft lip and palate and amelia. ***(For color version, see Plate 1)***

Courtesy: Dr Rajendra S Kulhari, SPMC, Bikaner.

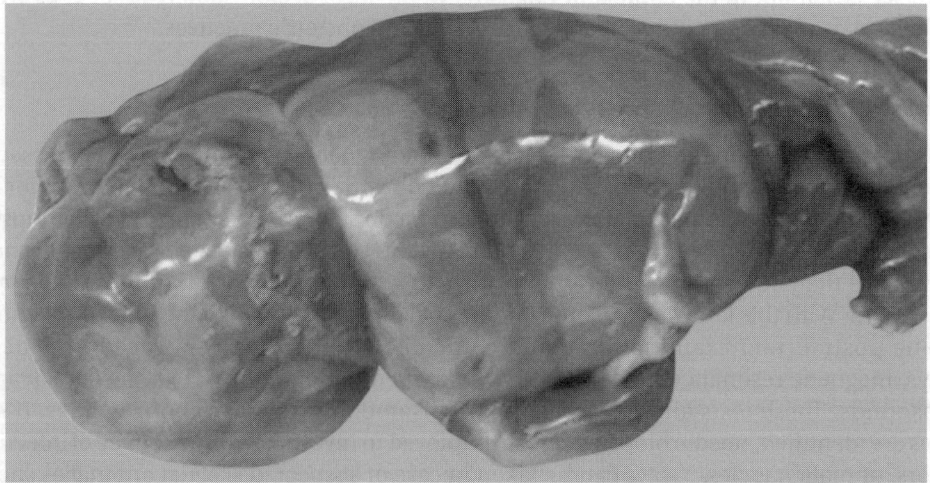

Fig. 29.1.2: Nonimmune hydrops fetal is showing generalized edema. ***(For color version, see Plate 1)***

Examination of the Fetus/Newborn

External Examination

By assessing the infant's weight, measuring their height (crown-heel length) and considering additional metrics (such as crown-rump length, head circumference, chest circumference, and foot length), it is possible to estimate the gestational age with a degree of accuracy **(Table 29.1.1 and Figs. 29.1.3A to D)**. Nevertheless, it is important to recognize that morphological measurements are not foolproof indicators of chronological age at any stage of life. Individual

Table 29.1.1: Gestational age based on physical parameters.

Weeks' gestation	*Features*
4	Length: 1–1.25 cm, weight: 2.5 g; eyes are seen as two dark spots and mouth as cleft
8	Length: 4 cm, weight: 10 g; eyes and nose recognizable, hands and feet are webbed; anus is seen as a dark spot; placenta is formed
12	Length: 9 cm, weight: 30 g; eyes are closed and pupillary membrane appears; nails formed on digits; placenta well formed; lanugo all over body; neck is formed. Hair formation begins in the 3rd month of fetal life
16	Length: 16 cm, weight: 120 g; sex can be recognized; lanugo hair is visible on body; pupillary membrane is visible; meconium is seen in the upper part of small intestine
20	Length: 18–25 cm, weight: 350–450 g; nails are distinct and soft, vernix caseosa appears on the body; fine hair on scalp; meconium at the beginning of large intestine; center of ossification for calcaneum appears
24	Length: 30 cm, weight: 700 g; eyebrow and eye lashes appear; eyelids are adherent and pupillary membrane is still present; skin is red and wrinkled for want of fat; testes are close to kidneys and scrotum is empty; meconium is seen in upper part of large intestine
28	• Length: 35 cm, 23–25 cm crown–rump, weight: 900–1,400 g, foot length of 8 cm; eyelids are open, pupillary membrane disappears; nails are thick but do not extend to the tips of fingers and toes; skin is dusky-red, thick and fibrous; meconium present in entire large intestine • Centre of ossification for talus appears (*fetal viability*) **(Fig. 29.1.4)**
32	Length: 40 cm, weight: 1.5–2.0 kg. Scalp hair is thick; nails reach the tips of fingers; skin is not wrinkled; lanugo hair on face; left testes in scrotum, right testes near the external inguinal ring
36	Length: 45 cm, weight: 2.5–3 kg. Scalp is covered with dark hair; lanugo hair is seen only in shoulders; vernix caseosa is present over the flexures of joints and neck folds; scrotum is wrinkled and contains both testes. In females, vulval labia close vaginal opening; meconium is near the end of large intestine; ossification centers for lower end of femur (36–37 weeks), cuboid and capitate appear
40 (full term)	Length: 48–53 cm, weight: 3–3.5 kg, 28–32 cm crown–rump, 33–38 cm head circumference; lanugo hair is absent or seen only over shoulders; head hair is about 2–3 cm long; nails project beyond fingertips **(Figs. 29.1.5A and B)** but reach only the tip of toes; rectum contains dark green or black meconium; six fontanelles are present. Ossification centers for lower end of femur always present (being about 6 mm in diameter); center of ossification for upper end of tibia appears (38–40 weeks, 80% of full-term fetus)

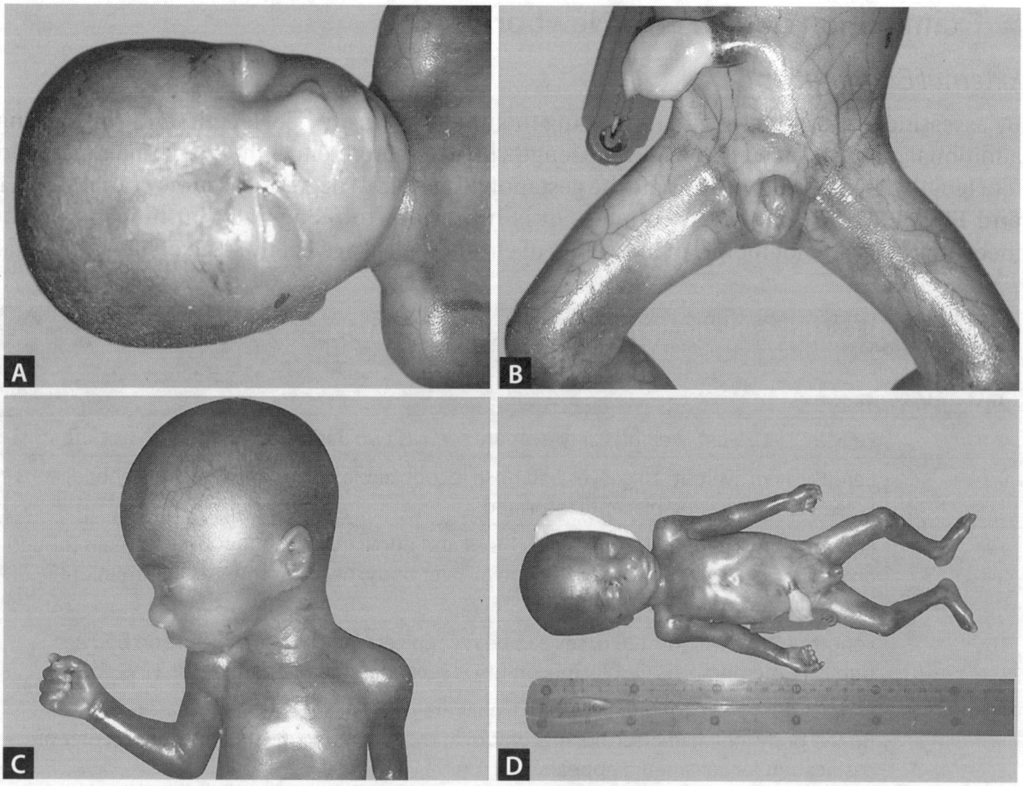

Figs. 29.1.3A to D: Fetus of 21–22 weeks' gestation (weight 365 g). ***(For color version, see Plate 1)***

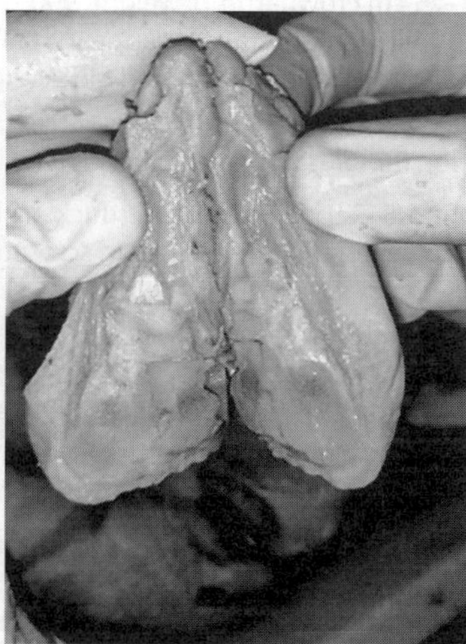

Fig. 29.1.4: Ossification centers of calcaneum (5th month) and talus (7th month). ***(For color version, see Plate 2)***

Courtesy: Dr Murugesa Bharathi, IGMC and RI, Puducherry.

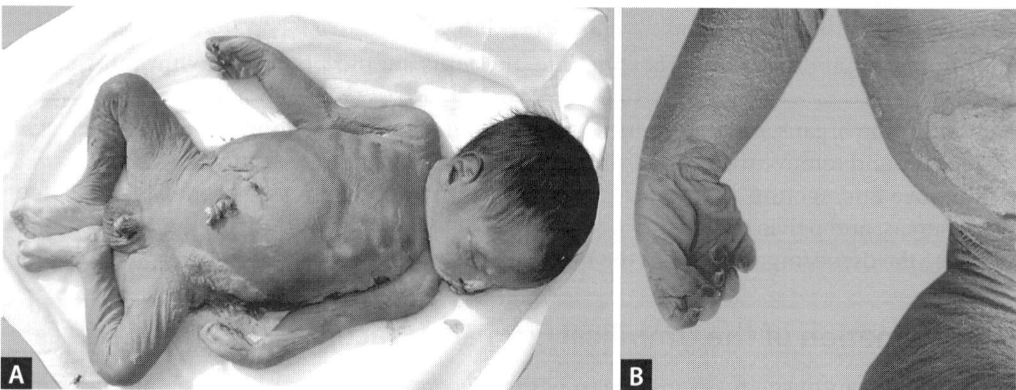

Figs. 29.1.5A and B: Post-term baby. Note the nails are beyond the fingertips. ***(For color version, see Plate 2)***

Courtesy: Dr Parmod Goyal, AIMSR, Bhatinda.

Box 29.1.2: Summary of fetal autopsy protocol.

- Photographs—front and back
- Radiographs, if indicated
- Careful inspection
- Autopsy
- Placenta and umbilical cord examination
- Placental cultures for suspected infection
- Fetal karyotype

differences are influenced by factors such as gender, ethnicity, and nutrition, which can introduce variability and affect precision. Furthermore, the previously held notion of uniformity in the timing of ossification center emergence is no longer universally accepted.

A set protocol may be followed to document the findings as follows ***(Box 29.1.2)***:

- Capture images of the head, face, entire body, hands, and feet. Ensure comprehensive photographs of the fetus/newborn are taken from front, back, and side angles. Document any anomalies by photographing and noting them.
- *Measurements*: Weight, length, head circumference, chest circumference, abdomen circumference, crown to rump, crown to heel, and foot length
- *Facial characteristics*: Positioning of ears, eyes, nose, mouth, and cranium
- *Neck, spine, and/or cranial irregularities*: Cystic hygroma, spina bifida, or unusual pigmentation
- *Skin*: Tone, maceration, or shedding
- *Umbilical cord attachment*: Central, marginal, or membranous
- Abdominal wall examination
- *Sex determination*: Ambiguous, female, or male
- Limbs, fingers and toes (clubbed, polydactyly, and syndactyly), and palm creases (simian)

Internal Examination

After the external examination is complete, the fetus should be opened with the Y-shaped incision:

- Identify the organs and determine if they are in the correct anatomic location.
- Identify and remove the gonads—it is done before any other dissection.
- Remove and section the organ (heart, lungs, thymus, kidneys, adrenals, liver, spleen, pancreas, and pelvic organs).
- Place the tissue/organs back in the body cavity.

Examination of the Umbilical Cord and Placenta

Apart from an autopsy, the examination of the placenta holds the utmost significance, often aiding in diagnosing approximately half of stillbirths or cases of neonatal demise.

A comprehensive analysis of both the umbilical cord and the placenta is conducted, with detailed observations recorded, including measurements. Visual documentation of the placenta and cord through photographs is recommended. Additionally, swabs are obtained from the placenta for culture, positioned between the chorionic and amniotic membranes, utilizing both aerobic and anaerobic culture swabs where appropriate. For cytogenetic investigations, segments of fresh skin are gathered and preserved in RPMI medium.

Reconstitute the membranes for completeness.

Determine the minimum distance between the membrane rupture site and the placental disk's perimeter. Document the type of membrane insertion, along with its color and texture. Measure both the greatest and smallest dimensions of the placenta, while also observing for any additional lobes or atypical configurations. Note any lesions found and take photographs of them.

Record the position and nature of the umbilical cord insertion by gauging the gap from the edge of the placental disc to the cord's attachment point. Observe the extent of exposed umbilical vessels, any intravascular umbilical blood clots, and the overall length of the umbilical cord. Document any false or true cord knots or twists and note if there is any cord edema, hemorrhage, laceration, or avulsion.

LIVE-BORN OR STILLBORN OR DEADBORN

The matter of whether a fetus/infant was delivered alive or not remains a subject of debate. For this reason, such deaths are quite difficult to deal with, particularly so in the setting of decomposition. In cases without decomposition, several factors are considered to address this query. There are essentially three potential scenarios:

1. The infant was born alive.
2. The infant passed away in the womb.
3. The infant expired during the birthing process.

Unfortunately, it is frequently not possible to differentiate between these possibilities.

Signs of Live Birth

In cases where a woman is charged with infanticide, the prosecution bears the responsibility of proving that the child existed as a separate entity. The autopsy surgeon is mandated to refrain from diagnosing live birth unless compelling evidence is present, such as fully expanded lungs, stomach content, or vital reaction in the umbilical cord's residual section. Convictions for infanticide have been overturned when any degree of uncertainty surrounds the question of whether the child was born alive. Live birth signifies the infant being alive after complete delivery or when at least a part of its body emerges from the mother's womb. The following indicators are considered as evidence of live birth:

- Audible crying of the baby—strongly supports the occurrence of live birth and respiration.
- Muscle twitches or limb movements
- Sneezing and yawning

The most reliable confirmation of live birth comes from an independent and credible witness who has observed the infant's movement or heard its cries. Presence of milk within the stomach signifies the infant's viability long enough to feed and partake in such actions. The drying and separation of the umbilical cord stump, a process typically occurring within 24–48 hours, along with histological evidence of tissue reaction, can be informative, although less so for deaths immediately following delivery.

In civil cases, any indication of life following the full delivery of a child is regarded as evidence of live birth. In criminal cases, the judge requires the medical witness to prove from postmortem examination that the child showed signs of life as a separate existence after it had wholly or partially emerged from its mother's womb. The most important sign is the establishment of respiration, which can be determined from examining the chest and the lungs.

Artificial resuscitation, chest compression, or administration of oxygen may artificially inflate the lungs in stillborn.

Ear Crepitus Test

If a small lung fragment is gently rubbed between the fingers near the ear and no crackling sound is heard (noncrepitant lungs)—the baby is considered as stillborn, and if crepitus is heard (crepitant lungs), then it is considered as live-born. This test is the most sensitive standard, yet it hinges on the extent to which the autopsy surgeon is convinced—after eliminating any potential for decomposition or resuscitation-related artifacts—that substantial respiration has taken place.

Hydrostatic or Flotation Test

One of the most time-honored tests used to assess whether respiration has occurred or not is the hydrostatic test. The hydrostatic or flotation test operates under the assumption that the lungs of an infant who has taken breaths will be expanded and infused with air, causing them to float when placed in water. This is in direct contrast to the lungs of a stillborn infant, which remain unexpanded and devoid of air, leading them to sink **(Fig. 29.1.6)**.

No matter the alterations introduced, the hydrostatic or flotation test retains restricted utility; at most, it offers an indirect indication rather than serving as a conclusive diagnostic tool. Regrettably, deciphering the results of this test is laden with challenges, given the prevalence of both erroneous positive and negative outcomes. Nevertheless, under the assumption that the body is recent, the combined buoyancy of the lungs and heart enhances the test's sensitivity.

Possible determinants of live birth are:

- Gestational age compatible with life (viability)
- No signs of maceration

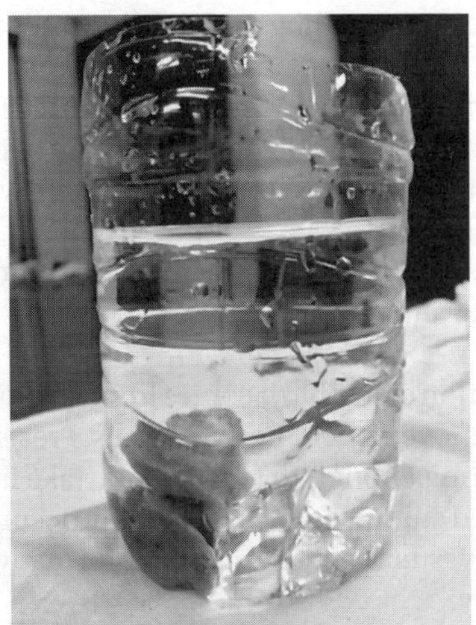

Fig. 29.1.6: Hydrostatic test showing sinking fetal lungs (negative test). ***For color version, see Plate 2)***

- No determinable reason for intrapartum death
- Air in lungs, middle ear, stomach, or gastrointestinal tract (GIT)
- Food in the stomach or extrauterine materials
- Inflation of the lungs—grossly or microscopically
- Positive ear crepitus test
- Positive hydrostatic test with no signs of putrefaction
- Vital reaction of umbilical cord

Stillborn Fetus (Intrapartum Deaths)

An alternative explanation for fatalities among newborns born without medical supervision or experiencing complications is that they died during the birthing procedure. Stillbirth can be attributed to various factors, including complications during labor, hypertension, diabetes, infection, congenital and genetic anomalies, placental dysfunction, and pregnancies that extend beyond 40 weeks. Among stillbirth cases, fetal growth restriction and placental irregularities stand out as commonly observed factors.

Indicators that lean toward an intrapartum death include the absence of maceration and the lack of lung aeration. Nevertheless, in the majority of cases, based solely on autopsy findings, it remains challenging to differentiate between these instances and deaths occurring before birth that have not yet displayed signs of maceration, or deaths occurring after birth where lung aeration is minimal or absent. Additionally, research has shown that in cases of rapid births, air can enter the lungs through chest compression, followed by swift chest expansion during passage through the birth canal, even if the infant does not actively inhale.

Deadborn Fetus

Important signs to identify deadborn fetus are the presence of maceration (skin slippage) **(Fig. 29.1.7)** and red-brown discoloration (normally yellow-tan color) of the umbilical cord stump along with primary atelectasis.

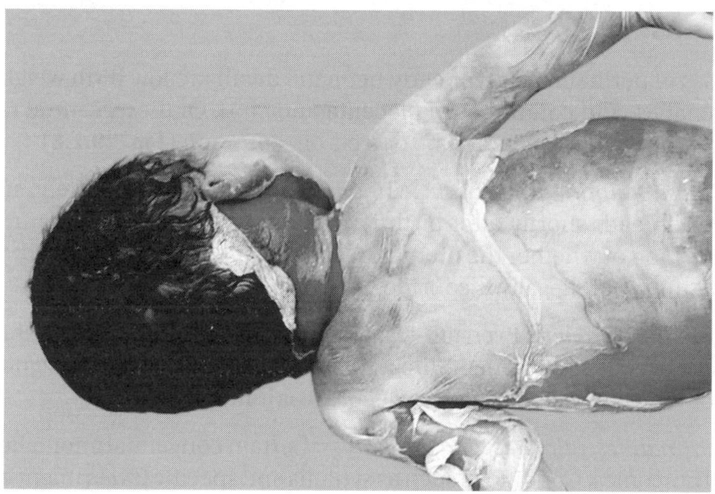

Fig. 29.1.7: Deadborn fetus showing skin maceration. ***(For color version, see Plate 2)***

Courtesy: Dr Joseph Prahlow, Kalamazoo, MI, US.

Various autopsy features may be analyzed to determine how long the fetus had been dead prior to delivery, which may be correlated to the time of assault. Important considerations are to the degrees and locations of desquamation of the skin of the fetus, nuclear basophilic changes of various organs, and death-related involutional changes in placenta.

While evaluating the timing of fetal death within first few days prior to delivery, features which are taken into considerations are assessment of desquamation/maceration of the fetus and loss of nuclear basophilia in myocardium.

In many cases, distinguishing between these scenarios can prove challenging. Solely relying on autopsy results does not offer a definitive means of distinguishing these instances from deaths that transpired before birth without significant decomposition or from postbirth deaths characterized by limited lung aeration. Moreover, in instances of abrupt deliveries, research has demonstrated that air can enter the lungs through the compression and swift expansion of the chest during passage through the birth canal, regardless of whether the infant inhales voluntarily. Confusion may arise, since a child who is born alive and taken few breaths or shallow breaths may have poorly inflated/expanded lungs, grossly and microscopically. Radiographs may show air in the lungs or stomach supporting breathing or swallowing, respectively. Putrefactive gases and air introduced during resuscitation will show on radiographs.

CAUSE OF DEATH

The factors behind these fatalities might be linked to complications during pregnancy, encompassing maternal or placental disorders, birth injuries, inherent health conditions, or external injuries—whether unintentional or intentional. However, a comprehensive exploration of these matters is not within the purview of this text. Some of the important causes are illustrated further. Finally, if a definitive cause of death cannot be determined, the phrase "intrauterine fetal demise of undetermined etiology" can be given.

Natural Causes

Important causes of perinatal death or early neonatal death are low birth weight, birth injury, congenital anomalies, and conditions of placenta and cord. Of these, central nervous system (CNS) anomalies, particularly neural tube defects are common **(Fig. 29.1.8)**.

Premature birth and criminal induction: When a child is born prematurely, survival is often compromised and death shortly after birth is common. In cases of premature births, there might arise a question of whether the premature labor was criminally induced. Under the IPC, inducing premature labor illegally is considered an offense.

Debility and underdevelopment: Even full-term infants can succumb to death shortly after birth due to inadequate overall development. These instances generally reveal no significant diseases, except for minor lung atelectasis caused by feeble respiration.

Congenital abnormalities, ailments, and anomalies: Certain congenital anomalies and diseases can lead to fatal outcomes. Conditions such as syphilis and specific fevers might cause the death of either the mother or the child due to toxic blood conditions. Among internal organ disorders, lung infections and hyaline membrane formation are observed. Easily identifiable conditions include anencephaly, severe spina bifida, encephalocele, hydrocephalus, and congenital diaphragmatic hernia with notable underdeveloped lungs. However, subtle cardiovascular or metabolic issues might be harder to diagnose **(Figs. 29.1.9A and B)**. It is crucial to note that even in the presence of monstrosity or malformation, ending the life of an infant is not justified.

Laryngeal spasms: Spasms of the larynx can result from mucus or meconium being aspirated into the larynx or due to thymus gland enlargement.

Erythroblastosis fetalis and isoimmunization: Erythroblastosis fetalis, caused by isoimmunization when a rhesus-(Rh)-negative woman carries a Rh-positive fetus, can lead to fetal death.

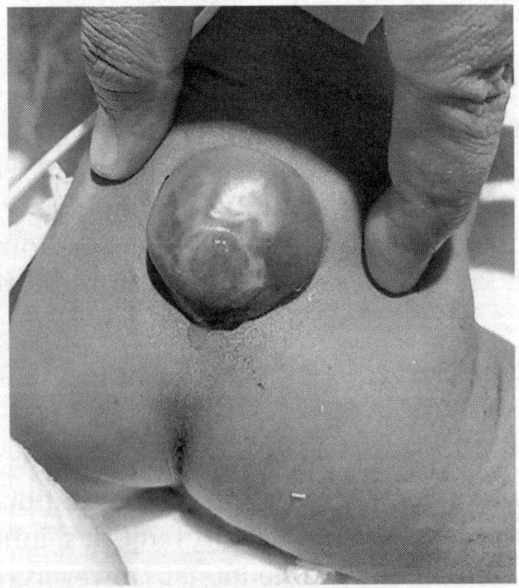

Fig. 29.1.8: Meningomyelocele. ***(For color version, see Plate 3)***

Courtesy: Dr Narinder S Bhatti, Jalandhar.

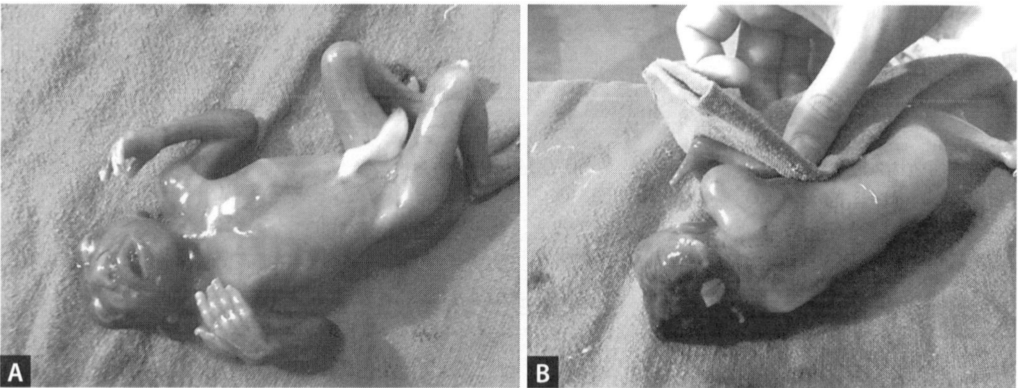

Figs. 29.1.9A and B: Anencephaly at 18 weeks' gestation. ***(For color version, see Plate 3)***

Courtesy: Dr Meenakshi, Jalandhar.

Accidental Causes

The process of delivery may itself be a traumatic event and cause a number of characteristic injuries to infants. Birth trauma encompasses various injuries that can occur during the birthing process. These injuries include fractures and dislocations of long bones when breech deliveries, malpresentation, or cephalopelvic disproportion (CPD) are involved. Additionally, there can be hemorrhage and edema within the scalp, which results in caput succedaneum, as well as subperiosteal hemorrhage known as cephalhematoma. In some cases, there might even be the rupture of the spleen and liver, as depicted in **Figure 29.1.10**. Regrettably, accidents leading to the unfortunate demise of the child can also take place either during the birthing process or in the postnatal period.

During the Childbirth Process

- *Prolonged labor*: It can lead to the child's demise due to blood leakage into the meninges or pressure on the head against the pelvis. When skull fractures occur, they usually involve slight fissures on the parietal and frontal bones or depression shaped like a spoon, without external scalp injuries. Prolonged labor often causes noticeable caput succedaneum and molding of the head.
- *Cord pressure or prolapse*: Asphyxia results from cord pressure or prolapse and postmortem examinations might reveal substances such as blood, meconium, amniotic fluid, or vernix caseosa in the bronchial tubes.
- *Cord knots or strangulation*: The fetus can be strangled before birth due to knots or loops tightening the cord or the cord wrapping around the neck during delivery.
- *Injuries*: Forceful impacts on a pregnant woman's abdomen using blunt objects, falls, or kicks from heights can cause fetal demise by causing brain concussion, skull fractures, ruptured blood vessels, or organ damage. External abdominal injury marks are not necessary.
- *Maternal death:* If the mother dies during delivery, the duration the child surviving in utero post mother's death depends on the cause. Slow death from hemorrhage offers little chance, but if a healthy mother suddenly dies from an accident, attempts to deliver within 25 minutes might save the child.

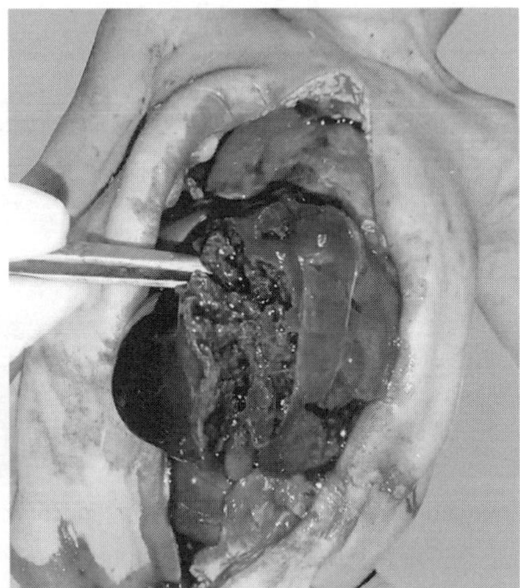

Fig. 29.1.10: Laceration of liver with hemoperitoneum. ***(For color version, see Plate 3)***

Courtesy: Dr Shalender K Saharan, SPMC, Bikaner.

- *Iatrogenic deaths*: These encompass a range of factors, from seemingly minor issues such as maternal body positioning, medication use (such as epidurals), to various medical procedures and surgical interventions. In rare cases of severe CPD, emergency attempts at removing the "stuck" fetus, using forceps or other instruments, with or without manual manipulation, can result in cervical vertebral column dislocation, or similar skeletal disruption, with associated lethal upper spinal cord or brainstem injury.

After Birth

Suffocation can occur when membranes cover the mouth and nostrils, or if the face becomes inadvertently pressed into clothing or submerged in substances such as blood, amniotic fluid, or meconium.

Likewise, precipitate labor, which is more frequent in women who have given birth multiple times, can also lead to the death of the newborn. Quick deliveries might result in asphyxia for small infants. If a mother delivers in a standing or squatting position with a long umbilical cord, there is a risk of the infant hitting the ground or floor, which can also lead to head injuries **(Fig. 29.1.11)**. This circumstance sometimes brings up the claim of unconscious delivery in cases of infanticide. Unconscious delivery might occur when a woman is under the influence of narcotics or intoxicating substances or if she is experiencing conditions such as syncope, asphyxia, coma, delirium, or eclamptic or hysterical convulsions.

Criminal Causes

When the forensic examiner establishes the separate existence of the newborn and verifies live birth, an additional responsibility emerges—to establish that the demise resulted from a deliberate action or a failure to act. The element of "intentionality" is a matter taken up by the prosecution, yet it rests upon the forensic examiner to substantiate fatal injuries or demonstrate negligence that led to the demise. This task is often exceedingly challenging. It is for this reason

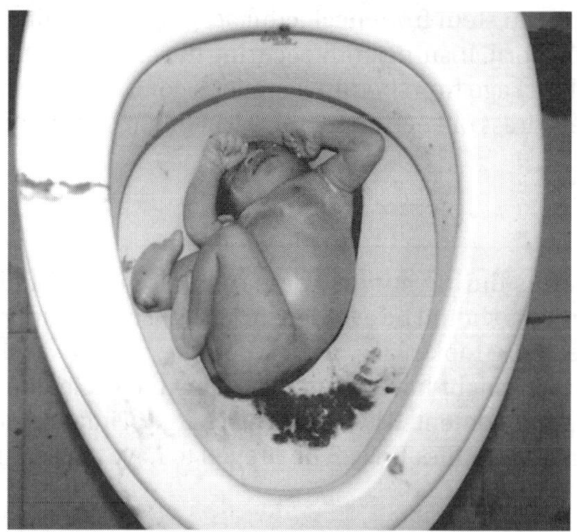

Fig. 29.1.11: Precipitate labor. ***(For color version, see Plate 3)***

Courtesy: Dr Viswakanth B, KIMS and H, Mangaluru.

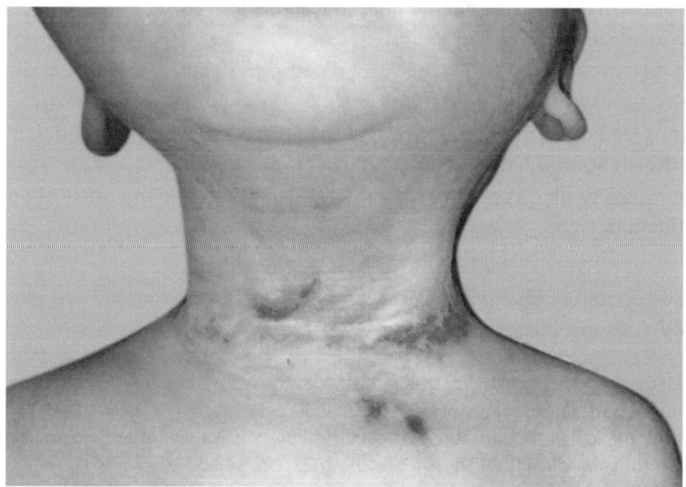

Fig. 29.1.12: Ligature strangulation. ***(For color version, see Plate 4)***

Courtesy: Dr Sandeep Haridas, Swami Ramanand Teerth Rural GMCH, Maharashtra.

that only a small proportion of suspicious neonatal deaths ever reach the court and even only few are convicted.

The most prevalent causes of these deaths often involve obstructed airways due to smothering or strangulation **(Fig. 29.1.12)**. A caregiver might cover an infant's nose and mouth in an attempt to stifle cries. Infants can suffocate when placed in plastic bags and concealed, while a mother tidies up postdelivery. Drowning can result if an infant is born into a toilet bowl and left there or submerged in a container of water. Instances of blunt head trauma may also arise. Occasionally, cut throats and stab wounds may be seen.

Furthermore, deaths can stem from neglectful acts, such as failing to provide appropriate care for a vulnerable newborn. Insufficiently securing the cut umbilical cord could lead to fatal blood loss and airway blockage from bodily secretions could impede breathing if not cleared. Neglecting to adequately dress or keep an infant warm might culminate in lethal hypothermia.

CONCLUSION

The examination of a fetus during autopsy demands careful and unhurried consideration. Rushing through the process should be avoided. In cases of uncertainty, it is imperative to state definitively that no breathing took place. Even when the forensic examiner leans toward the conclusion that respiration might have taken place, any lingering doubts should be explicitly expressed within the report's content. If live-born, no charge of infanticide can be brought, unless a willful act of omission or commission can be proved to have caused the death.

KEY LEARNING POINTS

- The forensic pathologist will have a good working knowledge of normal anatomy of fetus and legal sections (Sections 312–318 IPC) dealing with fetal deaths.
- Recognize the abnormal and preserve the anatomical relationships, as presence of malformations is often the major consideration.
- Determine the gestational age, sex, viability, and cause of death/congenital anomalies from gross external and internal examination with importance of associating histopathology.
- Detect conditions leading to manner of death of the fetus/baby whether natural or criminal, such as strangulation, drowning, and battered baby syndrome.
- Develop newer modality such as postmortem fetal MRI to determine the cause of death as part of the autopsy investigation.

BIBLIOGRAPHY

1. Atherton DS, McCleskey BC, Duncan VE. Utility of fetal autopsy findings to estimate time of intrauterine fetal demise in maternal trauma. Hum Pathol Rep. 2022;27:300586.
2. Biswas G (Ed). Infanticide and child abuse. Review of Forensic Medicine and Toxicology, 5th edition. New Delhi: Jaypee Brothers Medical Publishers (P) (Ltd).; 2021. pp. 348-67.
3. Biswas G, Sobti PC, Gulati R. Autopsy in Perinatal Deaths and its Medicolegal Implications. In: Biswas G (Ed). Recent Advances in Forensic Medicine and Toxicology, Volume 2. New Delhi: Jaypee Brothers Medical Publishers (P) (Ltd).; 2018. pp. 431-64.
4. Byard RW. Medicolegal problems with neonaticide. In: Tsokos M (Ed). Forensic Pathology Reviews, Volume 1. Totowa, New Jersey: Humana Press; 2004. pp. 171-88.
5. Chatterjee MS, Izquierdo LA, Nevils B, et al. (2002). Fetal foot: Evaluation of gestational age. [online] Available from https://thefetus.net/content/fetal-foot-evaluation-of-gestational-age/ [Last accessed May, 2024].
6. Cipriani N. (2019). Gross Pathology Manual: The University of Chicago Department of Pathology. Fetus. [online] Available from https://voices.uchicago.edu/grosspathology/peds-perinatal/fetus/ [Last accessed May, 2024].
7. Craig M. Perinatal risk factors for neonaticide and infant homicide: can we identify those at risk? J R Soc Med. 2004;97:57-61.
8. Das R, Mandal B, Das M, et al. Perinatal and fetal autopsies in Neuropathology: how I do it? Indian J Pathol Microbiol. 2022;65(5):207-17.

9. Illegal fetal age/viability deception scheme uncovered by operation rescue at Tiller's Abortion Clinic. [online] Available from http://www.operationrescue.org/noblog/illegal-fetal-ageviability-deception-scheme-uncovered-by-operation-rescue-at-tiller%E2%80%99s-abortion-clinic/ [Last accessed May, 2024].
10. Maslovich MM, Burke LM. Intrauterine Fetal Demise. In: StatPearls [Internet]. Treasure Island (FL): StatPearls Publishing; 2022.
11. Mattingly PJ, Joy S. Evaluation of Fetal Death. [online] Available from https://emedicine.medscape.com/article/259165 [Last accessed May, 2024].
12. Mishra S, Tiwari S, Misra S, et al. Fetal autopsy: A review. Medico-legal Update. 2016;16(1):66-9.
13. Prahlow J (Ed). Deaths in infancy and childhood. Forensic Pathology: For Police, Death Investigators, Attorneys, and Forensic Scientists. New York: Humana Press; 2010. pp. 501-38.
14. Saukko P, Knight B (Eds). Infanticide and stillbirth. Knight's Forensic Pathology, 3rd edition. London: Hodder Arnold; 2004. pp. 439-50.
15. Sharma L. (2020). Autopsy in Foetal Infant Deaths. Criminology and Post-Mortem Studies - Analyzing Criminal Behaviour and Making Medical Decisions. [online] Available from http://dx.doi.org/10.5772/intechopen.92673 [Last accessed May. 2024].
16. Shepherd R (Ed). Deaths and injury in infancy. Simpson's Forensic Medicine, 12th edition. London: Arnold; 2003. pp. 142-9.
17. Subrahmanyam BV (Ed). Infanticide. Modi's Medical Jurisprudence and Toxicology, 22nd edition. New Delhi: Butterworths; 1999. pp. 553-80.
18. Wikipedia, the free encyclopedia. Fetal viability. [online] Available from http://en.wikipedia.org/wiki/Fetal_viability [Last accessed May, 2024].

30

CHAPTER

Medicolegal Issues in Radiology

Tarvinder Bir Singh Buxi, Anurag Yadav, Astha Khushwah, Manisha Bhandari, Seema Sud, Samarjit Singh Ghuman, Kishan Singh Rawat

INTRODUCTION

Every doctor who enters into the medical profession has a duty to act with a reasonable degree of care and skill—this is what is known as "implied undertaking" that he would use a fair, reasonable, competent degree of skill. A man need not possess the highest expert skill [*State of Haryana versus Smt Santra (2000) 5 SCCI82: AIR 2000SC 3335*].

The last few decades have seen many ups and downs in the medical sciences. There are some undesirable changes, such as decreasing level of trust between patients and their physicians, decreasing values and morality, commercialization and corporate culture, and misuse of consumer protection laws by the patients for monetary gains. The scope and definition of understanding care as well as diagnostic efficacy has changed in the last two decades and will continue to change in upcoming years. However, what cannot be changed is the accuracy in diagnosis. The radiologist also comes from the same fabric as the rest of the society. If the patients are fearful and skeptical of doctors, the doctors reciprocate the apprehension in equal measure. The distrust is mutual and all encompassing.

Radiology is the first modality of choice in cases such as intracranial bleed, trauma, and pregnancy. Abundant scans are done in a year which play major role in patient's management and it has been observed that both under- and overutilization of radiology has an impact in the healthcare system in terms of delay in diagnosis and radiation exposure to the patient. For every study involving radiation, the radiologists have to practice the principle of ALARA—"As Low As Reasonably Achievable" by appropriately tailoring the study. As a corollary of this principle, all other radiological procedures should be carefully planned and meticulously executed. In every case, the study should fulfil the criteria of being "appropriate," which implies the possible adverse effects of the study outweigh the benefits of carrying out the study.

According to a study conducted in the United States (US), it was found that common cause of lawsuits against a radiologist is error in diagnosis rather than a delay in diagnosis. Apart from diagnostic radiology, the second most common cause of lawsuits is interventional radiology, especially due to miscommunication and procedural complications.

There are multiple studies conducted in various parts of world concluding that breast imaging is leading all the other imaging modality in lawsuits.

There are a set of rules for every country. Under the Consumer Protection Act, radiologists in India are held accountable in civil lawsuits brought by consumers. Patients are referred to as "consumers," while doctors are referred to as "service providers." Section 304A of the Indian Penal Code and Sec 106A of BNS, which addresses fatalities brought on by careless or reckless actions, is where cases of criminal negligence are launched.

Radiologists are responsible for not disclosing the gender of the fetus.

Under the Prenatal Diagnostic Techniques (Regulation and Prevention of Misuse) Act (PNDT), it is punishable to disclose the gender of baby to anyone; this law is enacted to prevent female feticide. Cases against radiologists can also be registered in the Medical Council of India/ National Medical Commission to warn, suspend, or revoke their license.

An improved understanding of the law and its ramifications may serve to prevent adverse legal effects found in the everyday practice of radiology. Legal issues also relate to the business aspects of radiology through radiologist's relationship to their group practice and the radiology group's relation to the outside world. These decisions range from business procedures that ensure a timely delivery of service to the choice and institution of quality assurance systems, to how to ensure that patients are informed results of radiological examination. Many actions of the physician in the practice of radiology have legal implications, not often recognized by the practicing radiologist.

CHANGES IN RADIOLOGY

The rapid advances in imaging technology have introduced a new accuracy into the diagnosis. Higher imaging resolution and faster scanning speeds of contemporary radiological modalities enable the performance of more examinations of higher caliber. As the need for radiological examinations expanded in current years, there is expansion in diagnostic imaging facilities as well. The clinical radiologist is certainly more closely involved with the patient than before and is thus more prone to litigation. Imaging not only helps in diagnosis, but now, it has become an integral part of modern drug programs. An excessive workload caused by the rapidly expanding number of imaging techniques increases the major risk factors for physician burnout and increases the likelihood of mistakes being made by the radiologist.

WHAT IS NEGLIGENCE IN RADIOLOGY?

An oversight in judgment is not negligence according to the law. A doctor must exercise a reasonable level of care that is consistent with their level of competence. Rather than necessarily providing "perfect care," a doctor is only required to provide "reasonable care." The mere fact that a mistake was made does not constitute medical malpractice.

The majority of the errors in radiology may be minor ones not resulting in significant damage, but the radiologists still have to be vigilant in this era of consumer empowerment and movement.

WHAT IS SPECTRUM OF NEGLIGENCE?

The Hon'ble Supreme court of India in its recent judgement has laid down guidelines to elaborate as to what constitutes Medical Negligence. In Neeraj Sud Vs Jaswinder Singh.

2024 SCC online SC 3069 the Hon'ble Apex court reiterated that actionable negligence in context of medical profession involves these constituents:

1. Duty to exercise due care
2. Breach of duty
3. Consequential damage

Further the Court stated that a simple lack of care, or error of judgment or an accident is not sufficient proof of Negligence on that part of the Medical professional, so long as the Doctor follows the acceptable practice of the medical profession in discharge of his duties.

The type of error/negligence committed may have a wide range or spectrum. The errors can be:

- *Perceptual errors*: They are almost a missed diagnosis, i.e., the abnormality though present is not perceived by the radiologist. A radiologist may review an X-ray using the degree of reasonable care but fails to detect an abnormality that, on an average, would have been reported by a radiologist. Radiologist simply cannot detect all abnormalities on all X-rays. Various reasons are responsible for these errors such as inability to perceive, overlooking another abnormality, difference in human anatomy, and limitations of equipment.
  The perceptual errors can be reduced by:
  - Proper exposure during procedure and positioning of the patient
  - Taking proper history and asking for previous radiographs (if available)
  - Reviewing the film for "second look" or discussing with referring clinician
  - Keeping the various possibilities or differential diagnosis in mind
  - Statistical probabilities should also be remembered.
- *Cognitive errors*: They are those in which the interpretation of the visualized abnormality is wrong. Often, a mistake is made in interpreting the films; it may have no effect on what eventually happened to the patient or may have serious clinical implications.
  The most commonly missed fractures can be those of cervical spine, scaphoid bone, and the neck of femur. Similarly, the dislocations of shoulder, tarsus, and carpus can be missed commonly.
  Missing of cervical spine fracture can, however, lead to serious and expensive errors as some of the patients may become paraplegic.

IS MISSED DIAGNOSIS (PERCEPTUAL ERROR) NEGLIGENCE?

Errors in perception may not always amount to negligence. It has been found that perceptual errors can be minimized and accuracy of diagnosis enhanced if proper history, clinical finding, and previous radiological reports are analyzed or interpreted simultaneously.

The fact that a mistake was made may constitute medical malpractice if the clinical outcome changed considerably due to error.

In Bandana Das versus Pratap Kesari Das case, a nursing home in Odisha failed to detect the physical deformities in the fetus even after conducting three ultrasonography (USG) tests on a pregnant woman and thus, the consumer court asked them to pay INR 10 lakhs in compensation for its failure to detect the physical deformities in the fetus. The woman may have terminated the pregnancy if she had known the fetus had a handicap. Because of the woman's faith in the nursing home and their findings, it is believed that she did not abort the pregnancy and gave birth to a boy kid with a physical disability. The radiologist who performed the ultrasound and wrote the reports may have seen the abnormalities in the fetus not once but three times. Giving false reports is a serious failing.

In Consumer Case No. 74 of 2009 Udayan & Ors. S/o Govind Shrouti, versus M/s Imaging Point & Ors., the medical negligence is attributed to the doctor and his Imaging Centre. The Opposite Parties' numbers 1 and 2 are directed to pay jointly INR 1.25 crore to the complainants.

The radiologist failed to diagnose the structural anomalies of the fetus at 17–18 weeks. The child was delivered via cesarean section (C-section) and the parents were shocked to see the grossly malformed baby as he had agenesis of fingers, right leg below knee, and left foot below ankle.

The principle of *res ipsa loquitur* applies in this situations, where carelessness is obvious and the complainant is not required to present any evidence because the item (res) speaks for itself. This is a well-established principle of justice.

Missing a fetal abnormality is the most frequent ultrasound-related legal dispute. The failure to advice pregnancy termination as a result of failing to diagnose the flaws at an early stage is the main cause of litigation.

There are cases, e.g., *R Sinha versus Dr A Mitra 11 (1995) CPJ 227,* where the computed tomography (CT) scan did not reveal any abnormality, but when patient went for surgery, there were evidences of uterine malignancy. The National Commission dismissed the appeal against radiologist by observing that it is important to explore the medical history in detail instead of relying totally on radiologist and in this case, the history was suggestive of a significant illness, amounting to cognitive error.

Many in the medical community, including radiologists, attorneys and lay people alike, believe that if a radiologist has missed an important finding that can be seen retrospectively, the miss cannot be considered anything but negligence.

OBSTETRIC RADIOLOGY

More than any other discovery, ultrasound has completely changed how obstetrics and gynecology are practiced today. The medicolegal hazards should be understood by practitioners, nevertheless.

Obstetric ultrasound is becoming more and more important in legal proceedings, whether it be as the center of attention in a case alleging wrongful birth in which an anomaly was not detected and the mother was denied the opportunity to terminate her pregnancy, or as a significant or contributing factor in a case of negligent obstetric care.

The American College of Obstetricians and Gynecologists (ACOG) and the American Institute of Ultrasound in Medicine (AIUM) are the organizations which issue the recommendations regarding the guidelines, documentation, quality control, and examination content.

The ACOG noted that doppler and diagnostic ultrasound are totally safe for the fetus.

There are indications for when to perform first- and second-trimester ultrasound and they clearly mention that if the patient is low risk and there is no indication for the radiologist to perform the ultrasound.

The AIUM and ACOG are using certain terminologies such as "standard," "limited," and "specialized" to explain the types of obstetric ultrasound.

The "standard" examination includes determining the fetal position, liquor, cardiac activity, etc. Presentation, amniotic fluid index (AFI), placenta, and biometry are components of standard USG. When the examination is done for specific indication, it is called limited examination. In specialized examination, doppler studies and fetal ECHO are used to answer a specific query related to fetal anomaly and it totally depends on the patient's condition and may vary from patient to patient.

How to Prevent from Getting Sued for Ultrasound?

There are a number of ways a radiologist can get sued for ultrasound, but the leading one is missing the finding, especially if it is related to fetal anomaly scan or misinterpreting it.

Taking care of good quality films, personal interaction with patient, taking detailed history by yourself, comparing patient's previous reports, advising follow-up scan or anomaly scan timely even if not advised by treating doctor, and completing your examination properly can save the radiologist from litigations. Patients with suspected anomalies, which are not understood by the sonologist, a proper reference should be given to an expert in writing for a second opinion.

Always make sure a female attendant is there with male radiologist while performing an ultrasound; convey the report to physician verbally in case of emergency as soon as possible.

Interventional procedures also form a large part of litigations in ultrasound such as vaginal bleeding or leaking after a procedure, abortions as a result of complication of procedure, not obtaining proper consent, or explaining the complications of procedure.

Ultrasound Alone is not Diagnostic for Fetal Anomalies! Why?

For diagnosing fetal anomalies, there are USG soft markers, combined tests, and integrated tests which are done in first trimester itself. These tests are followed by a level 2 scan which is also called anomaly scan.

Ultrasonographic soft markers include nuchal translucency, nuchal fold thickness, etc. Nothing is always pathological, but these have a strong correlation with chromosomal anomalies in the fetus. The likelihood ratio is elevated with increased nuchal translucency.

Similarly, for detecting trisomy 21, sensitivity of quadruple test is 72–83% and 90% for the combined tests. The above numbers show that nothing is 100% diagnostic and blaming a missed diagnosis on one will not solve the future diagnosis.

Chronic villous sampling provides a definitive diagnosis for chromosomal anomalies and can be performed at 11–14 weeks' gestation. So whenever in doubt, a comprehensive approach can be used for eliminating the risk of missing a congenital anomaly by looking at all the parameters.

Fetal magnetic resonance imaging (MRI) is the modality which is been used for detailed visualization of fetal structures. USG remains the primary modality for evaluation of fetal structures. However, it is limited by various factors such as maternal obesity and oligohydramnios. MRI provides better soft-tissue contrast resolution and large field of view. So it is advised that whenever there is doubt, fetal MRI should be done as it is a noninvasive modality and there is no radiation exposure.

Prenatal MRI can contribute in determining pregnancy outcome and therapy by displaying the fetal condition. MRI results can also assist physicians and expecting parents in understanding the severity of the problem and in making an educated choice about whether to continue or end the pregnancy. A fetal MRI should be advised whenever needed.

IS WRONG DIAGNOSIS (COGNITIVE ERROR) NEGLIGENCE?

A wrong diagnosis cannot be considered as deficiency in service, unless its genesis is in negligence or incompetence. It can still, however, be challenged in court as delay in treatment.

Shividhya Koteeswaran versus Dr Natasha Nanda (Radiologist) on April 30, 2019 alleged that patient did not receive proper treatment due to wrong reports and there was medical negligence.

Ultrasound was performed on two different days; the first one was reported as hydronephrosis instead of pyelonephritis and the second one was reported as pyelonephritis. Because of conflicting diagnosis on 2 days, there was no proper diagnosis and hence, the treatment was delayed.

Judgment was passed against the radiologist and compensation was demanded in terms of delay in diagnosis, leading to delay in its drainage and the "*lost chance doctrine.*"

A medical professional would only be held responsible if his actions fell short of those of a fairly qualified practitioner in his specialty.

The clinical history and other investigations can only help in differentiating between different entities. For example, soft-tissue stranding may be seen in the infection or inflammation or tissue injury. But two conditions may be present concurrently. Not everything is black or white, there are shades of gray.

AGE DETERMINATION: A MEDICOLEGAL ASPECT?

Age estimate of live people is crucial because it helps to verify the chronological age of a person whose age is unknown in the most precise manner feasible for both civil and criminal processes. For instance, the legal minimum age of criminal liability is 18 in several places. Therefore, it is crucial to check whether or not a person has achieved the age of legal consent, especially if it seems that they are forging their age.

In a recent ruling in the case *State of MP versus Anoop Singh [(2015) 7 SCC 773: (2015) 4 SCC (Cri) 208]*, the court emphasized that the ossification test should not be the sole determining factor for establishing a person's age. The court cited precedent cases such as *Babloo Pasi versus State of Jharkhand [(2008) 13 SCC 133: (2009) 3 SCC (Cri) 266]* and reiterated that the ossification test cannot be considered conclusive in the process of age determination.

"There are various criteria for age determination of an individual, of which eruption of teeth and ossification activities of bones are important. Nevertheless, age can usually be assessed more accurately in younger age group by dentition and ossification along with epiphyseal fusion."

Radiological examinations, while valuable in assisting age determination, are not definitively conclusive and indisputable. Courts that acknowledge this reality have taken judicial notice of the inherent margin of error associated with such evidence. Even if it is a very helpful guiding element, medical data about a person's age must be taken into account with other factors before passing a final judgment.

WHAT IS VICARIOUS LIABILITY?

The concept of vicarious liability is applicable in the cases related to radiology also. The National Commission in a case *Bombay hospital versus Sharifabai Ismail I (2008) CPJ 432 (NC)* held that consultant is liable for errors in interpreting report. Senior consultant is not expected to sign whatever junior staff suggests, without reading the same. The consultant radiologist who signed for the report is responsible for misreading/nonreading of MRI films correctly. The duty of the consultant does not end with correct interpretation of reports of film/scan. The radiologist is liable for the errors of the technologist employed under him. Similarly, the hospital management will be liable for the deficiencies of radiologist and other staff.

Medical staff working in radiology department does not only comprise doctors but also includes all the technicians, nurses, receptionist, anesthetist, and helpers.

The entire staff should be trained to have adequate medical and radiological skills to handle emergencies such as drug reactions and cardiopulmonary resuscitation (CPR). It should be an integral part of the teaching curriculum.

Reasonable degree of expertise is mandatory requirement for carrying out the investigations.

Standard operating procedures (SOPs) have to be instituted at every step of the radiology investigations to minimize errors and have a smooth workflow. These should come in play even before the patient enters the radiology department as prior instructions communicated by the receptionist. Identification of patients who need emergency investigations at a priority should be done judiciously for timely and appropriate diagnosis and minimize chances of negligence. Streamlining and close monitoring of these SOPs on a regular basis are essential for better management of the patients and safeguarding the radiology team.

RECORDKEEPING IN RADIOLOGY

Recordkeeping is becoming more crucial for providing excellent patient care as a result of the complexity of modern medicine. Whether it is a diagnostic report or a written summary of an interventional procedure, the radiological report is the radiologist's principal method of maintaining medical records. This can be in the form of a handwritten report in the patient records; however, electronic reports are growing more prevalent. The radiological information system then stores this computerized report.

In the radiology world, picture archiving and communication system (PACS) is the system for lifecycle management. Radiologists using PACS in all or part of their practice should develop and implement quality control mechanisms to ensure that all examinations performed are successfully transmitted in the PACS network and interpreted in a timely fashion.

In situations in which an entire study or key images are lost or when images cannot otherwise be interpreted, the referring physician or the patient should be promptly contacted to schedule a repeat study.

Destruction of Records

Before destroying the records, it is must that they are checked by authority person to confirm that the data is suitable for destruction.

CONTRAST MEDIA, CONSENT, AND PREANESTHETIST EVALUATION

Contrast media (CM) enhance the quality of images, revolutionizing the radiologist's ability to differentiate soft-tissue densities. The issue of informed consent, which entails a duty to inform patients about the nature of the procedure, the availability of alternative procedures, the severity of the risks associated with using CM, and finally the risks associated with refusing the procedure, is more prominent and potentially more significant. Failure to obtain proper informed consent is a frequent cause of lawsuit.

It is ethically required to obtain consent for all radiological CM procedures, regardless of the type of agent utilized or the likelihood and seriousness of any potential side effects.

Instead of relying solely on the patient, the radiologist who decides to use a contrast agent should find out if the patient has a history of allergies and elicit from the patient any information regarding allergies through specific questions, as the latter could overlook clinically significant details.

Premedication may be necessary in some situations, especially in patients who have previously experienced reactions to CM and for whom a pretreatment regimen is regarded to be safe, including administration of corticosteroids with or without antihistamines or other drugs. However, even when a patient is taking a prescription medication, acute adverse reactions (breakthrough adverse reactions) are known to happen.

The frequency and/or intensity of responses to CM have been reduced by a number of different premedication regimens. As additional safety measures, radiologists are advised to consider switching to alternative contrast agents and closely monitoring patients (20/30 minutes after the contrast medium injection, with resuscitation medications and equipment immediately available).

It is imperative to take an informed written consent of the patient and the attendant or the guardian in case of minor for any radiological procedure irrespective of the study. What is considered "*safe*" today may be proved to be "*not so safe*" at later date.

DOCUMENTATION AND REPORTING

Reporting

The final product, the essence of the radiologists' skills, is the radiology report. Therefore, it is crucial that radiology reports are created in a way that not only accurately reflect the knowledge and skills of radiologists but also takes any potential for unintended harm into account. An inaccurate report's most serious repercussion is harm to the patient. This risk can be reduced by being aware of any potential flaws in a radiological report. The possibility of legal action against the radiologist as a result of a poor report is a secondary disadvantage; thus, it is essential to understand the terminology used in the report in terms of its potential for litigation.

Poorly written or confusing radiology reports may cause the referring physician to make mistakes that could endanger the patient.

Regardless of the referring clinician's preference, a follow-up study should always be strongly and unequivocally advised when it is necessary for additional examination. The radiologist is considered the expert who is ultimately in charge of obtaining the best study in a court of law.

When in doubt, it is preferable to use straightforward, everyday language and terminology in a report, at least from a legal standpoint. After all, the jury or the board is made up of nonmedical individuals as well.

Comparison studies must be mentioned. It is necessary to document comparisons with pertinent references to earlier studies throughout the report; merely making comparisons is not sufficient.

Documentation

Care for patients includes accurate recordkeeping on a daily basis. This applies to all diagnostic specialties, including radiology, and it must be acknowledged that documentation should go beyond the confines of diagnostic report.

Verbal Communication

Radiologists often converse verbally with other medical professionals on a variety of clinical topics, including therapeutic advice that can have an effect on patient treatment. This therapeutic guidance offered to hospital doctors and practitioners is frequently seen as not requiring documentation. For instance, the rationale behind a choice to defer an imaging request or recommend an alternative is not always recorded. As with every clinical recommendation made by an expert, there is a chance that it may be disregarded or understood incorrectly, which might have major repercussions. Unfortunately, the radiologist has neither a record nor supporting documentation to function as a defense. Future patient treatment and continuity of care may suffer if this information is not recorded.

HOW CAN ARTIFICIAL INTELLIGENCE IMPACT THE LEGAL SYSTEM AND MALPRACTICE SUITS?

Many machine vision systems need intricate software models, whose functioning can occasionally be obscure even to their creators. This raises questions from doctors about their ability to depend on the judgment of a machine they do not completely comprehend.

This may also cause people to worry about malpractice lawsuits.

Artificial intelligence (AI) has a fast-growing range of applications in the medical field, with machine vision for medical imaging being one of the most promising of them. However, given the lack of relevant case law, the incorporation of AI technology into clinical practice raises difficult legal problems of culpability.

Machine vision models are "black boxes," making it challenging to understand why machine had made the particular diagnosis.

A radiologist can be asked to justify his/her diagnosis in court of law but a machine cannot.

A radiologist can correlate the diagnosis with history of the patient and highlight the most important and specific findings related to the pathology.

There are claims that machine vision models can also use heatmaps via which they can highlight the areas they are interpreting.

Initially, machine vision will probably be used as a computer-aided detection (CAD) product or as a triage tool for patient scans. The CAD will act as overread or second read to identify pathology and can help picking up the diagnosis which could have been missed and eventually decreasing the lawsuits.

Both contacting a qualified physician and using an accurate, understandable machine vision equipment satisfy the four criteria for a radiological consultation.

In machine vision ecosystem, the liability not only lies on the physician but also lies on the manufacturer under doctrine of "product liability."

There is Learned Intermediary Doctrine which states the if proper warning regarding the product risks is already given to the physician, then the responsibility lies on the physician to convey it to patient. But interestingly, there are two exceptions to this rule—first, if the manufacturer is in direct consumer marketing, he can use this rule as a defense. Second, if the system is designed such that it is taking the scan and making a diagnosis and the physician is not playing an active role in the diagnostic part, then the whole responsibility will lie on the manufacturer.

So the manufacturer will always want an active role of physician in making a diagnosis to exempt himself from the lawsuits.

In order to guarantee that incentives are appropriately aligned and that liability falls where it should, careful analysis is needed to identify how the legal system should handle machine vision and medical AI.

TELERADIOLOGY

Teleradiology is the electronic transmission of diagnostic imaging studies from one location to another for the purposes of interpretation and/or consultation. Teleradiology is now an integral part of the life of a radiologist because of the development of PACS and workplace communication.

Teleradiology should never hamper the patient care and it is advised that it should adhere to the American College of Radiology (ACR) technical standards for teleradiology. There are certain rules which must be followed for practicing teleradiology like a radiologist who is interpreting a scan should be licensed in transmitting country/state. Radiologist should interpret the reports generated outside independently and provide official authenticated report.

With the use of teleradiology, timely access of a radiologist can be provided to underserviced hospitals; however, teleradiology comes with limitations in terms of poor-quality images.

It is always advised to provide judicially adequate clinical information and in case of any doubt, a second opinion is always suggested.

Peer review-driven quality assurance is the cornerstone of effective teleradiology practice.

The radiologists need to be vigilant, compassionate, intelligent, and well trained to do full justice to the expectations from them. If in doubt, they should confer with their colleagues, seniors or specialists of a particular organ system before giving their final reports.

This would decrease "second opinion and multiple opinions" and instill more confidence in the patients.

CONCLUSION

In radiology not everything is black or white, there are lots of shades of gray.

Radiologist should act as a clinician and take full responsibility of the report generated after careful assessment of the patient and not be like a technologist who just interprets an image. An ideal scenario would be an integrated use of CAD, AI, radiologist, and clinician in perfect synchrony with the patient for a detailed and comprehensive detection and interpretation of disease pathology.

KEY LEARNING POINTS

- No single radiologist can have the highest level of expertise in all fields and therefore, second opinions should be considered to provide reasonable care to the patient.
- Medical science is never complete, it is always evolving. A drastic and phenomenal change is seen in the field of medical science in the last two decades and it will continue to evolve further in the upcoming years. So the best is yet to come

BIBLIOGRAPHY

1. ACOG Committee on Practice Bulletins. ACOG Practice Bulletin No. 58. Ultrasonography in pregnancy. Obstet Gynecol. 2004;104(6):1449-58.
2. American Institute of Ultrasound in Medicine. AIUM practice guideline for the performance of an antepartum obstetric ultrasound examination. J Ultrasound Med. 2003;22(10):1116-25.

3. Bhaktwani A. The PC-PNDT act in a nutshell. Indian J Radiol Imaging. 2012;22(2):133-4.
4. Biswas S, Biswas S, Awal SS, et al. Malpractice and lawsuits in radiology: what the radiologist should know. Egypt J Radiol Nucl Med. 2023;54:19.
5. Braithwaite JM, Morris RW, Economides DL. Nuchal translucency measurements: frequency distribution and changes with gestation in a general population. Br J Obstet Gynaecol. 1996;103(12):1201-4.
6. Darden v. Driscoll, No. 1:12-cv-01001-EPG (PC), 2016 U.S. Dist. LEXIS 174510 (E.D. Cal. Dec. 16, 2016).
7. Chervenak FA, Chervenak JL. Medicolegal Issues in Obstetric and Gynecologic Ultrasound. Donald School J Ultrasound Obstet Gynecol. 2012;6(1):9-13.
8. Cuckle H, Maymon R. Development of prenatal screening—a historical overview. Semin Perinatol. 2016;40(1):12-22.
9. Davenport MS, Cohan RH, Caoili EM, et al. Repeat contrast medium reactions in pre-medicated patients: frequency and severity. Radiology. 2009;253(2):372-9.
10. Gray H. Gray's Anatomy, 37th edition. Edinburgh: Churchill Livingstone; 1989. pp. 341-2.
11. Katzman GL. The legislative and working environment: clearing the muddied waters. In: Yousem DM, Beauchamp NJ, editors. Radiology business practice. Philadelphia (PA): W.B. Saunders; 2008. p. 444-62.
12. Supreme Court of India. *Neeraj Sud and Anr. v. Jaswinder Singh (Minor) and Anr.* Civil Appeal No. 272 of 2012 and Civil Appeal No. 5526 of 2012. 2024 Oct 25.
13. Halpin SFS. Medico-legal claims against English radiologists: 1995–2006. Br J Radiol. 2009;82:982-8.
14. Harned Z, Lungren MP, Rajpurkar P. (2019). Machine Vision, Medical AI, and Malpractice. [online] Available from https://jolt.law.harvard.edu/digest/machine-vision-medical-ai-and-malpractice [Last accessed May, 2024].
15. Harry E, Sinsky C, Dyrbye LN, et al. Physician Task Load and the Risk of Burnout Among US Physicians in a National Survey. Jt Comm J Qual Patient Saf. 2021;47:76-85.
16. Information Governance Alliance. Records Management Code of Practice for Health and Social Care 2016. London: Information Governance Alliance; 2016.
17. Nicolaides KH, Azar G, Byrne D, et al. Fetal nuchal translucency: ultrasound screening for chromosomal defects in first trimester of pregnancy. Br Med J. 1992;304(6831):867-9.
18. Pomara C, Pascale N, Maglietta F, et al. Use of contrast media in diagnostic imaging: medico-legal considerations. Radiol Med. 2015;120:802-9.
19. Saleem SN. Fetal MRI: An approach to practice: A review. J Adv Res. 2014;5(5):507-23.
20. Sanders RC. The effect of the malpractice crisis on obstetrics and gynecologic ultrasound. In: Chervenak FA, Glenn C, Isaacson GC, et al. (Eds). Ultrasound in Obstetrics and Gynecology. Boston: Little, Brown and Company; 1993. pp. 263-7.
21. Singh SS, Jayaram N. Medico-legal issues in radiology: Indian context. J Med Soc. 2015;29:129-34.
22. Srinivasa Babu A, Brooks ML. The malpractice liability of radiology reports: minimizing the risk. Radiographics. 2015;35(2):547-54.
23. The UK Government. Data protection act 1998. London: The Stationery Office; 1998.
24. van Breast Smallenburg V, Setz-Pels W, Groenewoud JH. Malpractice claims following screening mammography in the Netherlands. Int J Cancer. 2012;131:1360-6.
25. Webb JAW. Prevention of acute reactions. In: Thomsen HS (Ed). Contrast Media: Safety Issues and ESUR Guidelines. Berlin: Springer; 2006. pp. 11-9.
26. Yoshizato T, Kozuma Y, Horinouchi T, et al. Diagnosis of Fetal Abnormalities during the First Trimester. Kurume Med J. 2021;66(2):85-92.

31

CHAPTER

Medicolegal Issues in Dermatology

Pallavi Nigam Sethi, Pramod Kumar Nigam

INTRODUCTION

The skin is not only the mirror of the internal environment of the body, it also contributes significantly to the individual identity and shaping of self-esteem. Presently, dermatology is deeply invaded with cosmetic considerations and other means meant to improve the physical appearance of patients, besides managing chronic and serious skin illnesses. Recently, dermatology, dermatosurgery, and cosmetic surgery have recorded significant developments, especially in diagnostic and therapeutic techniques. Psoralen plus ultraviolet-A (PUVA) radiation therapy, lasers, immunohistochemistry, biologics, dermoscopy, Moh's surgery, etc., have significantly revolutionized the approach in this specialty. Simultaneously, dermatological patients have also become more and more aware of promoting and defending their rights, due to wider and easier access to information, thus making this specialty risky. Jena et al. considered dermatology as a specialty of "low risk" but not "worry-free." It was estimated that by 65 years of age, 75% of physicians in these "low-risk" specialties could expect to face a claim of malpractice. Dermatology is placed among the specialties which represent the "changing face" of medicine and also among high-risk specialties with a greater risk of litigation.

The law interacts with dermatology practice in myriad ways, including malpractice, use of medications, chemicals or devices, compliance with patient privacy laws, etc. The threat of malpractice is probably the most terrifying and direct means by which physicians are impacted by the law. Malpractice occurs when medical acts are in breach of the accepted standard of care. The notion of an accepted standard, which is a legal concept rather than a medical one, is used synonymously with correct technique, or more precisely, medical care that is reasonable, follows protocol, or would be provided by any well-trained physician under the same or similar circumstances. Medical malpractice litigation is a significant factor impacting healthcare costs, insurance rates, affordability, and availability of care.

COSMETICS

Cosmetics are defined as "articles intended to be rubbed, poured, sprinkled, or sprayed on, introduced into, or otherwise applied to the human body or any part thereof for cleansing, beautifying, promoting attractiveness, or altering the appearance." From a dermatologist's point of interest, the cosmetic may be skin care cosmetics (cleansing agents, moisturizing agents, etc.), hair care cosmetics (shampoos, hair colorants, styling agents, etc.), face care cosmetics (facial foundations, powders, eye shadows, mascara, lipsticks, etc.), nail care cosmetics (nail varnishes, paint removers, etc.), fragrance products (deodorants, aftershaves, perfumes, etc.), and ultraviolet (UV) light screening preparations. Cosmetics market in India, particularly in urban centers, is growing at a rapid pace, owing to several factors such as greater purchasing power because of higher incomes, the increasing influence of western culture, the desire to look better and more attractive, etc. An Environmental Working Group (EWG) survey found that an average adult uses nine cosmetic products daily. More than 25% of women use 15 or more.

Allergic contact dermatitis is the most common dermatological reason for hospital referrals and cosmetics, toiletries, and skin care products, including sunscreens are the most frequent offenders. The incidence of allergy to a cosmetic or one of its ingredients is 1–3% of the general population. It was observed that about 700 cases of reactions occurred out of 30,000 in an American survey. Various untoward reactions to cosmetics may occur in the form of acute toxicity, percutaneous absorption, skin irritation, eye irritation, skin sensitization and photosensitization, subchronic toxicity, mutagenicity/genotoxicity, and phototoxicity/photoirradiation. The adverse reactions may occur to one of the primary constituents of the cosmetic formulation or contamination or procedural misconduct. Preservatives are the second most common cause of skin reactions, besides fragrances. Most reactions are irritant rather than allergic in nature. Drugs associated with risk (such as methotrexate, antimalarial agents, biologics, retinoids, corticosteroids, sulfones, or propranolol) should be prescribed with extra care. Patient safety recommendations should also be followed when surgical or laser treatments are provided. In most cases, these are only mild or transient such as stinging and smarting and contact urticarial. Sometimes, reactions may be more severe, with redness, edema, dryness, and scaling.

COSMETIC DERMATOLOGY: LEGAL ISSUES

While cutaneous medicine mainly deals with the etiopathogenesis, diagnosis, treatment, and prevention of skin disease, cosmetic dermatology focuses on improving the physical appearance of the patients. "Medical therapeutic or cosmetic medical procedure, device, or treatment" means a treatment or procedure that uses any of these—if the procedure or treatment alters or damages or is capable of altering or damaging living tissue, to improve the patient's appearance or to achieve an enhanced aesthetic result, injection or insertion of a biologic or synthetic substance for soft tissue augmentation, application of a chemical substance, application of microwave energy, or application of an approved prescription device that uses waveform energy of any kind, including but not limited to lasers or intense pulsed light (IPL). Cosmetic dermatology is an exciting field that is constantly offering new procedures. The tools and methods available in cosmetic dermatology include *lasers, IPL, radiofrequency, resurfacing, liposuction, chemical peels, Botox, fillers,* and other topical treatment modalities such as retinoids. These procedures can also be combined for even better effects.

Cosmetic procedures are becoming increasingly popular in dermatological practice. Dermatologists are supposed to provide a certain duty of care to each patient that comes seeking treatment from them. Failure to provide this duty of care by acting in a manner that is negligent, improper, or insufficient results in the patient developing skin complications, making it possible for the patient to file a dermatologist malpractice lawsuit. Nearly all cosmetic procedures are voluntary and there is seldom a strong medical need driving a patient's decision to undergo treatment. The voluntary nature of these procedures adds an extra burden to disclose risks more fully. "Clearly nonessential cosmetic surgery requires a higher degree of disclosure than potentially life-saving cancer surgery." Hence, those clinicians who practice cosmetic dermatology mainly are at even greater risk of litigation.

Various factors, including physician gender, merit attention when weighing the possibility of risk of future malpractice suits in dermatology. A full-body examination may be medically justified for a patient who has sun-damaged skin, precancerous or melanocytic lesions, or a history of skin cancer but may be annoying for some patients. To avoid full nudity, examinations can be done in stages and are best carried out in the presence of a nurse or assistant, with informed consent. Although routine dermatological consultations usually do not require consent, any procedure or application of chemicals does require informed consent.

Informed Consent

Cosmetic procedures have become a regular part of dermatology practice. All available therapeutic and prognostic options, including their risks and benefits, must be disclosed and discussed with the patient before arriving at any management decision. Yet, the practice of informed consent is compromised if reasonable diagnostic or treatment options are withheld by the physician. Preprocedure and postprocedure checklists and disclosures are also vital for both excellent patient care and medicolegal protection for patients and practitioners. Competence is usually assumed for adult patients seeking cosmetic procedures. However, competence may be in question in patients with body dysmorphic disorder (BDD). This issue was raised in the case of Lynn versus Hugo, in which a cosmetic surgeon was sued by a patient who claimed BDD rendered her incompetent to give consent. This raises the risk that BDD may be a barrier to informed consent. BDD is characterized by a preoccupation of the mind with a minimal or nonexistent physical flaw and resultant distress that may inhibit normal daily functioning. Besides competence-related issues, BDD patients are also more prone to be dissatisfied with cosmetic result outcomes and are more likely to take legal action against dermatologists.

Mostly, cosmetic surgical procedures are subjective requirements and nonessential. Thus, cosmetic surgical procedures require a higher degree of information and disclosure to patients. It is always better to document those risks in the consent signed by the patient. Makdessian et al. observed that cosmetic patients remembered significantly more risks if they were disclosed in written format. Written information also enhances recall of risks and benefits. Patients are also becoming more knowledgeable and seeking more information about therapeutic options. There may be a lack of communication and understanding between the treating dermatologist and the patient if information is not conveyed and recorded properly. It has been suggested that physicians are reluctant to share much information in order to maintain supremacy over their patients. The ability of patients to make informed choices is enhanced if they are also appraised of the potential risks associated with each procedure.

Cosmetic products are frequently used off-label from their United States (US) Food and Drug Administration (FDA) indications and are acceptable medical practice. As long as the use of cosmetic medications and devices is consistent with standard care routinely performed by other physicians, medical liability is minimal.

In Rogers versus Whitaker, it was held that a medical practitioner has a duty to warn the patient of a material risk inherent in a proposed treatment, except in cases of medical emergencies.

In a judgment, Minnesota Supreme Court established two points of departure for the nascent doctrine of informed consent. First, the consent of the patient would be invoked only when the physician's care involved surgery and second, the physician retains near-absolute discretion as to the "method of treatment." The Supreme Court of Oklahoma elaborated on the second point in Rolater versus Strain and held that "the patient had the right to insist upon a strict performance" of the agreed parameters of consent.

In Hunter versus Burroughs, the patient was submitted to X-ray therapy to cure eczema and this treatment damaged the patient's skin. The court upheld "the duty of a physician in the exercise of ordinary care to warn a patient of the danger of possible bad consequences of using a remedy" only in a very limited sense.

In Pandiya versus Dr Trivedi and others, a 12-year-old boy who had exanthematous fever diagnosed initially as measles instead of a diagnosis of measles and bronchopneumonia was found guilty of negligence.

■ Keeping Records

Medical records are acceptable evidence in a court of law as per Section 3 of the Indian Evidence Act, 1872, amended in 1961. Any information in medical records should be clear, comprehensive, and documented in chronological order at the time the events happen or as soon as possible afterward on a daily basis. From a litigation point of view, even if everything was done correctly at the time of an incident, if it has not been documented chronologically, it has not been done. This makes even the best of doctors difficult to defend. The physician is liable, both medically and legally, for the proper maintenance, custody, and storage of the record of each patient for the required statutory period. Besides medicolegal importance in malpractice suits, properly maintained records of patients also help in the scientific evaluation of the patient treatment profile and in planning governmental strategies for future medical care. Even though the medical record is not the sole information upon which the courts will rely in determining negligence liability, it can serve as an important chronology of events of patient care. A properly documented case record can help protect a cosmetologist in case of negligence due to performed procedure. The indoor patient records should be maintained and preserved in standard pro forma for 3 years as per Medical Council of India (MCI)/NMC regulations. However, records of cases with medicolegal issues should be preserved till their final disposal.

Confidentiality of the patient's personal records is an important component of the rights of the patient. It is the responsibility of the treating dermatologist or the hospital to maintain confidentiality. Breach of confidentiality may always result in a case of negligence. However, negligence does not occur during referrals, or when legally required for insurance cases, or other government agencies.

The National Commission had held that if the patient has been provided a detailed summary note, the hospital is not bound to provide complete medical records and not liable for negligence unless it is required for a legal reason. However, in Raheja versus The Maharashtra Medical Council and Ors, the Bombay High Court held that if patient or his relatives demand medical records, the doctor or hospital has to provide them and they cannot withhold them on grounds of confidentiality.

In Trivedi versus Dr Satyanarayan Vishwakarma, a deficiency in service was observed as the doctor and hospital could not produce the case records before the court to refute the charges of poor care. In Quereshi versus PMHRC, the hospital was found guilty of suppressing facts by destroying the case records before the final disposal of the case.

In Dr Shyam Kumar versus Kachiya, it was held that it is the responsibility of the hospital to produce medical records in the court otherwise hospital may be held responsible for ill care.

In Force versus Ganeswara Rao, the doctor was held responsible for negligence as the case records were missing the proper history, investigations, and consent papers.

In Yeptomi versus Apollo Hospital, the hospital was held responsible for negligence as the human immunodeficiency virus (HIV) status of the patient was disclosed to others without taking the consent of the patient.

DERMATOLOGY IMAGES, CONFIDENTIALITY, AND THE LAW

Dermatology is basically a visual science and mostly depends upon visual observational changes. Digital images are commonly used in dermatology and assist in better and more efficient care of patients. These help in comparing the progress as well as help patient satisfaction, especially in cases with cosmetic surgery. These also help as important clinical records, especially in patients with cosmetic and Moh's surgery. It has been observed that clinical photographs of pre- and postprocedure always have more satisfaction with treatment than those without photographs. In today's modern era of digital transmission, images always help in several ways, especially by taking opinion and consultations from higher centers. Similarly, patients from remote areas may be provided health services through the digital transmission of images. These also help as clinical records and must be preserved as important clinical medical records like other records. As the identity of the patient may be disclosed, consent must always be taken before taking photographs. Intended use of photographs should always be discussed with patients and necessary written consent must always be taken for all present and future uses, if required, such as publication as research articles or teaching purposes. Consent is unnecessary and may not be required when nonidentifiable digital images are used for educational purposes. The patient may also demand their photographs and other digital image records. All legal issues regarding the application, sharing, and storing digital data and their implications should be kept in mind to protect the confidentiality of the patient. Health Insurance Portability and Accountability Act (HIPAA) defines confidentiality as any information that "identifies the individual or reasonably may be used to identify the individual" qualifies as "protected health information" (PHI).

In the year 2021, Forefront Dermatology, one of the big dermatology service providers in the USA, faced one of the largest healthcare data breaches, affecting about 2.4 million patients and paid a huge $3.75 million, one of the largest class action settlements for a lawsuit alleging negligence in protecting patient privacy.

The higher judiciary of the country has recognized the right to privacy as a right "implicit in the right to life and liberty guaranteed to the citizens of this country by Article 21." Indian law has made some exceptions to the rule of privacy in the interest of the public, especially subsequent to the enactment of the Right to Information (RTI) Act, 2005. The RTI Act makes an exception under section 8 (1) (j), which exempts disclosure of any personal information which is not connected to any public activity or of public interest or which would cause an unwarranted invasion of privacy of an individual. In 2011, India adopted new privacy regulations, known as the information technology (Reasonable Security Practices and Procedures and Sensitive Personal Data or Information) rules. These rules impose wide-ranging obligations on any "body corporate" (company) that "collects, receives, possesses, stores, deals, or handles" personal information.

There have always been legal concerns on the validity of using clinical images and other digital records as evidence as they may differ on digital screens or modified technologically.

In State versus Swinton, images were found manipulated. Court also recognized that all digital evidence must be authenticated by a jury of members.

In Stubbs versus NMMC, the clinical pictures of the cosmetic surgery of Stubb's nose were used for educational purposes without taking her consent. The physician was sued for breach of confidentiality and privacy and legal liability was fixed. On the other hand, in Anderson versus Mayo Clinic, an interview broadcasted by the Mayo Clinic was found to be valid as Anderson had already consented for use of her images.

TOPICAL ANESTHETIC USE IN DERMATOLOGY: LEGAL ISSUES

Topical anesthetics are widely used to anesthetize the skin for medical and cosmetic procedures such as laser and to relieve pain, burning, and itching due to a variety of medical conditions. These topical anesthetics contain various drugs such as lidocaine, benzocaine, prilocaine, etc., in a cream, ointment, or gel form. Topical lidocaine application may result in sensitization, potential ototoxicity, shock, and even death due to methemoglobinemia, cardiac arrest, or idiosyncratic reaction after systemic absorption. Applying topical anesthetic for a medical procedure is usually done in a clinic setting by a trained medical professional. As in unsupervised application, a patient may apply large amounts of topical anesthetics to their skin which can result in high levels of these chemicals in the blood, causing life-threatening side effects, such as an irregular heartbeat, seizures, and death. In one case, a 20-year-old Coast Guard cadet died as a result of an allergic reaction and cardiac arrest after a topical anesthetic was applied to his back prior to planned laser hair removal by a plastic surgeon. A wrongful death lawsuit was filed by his parents and the case was settled for $725,000. In another case involving the use of a topical compounded mixture of lidocaine and tetracaine applied to the legs under occlusion on a healthy 23-year-old woman resulted in a respiratory arrest and ultimately death.

BOTOX (BOTULINUM TOXIN A) AND ILLEGAL BOTOX SCAMMERS

Botulinum toxin A (BTX-A), a purified protein derived from the bacteria *Clostridium botulinum*, has been widely used in aesthetic dermatology. Though BTX-A was initially used by neurologists extensively for neurological conditions such as blepharospasm, dystonia, and spasticity, it has become popular among dermatologists and plastic surgeons for its cosmetic indications, mainly smoothening out frown and perioral lines to make them less visible.

Botulinum toxin A is an injectable drug and should be administered by a trained, qualified healthcare professional in an appropriate setting using sterile instruments. A nonphysician who is appropriately licensed and trained may also perform the injections under the supervision of a qualified physician. All Botox product labels now have a black box warning that the effects of the botulinum toxin may spread from the area of injection to other areas of the body, causing symptoms similar to those of botulism. Those symptoms, which have mostly been seen in children with cerebral palsy who received injections off-label for the treatment of muscle spasticity include potentially life-threatening swallowing and breathing difficulties and even death. In the USA, under federal law, no form of botulinum toxin may be commercially distributed for use on humans unless it has been approved by the FDA and healthcare professionals must make sure that they are using only an FDA-approved product purchased within the US. The benefits and risks must be fully explained to the patient before injecting.

Severe botulism poisoning and temporary paralysis have resulted after illegal botulinum toxin injections not approved by the FDA by Illegal Botox scammers. The doctor who injected the toxin had passed it off as Botox cosmetic, an FDA-approved drug to treat forehead wrinkles. In an investigation in the USA, 31 arrests and 29 convictions of individuals who purposely injected an unapproved, cheaper substitute ("For Research Purposes Only, Not For Human Use") toxin for FDA-approved Botox Cosmetic into nearly 1,000 unknowing patients. They were indicted for fraud, misbranding a drug, tampering with documents, and making false statements. Besides this, single-use medication vials used on more than one patient have also resulted in Botox lawsuits. It raised issues on injections for the unacceptable and unreasonable risk of serious and debilitating injuries and illnesses, including HIV and hepatitis B and C and according to the lawsuit, the part of the medication cannot be saved for later use on the same patient because once a vial is opened, it must be thrown away within 4 hours of first use. A federal jury has ordered the maker of Botox, Allergan, to pay $212 million to a man who allegedly suffered brain damage leading to disablement, following the use of the drug.

COSMETIC LASER SURGERY AND THE LAW

The word "laser" stands for light amplification by the stimulated emission of radiation. Lasers work on the principle of producing an intense beam of light that travels in one direction and cuts, seals, or vaporizes skin tissues and blood vessels. Lasers are being increasingly used by dermatologists as a part of their cosmetic procedures, including hair removal, nonablative treatments, resurfacing, as well as the removal of pigmented and vascular lesions. The American Medical Association's Policy H-475.988, laser surgery, opines that revision, destruction, incision, or other structural alteration of human tissue using laser is surgery. Laser surgery should be performed only by practitioners licensed to practice medicine and surgery or by those categories of practitioners currently licensed by the government to perform surgical activities. With new innovations and the availability of increasingly powerful laser technologies and safety applications, an increasing number of physicians and nonphysicians are performing these procedures. However, new technology also increases the potential for new problems, mainly negligence.

All cosmetic and surgical procedures and use of instruments must be carried out within a widely accepted clinical standard. Expert testimony may still be required to check for its relevancy. All instruments and medical devices such as lasers are regulated by FDA. However, new innovations and experimental procedures to achieve results are regularly tried by the surgeons and cosmetologists. These may, sometimes, result into a poor result. If done without taking prior consent, this may result into litigation.

MEDICOLEGAL ISSUES IN CRYOTHERAPY

Cryotherapy is an office procedure that is frequently carried out in general practice. The common indications include warts, corn, calluses, keratoses, etc. If the patients are selected carefully and appropriately and care is taken with the procedure, it offers many patients a speedy and efficient alternative to other complicated surgical procedures. In terms of the cryotherapy procedure, the risks could include recurrence, blistering, scarring, and varying degrees of pain.

All those carrying out cryotherapy in general practice should be up-to-date and adequately trained in the procedure and skills in accordance with national guidelines. Ideally, training schedules should be documented. Equipment should be regularly serviced and service records should be maintained. All staff-designated protocols should be clearly setting out their roles and responsibilities for the relevant procedure. Patients should be thoroughly explained about the procedure and warned about its risks. Informed consent must be taken and aftercare advice should be given and recorded. Risk management advice comprises avoiding the potential risk of complaints and claims following cryotherapy and to improve patient safety.

Although cryotherapy procedures are relatively safe and seldom lead to complications, lawsuit cases concerning cryotherapy can arise mainly from failures in practice procedures. At one center, 86% of claims relating to cryotherapy were from primary care, with the remainder arising from dermatological and ophthalmological practice. Extended use of a cryotherapy machine is associated with injuries including frostbite, skin damage, skin necrosis, nerve damage, gangrene, and more. Even amputation may result. A Californian woman has been awarded more than $12 million in compensatory and punitive damages after a lawsuit was filed over problems suffered during cryotherapy. In two cases, repeated cryotherapy was administered to lesions that later proved to be malignant and the resulting claims were settled for a total of £175,590. In another 13 cases, settlements were made totaling £194,530. In some of the settled claims, other indemnifiers also contributed to the compensation awarded to the claimant. These cases arose from failure in practice procedures because of faulty equipment or because the treatment that caused the injury was administered by an unindemnified employee at the practice.

MEDICOLEGAL CONSIDERATIONS IN THE MEDICAL SPA

The medical spa includes procedures that are incisionless, provide minimal discomfort, create little-to-no skin wounds, and are performed in less than 1 hour. The procedures that fit this model are mostly intended to promote antiaging, cellulite reduction, tissue tightening, acne treatments, and hair removal. The core procedures include microdermabrasion, chemical peels, medical facials, laser hair removal, photorejuvenation, botulinum toxin, and injectable fillers. Less common procedures include laser resurfacing, laser-assisted lipoplasty, sclerotherapy, photodynamic therapy, and cosmetic surgery. The spa business is booming worldwide. More and more spa facilities are opening up, almost on a daily basis. Dermatologists are the owners of some spas, but spas are often being run by other types of physicians or, more alarmingly, by people unfamiliar with treating skin conditions of any kind. The medicolegal considerations of the medical spa include failure in practice procedures, because of faulty equipment or because the treatment that caused the injury was administered by an unindemnified employee at the practice.

In Melissa Smith versus Patricia Dunwell, HCV 02484-2008, Supreme Court of Jamaica, the counsel claimed that the dermatologist did not properly advise of the risks involved in the peeling treatment for hyperpigmentation. The defendant submitted that the claimant was properly advised, both verbally and in writing, about the procedure, complications, and side effects involved. Informed consent was also taken. The case was dismissed as no negligence was found.

COSMETIC SURGERY ON CHILDREN: LEGAL IMPLICATIONS

Cosmetic surgery is defined as "procedures undertaken by a qualified medical practitioner to revise or change the appearance, color, texture, structure, or position of normal bodily features with the sole intention of improving the patient's appearance or self-esteem. The body image dissatisfaction frequently motivates the decision to have cosmetic surgery. There are concerns about the ethics and application of cosmetic surgery in children and this should be governed by what is in the "best interest" of the children. There is a lack of professional guidelines for cosmetic surgery in India. No relevant policy has been published by MCI or similar surgical bodies such as the Indian Society of Plastic Surgeons or the Indian Association of Pediatric Surgeons. Mathews highlighted certain factors that must be considered before conducting cosmetic surgery on children. Certain scientific bodies have suggested that children below 18 years of age should not have cosmetic procedures unless it is essential in their medical, physical, or psychological interests. Still, some suggest giving a cooling-off period of at least 3 months to reconsider the procedure and its essentiality. If the child is above 18 years of age and is mentally fit, he/she can give consent for medical and cosmetic procedures. However, if the child is younger, the child's parents can legally provide consent. The legal tests of "best interest" for the child are flexible and not well-defined; however, these must include his medical, psychological, and social interests. Views of the child should also be sought and considered. The timing of the procedure, especially whether waiting until the child becomes an adult, should also be considered. The best interests test dictates that the needs of each child be addressed individually, not the desires of parents or treating surgeons.

DRUG SAFETY: MEDICOLEGAL IMPLICATIONS FOR THE DERMATOLOGIST

The skin is the organ most frequently affected by adverse drug reactions (ADRs) followed, in order, by the hematological, gastrointestinal, nervous, cardiovascular, hepatic, endocrine and metabolic, respiratory, and renal systems. Thus, it results into huge implications for the dermatologist and dermatopathologist. Among adults 65 years of age or older, 40% take 5–9 medications and 18% take 10 or more daily. Such huge exposure to drugs further increases the chances of adverse drug effects. Cutaneous ADRs comprise between 18.4 and 23.5% of all ADRs' cases. A number of drugs have been removed from the marketplace over safety concerns and reported adverse events worldwide. Similarly, a few drugs with significant reports of ADRs have remained on the market with either a "black box" warning or strict prescribing guidelines. In many cases, the removal of drug from the market is preceded by the filing of one or more product liability lawsuits under claims of negligence, strict liability, breach of warranty, and consumer protection claims caused by life and financial loss. There are also certain drugs that remain on the market because their benefits outweigh the risks associated with their labeled usage. At the same time, there have been drugs that have been placed on the market with known defects or properties rendering their risk disproportionate to their benefit and resulting in significant morbidity and mortality.

Adverse cutaneous reactions to drugs are frequent, affecting 2–3% of all hospitalized patients. The incidence of adverse cutaneous drug reaction (ACDR) in developed countries range from 1 to 3% among patients, whereas in developing countries such as India, some studies peg it to 2–5% in patients. Watkarou et al. reported that approximately 2,216,000 Americans were harmed by ADRs each year, with an incidence rate of 6.7% (5.2–8.2%). They estimated that the number of deaths caused by these ADRs could be as high as 106,000 annually, leading to the fourth highest cause of death in the US. Liao et al. observed that the average increase in medical expenses among cutaneous ADR cases were 2.5-fold higher than the matched controls. Failure to adequately inform and warn the patient of those risks a reasonable person in the same situation would want to be shared with them, are cause of most of these litigations. The majority of claims in these litigation did not involve allegations against the prescribing physician but rather that "negligence" of the manufacturer involving a drug-related manufacturing defect, design defect, or did not adequately warn doctors and patients of potential side effects of the drugs. Drugs associated with risk (such as methotrexate, antimalarial agents, biologics, retinoids, corticosteroids, sulfones, or propranolol) should be prescribed with extra care. Patient safety recommendations should also be followed when surgical or laser treatments are provided.

In BK Ghosh versus Dr P Maulick, the complainant who was suffering from rheumatoid arthritis (inflammation of joint) was taken to the opposite party for treatment. The opposite party's doctor after examining her prescribed certain pathological and clinical tests and after reports of such tests were available, he prescribed a medicine called Myocrisin 10 mg in 0.5 mL. Since there had been disorientation of the eyeballs of the patient, he advised her to consult some eye specialist. Subsequently, the patient contacted doctor again with acute pain to know the procedure to be followed to combat her rheumatoid arthritis. The doctor examines her this time and prescribes another medicine "Imuran" without holding any prior investigation or test. Immediately, she had alopecia (complete hair loss on her head) and bone marrow suppression as a result of taking this medicine. Since then, the patient became completely bedridden and underwent extreme mental trauma with acute type of physical discomfort. The patient suffered this due to the side effect of the abovementioned two medicines which she took as per the advice of the doctor. It was observed that the doctor had applied the medicine Imuran to the patient without holding any prior test to ascertain her findings to take such medicine and certainly committed an act of gross negligence.

There are no specific guidelines on what adverse effects should be disclosed by the physician. However, some case laws suggest that the more uncommon and rare adverse effects are not required to be disclosed.

In Watkins versus US, the patient was prescribed quinacrine (an antimalarial drug) by his dermatologist for the treatment of discoid lupus erythematosus (DLE). The patient was warned of the possibility of his skin turning yellow, and eventually developed exfoliative dermatitis. On the issue of adequately warning the patient about side effects of the drug, the district court observed that the physician did warn about common side effects. The appellate court further held that "under the recognized standard in the medical profession and the specialty of dermatology, the physician was not required to warn the patient about rare side effects including exfoliative dermatitis and erythema multiforme."

In Akers versus Levitt, the patient developed cataracts secondary to the long-term use of potent topical corticosteroids for psoriasis. The court observed that the patient was informed of the material risks involved with the treatment of potent topical corticosteroids and even though the physician did not warn of the risk of cataracts. The court also noted that while there was disagreement regarding the length of use and potency levels of corticosteroids, there was expert testimony that the treatment met the standard of care.

In Woods versus Pommerening, a patient was treated with gold injection for DLE. The patient developed jaundice during the course of therapy. The court observed that it was not the customary standard of practice to inform the patient of jaundice and all the risks involved.

However, in Bowman versus Songer, the patient developed second- and third-degree burn after prolonged sun exposure after taking methoxsalen prescribed by the dermatologist. The court observed that the physician did not warn of the drug's potential to cause severe burns.

PRESCRIBING DERMATOLOGICAL MEDICATIONS IN PREGNANCY: MEDICOLEGAL ASPECTS

Dermatologists should take precautions in prescribing medicines to females of childbearing age. It has been observed that 86% of female patients take an average of 2.9 prescriptions per user during pregnancy. Care should be taken while prescribing certain potential high-risk medications, especially for acne, psoriasis, autoimmune diseases, connective tissue diseases, etc.

Antihistaminic diphenhydramine, although can be used safely in first two trimesters, may stimulate uterine contractions and cause retrolental fibroplasia in premature infants. Use of systemic retinoids in pregnancy may cause retinoid embryopathy and cardiac myopathy. Earlier studies hinted that topical application of retinoids during pregnancy may also cause side effects similar to systemic retinoids. Subsequent studies did not show these side effects and other major congenital birth defects with the topical application. However, it is better to avoid its use in pregnancy. Isotretinoin, an oral retinoid drug (pregnancy category X), is also known to cause fetal toxicity and congenital birth defects, such as microtia, cleft palate, hydrocephalus, and cardiac anomalies, when taken during pregnancy, especially in the first trimester. Acitretin, a pregnancy category X drug mainly used for the treatment of psoriasis, is also known to cause craniofacial, cardiac, and central nervous system anomalies. It has been suggested that women of childbearing age should avoid pregnancy for 3 years after discontinuing its use. Methotrexate, a folic acid antagonist and pregnancy category X drug used for the treatment of psoriasis, can cause hepatotoxicity, abortion, and congenital anomalies etc. Methotrexate should not be used for the treatment of dermatological disorders during pregnancy. Biologics (pregnancy category B), such as adalimumab, etanercept, infliximab, and ustekinumab, are immunosuppressants and are being increasingly used for the systemic treatments for moderate-to-severe psoriasis and many other skin disorders. Although limited studies have not revealed any increased frequency of congenital malformations, they should be used with caution in pregnancy after carefully weighing the benefits against the unknown risks to the fetus. Cyclosporine, a pregnancy category C drug, used in dermatology for the treatment of severe psoriasis and atopic dermatitis, is associated with serious maternal side effects such as hypertension. Oral corticosteroids are pregnancy category C drugs and are frequently used in various dermatological disorders. An increased risk of maternal morbidities including gestational diabetes, hypertension, preeclampsia and eclampsia, and even intrauterine growth restriction (IUGR) has been observed with their prolonged use in high doses. Immunosuppressant drugs, such as mycophenolate mofetil, used in atopic dermatitis patients, are also known to produce congenital malformations including microtia, external auditory canal atresia, cleft lip and/or palate, etc., and even an increased risk of first-trimester pregnancy loss and should be avoided during pregnancy.

Minoxidil, a pregnancy category C drug, commonly prescribed for the management of androgenetic and common diffuse alopecia, has been observed to be associated with cardiac defects and other congenital anomalies in infants born to mothers using topical minoxidil during pregnancy.

Hydroxychloroquine (pregnancy category C; HCQ) is used for the treatment of DLE and other dermatological conditions. It is observed that maternal use of HCQ does not increase the risk of congenital, neurological, or auditory abnormalities or miscarriage. Rather, the use of HCQ during pregnancy has been observed to reduce the daily dose of corticosteroid, as well as reduced the risk of developing cardiac neonatal lupus.

MELANOMA: MEDICOLEGAL PERSPECTIVE

There is an alarming increase in the incidence of malignant melanoma in the general population during the past few years. Today, >80% of all melanomas are diagnosed at an early stage and the 10-year survival for patients in this category is in excess of 90%. About 13% of all medical malpractice claims are alleged to relate to melanocytic neoplasia. One study suggested that melanoma was the second most common cause of malpractice litigation in the US. Significant morbidity and mortality resulting from mistaken underdiagnosis, nonrecognition, or delay in diagnosis of melanoma are the main causes of melanoma malpractice litigations. The distinction between melanoma and nevus can be challenging at the light microscopic level, and even at the molecular level just as it is at the clinical level. Further, studies have shown that even expert melanocytic lesion pathologists are unable to obtain a concordant view on one quarter to two-thirds of studied lesions.

OCCUPATIONAL DERMATOSES: MEDICOLEGAL ASPECTS

The application of new technological advances in the growth of industry, agriculture, mining, and manufacturing has been paralleled by the development of occupational diseases of the skin. Unfortunately, there is no accurate assessment of the number of cases, causal factors, time lost, or actual cost of occupational skin disease in most countries. The skin can react to a large number of mechanical, physical, biological, and chemical agents, acting alone or in combination, available in the occupational environment. The American Medical Association defined occupational dermatoses as a "pathological condition of the skin for which occupational exposure can be shown to be a major causal or contributory factor." In legal sense, there should be a clear, direct correlation of the skin disease with the occupation or work of the patient. In India, the Employees' State Insurance (ESI) Act 1948 defines occupational disease as if an employee employed in any establishment specified in Part A of the Third Schedule contracts any disease specified therein as an occupational disease peculiar to that employment, or if an employee employed in the employment specified in Part B of that Schedule for a continuous period of not less than six months contracts any disease specified therein as an occupational disease peculiar to that employment or if an employee employed in any employment specified in Part C of that Schedule for such continuous period as the corporation may specify in respect of each such employment, contracts any disease specified therein as an occupational disease peculiar to that employment, the contracting of the disease shall, unless the contrary is proved, be deemed to be an "employment injury" arising out of and in the course of employment. As regards with compensation, Sulzberger proposed a compensation law as "when an employee suffers from any skin condition, or from the sequelae of any skin condition, in which his occupation can be proved, beyond reasonable doubt, to be, directly or indirectly, a causal or contributory factor, such employee is entitled to compensation commensurate with: (a) the degree to which the occupation is responsible for the skin disease and/or its sequelae and (b) the extent and duration of the skin condition and/or sequelae, the resulting discomfort, disability and/or disfigurement. Such an employee is further entitled to the payment of the reasonable costs of adequate medical attention investigation and treatment, administered through qualified physicians, hospitals, etc., of his own choice."

Occupational dermatoses may present as eczematous and noneczematous dermatitis, photosensitivity dermatitis (phototoxic or photoallergic), folliculitis, acneiform eruptions of external chemical origin, leukoderma, vibration white finger, occupationally induced nail dystrophy and skin tumors, etc. Dermatitis that primarily originates from occupational exposure is influenced by many other factors such as constitutional factors and stress and may cause legal dispute. Occupational dermatoses constitute over 63% of all industrial diseases. Skin diseases constitute about 15–30% of all occupational diseases, mainly the contact dermatitis, urticaria, and infective conditions, and account for a huge loss of working hours. Among Indian studies, occupational dermatoses comprised 15–19% of all the cases. Cement is one of the most important causes of occupational disease in construction workers and potassium dichromate is the most common allergen, in 10–31.9%. The diagnosis depends upon occupational history, clinical examination, and in obtaining as detailed a picture as possible of what the patient actually does at work. Investigations needed include skin prick test/radioallergosorbent test (RAST), patch testing, chemical investigations, and even factory visiting. It is often necessary to withdraw a patient from work. The physician should specify as precisely as possible the estimated length of the disability period. Return to modified tasks will be postponed until the skin lesions have completely disappeared keeping in mind that full restoration of the epidermal barrier takes 4–5 weeks after the dermatitis is clinically cured. The legal forms that will allow the disabled worker to receive adequate compensation should be diligently filled out. Finally, the extent must be determined of permanent impairment or the presence of functional limitations, which may render a patient unfit to return to his former work and make him a candidate for rehabilitation. This will also allow workers to be adequately compensated.

Advertising in Dermatology

The practice of dermatology has significantly changed during the last few years. Advertisements, promotional pamphlets, and brochures and media services are being increasingly used to introduce and promote the service and products, which sometimes carry unreasonable and false claims and invoke unpleasant legal responses for unfair trade practices. An advertisement may claim the virtues of a cosmetic surgery as making you beautiful or a cosmetic procedure making you glow in a few days, but the results may be disappointing. The MCI/NMC Code of Medical Ethics Regulations 2002 has issued guidelines regarding advertising (6.1, 7.11, 7.12, 7.13). It prohibits advertising and calls it unethical and professional misconduct if a physician makes use of him/her (or his/her name) as subject of any form or manner of advertising or publicity through any mode either alone or in conjunction with others which is of such a character as to invite attention to him or to his professional position, skill, qualification, achievements, attainments, specialties, appointments, associations, affiliations, or honors and/or of such character as would ordinarily result in his self-aggrandizement. If the medical practitioner is found to be guilty of committing professional misconduct, the appropriate Medical Council may award such punishment as deemed necessary or may direct the removal altogether or for a specified period, from the register of the name of the delinquent registered practitioner.

Deletion from the Register shall be widely publicized in local press as well as in the publications of different Medical Associations/Societies/Bodies (Rule 8.2). Decision on complaint against delinquent physician shall be taken within a time limit of 6 months (Rule 8.2).

The Monopolies and Restrictive Trade Practices (MRTP) Act and the Consumer Protection Act also incorporate provisions relating to unfair trade practices. The Consumer Disputes Redressal Agencies (Consumer Forums) can order the return to the complainant of the price or charge paid and the discontinuation of the unfair trade practice. They can also direct that corrective advertisements be issued to neutralize the effects of the misleading advertisement and their expenses to be borne by the person responsible for issuing the misleading advertisement.

TELEDERMATOLOGY (E-DERMATOLOGY): MEDICOLEGAL IMPLICATIONS

Teledermatology (TD) or e-dermatology care is providing dermatological care through online consultations to patients remotely by means of the application of information and communication technology. TD has increased the availability of specialist dermatology care. This was observed during the crisis caused by the coronavirus disease 2019 pandemic, reducing unnecessary hospital visits and the possible exposure of patients, especially old age persons and children. The ability to observe, record, store, exchange, and analyze data and images at a distance using different means of communication, such as audio, video, and image, has put virtual consultations possible for dermatologic care, at least of mild and nonurgent diseases without exposing both patient or dermatologist to the risk of infection. It is estimated that now TD is being applied in 1% (0.3–3.0%) of dermatologic diagnoses. It is now considered to be a good solution for providing skin care to remote communities, where factors such as geographic isolation or transport times and costs are major factors affecting access to healthcare and also in certain social contexts, such as old age homes, catastrophes, and military conflict areas. However, these modalities should be approached cautiously because HIPAA compliance, security of data, photo and video quality, and accurate and adequate history may have legal implications for the dermatologist.

Teledermatology is also governed by the Professional Code of Ethics and the use of TD must ensure the right to the autonomy of the patient, doctor–patient confidentiality, data protection, and privacy. This requires an implicit will and consent by the patient or his legal guardian, and this must be recorded in the patient's medical records. Consent by the patient requires a clear and understandable demonstration of the working of telemedicine (TM), its advantages and disadvantages, and potential privacy concerns. The option of receiving distance care must be accepted by the patient. The virtual medium used to perform the consultation and the recommendations and medical treatment prescribed must be recorded in the patient's medical records. Any TD application must meet the confidentiality and privacy requirements set out in the law on the protection of personal data. Special attention must be paid to the encryption of photographs when they are included in the clinical records or when they are uploaded to make access by unauthorized users impossible.

Teledermatology may also be used as a useful educational tool for trainee specialists. It can contribute to improving dermatology training of primary care physicians and trainee specialists in both family medicine and dermatology.

CONCLUSION

Dermatologists, especially cosmetologists, should take due precautions while dealing with their patients. Patients should be informed about their illness and planning of management of their illness and their complications. Informed consent must be taken before doing any procedure or cosmetic surgery. Confidentiality of the data should be maintained. All the activities and progress in the management of the illness should be well documented in chronological order as deficient documentation can be detrimental. Due care must be taken while dealing with patients with BDD, pregnant females, and high-risk cases.

KEY LEARNING POINTS

- Recently, dermatology, dermatosurgery, and cosmetic surgery have recorded significant developments, especially in diagnostic and therapeutic techniques.
- Cosmetic procedures are becoming increasingly popular in both private dermatology clinics as well as in academic institutions. Mostly, the voluntary and subjective nature of these procedures puts an extra responsibility on dermatologists to disclose associated risks more completely.
- The physician must explain and disclose all significant alternative treatment options to the patient and must take an informed consent before any cosmetic procedure.
- Any information in medical records should be clear, comprehensive, and documented in chronological order.
- Digital images are frequently used in dermatology. Due care must be taken to keep confidentiality. The importance of obtaining patient consent, in particular when using images, especially for marketing, must be considered.
- Due care must be taken while prescribing dermatological medications in pregnancy and children.
- TD is also governed by the Professional Code of Ethics and due care must be taken in maintaining confidentiality, data protection, and privacy.
- Dermatology is now considered as a high-risk specialty with a greater risk of litigation.

BIBLIOGRAPHY

1. Abarientos C, Sperber K, Shapiro DL, et al. Hydroxychloroquine in systemic lupus erythematosus and rheumatoid arthritis and its safety in pregnancy. Expert Opin Drug Saf. 2011;10:705-14.
2. Accutane Products Liability, case No. 8:04-md-02523, in the U.S. District Court for the Middle District of Florida. [online] Available from https://mdl.law.uga.edu/sites/default/files/2005.09.01%2520-%2520111%2520-%2520PSC%2527s%2520Motion%2520for%2520Common%2520Benefit%2520Order.pdf [Last accessed May, 2024].
3. Adams RM. Medicolegal aspects of occupational skin diseases. Dermatol Clin. 1988;6:121-9.
4. Adler NR, Adler KA, Grant-Kels JM. Doctors' mental health, burnout, and suicidality: Professional and ethical issues in the workplace. J Am Acad Dermatol. 2017;77:1191-3.
5. Akers v Levitt, Ohio App LEXIS 300 (Ohio App. 1992).
6. Arimany Manso J, Taberner Ferrer R, Pidevall I, et al. Implicaciones bioéticas y médico-legales del uso de la fotografía en dermatología. Actas Dermosifiliogr. 2020;111:107-14.
7. Arlton v. Shraut, 936 N.E.2d 831 (Court of Appeals of Indiana, 2010).

8. Armstrong AP, Cole AA, Page RE. Informed consent: are we doing enough? Br J Plast Surg. 1997;50:637-40.
9. Arulmani R, Rajendran SD, Suresh B. Adverse drug reaction monitoring in a secondary care hospital in South India. Br J Clin Pharmacol. 2007;65:210-6.
10. B.K. Ghosh v. Dr. (Prof) P Maulick. 2005(I) CPJ 737 (West Bengal, SCDR).
11. Bar Oz B, Hackman R, Einarson T, et al. Pregnancy outcome after cyclosporine therapy during pregnancy: a meta-analysis. Transplantation. 2001;71:1051-5.
12. Beauchamp TL, Childress JF (Eds). Principles of Biomedical Ethics, 5th edition. Oxford: Oxford University Press; 2001. pp. 454.
13. Bercovitch L, Long TP. Dermatoethics: A curriculum in bioethics and professionalism for dermatology residents at Brown Medical School. J Am Acad Dermatol. 2007;56:679-82.
14. Birmingham DJ. (2011). 12. Skin diseases: Overview: Occupational skin diseases. [online] Available from https://www.iloencyclopaedia.org/part-i-47946/skin-diseases/item/467-overview-occupational-skin-diseases [Last accessed May, 2024].
15. Brendel RW, Schouten R. Legal concerns in psychosomatic medicine. Psychiatr Clin North Am. 2007;30: 663-76.
16. Brown JP. Toward an economic theory of liability. J Legal Stud. 1973;2:323-49.
17. Bruguera M, Gómez-Durán EL, Arrizabalaga P, et al. Reclamaciones por presunta malapraxis. ¿Existen diferencias entre médicos varones y mujeres? Med Clin. 2014;143:420-1.
18. Buendía-Eisman A, Arias-Santiago S, Molina-Leyva A, et al. Análisis de los diagnósticos realizados en la actividad ambulatoria dermatológica en España: muestreo aleatorio nacional DIADERM. Actas Dermosifiliogr. 2018;109:416-23.
19. Calnan CD, Rycroft RJG. Rehabilitation in occupational skin disease. Trans Coll Med S Afr. 1981;25:136-42.
20. Campbell L. $212M Jury Award Ordered in Allergan Botox Brain Injury Lawsuit. [online] Available from http://www.lawyersandsettlements.com/settlements/15771/212m-settlement-reached-with-allergan-over-botox.html [Last accessed May, 2024].
21. Carroll KA. Dermatology and the changing face of medicine, Virtual Mentor, Am Med Assoc J Ethics. 2006;8:493-4.
22. Cereza G, Agusti A, Pedros C, et al. Effect of an intervention on the features of adverse drug reactions spontaneously reported in a hospital. Eur J Clin Pharmacol. 2010;66:937-45.
23. Clowse ME, Magder L, Witter F, et al. Hydroxychloroquine in lupus pregnancy. Arthritis Rheum. 2006;54: 3640-7.
24. Coenraads P-J, Diepgen T, Uter W, et al. Epidemiology. In: Frosch PJ, Menné T, Lepoittevin J-P (Eds). Contact Dermatitis, 4th edition. Berlin: Springer; 2006. pp. 135-63.
25. Consejo General de Colegios Oficiales de Médicos. (2011). Código de Deontología Médica Guía De Ética Médica. [online] Available from https://www.cgcom.es/sites/main/files/files/2022-03/codigo_deontologia_medica.pdf [Last accessed May, 2024].
26. Corona R, Mele A, Amini M, et al. Interobserver variability on the histopathologic diagnosis of cutaneous melanoma and other pigmented skin lesions. J Clin Oncol. 1996;14:1218-23.
27. Crowson AN. Medicolegal aspects of neoplastic dermatology. Mod Pathol. 2006;19:S148-54.
28. Das S, Chatterjee T. Pattern of skin diseases in a peripheral hospital's skin OPD: A study of 2550 patients. Indian J Dermatol. 2007;52:93-5.
29. De Groot AC, Beverdam EGA, Tjong Ayong Ch, et al. The role of contact allergy in the spectrum of adverse effects caused by cosmetics and toiletries. Arch Dermatol. 1988;124:1525-31.
30. De Groot AC. Labelling cosmetics with their ingredients. Br Med J. 1990;300:1636-8.
31. Dhingra J, Arora G, D'Souza P. A Study of Pattern of Medico-Legal Cases in a Premier Hospital in Delhi. JMSCR. 2014;2(5):1006-10.
32. Dr. Shyam Kumar vs Rameshbhai Harmanbhai Kachiya, 2002;1 CPR 320 I (2006) CPJ 16 (NC).
33. Dr. Tokugha Yeptomi Vs. Apollo Hospital Enterprises Ltd. and Anr. III. 1998 CPJ 132 (SC).
34. Echeverría-García B. La teledermatología como herramienta al servicio del médico de familia en poblaciones aisladas. Actas Dermosifiliogr. 2019;110:623-5.
35. Eiermann HJ, Larsen W, Maibach HI, et al. Prospective study of cosmetic reactions:1977-1980. J Am Acad Dermatol. 1982;6:909-17.
36. Farmer ER, Gonin R, Hanna MP. Discordance in the histopathologic diagnosis of melanoma and melanocytic neoplasms between expert pathologists. Hum Pathol. 1996;27:528-31.

37. FDA Consumer Health Information. (2009). FDA Law Enforcers Crack Down on Illegal Botox Scammers. [online] Available from http://www.cosmeticsurgeryspecialists.org/images/TRI_BOTOX_scam.pdf [Last accessed May, 2024].
38. Federal Food, Drug, and Cosmetic Act, 21 U.S.C.A. §301. [online] Available from https://uscode.house.gov/view.xhtml?req=(title:21%20section:301%20edition:prelim) [Last accessed May, 2024].
39. Fischer AA (Ed). Cutaneous Reactions to Cosmetics, 2nd edition. Philadelphia: Lea & Febiger; 1973. pp. 217-41.
40. Foley P, Nixon R, Marks R, et al. The frequency of reactions to sunscreens: results of a longitudinal population based study on the regular use of sunscreen in Australia. Br J Dermatol. 1993;128:512-8.
41. Force v. M Ganeswara Rao. 1998;3 CPR 251; 1998 (1) CPJ 413 (AP SCDRC).
42. Galvan-Banqueri M, Marin Gil R, Santos Ramos B, et al. Biological treatments for moderate-to-severe psoriasis: indirect comparison. J Clin Pharm Ther. 2013;38:121-30.
43. Geier J, Schnuck A. A comparison of contact allergens among construction and non-construction workers attending contact dermatitis clinics in Germany: results of the Information Network of Departments of Dermatology from November 1989 to July 1993. Am J Contact Dermatitis. 1995;6:86-94.
44. Gillenwater G. (2008). 16 deaths linked to Botox. [online] Available from http://www.lawyersandsettlements.com/features/botox-death-paralysis/botox-deaths.html [Last accessed May, 2024].
45. Gimeno-Vicente M, Alfaro-Rubio A, Gimeno-Carpio E. Teledermatología por WhatsApp en la Comunidad Valenciana. Características de esta teleconsulta y su repercusión en la vida del dermatólogo. Teledermatology by WhatsApp in Valencia: Characteristics of Remote Consultation and Its Emotional Impact on the Dermatologist. Actas Dermosifiliogr. 2020;111(5):364-80. [English, Spanish].
46. Gimeno Carpio E. ¿Es la teledermatología una herramienta útil para médicos, pacientes y administración? Actas Dermosifiliogr. 2018;109:577-8.
47. Goldberg DJ. Lasers and the Law: What the Dermatologist Needs to Know. Seminars. Cut Med Surg. 2013;32:205-8.
48. Goldberg DJ. Legal ramifications of off-label filler use. Dermatol Ther. 2006;19:189-93.
49. Goldsmith LA, Bolognia JL, Callen JP, et al. American Academy of Dermatology Consensus Conference on the safe and optimal use of isotretinoin: summary and recommendations. J Am Acad Dermatol. 2004;50:900-6.
50. González Coloma F, Sandoval Garcés M, Gedda Quiroga V, et al. Teledermatología aplicada en zonas extremas: experiencia de 4 centros asistenciales chilenos en ámbito rural y aislamiento extremo. Actas Dermosifiliogr. 2019;110:653-8.
51. Grief M, Maibach HI. Cosmetic ingredient labelling. Contact Dermatitis. 1977;3:94-8.
52. Gupta R, High WA, Butler D, et al. Medicolegal Aspects of Prescribing Dermatological Medications in Pregnancy. Semin Cutan Med Surg. 2013;32:209-16.
53. Hales M. (2022). Forefront Dermatology Pays $3.75 Million Settlement. [online] Available from https://thehipaaetool.com/forefront-dermatology-pays-3-75-million-settlement/ [Last accessed May, 2024].
54. Hollabaugh ES, Wagner RF Jr, Weedn VW, et al. Patient personal injury litigation against dermatology residency programs in the United States, 1964-1988. Implications for future risk-management programs in dermatology and dermatologic surgery. Arch Dermatol. 1990;126:618-22.
55. Hsueh MT, Eastman K, McFarland LV, et al. Teledermatology patient satisfaction in the Pacific Northwest. Telemed J E Health. 2012;18:377-81.
56. India Code. (2011). Information Technology (Reasonable security practices and procedures and sensitive personal data or information) Rules, 2011. [online] Available from https://www.indiacode.nic.in/handle/123456789/1362/simple-search?query=The%20Information%20Technology%20(Reasonable%20Security%20Practices%20and%20Procedures%20and%20Sensitive%20Personal%20Data%20or%20Information)%20Rules,%202011.&searchradio=rules [Last accessed May, 2024].
57. In the Supreme Court of Judicature of Jamaica Claim No. 2008 HCV 02484. [online] Available from https://www.supremecourt.gov.jm/sites/default/files/judgments/Smith%2C%20Meliss%20v%20Dunwell%2C%20Patricia.pdf [Last accessed May, 2024].
58. Jackson I. (2012). Polar Care Cold Therapy Lawsuit Results in $12M Verdict. [online] Available from http://www.aboutlawsuits.com/polar-care-cold-therapy-lawsuit-verdict-31493/ [Last accessed May, 2024].
59. Jayendra Maganlal Pandiya V. Dr. Lalit P Trivedi & Others. 1997(1) CPJ 11.
60. Jena AB, Seabury S, Lakdawalla D, et al. Malpractice risk according to physician specialty. N Engl J Med. 2011;365:629-36.

61. Johnston JC, Sartwelle TP. The expert witness in medical malpractice litigation: through the looking glass. J Child Neurol. 2013;28:484-501.
62. Jones B. Legal aspects of consent. BJU Int. 2000;86:275-9.
63. Kaliyadan F. Digital photography for patient counseling in dermatology—a study. J Eur Acad Dermatol Venereol. 2008;22:1356-8.
64. Kanaiyalal Ramanlal Trivedi v Dr. Satyanarayan Vishwakarma. 1996; 3 CPR 24 (Guj); I (1997) CPJ 332 (Guj); 1998 CCJ 690 (Guj).
65. Karim A, Ahmed S, Siddiqui R, et al. Methemoglobinemia complicating topical lidocaine used during endoscopic procedures. Am J Med. 2001;111:150-3.
66. Kim M, Rostas S, Gabardi S. Mycophenolate Fetal Toxicity and Risk Evaluation and Mitigation Strategies. Am J Transplant. 2013;13(6):1383-9.
67. Kunde L, McMeniman E, Parker M. Clinical photography in dermatology: ethical and medico-legal considerations in the age of digital and smartphone technology. Australas J Dermatol. 2013;1-6.
68. Lakdawala N, Fontanella D, Grant-Kels JM. Ethical considerations in dermatologic photography. Clin Dermatol. 2012;30:486-91.
69. Lane JE. Image registration of sequential transparent photographs to localize and detect new versus recurrent tumors in dermatologic and Mohs micrographic surgery. J Am Acad Dermatol. 2011;64:786.e1-2.
70. Las Vegas Review Journal. (2009). Botox lawsuit raises issues on injections. [online] Available from https://www.reviewjournal.com/news/botox-lawsuit-raises-issues-on-injections/#:~:text=The%20Botox%20business%20model%20%22created,the%20Central%20District%20of%20California [Last accessed May, 2024].
71. Lau CK, Schumacher HH, Irwin MS. Patients' perception of medical photography. J Plast Reconstr Aesthet Surg. 2010;63:e507-11.
72. Leachman SA, Reed BR. The use of dermatologic drugs in pregnancy and lactation. Dermatol Clin. 2006;24:167-97,vi.
73. Ley 41/2002, de 14 de noviembre, básica reguladora de la autonomía del paciente y de derechos y obligaciones en materia de información y documentación clínica. BOE núm. 274. 2002. pp. 40126-32.
74. Liao Pradaxa-J, Shih C-P, Mao C-T. The cutaneous adverse drug reactions: risk factors, prognosis and economic impacts. Int J Clin Pract. 2013;67:576-84.
75. Liden C, Bruze M, Menne T. Metals. In: Frosch PJ, Menne T, Lepoittevin JP (Eds). Contact Dermatitis, 4th edition. Germany: Springer; 2006. pp. 537-68.
76. Lin BB, Taylor RS. Digital photography for mapping Mohs micrographic surgery sections. Dermatol Surg. 2001;27:411-4.
77. Linda B, Sedlewicz BS. Cosmetic Preservatives: Friend or Foe? Skinmed. 2005;4:98-100.
78. Lipson AH, Collins F, Webster WS. Multiple congenital defects associated with maternal use of topical tretinoin. Lancet. 1993;341:1352-3.
79. Lowenstein EB, Lowenstein EJ. Isotretinoin systemic therapy and the shadow cast upon dermatology's downtrodden hero. Clin Dermatol. 2011;29:652-61.
80. Maibach HI, Johnson HL. Contact urticaria syndrome. Arch Dermatol. 1975;111:726-30.
81. Makdessian AS, Ellis DA, Irish JC. Informed consent in facial plastic surgery: Effectiveness of a simple educational intervention. Arch Facial Plast Surg. 2004;6:26-30.
82. Markus PA, Zuiker ES. (2009). Cell phone camera use in healthcare facilities: shutter it. Available from http://www.smithmoorelaw.com/files/Publication/0b479c5a-08e8-4754-bff6487214574a66/Presentation/PublicationAttachment/6cd8d168-6601-4464-b3eb-4a2d1e16dfee/20090129-hitnews-markuszuiker.pdf [Last accessed May, 2024].
83. McCall BP, Horwitz IB, Feldman SR, et al. Incidence rates, costs, severity, and work-related factors of occupational dermatitis: a workers' compensation analysis of Oregon, 1990–1997. Arch Dermatol. 2005;141:713-8.
84. Meyer DJ, Simon RI. Psychiatric malpractice and the standard of care. In: Simon RI, Gold LH (Eds). The American Psychiatric Publishing Textbook of Forensic Psychiatry. Washington, DC: American Psychiatric Publishing; 2004. pp. 185-203.
85. Moreno-Ramírez D, Romero-Aguilera R, Pasquali P, et al. Posicionamiento de la Academia Espanola ˜ de Dermatología y Venereología sobre la teledermatología. Actas Dermosifiliogr. 2018;109:4-5.

86. Nayak S, Acharjya B. Adverse cutaneous drug reaction. Indian J Dermatol. 2008;53:28.
87. Panchaud A, Csajka C, Merlob P, et al. Pregnancy outcome following exposure to topical retinoids: a multicenter prospective study. J Clin Pharmacol. 2012;52:1844-51.
88. Piepkorn M, Odland PB. Quality of care in the diagnosis of melanoma and related melanocytic lesions. Arch Dermatol. 1997;133:13936.
89. Poona Medical Foundation v Marutirao Titkare. 1995;1 CPR 661(NC).
90. Roberts K. Medico-legal issues in cryotherapy. [online] Available from http://www.mims.co.uk/news/670081/Medico-legal-issues-cryotherapy/ [Last accessed May, 2024].
91. Romero-Aguilera G, Ferrandiz L, Moreno-Ramírez D. Teledermatología urbana: concepto, ventajas y desventajas. Actas Dermosifiliogr. 2018;109:471-5.
92. Ryan M. Medical malpractice: A review of issues for providers. Hematol Oncol Clin North Am. 2002;16:1331-50.
93. S.A. Quereshi v Padode memorial Hospital and Research Centre II. 2000. CPJ 463 (Bhopal).
94. Sasseville D. (2011). 12. Skin diseases: Occupational Contact Dermatitis. Available from https://www.iloencyclopaedia.org/part-i-47946/skin-diseases/item/470-occupational-contact-dermatitis [Last accessed May, 2024].
95. Schaefer C, Peters PWJ, Miller RK. Drugs During Pregnancy and Lactation: Treatment Options and Risk Assessment, 2nd edition. Amsterdam: Elsevier Academic Press; 2007.
96. Scheinfeld N. Legal considerations in the application of topical lidocaine. [online] Available from https://iacdworld.org/medical-legal/legal-considerations-in-the-application-of-topical-lidocaine/ [Last accessed May, 2024].
97. Schouten R. Informed Consent: Resistance and Reappraisal. Crit Care Med. 1989;17:1359-60.
98. Shapiro J. Safety of topical minoxidil solution: a one-year, prospective, observational study. J Cutan Med Surg. 2003;7:322-9.
99. Shriner DL, Wagner RF Jr, Weedn VW, et al. Informed Consent and Risk Management in Dermatology: To What Extent Do Dermatologists Disclose Alternative Diagnostic and Treatment Options to Their Patients? J Contemp Health Law Policy. 1992;8:137-62.
100. Silas KR. Camera phones, patient privacy, and HIPAA: the growing problem of camera phone abuse in health-care facilities. La B J. 2011;59(3):181-3.
101. Sullivan M. How to protect yourself from melanoma claims. Skin Allergy News. 2005:24-5.
102. Sulzberger MB. Medico-legal aspects of occupational dermatoses. Am J Surg. 1935;3:531-54.
103. Tonkovic Capin M, Riddle CC, Schweiger ES, et al. Brief Discussion: Medicolegal Aspects of Consent and Checklists for Common Cosmetic Procedures. Cosmetic Dermatol. 2007;20(5):291-4.
104. Troxel DB, Sabella JD. Problem areas in pathology practice. Uncovered by a review of malpractice claims. Am J Surg Pathol. 1994;18:821-31.
105. Turner S, Carder M, van Tongeren M, et al. The incidence of occupational skin disease as reported to The Health and Occupation Reporting (THOR) network between 2002 and 2005. Br J Dermatol. 2007;157:713-22.
106. Tyler KH, Zirwas MJ. Pregnancy and dermatologic therapy. J Am Acad Dermatol. 2013;68:663-71.
107. Watkarou J, Pomeranz BH, Corey PN. Incidence of adverse drug reactions in hospitalized patients: a meta-analysis of prospective studies. JAMA. 1998;279:1200-5.
108. Wilson JB, Arpey CJ. Body dysmorphic disorder: suggestions for detection and treatment in a surgical dermatology practice. Dermatol Surg. 2004;30:1391-9.

Legal Issues in HIV

Ira Shah, Zahabiya Nalwalla

INTRODUCTION

Since the early 1990s, human immunodeficiency virus–acquired immunodeficiency syndrome (HIV/AIDS) has evolved from a definite death sentence to a chronic manageable illness. Although the prevention of spread of the virus remains a priority for health professionals, policy makers, and the public, there is also is a need to ensure effective medical care and secure the human rights of all persons, including children living with the disease.

Statistics showed approximately 81,430 children living with HIV in 2020; and approximately 10% of the total new HIV infections were observed among children (<15 years). With such a large number of children living with HIV, apart from special medical care, legal protection and safety remains a top priority for the Government of India (GOI) and pediatricians as well. On this basis, the GOI established the Human Immunodeficiency Virus and Acquired Immune Deficiency Syndrome (Prevention and Control) Act, 2017, applicable to all individuals living with HIV.

Before proceeding to the provisions for legal security, it is necessary to know the definitions as described by the Act.

a. "AIDS" means acquired immune deficiency syndrome, a disease caused by human immunodeficiency virus (HIV), characterized by weakened immune system which leads to increased susceptibility to life threatening infections.
b. "capacity to consent" means the capability of an individual to make an informed decision regarding any action after understanding the consequences and nature of the action.
c. "child affected by HIV" means an individual <18 years, who is HIV-positive or whose parent or guardian is HIV-positive (with whom he/she resides); or has lost a parent or guardian due to AIDS (with whom he/she were residing) or lives in a household fostering children orphaned by AIDS.
d. "discrimination" means any act or omission which enforces an obligation, burden, liability, disability, or a disadvantage; directly or indirectly; on any individual on HIV-related grounds. It also includes denial of benefit or opportunity to an individual on the basis of these grounds.
   Either an HIV positive individual or any individual living with a seropositive person are included in the terminology of "HIV related grounds".
e. "informed consent" means consent given by any individual or his representative, in the language understood by them, without any influence, fraud, coercion, mistake or misrepresentation; and the consent obtained is understood by the individual or their representative.

In this chapter, we will try to deal with most of the common medicolegal issues faced when dealing with HIV-infected persons.

CONSENT FOR HUMAN IMMUNODEFICIENCY VIRUS TESTING

The provisions for consent are described in Chapter III of the Act. HIV testing can be performed only after obtaining informed consent from a person or his/her representatives. The informed consent for HIV test is accompanied with pre and post-test counseling. A written informed consent in the language understood by the person/person's representative should be taken.

The patient needs to be informed about the implications of HIV testing and the necessity for conducting the tests. For adults, the patient himself/herself has to give the consent. In children <12 years, the consent has to be given by the person's parent or legal guardian. For children between 12 and 16 years of age, consent can be given by the patient or if the concerned healthcare provider assesses in writing that the patient lacks the capacity to consent, then the consent can be given by the parent or legal guardian.

Informed consent is not required in the following circumstances:
- Where a court decides it is part of a medical examination or determination of other issues.
- For acquiring, processing, or circulation of a human body or part (blood, tissues, semen, or any bodily fluids) for medical therapy or research. (the donor should undergo counseling at the voluntary counseling and testing center in case he/she requests the results of the test).
- Where HIV testing is anonymous and for surveillance or epidemiological purposes. The person should be informed about the purpose of the study
- Screening purposes in blood banks

Consent for Research or Clinical Trials in HIV/AIDS Patients

As per the guidelines issued by the Indian Council of Medical Research, research subjects should be informed about the type of research, the risk involved, about their right to withdraw from research, voluntarily enlist, and then written informed consent should be taken.

Confidentiality of Patients Living with HIV

Data protection measures such as security systems for protection of confidentiality of all individuals with HIV, official procedure for accessing information, and a system to ensure liability of individuals in the institution should be adopted by every establishment keeping records of HIV-related information. A simple example of such a process would be prescribing sequential numbers to person living with HIV (PLHIV) and calling the persons out by numbers instead.

DISCRIMINATION AGAINST PEOPLE LIVING WITH HIV

Chapter II of the Act clearly lays down strict measures to prevent discrimination of PLHIV. No HIV-infected person should be denied or terminated from school/work place, educational/professional services, right to reside, and right to treatment solely on the basis of his HIV-positive status. This would not be applicable if the individual poses a risk of transmission of the virus to other people or is unfit to perform duties of the job. This requires an assessment by a qualified and competent healthcare provider with a written certificate for the same.

The Act also prohibits any feelings of animosity against any protected individuals or a group of such individuals in the form of words, publications, advocate, visual representations, or broadcast messages, which is likely to display hatred, discrimination, or physical violence.

Disclosure of HIV Status

This has been described in Chapter IV of the Act. On testing a person after informed consent for HIV, the results of tests should be kept strictly confidential and should only be disclosed to the person. They should be disclosed to other family members only after his/her consent after proper counseling. For children, the results of the test may be disclosed to the child's representative who has given the consent. Confidentiality also has to be maintained even after death of the patient.

Doctors should not disclose HIV-related information or any private information of a patient except in court when commanded by the governing judge. Doctor may provide the same information to another healthcare professional when necessary to provide care and treatment for the HIV-infected person.

The doctor may inform partner of the HIV-infected person under their care about the HIV status without consent of the patient if the healthcare provider believes that the partner is at significant risk of transmission of HIV from the patient and the doctor believes that patient will not inform the partner even after being counseled to inform for the protection of the partner with appropriate counseling. This may be the situation in discordant couples where one partner may be HIV positive and the other partner is HIV negative and the doctor may need to safeguard the interests of the HIV-negative person. The disclosure should be done only to the partner and not to anyone else. This is called partner notification. Disclosure can also be made if the HIV-infected person has suicidal thoughts and thus one may need to disclose his/her status to the partner or the health physician taking care of the patient to safeguard the patient's life.

Duties of Person Living with HIV

This brings us to learn about the duties of a PLHIV. All PLHIV should be counseled regarding the nature of the disease and the mode of transmission. They should be well aware of the guidelines related to the disease. They should practice all possible strategies to reduce the risk of transmission, which include prevention during sexual contact, prevention of sharing of needles, and they should not donate blood. They should inform their partner their seropositive status in advance prior to any sexual act. An HIV-infected person cannot deliberately or negligently spread HIV to noninfected people and can be criminally liable under the Indian Penal Code section 269 and section 270.

The Bharatiya Nyaya Sanhita (BNS) is the new criminal code of India, established in 2023. Although are no specific sections directly addressing HIV/AIDS, section 271 of BNS is similar to section 269 and 270 of IPC. Section 271 of chapter XV in BNS deals with negligent acts likely to spread infection of disease which is dangerous to life. Those prosecuted under this act, can be punished with fine, or imprisonment or both, extending up to 6 months.

Diagnosis and Management of Person Living with HIV

Chapter VI and VII of the Act establish guidelines for the management of PLHIV. The Central and State governments are responsible for publishing and executing protocols for prevention of HIV/AIDS, diagnosis of HIV/AIDS, and guidelines for antiretroviral therapy (ART) and opportunistic infection (OI) management of PLHIV. They are responsible for dissemination of this information to the public. Keeping these chapters in mind, the National AIDS Control Organization (NACO) publishes guidelines, with the most recent update in 2022.

All tests for HIV are not 100% sensitive or specific. Thus, enzyme-linked immunosorbent assay (ELISA) and polymerase chain reaction (PCR) test can be false positive and false negative. Also, sometimes results may be indeterminate. In children <18 months born to HIV-positive mothers; maternally transmitted HIV antibodies may interfere with the ELISA test. Thus, for children <18 months, HIV PCR test is done to determine the HIV status, whereas in children >18 months, the ELISA test can be done. However, no patient should be diagnosed on the basis of one positive result. For children <18 months, one positive HIV PCR should be confirmed with another PCR test as soon as possible or by an HIV ELISA test after 18 months of age. A single positive HIV ELISA test in a child >18 months or in adults can be confirmed by a Western blot test or by at least two positive results on three HIV ELISA tests using three different kits. A detailed diagnosis algorithm is described in the latest NACO guidelines and clinicalinfo.hiv.gov.

Treatment of HIV-infected Persons

No HIV-infected person can be refused treatment solely on the grounds of his/her HIV status and amounts to violation of Article 21 of the Constitution of India. It includes various rights such as right to live with dignity and right to be given immediate medical aid in injury cases. The Indian Medical Council/NMC Regulations, 2002 also forbids refusing treatment of a patient on the basis of discrimination.

However, when a patient is suffering from a disease, which is beyond the skill set and experience of the treating physician, the physician may refuse the treatment and refer the patient elsewhere. Similarly, surgery and intensive care treatment in an HIV-infected person cannot be refused solely on the grounds of his/her HIV status. However universal precautions, disposable ventilator equipment, and adequate sterilization of scopes may be needed to prevent transmission of HIV to other patients too.

HIV in Pregnancy

Vertical transmission of HIV is the most common mode of transmission of HIV in children. Thus, screening of pregnant women for HIV would be needed to diagnose HIV in pregnant women and thus ensure prevention of parent-to-child transmission (PPTCT) of HIV. Pre- and post-test counseling are required for pregnant women prior to HIV testing. Every HIV-positive pregnant woman has the right to receive such information and counseling and information to enable her to make a decision about her pregnancy, whether or not to undertake HIV-related treatment and regarding PPTCT. No HIV-infected pregnant woman should be forced to sterilization or abortion. The HIV-infected woman should exercise her right regarding abortion, treatment with antiretroviral agents, the mode of delivery as well as feeding practices after discussion with the doctor regarding benefits and risks to her and her fetus. Guidelines for the same are described by the NACO, World Health Organization (WHO), and Clinical Info-HIV.

Blood Transfusion and HIV

All persons receiving blood transfusion should be given blood that has been tested for HIV-1 and -2 and is free from HIV antibodies. Ideally, the PCR should be the test to detect the virus. However, due to cost factors, HIV-1 and -2 antibodies are tested by the ELISA test. Any blood that has presence of HIV-1 or -2 antibodies should be discarded and not transfused. However, transmission of HIV may still take place if the donor was in the window period and even if blood is free of HIV antibodies in which case doctor is not liable for the transmission if it occurs.

Safe Working Environment

Chapter VIII of the HIV Act lays down regulations for a safe working environment where there is a significant hazard of occupational exposure. It ensures the establishment of universal precautions for all people working in such an environment, training for the use of universal precautions, postexposure prophylaxis (PEP) to all people working in such an environment, and education of all persons working in the environment regarding universal precautions and PEP.

HIV and Gay Law

Compared to the national average of 0.26%, the prevalence of HIV in men who have sex with men (MSM) in India is 2.7% and among transgender strata is 3.1%. Every 3rd and 4th gay individual and transgender out of a cohort of 10 in India do not know their HIV status. On 5th September 2018, a five judge bench invalidated a part of section 377, which criminalizes homosexuality.

This has been a landmark decision, alleviating the stigma pertaining to LGBTQ (lesbian, gay, bisexual, transgender, queer or questioning) persons. This has opened an arena of early detection, treatment, and prevention of transmission of HIV virus among the LGBTQ community as they can readily seek healthcare services without being legally and socially stigmatized.

CONCLUSION

Human immunodeficiency virus/acquired immunodeficiency syndrome has gradually progressed from an incurable disease to a chronic manageable illness. Awareness of the laws pertaining to the disease are essential for every individual working in healthcare services, especially when dealing with consent, disclosure of HIV status, and prevention of HIV transmission.

KEY LEARNING POINTS

- HIV testing can be performed only after obtaining informed consent from a person or his/her representatives. The informed consent for HIV test is accompanied with pre- and post-test counseling.
- No HIV-infected person should be denied or terminated from school/workplace, educational/professional services, right to reside, and right to treatment solely based on his HIV-positive status.
- On testing a person after informed consent for HIV, the results of the tests should be kept strictly confidential and should only be disclosed to the person.

- An HIV-infected person cannot deliberately or negligently spread HIV to noninfected people and can be criminally liable under Indian Penal Code section 269 and section 270.
- No HIV-infected person can be refused treatment solely on the grounds of his/her HIV status and amounts to violation of Article 21 of the Constitution of India.
- No HIV-infected pregnant woman should be forced to sterilization or abortion. The HIV-infected woman should exercise her right regarding abortion, treatment with antiretroviral agents, and the mode of delivery as well as feeding practices.

BIBLIOGRAPHY

1. Clinicalinfo.HIV.gov. Antiretroviral management of newborns with perinatal HIV exposure or HIV infection. [Online] Available from https://clinicalinfo.hiv.gov/en/guidelines/perinatal/antiretroviral-management-newborns-perinatal-hiv-exposure-or-hiv-infection [Last accessed May, 2024].
2. Clinicalinfo.HIV.gov. Maternal HIV Testing and Identification of Perinatal HIV Exposure. Available from https://clinicalinfo.hiv.gov/en/guidelines/perinatal/maternal-hiv-testing-and-identification-perinatal-hiv-exposure?view=full [Last accessed May, 2024].
3. Government of India. HIV and AIDS Act. [Online] Available from http://naco.gov.in/sites/default/files/HIV%20and%20AIDS%20Act-%20English.pdf [Last accessed May, 2024].
4. NACO. (2021). National Guidelines for HIV Care and Treatment_2021. [Online] Available from http://naco.gov.in/sites/default/files/National_Guidelines_for_HIV_Care_and_Treatment_2021.pdf [Last accessed May, 2024].
5. Parliament. THE BHARATIYA NYAYA SANHITA, 2023 [Internet]. THE BHARATIYA NYAYA SANHITA. 2023. Available from: https://www.mha.gov.in/sites/default/files/250883_english_01042024.pdf

33

CHAPTER

Medicolegal Issues in Ayurveda

Amrita Mishra

INTRODUCTION

Ayurvedic practitioners are subjected to several medicolegal issues. Taking into consideration, the immense need of medical practitioners and facilities at various levels of society, these issues should be taken up with outmost priority. Time has come to prioritize the problems faced by Ayurvedic students and practitioners, taking into account a huge number of these registered practitioners working at primary health centers, rural hospitals not excluding urban set ups. The Central Council of Indian Medicine (CCIM) is the apical body and there are various state governing bodies. Apart from that, Department of Health and Family Welfare, Government of India has laid the concerned responsibility on AYUSH (Ayurved, Unani, Siddha, Homeopathy), which deals with the formulation, implementation and decides on various issues related to Ayurved.

Ayurved undergraduate curriculum includes Ayurvedic and modern knowledge of Anatomy, physiology, preventive and social medicine, toxicology, surgery, gynecology, medicine and other subjects. Ayurvedic postgraduation includes detailed knowledge of the concerned subjects. The curriculum is structured in such a manner that by the end of it, student acquires skill and knowledge of Ayurved and modern science in the concerned theoretical or clinical subject. Still they are subjected to various legal issues during their practice.

THE ISSUE OF CROSSPATHY

The major issue is that of Ayurvedic or Homoeopathic doctors prescribing the drugs of modern medicine. The Hon. Supreme Court in, Poonam Varma vs. Ashwin Patel (AIR 1996 SC 2111) has observed that, a person who does not have knowledge of a particular system of medicine but practices in that system is a quack and a mere pretender to medical knowledge or skill, or to put it differently, a charlatan. The reason for this was that it was construed that Ayurvedic curriculum does not provide adequate allopathic knowledge and that they are expected to practice their basic pathy, i.e., Ayurved. Although, the argument of practicing one's basic pathy is undisputed, but taking into account the huge number of patients that Ayurvedic doctors are dealing with, at rural and urban, private and government setups, it is for the health benefit of population, that Ayurvedic doctors are allowed to practice both pathies depending on the need of the patient. Taking into account the importance of need based medicine and the extent knowledge of both the pathies, acquired by Ayurved doctors, Maharashtra State

Government, has granted them the permission to practice allopathy. The official publication dated 25/11/1992, Department of Medical education and Drugs, Mantralaya, Mumbai, as per the provisions of Maharashtra Medical Practitioners Act, 1961 legalizes Ayurvedic doctors graduated from CCIM approved institutes, to practice Allopathy, to the extent of the training they received in that system. As per the notification of the Central Council of Indian Medicine dated 30/10/96 "Institutionally qualified practitioner of Indian System of Medicine (ISM) are eligible to practice Indian system of medicine and modern medicine including surgery, obstetrics, and gynecology based on their training and teaching which are included in syllabi. It was further clarified that the rights of practitioners of Indian system of medicine to practice modern system are protected under section 17(3) of IMCC Act 1970". As per the notification dated, 22/1/2004; the Government of India from time and again have asked the council to improve the syllabus by including subjects with regard to National Programs like National Malaria Eradication program, RCH program, Immunization, AIDS, and Cancer related program, etc., and accordingly the council has strengthened the syllabus of all the system of medicine.

The four autonomous boards have been constituted by Central Government as per the provisions of National Commission for Indian system of Medicine (NCISM) Act 2020. The medical standards provisions, rules and regulations as per The Indian Medicine Central Council (IMCC) Act 1970 (Now repealed) shall continue to be in force till the new regulations are finalized.

The letter from Ministry of Health and Family Welfare dated 29th May 2013; states that many PHCs in remote areas are being already run by AYUSH doctors and the states have expressed their satisfaction about the services being provided by such doctors at PHCs and under various National Health programs. The Department of AYUSH has taken an in principle approval from the hon. HFM to empower ISM qualified doctors to practice modern system of medicine in a limited way and constituted a committee to examine the issue.

Many private hospitals including multispecialty hospitals appoint ayurvedic or homoeo pathic graduates as medical officers. These graduates look after not only the routine patient care but also manage the emergency care and follow-up under the supervision of a modern medicine consultant or expert.

Furthermore, Maharashtra University of health sciences is taking effective steps in the direction of integrating Ayurved, Homeopathy and Modern medicine. It has made Ayurved OPD's mandatory in every medical college. Also, there is almost equal representation of Ayurved, Homeopathic doctors in Executive Council, Board of Studies and other important platforms or decision-making bodies or committees. It is also laying emphasis on research in Ayurved.

Several modern medicine books have included chapters on Ayurvedic preparations. Allopathic doctors prescribing Ayurvedic medicines like Live 52, M2 Tone, Septilin, Cystone, etc., is also a common practice these days. Large number of population, nationally and internationally, is opting for Ayurvedic medicines and therapies like PANCHAKARMA.

So, if university is emphasizing the integration of pathies and the similar need is reflected in students and masses, the obvious question that arises is that why government and judiciary is not taking necessary steps in this regard? If Ayurved graduate is almost equivalent (as far as eligibility and duration of course) to Allopathy, then the issues mentioned above should be definitely sorted out. For, if these issues exist, the society is being kept devoid of major health benefits.

ARE AYURVEDIC AND MODERN MEDICINE COURSES EQUIVALENT?

Another issue is that of Ayurvedic doctors not eligible for selection in defense hospitals as medical officers or similar posts. The thought that needs to be provoked is that if Government has recognized efficiency and need of Ayurvedic graduates, why they should be refrained from serving in defense setups? In fact Ayurved being anciently routed to India, it should be prioritized in defense set ups.

The Ministry of Ayush and Department of Ex-servicemen Welfare and ECHS, Ministry of Defence signed MoU for integrating Ayurveda in ECHS Polyclinics and various defense establishments initially as OPD services for 5 years. Ministry of Ayush and Defence Ministry have strengthened their association for providing Ayush services. There will be requisite infrastructure, AYUSH specialists, pharmacist and paramedical staff in ECHS dispensaries.

Similarly, they are not allowed to perform postmortem and medicolegal cases. If the reason is insufficient knowledge of the concerned subject, it can be included in the existing Ayurvedic curriculum of the concerned subject, which will also help in dealing with the scarcity of eligible doctors.

Another most important and talked about issue is that of legalizing Ayurvedic surgeons to perform surgeries independently. Existing postgraduate curriculum has made inculcation of surgical skills mandatory for the Postgraduate students in surgical subjects like surgery, gynecology, etc. The students are required to perform a minimum number of listed important surgeries, deliveries, MTPs and sterilization procedures as a part of their curriculum. This has certainly contributed in the improvement of surgical knowledge and skill in the necessary set up. The necessary amendment in this regard is waited from the Government of Maharashtra and later on it can be extended to other states of the country as well.

Also, multinational companies opt only for Allopathic doctors and not Ayurvedic one's in their set ups. The reason is obviously the belief that Ayurvedic doctors do not possess adequate knowledge and skills to be able to deal with the health issues of their employees; this can be considered a myth, taking into account the curriculum of Ayurved.

The Department of AYUSH, Government of India in an official memorandum dated 3/12/2008 has clarified that as per the provisions of Section 17(2)© of Indian Medical Central Council Act 1970, AYUSH registered degree holder doctors are authorized to issue medical or fitness certificate for a person for any official purpose including grant of armed license.

CONCLUSION

The practice of Ayurved as discussed earlier; is not only ancient but is also supposed to be spiritual as far as India is concerned. In fact it is considered as medicine practiced by god, *rishi-munies* and our ancestors. In most of the part of our country especially the villages or rural areas there is paucity of qualified graduates of modern medicine. The patient has to either suffer because of lack of health care facilities or has to travel long distance before he can consult a qualified modern medicine graduate. As against this many doctors trained in Indian system of medicine may be available in remote areas. Hence, there is need to have coordination, cooperation and integration as far as different pathies of medical services are concerned.

Note: The IMCC Act 1970 is repealed by constitution of NCISM Act 2020 by the Central Government. The readers are suggested to refer the NCISM Act for recent updates, guidelines or rules/regulations.

KEY LEARNING POINTS

- Ayurvedic practitioners are subjected to several medicolegal issues.
- Ayurved UG curriculum includes Ayurvedic and modern medicine.
- Maharashtra Medical Practitioners Act, 1961 legalizes Ayurvedic Doctors graduated from CCIM approved institutes, to practice Allopathy as per their training during UG course.
- Many private hospitals including multispecialty hospitals appoint ayurvedic or homoeopathic graduates as medical officers.
- Maharashtra University of health sciences is taking effective steps in the direction of integrating Ayurveda, Homeopathy and Modern medicine.

BIBLIOGRAPHY

1. MoU signed between Ministry of Ayush and Department of ex-servicemen welfare, Ministry of Defence. https://www.pib.gov.in/PressReleaseIframePage.aspx?PRID=1910364#:~:text=According%20to%20this%20MoU%20Ayurveda,support%20as%20may%20be%20required.&text=Both%20ministries%20have%20agreed%20to,Forces%20Medical%20Services%20(AFMS) Accessed 24 May 2025.
2. National Commission for Indian System of Medicine. https://ncismindia.org/Accessed 24 May 2025.

34

CHAPTER

Medicolegal Issues in Homeopathy

Rajneesh Kumar Sharma

INTRODUCTION

Mahatma Gandhi said, "*Homeopathy cures a larger percentage of cases than any other methods of treatment and is beyond doubt safer, more economical, and most complete medical science*". According to the World Health Organization (WHO), homeopathy is the second largest system of medicine in the world. It is the medicine of choice among a great number of people due to the tenderness of its cure and no side effects. Homeopathy is a separate medical specialty and is used all over the world. It is a recognized medical stream in India and was controlled formerly by Homeopathy Central Council Act, 1973 and now by the National Commission for Homoeopathy Act, 2020.

Homeopathic remedies are used by a large number of people for numerous ailments, especially viral diseases, allergies, skin disorders, psychiatric problems, and numerous chronic diseases. It is effective in many ailments where there is less efficacy in other medical systems. Homeopathy is mainly used for women and children's diseases, metabolic diseases, hormonal disorders, pain and palliative care, and infertility. Likewise, it is of great value as an adjuvant therapy in cancer, chronic obstructive pulmonary disease (COPD), and diabetes and its complications. As preventive care, homeopathic medicines are used based on a unique concept of "Genus epidemicus", as in the coronavirus disease (COVID) pandemic, homeopathy was adopted as the second-line preventive by the Ministry of Ayush.

Despite the equality in rules, regulations, and syllabi of all the recognized medical curriculums, the homeopathic system of medicine is often ignored and deprived of certain rights it must have.

Ancient medical knowledge as well as Hippocratic writings have two assorted principles of treating diseases. Hippocrates was known to have said, "*Through the like, disease is produced, and through the application of the like it is cured.*" Homeopaths generally refer this as "similia similibus curentur", i.e., like be treated with likes.

Homeopathic system was introduced by German physician Dr Christian Friedrich Samuel Hahnemann. The word "Homeopathy" is derived from two Greek words hómoios (similar) and páthos (suffering). Homeopathy treats natural diseases with substances that produce effects in healthy individuals like sufferings. Homeopathy is the dynamic, vitalistic, and holistic system of therapeutics, based on the law of similar, the theory of individualization, and the law of minimum doses. Theory of chronic diseases, direction of cure, susceptibility, idiosyncrasy, individualization, and theory of miasms are the basics of homeopathy. It is well capable to cure the diseases that are curable, and it certainly relieves symptoms of incurable flora.

CRITERIA FOR ADMISSION IN HOMEOPATHY COURSES IN INDIA

Admissions take place as per "the National Commission for Homoeopathy Act, 2020".

National Examination

Rule 14. (1) There shall be a uniform National Eligibility-cum-Entrance Test, for admission to the undergraduate in Homeopathy in all medical institutions governed under this Act.

(3) The Commission shall specify by regulations the manner of conducting common counselling by the designated authority for admission to all the medical institutions governed under this Act:

Provided that the common counselling shall be conducted by the designated authority of—

(i) The Central Government, for All India seats; and

(ii) The State Government, for the remaining seats at the State level.

Rule15. (1) A common final year undergraduate medical examination, to be known as the National Exit Test, shall be held for granting license to practice as medical practitioner of Homoeopathy and for enrolment in the State Register or National Register, as the case may be.

(4) Any person with a foreign medical qualification shall have to qualify National Exit Test for the purpose of obtaining license to practice Homoeopathy as medical practitioner of Homoeopathy and for enrolment in the State Register or the National Register in such manner as may be specified by regulations.

Rule 16. (1) A uniform Post-Graduate National Entrance Test shall be conducted for admission to post-graduate courses in Homoeopathy in all medical institutions governed under this Act.

Rule17. (1) A National Teachers' Eligibility Test shall be conducted separately for the post-graduates of Homoeopathy who desire to take up teaching profession in that discipline.

DUTIES OF HOMEOPATHIC PRACTITIONERS TO THEIR PATIENTS

From the rulings laid down by the Central Council of Homeopathy:

10. Patient is not Neglected

A practitioner of Homoeopathy is free to choose whom he will serve provided he shall respond to any request for his assistance in an emergency or whenever temperate public opinion expects the service.

Non-homoeopath cannot judge negligence of a Homoeopath.

His acts of commission or omission shall not be judged by any non-Homoeopathic standards or professional service expected of him but by those standards as are expected from a Homoeopath of his training, standing and experience. [paragraph 3 of Central Council of Homoeopathy (CCH) rule].

12. Acts of Negligence

(4) A practitioner of Homoeopathy shall use any drug prepared according to Homoeopathic principles and *adopt other necessary measures as required.*

Necessary Measures Other than Medicine

Necessary measures other than medicine include the following:

- Rectification and maintenance of airways, breathing, and circulation (ABC)
- Maintenance of blood pressure, fluid volume, and electrolytes balancing by IV fluids and homeopathic remedies
- Supplementation by oxygen, blood transfusion, and nutrients
- Minor surgeries as first aid and stoppage of bleeding before referral to a concerned specialist
- Fixation of fractures prior to referral to the concerned specialist
- Conduction of normal labor and maintaining the complicated obstetric patient prior referring to a concerned specialist
- Cardiopulmonary resuscitation (CPR), defibrillation, shock management, bilevel positive airway pressure (BiPAP), continuous positive airway pressure (CPAP), and ventilator use

Some Restrictions in Adopting So-called Necessary Measures

There are some rumble strips in the way of modernized homeopathy. It seems homeopaths are deprived of several rights. Some examples are:

- Most government officials and the public think that the IV use of saline, supplements, and blood transfusion, etc., is not homeopathic.
- The use of Ryle's tube, Foley's catheter, ventilator, minor surgical procedures, even fine-needle aspiration cytology (FNAC) and biopsies, etc., are not supposed to be related to homeopathy.
- Radiological investigations, pathological tests, and cardiac examinations like treadmill test (TMT) and echocardiography are not thought to be of any importance in homeopathy.

HOMOEOPATHIC PHYSICIANS OBEY LAW AND REGULATION

Almost all the acts and regulations are applicable to homeopaths as those to other medical practitioners. Even then there are certain diplomatic rules. Here are some points from CCH rulings:

A physician:

- Shall not act contrary to the laws regulating the practice of homeopathy
- Shall not assist others to disobey the law regulating the practice of homeopathy
- Shall act in aid of the enforcement of sanitary laws and regulations in the interest of public health
- Shall comply with the provisions of the Drugs and Cosmetics Act 1940 (23 of 1940), Drugs and Cosmetics Rules, 1945, the Pharmacy Act 1948 (8 of 1948), the Narcotic Drugs and Psychotropic Substances Act 1985 (61 of 1985), the Medical Termination of Pregnancy Act 1971 (34 of 1971), the Transplantation of Human Organ Act 1994 (42 of 1994). the Persons with Disabilities (Equal Opportunity and Full Participation) Act 1995 (1 of 1996), Biomedical Waste (Management and Handling) Rules 1998, and such other related Acts, Rules, of the Central Government or the State Government or the Local Administrative Bodies relating to protection and promotion of public health (paragraph 12A. CCH rule).

Some Limitations of Homeopaths

There are certain so-called limitations of Homeopaths. They have learned equal skills and gathered the same level of knowledge by studying the same textbooks and doing practicals as other streams of medicine. However, the Government has different rules and regulations with homeopaths.

No Right to Do Radiological or Pathological Investigations

In Pre-Conception and Pre-Natal Diagnostic Techniques (PCPNDT) act, there is no provision for Ayurveda, Yoga and Naturopathy, Unani, Siddha, and Homeopathy (AYUSH) doctors to get registration. Though the minimum qualification for the same must be a radiologist degree or diploma, numerous MBBS degree holders are registered with the act and doing their practice as full-fledged sonologist or radiologist **(Fig. 34.1)**.

SOME RIGHTS OF HOMEOPATHS

Rulings by the Government of India clearly define the rights of homeopaths as under:

34. (1) No person other than a person who is enrolled in the State Register, or the National Register shall—
    (a) be allowed to practice Homoeopathy as a qualified practitioner;
    (b) hold office as a physician or a surgeon or any other office, by whatever name called, which is meant to be held by a physician or surgeon, as the case may be.

Right to Issue a Medical Certificate

From the rulings in CCH law:

(c) be entitled to sign or authenticate a medical or fitness certificate or any other certificate required by any law to be signed or authenticated by a duly qualified medical practitioner.

List of medical certificates which can be issued by any homeopath:

- Certificate of birth or death or disposal of dead under various Central or State Acts
- Certificates of lunacy and mental illness under the Mental Health Act 1987
- Certificates under education acts
- Certificates under public health acts and the orders made thereunder
- Certificates under the acts and orders related to the notification of infectious diseases
- Certificates under Employee's State Insurance Act, 1948
- Certificates in connection with sick benefit insurance and friendly societies
- Certificates for procuring or issuing passport
- Certificates of illness for seeking exemption from attending the court of justice, in public services, in public offices or in private employment
- Certificates under the control of the Department of Pension
- Certificates for procuring a driving license.

To

Sh. Rajneesh Kumar Sharma,
Homoeo Cure and Research Institute,
NH-74, Moradabad Road,
Kashipur, Uttarakhand- 244713

Subject: Information sought under RTI ACT, 2005.

Sir,

I am directed to refer to your online RTI application dated 18.01.2018 received from Online RTI portal on 08/02/2018 under the RTI Act, 2005, seeking information from this Ministry. With regard to your RTI application, point no. 4 pertains to PNDT Division, the requisite information is as under:-

Information Sought	Information
Point no. 4	Qualification to perform Ultrasonography has been prescribed under the PC & PNDT Act, 1994 and Rules made thereunder. You may please refer Section 2 of the Pre-conception and Pre-natal Diagnostic Techniques (Prohibition of Sex Selection) Act, 1994 and Rule 3(3) of the PC & PNDT (Prohibition of Sex Selection) Rules, 1996.
	Further, it is to state in this regard that non existing information is not covered under the definition of 'information' in the RTI Act, 2005. Under the RTI Act, 2005 information available in material form can be provided to the applicant. The Public Information Officer is not required to furnish information which requires drawing of inference and/or making assumption; or to interpret information; or to solve the problems raised by the applicants; or to furnish replies to hypothetical question.

2. . The First Appellate Authority in this matter is Smt. Bindu Sharma, Director (PNDT), Room No. 209 D, Ministry of Health & Family Welfare, Nirman Bhawan, New Delhi.

Yours faithfully,

(Ajay Kumar)
Under Secretary to the Govt. of India & CPIO
Tel: 23061883

Fig. 34.1: Answer by Central Council of Homoeopathy (CCH) to the author in a Right to Information (RTI) application.

Right for Evidence

(d) shall be entitled to give evidence at any inquest or in any court of law as an expert under section 45 of the Indian Evidence Act, 1872 on any matter relating to Homoeopathy (1 of 1872).

Right to Conduct Normal Deliveries

24. Engagement in an obstetrics case
   (1) If a practitioner of Homoeopathy is engaged to attend to a woman during her confinement, he shall do so. Refusal to do so on an excuse of any other engagement

shall not be considered ethical except when he is already engaged on a similar or other serious case.(CCH rule 24-1)

(2) When a practitioner of Homoeopathy who has been engaged to attend on an obstetrics case is absent and another is sent for and delivery is accomplished, the acting practitioner of Homoeopathy shall be entitled to his professional fees; provided that he shall secure the patient's consent to withdraw on the arrival of the practitioner of Homoeopathy already engaged. (CCH rule 24-2)

Right to Attend and Treat Emergencies

23. (1) The practitioner of Homoeopathy called in an emergency to visit a patient under the care of another practitioner of Homoeopathy shall, when the emergency is over, retire in favour of the latter; but he shall be entitled to charge the patient for his services. (CCH rule 23-1)

Right to Treat Epidemics/Pandemics

36. *Public Health*

Practitioners of Homoeopathy engaged in public health work, shall enlighten the public concerning quarantine regulations and measures for the prevention of epidemic and communicable disease. At all times the practitioners shall notify the constituted public health authorities of every case of communicable disease under their care, in accordance with the laws, rules and regulations of the health authorities. When an epidemic prevails, the practitioner of Homoeopathy shall continue his labors without regard to the risk to his own health. (CCH rule 36)

Right to Use Supplementation and Routine Diagnostic Methods

Homeopaths are taught every subject except pharmacology in their syllabus, but their studies are not accepted at certain times. For example, pathology, radiology, forensic medicine, surgery, gynecology and obstetrics, community medicine, etc., are not supposed to be at par with other systems of medicine. The government has provided certain rights and exemptions to the homeopaths. The Government officials are not aware of these laws related to homeopathy. For example, homeopaths can use all the necessary measures in treating a critical patient **(Fig. 34.2)**.

Question in Treating the Coronavirus Disease 2019 (COVID-19) Patients

The government is training homeopaths for COVID-19 treatment as well as issuing certificates as "Trained COVID-19 practitioners" to the homeopaths, but local authorities raise queries if a homeopath treats a COVID-19 victim.

Right to Prepare and Dispense His/Her Own Prescriptions

Dispensing: A practitioner of homeopathy has a right to prepare and dispense his own prescription. (CCH rule 37)

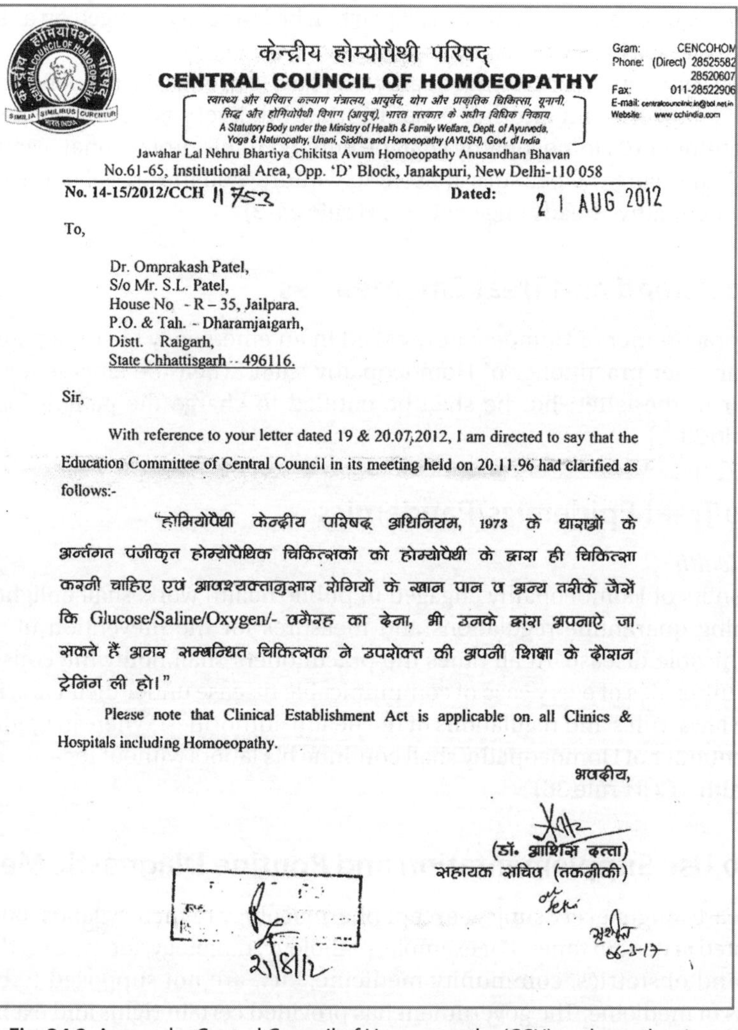

केन्द्रीय होम्योपैथी परिषद्

CENTRAL COUNCIL OF HOMOEOPATHY

स्वास्थ्य और परिवार कल्याण मंत्रालय, आयुर्वेद, योग और प्राकृतिक चिकित्सा, यूनानी, सिद्ध और होमियोपैथी विभाग (आयुष), भारत सरकार के अधीन विधिक निकाय

A Statutory Body under the Ministry of Health & Family Welfare, Deptt. of Ayurveda, Yoga & Naturopathy, Unani, Siddha and Homoeopathy (AYUSH), Govt. of India

Jawahar Lal Nehru Bhartiya Chikitsa Avum Homoeopathy Anusandhan Bhavan

No.61-65, Institutional Area, Opp. 'D' Block, Janakpuri, New Delhi-110 058

Gram: CENCOHOM
Phone: (Direct) 28525582
28520607
Fax: 011-28522906
E-mail: centralcouncilnic.in@bol.net.in
Website: www.cchindia.com

No. 14-15/2012/CCH 11753 Dated: 21 AUG 2012

To,

Dr. Omprakash Patel,
S/o Mr. S.L. Patel,
House No - R – 35, Jailpara.
P.O. & Tah. - Dharamjaigarh,
Distt. Raigarh,
State Chhattisgarh - 496116.

Sir,

With reference to your letter dated 19 & 20.07,2012, I am directed to say that the Education Committee of Central Council in its meeting held on 20.11.96 had clarified as follows:-

"होमियोपैथी केन्द्रीय परिषद अधिनियम, 1973 के धाराओं के अर्न्तगत पंजीकृत होम्योपैथिक चिकित्सकों को होम्योपैथी के द्वारा ही चिकित्सा करनी चाहिए एवं आवश्यक्तानुसार रोगियों के खान पान व अन्य तरीके जैसें कि Glucose/Saline/Oxygen/- वगैरह का देना, भी उनके द्वारा अपनाए जा सकते हैं अगर सम्बन्धित चिकित्सक ने उपरोक्त की अपनी शिक्षा के दौरान ट्रेनिंग ली हो।"

Please note that Clinical Establishment Act is applicable on all Clinics & Hospitals including Homoeopathy.

भवदीय,

(डॉ. आशिश दत्ता)
सहायक सचिव (तकनीकी)

21/8/12

Fig. 34.2: Answer by Central Council of Homoeopathy (CCH) to the author in a Right to Information (RTI) application.

GOVERNMENT ORDER (GO) REGARDING EXEMPTION OF HOMEOPATHS FROM BIOMEDICAL WASTE TREATMENT TIE-UP

The government has provided certain rights and exemptions to the homeopaths. Government officials are not aware of these laws related to homeopathy. For example, homeopaths can use all the necessary measures in treating a critical patient. They are exempted from biomedical waste treatment tie-up if not running indoors (most homeopaths do not have indoors) **(Fig. 34.3)**.

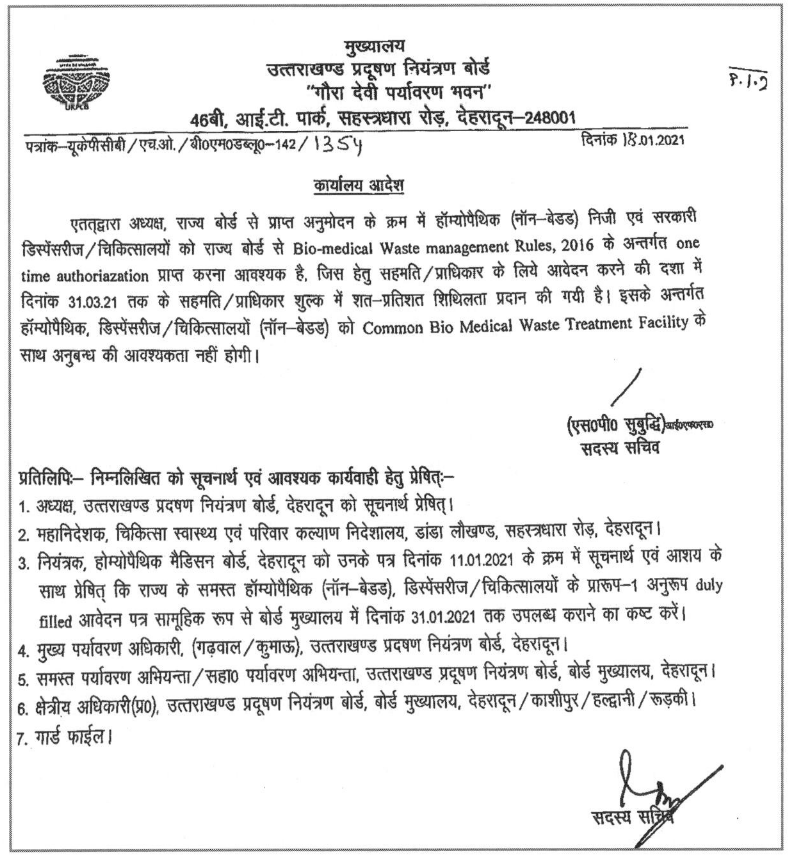

मुख्यालय
उत्तराखण्ड प्रदूषण नियंत्रण बोर्ड
"गौरा देवी पर्यावरण भवन"
46बी, आई.टी. पार्क, सहस्त्रधारा रोड़, देहरादून–248001

पत्रांक–यूकेपीसीबी / एच.ओ. / बी0एम0डब्लू0–142 / 1354 दिनांक 18.01.2021

कार्यालय आदेश

एतत्द्वारा अध्यक्ष, राज्य बोर्ड से प्राप्त अनुमोदन के क्रम में हॉम्योपैथिक (नॉन–बेडड) निजी एवं सरकारी डिस्पेंसरीज / चिकित्सालयों को राज्य बोर्ड से Bio-medical Waste management Rules, 2016 के अन्तर्गत one time authoriazation प्राप्त करना आवश्यक है, जिस हेतु सहमति / प्राधिकार के लिये आवेदन करने की दशा में दिनांक 31.03.21 तक के सहमति / प्राधिकार शुल्क में शत–प्रतिशत शिथिलता प्रदान की गयी है। इसके अन्तर्गत हॉम्योपैथिक, डिस्पेंसरीज / चिकित्सालयों (नॉन–बेडड) को Common Bio Medical Waste Treatment Facility के साथ अनुबन्ध की आवश्यकता नहीं होगी।

(एस0पी0 सुबुद्धि)आई0एफ0एस0
सदस्य सचिव

प्रतिलिपिः– निम्नलिखित को सूचनार्थ एवं आवश्यक कार्यवाही हेतु प्रेषित:–

1. अध्यक्ष, उत्तराखण्ड प्रदषण नियंत्रण बोर्ड, देहरादून को सूचनार्थ प्रेषित्।
2. महानिदेशक, चिकित्सा स्वास्थ्य एवं परिवार कल्याण निदेशालय, डांडा लौखण्ड, सहस्त्रधारा रोड़, देहरादून।
3. नियंत्रक, होम्योपैथिक मैडिसन बोर्ड, देहरादून को उनके पत्र दिनांक 11.01.2021 के क्रम में सूचनार्थ एवं आशय के साथ प्रेषित् कि राज्य के समस्त हॉम्योपैथिक (नॉन–बेडड), डिस्पेंसरीज / चिकित्सालयों के प्रारूप–1 अनुरूप duly filled आवेदन पत्र सामूहिक रूप से बोर्ड मुख्यालय में दिनांक 31.01.2021 तक उपलब्ध कराने का कष्ट करें।
4. मुख्य पर्यावरण अधिकारी, (गढ़वाल / कुमाऊ), उत्तराखण्ड प्रदषण नियंत्रण बोर्ड, देहरादून।
5. समस्त पर्यावरण अभियन्ता / सहा0 पर्यावरण अभियन्ता, उत्तराखण्ड प्रदूषण नियंत्रण बोर्ड, बोर्ड मुख्यालय, देहरादून।
6. क्षेत्रीय अधिकारी(प्र0), उत्तराखण्ड प्रदूषण नियंत्रण बोर्ड, बोर्ड मुख्यालय, देहरादून / काशीपुर / हल्द्वानी / रूड़की।
7. गार्ड फाईल।

सदस्य सचिव

Fig. 34.3: A Government order from Uttarakhand Pollution Control Board served to the author.

STATUS OF HOMEOPATHIC MEDICINES UNDER DRUGS AND COSMETIC ACT, 1940 AND RULES 1945

Homeopathic medicines are covered under the provisions of Drugs and Cosmetic Act, 1940 and the Rules made thereunder.

Some important provisions are:

- Homeopathic medicines are defined under Rule 2 (DD) of the Drugs and Cosmetics Rules, 1945.
- Standards of homeopathic medicines to be complied with for manufacture, sale, distribution. or import are defined under the Second Schedule of the Drugs and Cosmetics Act (item N.4a).
- New homeopathic medicines are covered under Rule 30AA.
- Minimum requirement for good manufacturing is included in Schedule M-1.
- Ophthalmic preparations, standards, and conditions for preparation thereof are covered under Schedule FF (Rule 126A).

- Homoeopathic Pharmacopoeia Laboratory, Ghaziabad is to function as Central Drugs Laboratory with respect to homeopathic drugs, under section 6 of the act under sub-rule 7 of rule 3A.
- Anybody can get medicines tested under Section 26.
- Under Section 26A, the Central Government can cancel the license for manufacturing a drug, if therapeutic claims are not genuine.
- Procedures for labeling and packing of homeopathic medicines are covered under Rule 32A, Rule 106A, and 106B (Part IXA).
- Rule 85B covers the manufacture of mother tinctures, potencies, or potencies from back potencies. Application for which is made under form 24C.
- Rule 85C and 30AA covers the manufacture of new homeopathic drugs.
- Individual pharmacists (shopkeepers) are allowed to manufacture potencies only and, that only from back potencies, under Rule 85D.
- Retail is covered under Rule 67C. Application be made under form 20C.
- Though wholesale is covered under Rule 67C, but application is made under form 20D.
- Licensing authority for the issue of licenses for homeopathic medicines lies with the State Government as per Rule 67A and 85B.

BITTER TRUTHS ABOUT HOMEOPATHY

There are certain bitter truths about homeopathy, which are given as follows:

- When a homeopath fails to treat a case, this is assumed that homeopathy fails (not that individual homeopath).
- Whenever a classic case is cured with homeopathy, it is presumed that homeopathy often does such a miracle, there is no special role of that homeopathic physician.
- At any time, if a homeopath fails to establish a perfect diagnosis, it is believed that this system of healing art deals with the sick person, not the disease.
- Whenever a homeopath treats a patient and the case is deteriorated or is complicated further, the complete system of homeopathy is blamed, not that homeopath.
- If a doctor of so-called modern medicine or a super-specialist in a particular field fails in curing a condition, nothing happens. Very rarely, negligence may be confirmed.
- If a homeopath is treating a usually benign condition (which rarely turns into malignancy), and the condition, by chance, is turned into malignancy, the homeopath is punished and declared as if he/she is not authorized to treat such conditions. One such example is given as follows:
    - *Case—Maldah*: Holding that a homeopathy doctor is not an oncologist and cannot treat a carcinoma patient, the District Consumer Disputes Redressal Commission, Maldah has directed a homeopathy doctor to pay a compensation of ₹50,000 for gross negligence in the treatment of a patient suffering from carcinoma. The case concerns a patient who visited the homeopath in 2016 for the treatment of a cyst.

CONCLUSION

The duration of study and syllabi by various Government Councils are the same for all the bachelor-level medical courses recognized by the Government of India, except only one subject, i.e., pharmacology. In each system of medicine, the concerned pharmacology is taught. There is no difference in study regarding basic subjects like anatomy, physiology, biochemistry, pathology, forensic medicine and jurisprudence, social and preventive medicine, surgery, gynecology and obstetrics, practice of medicine, etc., except their own pharmacology as per respected streams. In reading different body scans like magnetic resonance imaging (MRI), computed tomography (CT) scan, positron emission tomography (PET) scan, X-rays, ultrasonography (USG), echocardiography (ECHO), TMT, pathology, electrocardiography (ECG), electroencephalogram (EEG), electromyography (EMG) or many other diagnosing modalities, there is no role of different types of pharmacology.

Further, in the new Bachelor of Homeopathic Medicine and Surgery (BHMS) syllabus, the introduction to allopathic pharmacology has been added. This is only to make a homeopath acquainted with basic knowledge of modern pharmacology. This will help them to understand the prescriptions of other doctors and to make their prescriptions in accordance with them so that inter-reactions among different prescriptions, if must be used simultaneously, may be avoided.

There are so many restrictions to AYUSH system of medicine in utilizing many of them. Why do PCPNDT, Atomic Energy Regulatory Board (AERB), etc. have different moods with AYUSH system? Why is registered medical practitioner's definition always restricted to the schedules of the India Medical Council Act only? Every medical council registers their candidates in their respected schedules certifying him/her a registered medical practitioner, then why is there such a nonuniformity? While there is consistency in the syllabi and duration of study in all the medical streams, the rules for all of them should be identical.

KEY LEARNING POINTS

- Homeopathy is a holistic system of medicine.
- Homeopathy is well recognized in India and several other countries with specific rights.
- In India, Homeopathy is kept under AYUSH group of medical streams and has equal rights and privileges as the other systems of medicines do. The National Medical Commission governs every medical education as well as practice in India, including homeopathy under AYUSH banner.
- There are certain restrictions on homeopaths, which prevent them to opt during their clinical practice.
- There are certain things that every homeopath must know, e.g., their rights, domain, and their limitations in the medical field.
- While having similar syllabi and standards of studies in Homeopathy and other systems, the rights to use their specialties in homeopathy is not at par with others, e.g., to open a small-scale laboratory, recognition as sonologist, etc.
- Further proceedings are needed to make homeopaths at par with medical practitioners qualified in other medical streams.
- All the recognized medical streams must be uniformly treated and honored.

BIBLIOGRAPHY

1. Central Council of Homoeopathy. The Gazette of India, Extraordinary, Part III—Section 4. [online] Available from https://nch.org.in/upload/Code_of_Ethics_2March_1982.pdf [Last accessed May, 2024].
2. MD Bureau. Medical Dialogues. (2021). Homeopathy Doctor held liable for gross negligence in treating carcinoma patient, told to pay compensation. [online]. https://medicaldialogues.in/news/health/medico-legal/homeopathy-doctor-held-liable-for-gross-negligence-in-treating-carcinoma-patient-told-to-pay-compensation-74943 [Last accessed May, 2024].

3. Ministry of Law and Justice. (2020). The Gazette of India, Extraordinary. Part II—Section 1. The National Commission For Homoeopathy Act. [online] Available from https://www.livelaw.in/pdf_upload/pdf_upload-381801.pdf [Last accessed May, 2024].
4. National Commission for homoeopathy. (2022). Homoeopathy Degree Course–B.H.M.S.) Regulation-2022. [online]. Available from https://nch.org.in/upload/Homoeopathy%20Degree%20Course%20-%20B.H.M.S.%20Regulations-2022.pdf [Last accessed May, 2024].
5. National Commission For Homoeopathy. (2024). NCH Acts & Amendments. [online] Available from https://nch.org.in/nch-acts-amendments [Last accessed May, 2024].
6. Ramanayake RP, Ranasingha S, Lakmini S. Management of emergencies in general practice: role of general practitioners. J Family Med Prim Care. 2014;3(4):305-8.
7. Sharma RK. Need of modern diagnostic tools in Homoeopathy: Legal Aspects. JIMLEA. 2021;9(2):45-54.

35

CHAPTER

Issues Related to Crosspathy and Cross-specialty Practice

Ravishankar TN

INTRODUCTION

Medical sciences have been growing for centuries. The past five decades have seen a rapid advances in science so also in medical science. The age-old medical science in our country had been Ayurveda, Siddha and Unani. The growth of such medical science had not matched with the growth of modern or the so-called Western medicine.

Biotechnology have given a big leap for modern medical science. AYUSH system of Medicine has not concentrated on the growth of their respective system for the past two to three decades and have been left behind on providing the expectation of the population. Hence, it was the only option for these systems to adopt or mix their system with the ever growing modern medical science.

It is not adaptation, but to be clear crossing their limits in pharmacopeia and providing the gist for crosspatch. No modern medical practitioners have ever prescribed any of the AYUSH medication except for one or two products in the 70" or 80" when specific treatments were not available for a few diseases. The rapid growth of modern medical science and the medical code which prevented modern medical science from crossing their pharmacopeia restrained them and today AYUSH pharmacopeia are never used by the modern medical practitioners. However, the same in not vice versa, as the respective councils made provisions in their Code of Ethics for crossing the pharmacopeia.

Healthcare is provided in our country by qualified personals in the various systems that are been followed in our country. The vast majorly as followed in the Universe in the Western medical science or Allopathy practice has described in the Indian Medical Degrees Act 1916. There are the traditional system, such as Ayurveda, Unani, Siddha from our country and Homeopathy a system conceived from the European continent Germany. Each system has their own scientific principle and pharmacopoeia while the Western medical science or Allopathy has been evolving on research and never overran the other systems. Nomenclature as AYUSH by the Government of India is also following to an extent for a variation in the society with their existing pharmacopoeia. There are a lot in the Indian population who are quite satisfied with AYUSH system of medical management, and it is a common belief that chronic ailments are under control or cures with least side effects. Western medical science has been evolving in surgical intervention from Stenting to Replacing and Transplanting. This scientific advancement for total cure could not be replicated by the other systems since surgery has never been part of Ayurveda, Unani or for the fact never in Homeopathy. All these systems have been surviving or advising on the alternate for surgery for several conditions. With the advancement of science been adopted by the population all other pathy except Homeopathy are gradually adopting the surgical procedures. When hemodialysis was firmly objected, and medicals management was advocated by AYUSH today transplant is hearty accepted by them.

Poor doctor-patient ratio the shield for crosspathy: There have always been a hue and cry on the large disparity on the availability of doctor-patient ratio in our country as envisaged by the WHO. 1 for every 1000 population. And this was the basis for the Governments to pass orders for the AYUSH practitioners to prescribe Allopathic drugs. In June 2022 the statutory WHO's health index was almost on target in the Indian scenario. If one consider the 6 lakhs odd AYUSH practitioners along with the 11 lakhs odd Allopathic Practitioners, the WHO health index have been achieved. The disparity of Urban versus Rural in doctor-patient ratio is always there but it has narrowed down of late. The distribution of qualified practitioners in certain states of our country are at a satisfactory level. The distribution of qualified allopathic practitioners is insufficient in some states and these are the states that passed Government order allowing non-Allopathic to prescribe, Allopathic drugs.

The Homeopathy Central Council Act 1973 was constituted for the Homeopathy practitioners. The Central Council of Indian Medicine (CCIM) was constituted as a statutory body under the Ministry of Health and Family Welfare governing the AYUSH. Government of India has brought National Medical Commission for Indian System of Medicine replacing the CCIM. They now come under the Ministry of AYUSH and have their own set of rules and regulation for the medical institution and graduates produce from these institutes.

The Pharmacy Act 1948 has framed rules for the medical's shops established in our country to follow. It not only has a set frame of rules to establish a pharmacy, but also rules to whose prescription the medicines are to be dispensed. Section 4. (e) clearly defines the scope of the medical qualification of the person.

"Medical practitioner" means a person—

Holding a qualification granted by an authority specified or notified under Section 3 of the Indian Medical Degrees Act, 1916 (7 of 1916), or specified in the Schedules to the Indian Medical Council Act, 1956 (102 of 1956).

It has a provision 5 (iii) that the State Government has powers to pass Government order to enable the law to authorize other set or qualified personals to prescribe Allopathy drugs as stored within the legal compliance of Pharmacy Act 1948. As health is a state subject as per the constitution such a clause is there for states to decide.

JUDICIAL ORDERS ON CROSSPATHY

In a significant order, the High Court of Delhi on April 8, 2016, on the Writ Petition No. 7865/2010 pronounced that qualification of Indian System of Medicine or of Homeopathic Medicine has no legal authority to prescribe allopathic medicines. This was based on the Public Interest litigation filed by Delhi Medical Association, under Article 226 of the Constitution of India.

The Civil Appeal No. 89 of 1987 Dr Mukhtiar Chand and other versus State of Punjab and others categorically pronounced that qualified practitioners of Ayurveda, Unani, Siddha, and Homeopathy systems cannot prescribe Allopathic drugs. The Judgment passed in 1987 still stands good for quoting as it was a detailed in-depth judgement after studying the curriculum of the respective system of medicine and the consequence for the society if crosspathy is legalised. According to Section 2 (ee) of the Drugs and Cosmetics Rules, 1995, Registered Medical Practitioner means a person:

i. Registered or eligible for registration in a medical register of a state meant for the registration of persons practicing the modern scientific system of medicine (excluding the Homeopathy system of medicine); or
ii. Registered in a medical register (other than a register for the registration of homeopathic practitioners) of a state, who although not falling within sub clause (i) or subclause (ii) is declared by a general or special order made by the State Government in this behalf as a person practicing the modern scientific system of medicine for the purposes of this Act.

Honourable Supreme Court of India upheld the validity of Rule 2 (ee) (iii), as well as the notifications issued by various State Governments there under allowing Ayurveda, Siddha, Unani, and Homeopathy practitioners to prescribe allopathic medicines. In view of the above judgment, Ayurveda, Siddha, Unani, and Homeopathy practitioners can prescribe allopathic medicines under Rule 2 (ee) (iii) only in those states where they are authorized to do so by a general or special order made by the concerned State Government in that regard. Practitioners of Indian Medicine holding the degrees in integrated courses can also prescribe allopathic medicines if any State Act in the state in which they are practicing recognizes their qualification as sufficient for registration in the State Medical Register.

Since the Central council of Indian Medicine order more than ten states with low doctor-patient ratio have enacted the Government order allowing AYUSH to prescribe Allopathic drugs.

Writ Petition No. 5896/2000 titled Dr Mehboob Alam versus State of Uttar Pradesh visibly passed the order debarring the AYUSH practitioners from prescribing Allopathic pharmacopeia as it is not included in their curriculum. It further authorised to prescribe only their pharmacopeia.

The High Court of Madras, in Writ Petition No. 2907/2002 titled Dr K Abdul Muneer versus State of Tamil Nadu has remarked that it cannot authorise AYUSH to prescribe Allopathic drugs as their syllabus do not have the pharmacopeia of Allopathic.

The above verdicts are clear that one cannot cross their qualification and prescribe other speciality pharmacopeia. But it has been over exonerated with the Government orders based on Section 17 (3) (b) of the Central Council of Indian Medicine.

The Allahabad High court in a Special appeal No. 320/2004 went to the extent of directing the State government to ensure that the health of the individual is not abused by unauthorized prescription of unqualified practitioners.

Central council of Indian Medical order paving the way for legalizing crosspathy is:
Section 17 Rights of persons possessing qualifications included in Second, Third and Fourth Schedules to be enrolled.

(1) Subject to the other provisions contained in this Act, any medical qualification included in the Second, Third or Fourth Schedule shall be sufficient qualification for enrolment on any State Register of Indian Medicine.

(2) Save as provided in Section 28, no person other than a practitioner of Indian medicine who possesses a recognized medical qualification and is enrolled on a State Register or the Central Register of Indian Medicine.

(3) (2) (a) the right of a practitioner of Indian medicine enrolled on a State Register of Indian Medicine to practise Indian medicine in any State merely on the ground that, on the commencement of this Act, he does not possess a recognized medical qualification;

(b) the privileges (including the right to practice any system of medicine) conferred by or under any law relating to registration of practitioners of Indian medicine for the time being in force in any State on a practitioner of Indian medicine enrolled on a State Register of Indian Medicine.

All the above Sections were subsequent to several judgements that had restrictions on the AYUSH to provide healthcare on par the Allopathic in providing certificates on health condition of their patients, evidence in the courts. Section 17 (3) (b) was enacted to make states provision to enable the AYUSH prescribe Allopathic drugs.

National Medical Commission Draft to Curb Crosspathy

The Ethics and Medical Registration Board of the National Medical Association has released a draft of the Registered Medical Practitioner (Professional Conduct) Regulation, 2022 for public consultation on May 30th 2022.

The regulation proposed that every Registered Medical Practitioner (RMP) would only be allowed to practice the system of medicine in which they have been trained and certified.

"Every RMP shall practice the system of medicine in which he/she has trained and certified (for this purpose referred to as modern medicine or allopathic medicine) and shall not associate professionally with any unqualified person to perform any treatment, procedure, or operation," the draft said.

It also proposed that a person qualified in more than one system of medicine should decide which system he or she wants to practice.

"Once licensed to practice modern medicine under the NMC Act, they shall not practice another system of medicine simultaneously," said the draft regulation, adding that short courses in other systems of medicine do not qualify a practitioner to practice and prescribe medicines used in that system.

The above order if passed by the Parliament must be taken up by the medical associations and responsible citizens in all system of pathy and all walks of life and implement it legally which will prevent crosspathy in the country. The NMC order can only bind the Allopathic practitioners. If the order has to get its full powers CCIM, Pharmacy Act 1948 and the Drugs and Cosmetic Act must be in unanimity to prevent crosspathy. As such the present status allows AYUSH to prescribe Allopathy in those states where the Government order are prevailing allowing AYUSH to prescribe.

CROSSPATHY IN DIAGNOSTIC TECHNIQUES

Diagnostic inventions are the reflection of the growth of science and community. However, the science and fundamentals of AYUSH has been always nonintervention on the Human system. With advancement of Biotechnology the same diagnostic tools have been adopted by the AYUSH system that their syllabus now do have Pathology, Biochemistry, and Radiology, etc. Central council of Indian medicine area by notification F. No 8-5/2002 (mm) dated 22.01.2004 clarified to include in the syllabus of India medicine, Ashtang Ayurveda, Siddha and Unani Tibb such subjects with regards to National Programs like malaria eradication, TB, Leprosy, Family Welfare programs, Immunization program, AIDS, Cancer, etc. It enabled them to prescribe Allopathic medicines in all the above national program with the right to prescribe for Indian Medicine

Council Registered candidates. It also indirectly gave the hidden fact that the respective system does not have complete cure for such ailments; hence, Government of respective states have adopted this short cut option. It prevented the different system for venturing into research for new molecules with their framework.

Imaging technology and evaluation of molecular biology, immune chemistry and such inventions with the involvement of Allopathy has been adopted and accepted by Indian Medicine system with No.V.26011/4/70 Ay Desk. New Delhi date. 13.09.1976.

Pharmacopoeia of modern medicine and biotechnology growth with Government order from respective states and Section 17 of Indian Medical Central Council Act 1970 provides legal authorities more than immunity to Practice Modern Medicine Allopathy.

The government orders have only allowed to prescribe, and no limitation or schedule of drugs are ever mentioned. The legal fact is one should qualify from specific Pharmacopoeia to prescribe the drugs which is the fundament rule also was quoted in the same judgment. But it has been bypassed with Section 4 (e) of The Pharmacy Act 1948. Also, if the Government is concern about the shortage of health care workers in rural region, only certain specific drugs for first aid, rehabilitation and supportive should have been allowed. A blanket government order to prescribe allopathic is assured to be misused and the same is in practice in our country. Even a qualified under graduate of Allopathic cannot legally and scientifically prescribe certain schedule drugs. When such is the law Government orders all over the country are silent on this general government order.

CROSS-SPECIALTY

Has been restricted by Section 7.20 of code of ethics and Etiquette of the National Medical Commission which is total adoption of the Medical Council of India's code. Unless qualified recognized by the National Medical commission one cannot treat a patient crossing the specialty one is qualified. An undergraduate who is aware and qualified in all branches of medicine and surgery is eligible legally to provide treatment as well do first aid and treatment to the extent it is known to one's knowledge and skill in emergency. But even in emergency an undergraduate cannot put his knife beyond the skin of his patient. If one had to go beyond the skin to the specific organ, one needs to acquire a postgraduate qualification in that specialty. A general medicine and general surgery have the legal sanction to treat to the extent, he has knowledge and skill. Even in this situation, when there is negligent as claimed by the patient the question of qualification is put across in the court. A complicated medical or surgical care involving, Cardiology, Neurology and such super specialty at the onset of treatment will necessitate the respective super specialty in the field of treatment. As long as the patient is satisfied and cured without any legal morbidity or mortality, the question of crossing specialty or inadequately qualified is not questioned.

Courts in several judgments have found fault on hospitals when thy have engaged non-allopathic qualified personal in their hospitals as Duty medical officers or Intensive care physicians. The landmark judgment of Poonam Verma vs Ashwin Patel and others is one such case dates back to 1997. Courts pronounce their judgments based the facts and documents that are put up in the case on their file. Government order are considered based on society's need logically, henceforth to implement National health programmes for citizen's welfare.

CONCLUSION

Crosspathy indicates that the liable elements cross each other. The above analysis of the events that is happing in the country, the various laws and code of ethics of the different system of medicine do not reflect that crosspathy is happing in the country.

All the judgments pronounced since 1990 have uphold that crossing one's system of pharmacopeia is illegal. The Pharmacy act have defined the content of prescription to be prescribed by the respective system of practitioners limiting them within their relevant pharmacopeia. The provision in CCIM and the various Government orders have allowed that AYUSH may be allowed to prescribe modern medicine to mitigate the poor doctor-patient ratio as formulated by the WHO.

It is clear that there is no crosspathy, but only violation and illegal use of modern medicine @Allopathy by all the system of medicine. It also proves that the value and need of modern medicine by the patients seeking cure and opting for preventive medicine. Allopathy or the so-called modern medicine is the one which provides the need of the population, hence, the illegal use of the same is practiced in the country with Governments order to provide healthcare to all with equality. Equality is also followed in the various system of medicine engulfing modern medicine for the practitioners to survive. Thus, it prevents the AYUSH from the research and hinder their growth and in due course to be swamped by Allopathy and not aiding for the growth of the AYUSH.

KEY LEARNING POINTS

- Every system of medicine have their own regulatory council to monitor the respective qualified practitioner in India.
- The Pharmacy Act 1948 revised from time to time have framed rules to be followed for the different system of medicines to be dispensed based on the qualification.
- Several judgments in our country have continued and reemphases that crosspathy is illegal and the said qualified personals registered in the respective council alone have the authority to prescribe the respective system drugs.
- Central council of Indian Medicine enacted a clause in their rules providing the right for the state government to pass Government order to enable AYUSH to prescribe modern medicines to match the disparity and nonavailability of qualified modern medicine practitioners.
- The legal immunity was thus provided and crosspathy is practiced in our country.
- Cross-specialty with modern medicine practitioner have been restricted by the Code of Medical Ethics and Etiquette of National Medicine Commission as well as several judgments have upheld the same.

BIBLIOGRAPHY

1. Doctor-patient ratio in India less than WHO-prescribed norm of 1:1000: Govt [Internet]. ET Healthworld. com. 2019 [cited 8 July 2021]. Available from: https://health.economictimes.indiatimes.com/news/industry/doctor-patient-ratio-in-india-less-than-who-prescribed-norm-of-11000-govt/72135237.
2. The Indian Medicine Central Council Act, 1970.
3. The Pharmacy Act, 1948.
4. The Drugs and Cosmetic Act, 1940.

5. Kumar R, Roy P. Deregulation of Allopathic prescription and medical practice in India: Benefits and pitfall. J Family Med Prim Care. 2016;5(2):215-9.
6. Supreme Court of India, Poonam Verma vs Ashwin Patel & Ors on 10 May, 1996 . "http://www.indiankaoon.com/"
7. Supreme Court of India. Mukhtiar Chand & Ors vs The State Of Punjab & Ors on 8 October, 1998, "http://www.indiankaoon.com"
8. Allahabad High Court Mehboob Alam vs State of U.P. on 16 September, 2019 "https://indiankanoon.com

36

CHAPTER

Medicolegal Issues in Psychiatry

Ravisankar TN

INTRODUCTION AND BACKGROUND

Besides the laws that regulate the practice of medicine generally, mental healthcare has a special act governing the practice of psychiatry.

The Mental Healthcare Act (MHCA), 2017 (Act 10 of 2017), has substantially impacted the delivery of mental healthcare services as it was traditionally delivered to the patients.

India, having ratified the Convention on Rights of Persons with Disabilities and its Optional Protocol, on October 1st, 2007, was obliged to ensure that the existing laws in the country were enacted or modified to be in harmony with covenant.

This chapter shall restrict discussion to the medicolegal issues that are relevant to the practice of psychiatry in India. The medicolegal issues such as privacy, confidentiality, issues related to violence, Protection of Children from Sexual Offences (POCSO), Narcotic Drugs and Psychotropic Substances (NDPS), etc., are as in other specialties, with the same legal obligations on the part of the practicing psychiatrist.

The Act extends to whole of India and includes all mental health establishments (MHE) where persons with mental illness (PMIs) are admitted, or reside in, or are kept in, "by whatever name called. A family residential place where a PMI resides with relatives or friends is excluded from the definition of a mental health care establishment.

Mental healthcare, as per the Act, not only consists of treatment, care, and rehabilitation but also includes analysis and diagnosis of a person's mental illness or suspected mental illness, thereby bringing outpatient department (OPD) services and psychological testing within its ambit.

DEFINITIONS

The MHCA, 2017, defines mental illness as a substantial disorder of thinking, mood, perception, orientation, or memory that grossly impairs judgment, behavior, capacity to recognize reality or ability to meet the ordinary demands of life, mental conditions associated with the abuse of alcohol and drugs, and specifically excludes mental retardation.

Mental illnesses will be determined in accordance with such nationally or internationally accepted standards, as may be notified by the Central Government.

The 11th revision of the International Classification of Diseases (ICD-11), which was issued in 2018, defines mental, behavioral, and neurodevelopmental disorders as disorders characterized by clinically significant disturbance in an individual's cognition, emotional regulation, or behavior that reflects a dysfunction or biological or developmental processes that underline mental and behavioral functioning. These disturbances, the manual states, are usually associated with distress or impairment in personal, family, social, educational, occupational, or other important areas of functioning.

This revision of the ICD has not yet been accepted for classification by the Government but will be the system in vogue soon. It is obvious then that while there is broad consensus on what constitutes a mental illness, the specifics may differ from patient to patient. This juxtaposed on the conditions required to assess, evaluate, and manage PMIs is a fertile ground for medicolegal issues to arise in the practice of psychiatry.

CAPACITY

The Act presupposes that every person, including a PMI, shall be deemed to have capacity to make decisions regarding his mental healthcare or treatment.

Capacity assessment is based on:
- The ability to understand the relevant information in order to take a decision on the treatment or personal assistance
- The ability to appreciate reasonably foreseeable consequences of a decision or lack of the decision
- The ability to communicate the decision by means of speech, expression, gesture, or any other means

A decision that is perceived by others to be inappropriate or wrong is not indicative of a lack of capacity on the part of the PMI.

While the assessment of capacity is the responsibility of the medical personnel, the determination of a person's mental illness alone is not enough to mean that a person is of unsound mind unless so declared by a Court. Mental capacity is considered to be time and task specific and dynamic. The Mental Capacity Act of England and Wales of 2005 guidelines have done so more elegantly and do not assess solely on appearances and behavior.

ADVANCE DIRECTIVE AND NOMINATED REPRESENTATIVE

All adults who have executed an Advance Directive (AD) are to be cared for and treated for a mental illness in the manner specified in the AD. The AD shall only be invoked when the person is incapacitated to make mental healthcare decisions. The AD does not take precedence over a PMI who has capacity and can be revoked, amended, or cancelled at any time.

The AD does not apply to emergency treatment.

All adults have also been given the right to appoint a nominated representative (NR) who are:
- An individual
- A relative
- A caregiver
- A suitable person appointed as such by the concerned board
- Director, Department of Social Welfare

ADMISSION AND TREATMENT

An adult person may be admitted in a MHE if he consents to the same. Form C of the Mental Healthcare (Rights of Persons with Mental Illness) Rules, 2018 must be filled in for the same. The mental health professional must determine that the illness is of a severity requiring in-patient care which shall benefit the PMI. The PMI should have the capacity and should be able to give informed consent.

A minor may be admitted only after a NR applies for admission. The admission can occur only after two psychiatrists or one psychiatrist and one mental health professional or one psychiatrist and one medical practitioner have independently examined the minor on the day of admission or in the preceding 7 days.

The examiners should have concluded that the severity of the illness is such that it requires in-patient management which shall be beneficial and is the only option after community-based intervention have been exhausted. Mental Health Review Board has to be informed of the admission within 72 hours. Electroconvulsive therapy (ECT) in a minor is prohibited, unless informed consent of the guardian has been obtained and permitted by the Board.

If the PMI is unable to give informed consent, or is otherwise incapacitated, and requires admission, he shall be admitted for up to 30 days as PMI having high support needs.

The person can be admitted on the application by the NR, if the PMI who has been independently examined on the day of admission or in the preceding 7 days by a psychiatrist and the other being a mental health professional or a medical practitioner. At the end of the examination, both conclude that the PMI has recently threatened or attempted to cause bodily harm to himself or has behaved violently toward another person or may cause bodily injury or is unable to take care of himself.

The psychiatrist, with due regard to the AD, needs to certify that in-patient evaluation at a MHE is the least restrictive care option possible in the circumstances and that the PMI is ineligible to be admitted as an independent admission due to his mental incapacity or needs support from the NR. The psychiatrist must inform the board of such an admission, within 3 days if the PMI is a woman or a minor or within 7 days of other admissions.

In case of an emergency, medical treatment may be provided by any registered medical practitioner either at a health establishment or in the community. The physician shall obtain informed consent of the NR, if available.

The emergency treatment is needed immediately to prevent death or reversible harm to the PMI or the PMI harming himself or others or damaging property as a result of his mental illness.

The emergency intervention includes the period required to transfer the PMI to a MHE and is to be limited to the management of the mental illness. The psychiatrist is prohibited from using ECT as a modality of treatment. Emergency admissions are limited to 72 hours or till he has been assessed at a MHE. The duration of admission can be extended to 7 days if a disaster or emergency has been declared.

Unmodified ECT, ECT for minors, sterilization, chaining or restraining, and psychosurgery are included in the list of prohibited procedures.

The Act lays down an elaborate procedure prior to discharging a PMI. The PMI, NR, and the psychiatrist to whom the PMI is to be handed over have to be consulted and treatment required or services provided are to be planned.

PSYCHIATRIST AS AN EXPERT WITNESS

Besides the professional duties, a psychiatrist may be summoned as an expert witness by a Court.

As an expert witness, a psychiatrist is permitted to submit his opinion. However, he will have to face examination in chief, cross-examination, and reexamination as any other witness.

Prior to deposing, the psychiatrist should study the documents, be dignified, acknowledge limitations, and explain the answers. He should not be browbeaten by the lawyers, should not take sides, and be objective.

CONCLUSION

The MHCA, 2017, was enacted with an emphasis on the rights of PMI. The Act has lofty ideals, aiming to ensure access to mental healthcare to all persons. It also provides the right to privacy, right to information about their illness, protection from inhuman treatment, right to decide manner of intervention, right to appoint a NR, etc. A PMI has the right to live in a safe, hygienic, sanitary environment, to be protected from any abuse, and to have adequate facility for recreation and education.

BIBLIOGRAPHY

1. Jiloha RC, Kukreti P, Kataria D. Forensic Psychiatry: An Indian Perspective. New Delhi: Jaypee Brothers Medical Publishers (P) Ltd.; 2019. pp. 505.
2. Legislation.gov.uk. Mental Capacity Act 2005. [online] Available from https://www.legislation.gov.uk/ukpga/2005/9/contents [Last accessed July, 2024].
3. Ministry of Health & Family Welfare, Government of India. (2018). Rights of Persons with Mental Illness. [online] Available from https://main.mohfw.gov.in/sites/default/files/Rights%20of%20Persons%20with%20Mental%20Illness_0.pdf [Last accessed July, 2024].
4. Ministry of Law and Justice. Government of India. (2017). The Mental Healthcare Act, 2017. [online] Available from https://prsindia.org/files/bills_acts/acts_parliament/2017/the-mental-healthcare-act,-2017.pdf [Last accessed July, 2024].
5. United Nations. (2007). Convention on the Rights of Persons with Disabilities. [online] Available from https://social.desa.un.org/issues/disability/crpd/convention-on-the-rights-of-persons-with-disabilities-crpd#:~:text=The%20Convention%20on%20the%20Rights,signature%20on%2030%20March%202007 [Last accessed July, 2024].
6. World Health Organization. International Classification of Diseases, 11th Revision. The global standard for diagnostic health information. [online] Available from https://icd.who.int/en [Last accessed July, 2024].

36.1 Mental Healthcare Act

Amitabh Shanker Saxena

INTRODUCTION

The Mental Healthcare Act (MHCA), 2017, was a seminal law that was necessitated to harmonize Indian laws after India ratified the Convention on Rights of Persons with Disabilities and its optional protocol in 2007. It replaced the Mental Health Act, 1987. The Act has revolutionized both in- and outpatient practice of psychiatry. The knowledge of the law is essential to every psychiatrist and is desirable for each medical administrator. The nuances of the law are discussed.

HISTORY

Indian lunacy laws prior to independence were primarily derived from laws prevalent in the parent nation, modified cosmetically to suit and favor the colonial masters.

Since the colonization was considered a burden of the white man, the British could not be seen to be falling prey to mental ailments. The East India Company, therefore, evolved a simple plan for them. The mentally ill white persons were simply repatriated to the mother nation. By removing them from India, the Company rid itself of any medicolegal or administrative problems that might arise. However, legislation in three presidencies of Bombay, Calcutta, and Madras were disparate and in need of harmonization, and the stage was then set for mental health-related legislation in India.

In 1845, a Lunatics Act was passed. The Act increased protection for the mentally ill from being detained in the asylums and also introduced safeguards to certify them.

In 1849, the Indian Legislative Council passed "An Act for the Safe Custody of Criminal Lunatics" in 1849 (Act IV of 1849).

The Act was undoubtedly influenced by the first draft of the Indian Penal Code that had been submitted by Lord Macauley in 1837.

The Act provided for the safety of the mentally ill persons who were accused of criminal offences by putting them in safe custody or protective detention. The Act also recognized insanity as a ground for acquittal. The Act was, in all probability, fathered by John Elliot Drinkwater Bethune, a law member of the Governor Generals Council. Bethune was an Anglo-Indian lawyer and had been appointed to the Council only a year prior to the passage of the Act.

This Act was followed by a Parliamentary Act in 1851—the Lunatics Removal (India) Act (14 and 15 Vict. c. 81) and in 1884, the Criminal Lunatics Act (47 and 48 Vict. c. 64).

The Acts read together concerned themselves with empowering the provincial governments in India for safe custody of the mentally ill criminals and their repatriation and the reimbursement of expenses for the same.

In the interim, Acts for persons other than the criminal lunatics were passed by the Legislative Council in 1858, relating to better provisions for the care of the estate of Lunatics. Another Act passed the same year codified the procedure for reception and detention lunatics in asylums. As per the Act, it was the police officers' responsibility to inform the concerned magistrate if a lunatic was neglected or otherwise treated cruelly. The word "lunatic" was to mean "every person found by due course of law to be of unsound mind and incapable of managing his affairs."

Both Acts also mirrored the Acts in parent country. The latter provided the basis for establishing asylums in India and to prevent illegal detention of the mentally ill in asylums. The Act was amended twice in 1886 and 1889 but remained virtually unchanged till the Indian Lunacy Act was passed in 1912.

Thus, the seed of mental health legislation was planted in 1858. The Acts in force, when examined through the prism of prevailing Victorian norms, were indeed revolutionary.

The Indian Lunacy Act, 1912, was enacted to govern the reception, detention, and care of lunatics. The Act provided the legal authority to safeguard the rights of the mentally ill and rehabilitate them. However, the Act gravitated toward institution-based treatment of mental illness.

The Mental Health Act, 1987, was passed on May 22, 1987, but came into force only in April 1993. The Act defined mental illnesses in consonance with the prevailing norms. It emphasized management and provided protection to the rights of the mentally ill.

The United Nations (UN) Convention on the Rights of People with Disabilities (UNCRPD) and its Optional Protocol was adopted by the UN General Assembly on December 13, 2006. India signed the convention in March 2007 and ratified it in October 2007.

The Convention signaled a paradigm shift from generosity and welfare to legally enforceable rights and empowerment. The onus was on the signatories to modify the prevailing laws to conform to the UNCPRD. The Mental Health Act, 1987, therefore gave way to the Mental Healthcare Act, 2017.

MENTAL HEALTHCARE ACT, 2017

The Act received presidential assent on April 07, 2017, and came into force on July 07, 2018.

The Act comprises the chapters and the sections and some of the important provisions and salient features are as follows:

- There can be no doubt that this Act is much ahead of its time. It not only emphasizes the role of the state in mental healthcare delivery and implementation, but there is also a discernible shift from institution based to community care.
- The Act is replete with provisos that mark a pronounced departure from its predecessors.
- The Act defines mental illness as a substantial disorder of thinking, mood, perception, orientation or memory that grossly impairs judgment, behavior, capacity to recognize reality or ability to meet the ordinary demands of life, and mental conditions associated with the abuse of alcohol and drugs but does not include mental retardation which is a condition of arrested or incomplete development of mind of a person, specially characterized by subnormality of intelligence.
- The Act is applicable to all mental health establishments, including those established by practitioners of alternative, complementary medicines, as well as AYUSH (Ayurveda, Yoga and naturopathy, Unani, Siddha, and Homeopathy) and units established by the central and state governments.
- The Act presupposes that the person with mental illness (PMI) has the capacity to make decisions regarding his mental healthcare. It therefore distinguishes between medical and legal insanity.
- The Act authorizes the PMI to make an Advance Directive (AD) signifying not only the way he would like to be treated but also specifying what forms of intervention which may not be used to manage him. The PMI may also specify the healthcare facility where he would

like to be managed. The PMI may also specify Nominated Representative (NR) who is authorized to take decisions regarding the care of the PMI in case the PMI is unable to take the decisions. The AD is to be maintained online by the Board and made available to the mental healthcare professional. The AD may be cancelled, revoked, or amended by the person who made it at any time.

- The AD is not applicable to emergency treatment. In case a mental health professional desires not to follow the AD, he has applied to the concerned board for reviewing, altering, or modifying the AD. The Central Authority is to review the AD periodically. The medical professional is indemnified of the consequences of following a valid AD.
- An adult PMI can appoint a NR, who is responsible for taking healthcare decisions on behalf of the PMI, when the PMI is unable to do so. The NR is responsible for providing support, is involved in discharge planning and authorizing inpatient care during emergencies, and ensures that the rights of PMI are not violated.
- The Act obliges the State to provide mental healthcare for PMI. The appropriate government is to ensure facilities for the same, without discrimination. The Act stresses on community care of the PMI, rather than institutional care, and has provisions to prevent the PMI from suffering inhuman practices. The Act permits visitors and telephone calls and allows the PMI to seek legal aid.
- The PMI or his NR also has a right to know about the illness and the proposed plan of treatment and discharge, as well as confidentiality regarding the same. The mental health professional may withhold the disclosure of records in case he feels that the information may cause serious harm to the PMI and to other persons.
- The State is mandated to initiate preventive and educative programs and take measures for resource development, training, and coordination. The State is also to establish and ensure the functioning and the roles of the Central and State Mental Health Authorities.
- All mental health establishments need to be registered with the Central or State Mental Health authorities, depending upon which government controls the establishment. The Act lays down the procedure and fees for the same.
- The Act contains provisos for establishment of mental health review boards which are authorized to adjudicate complaints from PMI or NR or a nongovernmental organization (NGO) who may be aggrieved by a decision of any mental health establishment.
- The Act classifies adult admissions as independent and with high support needs. The latter is limited to 30 days. For admissions beyond 30 days, or readmission within 7 days of discharge, the Act has built-in safeguards. The maximum duration of admission for a readmission is 180 days, with the concurrence of the concerned mental health board.
- Admission for emergency treatment under the Act is limited to 72 hours, and the mental health professional is barred from administering electroconvulsive therapy or any other intervention not directly related to the emergency.
- The list of prohibited procedures includes unmodified electroconvulsive therapy (ECT), ECT for minors (without permission of the Board), sterilization, chaining, and psychosurgery. The PMI is not to be subjected to seclusion or restraints except in specified circumstances.
- The Act regulates research, specifies the responsibilities of police while dealing with the wandering/homeless PMI, as well as any PMI whom the police have reason to believe has been mistreated.

- A magistrate is empowered to transfer a person suspected of having a mental illness or a PMI to the nearest mental health establishment for assessment. The PMI or a person suspected of having a mental illness can also be admitted for up to 10 days to enable the medical officer or mental health professional in charge of the mental health establishment to carry out an assessment of the person and to plan for necessary treatment, if any.
- The question of any person suffering from a mental illness is alleged during a judicial process, the same shall be referred to the concerned board for an opinion. Mental health professionals and medical practitioners are barred from cross pathy.
- The Act prescribes monetary penalties as well as imprisonment for up to 2 years for infringements. The Act has liberal timelines for admission in respect of persons residing in the north-eastern states, as well as states of Uttarakhand, Himachal Pradesh, and the union territory of Jammu and Kashmir, as well as the island territories.
- The Act presupposes severe stress as a precursor to attempted suicide and bars any proceedings against the person under Section 309 of the Indian Penal Code. Rather, the Act enjoins the state to provide care, treatment, and rehabilitation to a person so as to reduce the risk of recurrence.
- The Act has an overriding effect on all other Acts or instruments in force. The rule flows from the maxim "*generalia specialibus non derogant*" which is a settled principle of law. It means that when two statutes appear to be contradicting each other, the provisions of a specific law override that of the general Act.

Compared to its predecessors, MHCA, 2017, is indeed a breath of fresh air as far as intentions are concerned. The objectives of the Act are indeed noble as they empower the PMI, prevent them from exploitation and inhumane treatment, and make the State responsible for providing mental health services to the PMI. The Act precludes cross pathy and regulates the establishment and management of mental health establishments. By encouraging community care, the Act aims to integrate PMI in the society.

ARE THERE SOME INADEQUACIES/LIMITATIONS IN THE ACT

The Act is in synch with the UNCRPD as well as the legislation of developed countries across the globe.

Therein lies the flaw of the Act. The Act ignores the prevailing societal norms of our nation. India is a country where the stigma associated with mental illness is rampant. The pathway to definitive care for a PMI often is long and arduous, and in most occasions, one that never reaches the destination.

A PMI and his family members usually consult practitioners of alternate and complimentary medicine and then various medical and surgical specialties before he is finally sent to the psychiatrist as the last resort.

The Act, by presupposing capacity to every PMI, equates mental ailments with physical ailments. However, it is a fact that a significant number of PMI is not competent as a result of their altered sense of reality to understand the consequences of their decisions. It is also a fact that in a country such as India, where the governmental healthcare facilities are overwhelmed with sheer numbers of patients, it is not humanely possible for the medical practitioners to devote time and energy to provide adequate information to patients. This negates the very basis of informed consent.

The concept of NR for PMI is a novel concept but is again fraught with difficulties. The Act bestows the NR with adequate knowledge and neutrality to be able to take a dispassionate decision in the best interest of the PMI. The same may not hold true in all cases at all times.

In the absence of funds to operationalize the community aspects of the Act, it is not clear as to how the noble ideals of management in the least restrictive setting would be achieved. Even after a sufficient duration since the passage of the Act, the Central Mental Health Authority is yet to be established and not all states have constituted the State Mental Health Authority. In the absence of definitive fund allocation, it is not clear as to how the State shall discharge its obligations toward the homeless and the poor, mentally ill persons.

The review boards are also conspicuous by their absence. It is not clear as to how the functions of the board are to be carried out till the time the boards are constituted.

It is a proven fact that ECT is the most effective modality of treatment in various psychiatric emergencies. The directive to bar ECT as an emergency treatment flies in the face of scientific evidence.

The decriminalizing of attempts at suicide is indeed noble. However, the scourge of dowry deaths, horror killings, and other societal evils, where murder is often labeled as suicide may be provided with a modicum of relief by the Act.

The disposal of property, rights of inheritance, divorce and guardianship related to the PMI are conspicuous by their absence. The Act is ambiguous about mental disorders arising as a result of substance abuse and intoxication. There is no mention of personality disorders in the Act. Termination of pregnancy is not mentioned in the Act.

The Act has shades of the developed nations' notions of autonomy and human rights. It places the patient first and gives enormous rights to the PMI and his family members. However, the Act appears to cast the mental healthcare professionals as violators of law and seeks to regulate evaluation, admission, and intervention, which is indeed unfortunate.

CONCLUSION

The Acts is both transformational and aspirational. There is, however, a need to adapt this revolutionary step to the prevailing social conditions of the country and more in tune with the socioeconomic and cultural milieu. The Act may be considered a benchmark which needs to be achieved by environmental and societal manipulation. However, the process would require capacity building, training, allocation of human and financial resources, as well as sensitization of the stake holders, which includes the executive, judiciary, and the bureaucracy.

CASE LAWS

- Accused X vs. State of Maharashtra Criminal Appellate Jurisdiction Review Petition (Criminal) No. 301 of 2008 in Criminal Appeal No. 680 of 2007
- Gaurav Kumar Bansal vs. Union of India WP (C) No.001496/2018
- Pushpa M Rawtani vs. Madhya Pradesh SC Order CRLMP No(s). 8154-8155/2017
- Suchita Srivastava vs. Chandigarh Administration AIR 2010 SC 235

KEY LEARNING POINTS

- The evolution of laws related to the treatment of the mentally ill reflects the attitudes of the society toward these patients.
- The laws have gradually moved from institutionalized care to patient autonomy and care in the community rather than asylum-based treatment.
- Besides the psychiatrists, the patient themselves, their caregivers, and civil society have been provided a role in management and treatment of the mentally ill.

BIBLIOGRAPHY

1. Behere Prakash B, Rathod Anupam V, Behere Aniruddh P. A Journey from Indian Lunacy Act 1912 to Indian Mental Health Act 1987 & Draft Amendment. Indian J Forensic Med Pathol. 2010;3(4).
2. Bhattacharyya A. (2013). Indian Insanes: Lunacy in the 'Native' Asylums of Colonial India, 1858-1912. [online] Available from https://core.ac.uk/reader/28945160 [Last accessed September, 2024].
3. Duffy RM, Kelly BD. Concordance of the Indian Mental Healthcare Act 2017 with the World Health Organization's Checklist on Mental Health Legislation. Int J Ment Health Syst. 2017;11:48.
4. Indian Mental Health Act, 1987 (Act 14 of 1987).
5. Mental Healthcare Act, 2017 (Act 10 of 2017).
6. Ranganathan G. Mental Healthcare Act, 2017: An Evaluation. NLUJ LR. 2017;59.
7. Somasundaram O. The Indian Lunacy Act, 1912. The historic background. Indian J Psychiatry. 1987;29(1): 3-14.
8. The Mental Healthcare (Central Mental Health Authority) Rules, 2018.
9. The Mental Healthcare (State Mental Health Authority) Rules, 2018.
10. United Nations Convention on the Rights of Persons with Disabilities, 2006.

SECTION

5

Miscellaneous

Section Editors: Atul Bhargava, Dnyanesh DK, Rohini Deshpande

Section Outline

37

CHAPTER

Legal Issues in Immunization

Kritika Tiwari, Satish Tiwari

INTRODUCTION

We are living in an era where health is considered as one of the basic necessities of the human life. In fact, health is guaranteed as one of the fundamental rights in the constitution of the nation. This does not include only rights to life but also quality of life. Though we claim that we are living in a modernized era, most of the world inhabitants are still exposed to age old infectious disease-related illnesses, which result in significant mortality and morbidity. It is said that an ounce of prevention is better than pound of treatment. Immunization is one of the most cost-effective ways of protection from the infectious diseases. Vaccination is supposed to be a "*magic bullet*" of medical science against many communicable diseases, which are to be stored at normally 2°–8°C. Some are stored at –15° to –50°C.

WHETHER TO IMMUNIZE OR NOT

Though we are living in the third millennium, there are many misconceptions related to infectious diseases/immunization. As the modern medicine is developing and becoming evidence based, many newer side effects associated with drugs or vaccines are becoming more and more obvious. Access to internet has added fuel to the fire. Many parents now question the authenticity and side effects associated with modern drugs/vaccines. Even some of the modern medicine graduates are now discussing the need of the vaccines (especially as multinationals are coming out with newer and newer vaccines). Thus, there is obvious "*Cleavage of opinion*" and different schools of thoughts regarding immunization. Many of us also believe that the population in developing nations is being used as "guinea pigs" for these "*under trial vaccines*."

The aim of immunization is to protect the children against various communicable diseases so as to improve the quality of life and to prevent long-term morbidity and mortality. This raises the issues that whether all the vaccines, those are available in market, shall be administered to each and every child or there shall be selection bias.

COMPULSORY IMMUNIZATION

The compulsory vaccines are those which must be administered to all the children irrespective of their needs, affordability, socioeconomic status, etc. Most of the government schedules do not include these vaccines [such as measles-mumps-rubella (MMR) and typhoid] and this raises the very important issue that what about those children who are economically deprived. Should they be allowed to suffer only because of paucity of funds? Whether we want to run these programs for "classes or masses?" *Can we nationalize the healthcare and immunization services?*

OPTIONAL IMMUNIZATION

Another issue is to have the choice of the parents and immunize the children as per the options available with the parents. This in fact is based on the principle of "informed consent." Both transparency of policies and close engagement with communities are imperatives for maintaining trust. We are in the era of judicial activism and as per the present thinking, it is the right of the child or parent to take their own decisions after getting proper information.

NEED OF THE INDIVIDUAL

While selecting the vaccines, of course, we have to keep in mind the need of the individual, the disease to which he is going to be exposed or already exposed, the economic background of the family, etc. The treatment costs of serious illnesses pull many families below poverty line; hence, disease prevention is also poverty alleviation.

The term "child abuse" refers to any act or failure to act that violates the right of the child that endangers his or her optimal health, survival or development, and the failure of child's caretaker to provide adequate food, clothing, shelter, supervision, and medical care. So, does it amount to child abuse or neglect if a parent or family cannot immunize their children as per the recommendations. Should this lead to punishment to the child or parents? Will such action amount to violation of human rights under Article 21 of the constitution?

NEED OF THE COMMUNITY

Some diseases may be more prevalent in particular community or society. This will also depend on the "herd immunity." The individual's choice (whether to vaccinate or not to vaccinate) has an impact on community and successful vaccination requires families to be proactive rather than reactive. Therefore, immunization requires higher level of motivation among families and communities and this can be achieved through health education and proper information. It has been found that there are considerable inequities in childhood vaccination based on child's gender, birth order, area of residence, education of parents, religion, caste, access to healthcare, etc.

NEED OF THE COUNTRY

Similarly, the needs of the countries may also vary. The factors that will determine the need of the countries include epidemiology, transmission pattern, efficacy, safety profile, and cost-effectiveness, etc. Immunization against such diseases will be on priority list of that specific country. In order to achieve high routine immunization rates, there should be innovative methods, proper monitoring, improving operational efficiency, "reaching every community," adverse events following immunization (AEFI) monitoring, and post marketing surveillance. The full benefits of immunization should be extended to all people, regardless of where they are born, who they are, or where they live. In a situation where there is abundance of new and expensive vaccines on one hand and limitations of resources on the other, it becomes imperative that use of vaccines through government programs as well as in free market is done through a decision-making which confers positive health and economic benefits to society.

NEED OF THE WORLD

Though the immunization or healthcare is the program or agenda of the individual country depending upon their needs, infrastructure, policies, and financial situation, we should not forget that we are living in the era of globalization. Because of the international mobility and movement of population, each and every part of the world is under the fear of disease transmission and outbreak of an epidemic due to lack of proper measures of quarantine or disease control. An entry of a single infected individual can create havoc on the fertile virgin land of country where the particular infection may not be prevalent or known for many years. Hence, the international exposure has to be kept in mind before deciding the immunization needs of the world.

The coronavirus disease 2019 (COVID-19) pandemic was very distressing for the human race. Many vaccines were introduced by many countries during this pandemic. But unfortunately, there are lots of controversies and doubts regarding the dose, duration of protection, untoward side effects, and overall efficacy of different corona vaccines.

AGE OF IMMUNIZATION

Though immunization is the one of the most cost-effective ways of preventing the various infectious diseases, there is lot of discussion regarding age of vaccination and duration or interval between two vaccines, especially the live ones. It is agreed that the baby's immune system is best developed after 3 months of age, but many vaccines may be injected at an earlier age because of genuine practical difficulties. The ideal time for giving Bacillus Calmette–Guérin (BCG) may not be at birth, but still it is given usually before the discharge of patient. Similarly, the ideal interval between two doses of most of the vaccines is 6–8 weeks, but we have to inject diphtheria, pertussis, and tetanus (DPT) (now Penta), polio, hepatitis B, etc. at the fixed interval of 4 weeks. Can we think of deviating from the World Health Organization (WHO) recommended 6, 10, and 14 weeks' schedule and consider the sounder and more appropriate 2, 4, and 6 months' schedule? Thus, there are lots of ifs and buts regarding interval between these vaccines. Alternatively, ***a newer schedule*** Penta + Rota vaccine can be given at 6, 14, and 22 weeks and pneumococcal + inactivated polio vaccine (IPV) + oral polio vaccine (OPV) can be given at 10, 18, and 26 weeks. This will have immunological superior response (meaning better protection) and better follow-up for nutritional advice and growth monitoring and it will also help to reduce the large gap and hence the dropout rates.

The needs and trends in adolescent age need lots of discussion as the epidemiological shift for many infections has been altered due to immunization practices in childhood.

HISTORY TAKING

The history, especially that of adverse reactions, is very important as it may decide whether to inject a particular vaccine or not. History of allergy to the components or ingredients of vaccine is also vital to prevent severe reactions during or after vaccination. In cases of vaccine-related encephalopathy, shock, etc., relatives shall be informed of possible complications (written consent is preferred). Proper history of any previous complications must be recorded in writing, for example, before giving DPT/Penta vaccine, take history of any neurological complications, existing neurological deficits, excessive irritability with previous dose, etc. In *Tapankumar Nayak vs. State of Odisha II (1997) CPJ 14 NC*, a child developed severe reaction and brain damage after a triple vaccine. No other child suffered such complications. The National Commission, while confirming the order passed by Odisha State Commission that there was no scope for awarding relief to the complainant under the Consumer Protection (CP) Act, strongly recommended to the State Government to render all possible assistance in proper rehabilitation of the child.

It is also important to record the history of any immunosuppressive disorder or drug which the child may be having as this may alter the schedule or some of the vaccines may be contraindicated.

CONSENT

In the present era of technical advances, especially with availability of information on internet or websites, it is important that basic information related to immunization should be given to the parents or relatives. Judiciary and various courts are also of the opinion that health is the fundamental right of an individual including the right of refusal for trial or treatment. Hence, an informed consent may be considered as one of the prerequisites before vaccinating a child. An informed consent in relation to immunization may include information regarding need of the vaccine, its cost, what the consequences are of not taking a particular vaccine, and also the known adverse effects (a model consent form is attached in the form of appendix). It is also important to inform that in some cases, disease can result even after successful vaccination. The Center for Disease Control and Prevention (CDC) requires that even the vaccination information statements (VIS) should be given to parents in advance. At present, there is no such law in India, but remember that most of us including judiciary/government are following western countries.

DOCUMENTATION

An informed consent is not only a prerequisite, but it is important to document it, preferably in writing. It is equally important to document a *"negative consent"* if the relatives are not willing to take some vaccines for the reasons of costs or adverse reactions. The documentation is also important because the parents or individual may need a certificate at the time of travel or school admissions in the future life.

It is a well-known fact that a natural infection of typhoid may not induce lifelong immunity. Hence, a child recovering from typhoid shall be advised vaccination 6–8 weeks after the discharge, not doing so may amount to negligence on the part of treating pediatrician.

SIDE EFFECTS

The various side effects shall be informed before vaccinating the child. It is advisable to inform common as well as remote adverse reactions. The adverse reactions associated with vaccines shall also be reported to government or state agencies assigned with investigating this aspect of immunization. Various adverse reactions must be diagnosed and treated within proper and adequate time to avoid allegations of deficiency or negligence. Oxygen, adrenaline, intravenous (IV) fluids, and steroids shall be available in case reaction occurs. Various facilities needed to tackle or manage such adverse reactions shall be available in the hospital in case need arises.

The use of Rota vaccine by GlaxoSmithKline (GSK) was temporarily suspended by the United States Food and Drug Administration (US FDA) on the issue of contamination of the vaccine with porcine circovirus type-1. But after reviewing the details, it was finalized that at present, there is no need to modify the recommendations as there was no definite threat to the children. The rotavirus vaccine was also found to be associated with increased risk of intussusceptions for a short period of first dose in some of the population. After reviewing the recent data in India, it has been concluded that there is definite albeit a small risk of acute intussusception. The committee urges the manufacturers to actively monitor this risk as the usage of this vaccine is bound to go up.

The Government of India had to suspend two studies on human papillomavirus (HPV) vaccine on account of alleged deaths, sending alarm signals to all the concerned. All these will require strengthening of AEFI surveillance in the country.

EXPIRY DATE VACCINES

Sometimes, an expiry date vaccine may be administered inadvertently. Hence, it is important to be careful in preventing this medical error. One of the simplest ways to prevent this is to follow the principle of "*First in: First out*," i.e., the vial which goes first in refrigerator shall be used first for vaccination. If error has occurred, it is better to accept it as most of the times expiry date vaccine may not cause any major adverse reaction or side effects. One of the problems with expiry date vaccine may be that it has lost its potency. This deficiency can be easily solved or corrected by giving an extra dose, may be free of cost.

WHAT AMOUNTS TO NEGLIGENCE?

Medical negligence in vaccination can be alleged if there is deficiency or damage because an act of commission or omission is associated with the process of immunization. Sometimes, a wrong drug may be administered because of similar packing, size, shape, or color of the ampoule or vials. This can be easily prevented by remaining more vigilant or using separate fridge for vaccines and other medicines in the hospital. Hence, we shall take all the precautions in order to avoid any such deficiencies or allegations.

VICARIOUS LIABILITY

Vicarious liability involves the acts of staff members, partners, locum, etc. in different situations. Vaccine sometimes may be administered by politicians, celebrities, government officials, or social workers, especially during camps or immunization programs. The issue is can they do this? If yes, then whether it should be under the supervision of a qualified medical graduate or even in the absence of qualified staff? If any adverse reaction occurs, who shall be held responsible? All these issues need discussion and clarification.

IS IMMUNIZATION CROSSPATHY?

The vaccines are very commonly administered even by Ayurvedic or homeopathic graduates. It is often noticed that various vaccination camps are organized by these graduates as a fund-generating activity. Hence, if the vaccines are considered as a part of modern medicine, all such camps become part of cross pathy for those who are not trained in modern medicine. The fact is vaccines are a unique class of pharmaceutical products that meet the statutory definition of both a drug and biological products. By definition, it is a biological agent.

WHO IS RESPONSIBLE FOR INADEQUATE PROTECTION?

If a serological correlates of protection are not known for a vaccine, one has no choice but to conduct a field efficacy trials to prove noninferiority compared with the existing licensed vaccine, example of such vaccine being pertussis vaccine for which huge and expensive field efficacy trials were conducted by most manufacturers. The onus of conducting a scientific and authentic field efficacy trial lies on the manufacturer (that too before marketing), and not the doctors, the end users. The role of vaccine manufacturing industry is debated and always under scanner as far as their approach toward immunization is concerned. The need of vaccine, the way of promotion, the vaccine-related research, and various ethical issues are constantly debated. The outbreak of pertussis in some of the western countries needs lots of self-introspection, self-discipline, and soul-searching. The acellular pertussis vaccine was projected as superior, side effect-free magic remedy for the control of the whooping cough. But over time, it is now discussed that the DTaP vaccination was a risk factor for vaccine failure as compared to the traditional whole-cell vaccines. This means that the earlier trials of acellular vaccines were concocted, manipulated, and aimed at increasing the sales of the vaccine. The issue is who should be held responsible for these outbreaks and sufferings of the innocent children all over the world. Is it the manufacturers who promoted it in order to fill their *"ever-empty wallet,"* those academic organizations who without adequate evidence-based data supported these vaccines simply as a *"norm of reciprocity"* for the favors or kickbacks from vaccine industries, the modern age parents who wanted that their child should not have even slightest amount of discomfort associated with age old whole-cell vaccine or the policy makers who badly failed in their responsibility?

SOME SPECIFIC ISSUES RELATED TO IMMUNIZATION

Immunization during Travel

Travel, *especially people migrating internationally*, may result in exposure to many newer microorganisms worldwide. Because of this, there is need for strict vigilance and measures to control the spread of infections. Though this has the international significance, the needs may be country specific. There may be need for specific or special schedules or extra doses of particular vaccine depending upon the disease prevalence or herd immunity.

Specific Diseases (Sickle Cell and Thalassemia)

Some diseases may alter the body immune response depending upon the various changes in body or immune-regulating system. Nowadays, there are many programs for the benefit of children suffering from specific illnesses. There is need to provide special vaccination schedules to those who are prone to various infections but are economically deprived to afford costly vaccines.

Preterm/Small-for-dates

There are also lots of discussions regarding the child's gestation and the weight at the time of vaccination. Both of these parameters can affect the take-up of the vaccines and may ultimately decide the failure rates, effectiveness, or the protection levels. This will also decide the need for extra doses or secondary vaccination. Sometimes, we also have to consider the other options such as immunoglobulins or passive vaccination if active immunization is not possible due to extreme prematurity or low birth weight.

Immunosuppressive Disorders

Children suffering from immunosuppressive disorders may need modification in their vaccination schedule. Some of the live vaccines may be contraindicated while some vaccines can be given depending upon the severity of immunosuppression. Thus, it may need specific discussion and evidence-based approach in such a situation. If an immune-compromised child develops vaccine-associated paralytic poliomyelitis (VAPP), does it amount to medical negligence or it is an unexpected outcome? This issue needs discussion and debate.

Immunosuppressive Medicines

Similar situation may arise if the child is on immunosuppressive drugs. The schedule may need modification or temporary withdrawal of vaccines till the child is receiving such medicines.

Epidemics (Polio, Flu, and Cholera)

If there are epidemics in the community, the needs of individual or community may change. This may generate lots of controversies and discussions regarding efficacy and availability of the vaccines. The introduction of injectable polio vaccine and discontinuation of oral polio vaccine is the latest example of this. Possibility of benefit versus vaccine-associated adverse reaction may also be debated during epidemics.

Fear of Epidemics *(Kumbh Mela)*

A fear of epidemics during Kumbh Mela, Haj pilgrimage, etc. also raises the issue of vaccination during such gatherings. Even a single infected individual can spread the infections to many other individuals who are not immune to a particular disease. Infections such as cholera, typhoid, and hepatitis A can cause havocs in such situations as these illnesses are waterborne. We have vaccines against all these diseases, so it raises pertinent issue that whether these vaccines must be made mandatory to all those who are going to attend such gatherings. Should the government or organizers give it free of cost? What about those innocent people who are exposed to these infections?

ETHICAL ISSUES IN IMMUNIZATION

The developing world is still reeling under the morbidity and mortality due to infectious diseases. Vaccination was introduced as an evidence-based program to check the spread of communicable diseases, but it seems that ultimately this is going to end in commercialization of health packages full of ethical and legal queries. The vaccination market is the latest example of ethical dilemmas in pediatrics. Do our children need all the vaccines? How many of us can afford the newer and newer vaccines? Should we use them at the cost of nutrition, education, or other basic necessities of life? All these questions need a genuine and scientific discussion.

One of the world's largest drugs and vaccine manufacturing company (GSK) was ordered to pay $3 billion in the largest healthcare fraud settlement in the US history for its use of kickbacks, misbranding, and other misconduct to market drugs. The agreement is the largest healthcare fraud settlement which is "unprecedented in both size and scope," in history, spanning nearly every state, according to the Justice Department. The British company illegally marketed the drug, even sponsoring dinners and spa programs in the drug's name. Glaxo also used sham advisory boards and speakers at lavish resorts to promote the drug. The government also accused GSK of offering kickbacks to medical professionals, dangling cash, trips to Florida, and tickets to basketball games as an incentive. GSK was accused of withholding important safety information about the drug and illegally promoting drugs for unapproved uses. The goal was a culture of greed where patient safety took a back seat to profit and where drugs were promoted for disorders, though there was no medical evidence that these would help. There should be a limit to our dependence on pharmaceutical companies. Are we willing to sweep under the carpet serious ethical misadventures by accepting statements of inadvertent errors and apology issued by the industry? There must be a "*code of conduct*" on which the academia–industry relationship must subsist.

IMMUNIZATION CERTIFICATE

The immunization certificate may be a legal necessity during international travel. A certificate of appropriate corona immunization was mandatory during the COVID-19 pandemic. It is also accepted that immunization shall be made mandatory before the entry of individual in a school. All these will need a valid certificate from a competent authority. There is every possibility that a false certificate may be issued on many occasions. It is preferable that a fake or false certificate should not be issued as an unimmunized person may cause outbreak of an epidemic in the community. The better option in such a situation shall be to immunize the child with some of the vaccines and issue certificate for the same with the note that the remaining doses can be taken subsequently. Later on, the honorable Supreme Court upheld both right of individual against forcible vaccination and the government's current vaccination to protect communitarian health.

CONCLUSION

Adequate immunization is one of the most important preventive health services that can be provided to children, particularly from the poor and marginalized communities. The role of immunization in preventing diseases has been time-tested, and it is important that science prevails over misguidance. Now is the time to seize this momentum and commit to achieve immunization's full potential. There is need to have quality control in the manufacture, transport, and storage of vaccines. The government should take disease control seriously. Epidemiology, economics, and ethics demand that the policy makers and the health professionals should join hands to alleviate the misery caused by various diseases. There is need for a well-designed, ethical research regarding vaccines as they can prevent many diseases, thus decreasing the financial burden on family, exchequer, government, and policymakers. There must be extensive research before recommending any vaccines for community because if the vaccine is not cost-effective or there are major side effects, the entire planning will get defeated. Immunization is, and should be recognized as, a core component of the human right to health and a personal and collective ethical, legal, and moral responsibility. There is need to understand the various legal issues related to this aspect, otherwise many allegations may be leveled if we fail in controlling the vaccine-preventable diseases. There is a need for the medical graduates to keep themselves updated with the recent advances in the field of immunization. The physicians or doctors should have clear conscious and do right things so that the future generation can live a healthy life.

KEY LEARNING POINTS

- Vaccination can be one of the cost-effective measures to prevent infections.
- Immunization schedule shall be made depending upon the need of the individual, community, and the country.
- The schedule can be modified keeping in mind the risk factors or chances of epidemics.
- Inform the side effects to appropriate authorities.
- Do not issue false certificate for vaccination.

BIBLIOGRAPHY

1. Baldwa M, Tiwari S. Punishment for refusing OPV. Indian Pediatr. 2009;46:540-1.
2. Berman P, Ahuja R, Bhandari R. The impoverishing effects of health care payments in India: New methodology and findings. EPW. 2010;45:65-71.
3. Centers for Disease Control and Prevention (CDC). (2023). Vaccines and Immunizations: Current VISs. [online] Available from http://www.cdc.gov/vaccines/pubs/vis/default.htm [Last accessed September, 2024].
4. Cherry JD. Comparative efficacy of acellular pertussis vaccines: an analysis of recent trials. Pediatr Infect Dis J. 1997;16:S90-6.
5. Choudhury P, Jacob John T. Human Papilloma virus vaccine and current controversy. Indian Pediatr. 2010;47:724-5.
6. Gupta P, Vashishtha V. The game industry plays. Indian Pediatr. 2012;49:699.
7. Indian Academy of Pediatrics Committee on Immunization (IAPCOI). Consensus recommendations on immunization and IAP immunization Timetable 2012. Indian Pediatr. 2012;49:549-64.
8. Jesani A, Johari V. Ethical and legal challenges of vaccines and vaccination: Reflections. Indian J Med Ethics. 2017;2(2):72-4.

9. Lavin J, Broutin H, Harvill ET, et al. Imperfect vaccine-induced immunity and whooping cough transmission to infants. Vaccine. 2010;29:11-6.
10. Mathew JL. Inequity in childhood immunization in India: A Systematic review. Indian Pediatr. 2012;49:203-23.
11. Mittal SK, Mathew JL. Expanded program of immunization in India: time to rethink and revamp. J Pediatr Sci. 2010;5:e43.
12. Nair MKC. Child abuse. Indian Pediatr. 2004;41:319-20.
13. Paul Y, Tiwari S. Ethical issues in Immunization. In: Vashishta VM, Kalra A (Eds). IAP Textbook of Vaccines, 2nd edition. New Delhi: Jaypee Brothers Medical Publishers (P) Ltd.; 2020. pp. 819-23.
14. Paul Y. Medical Negligence & Vaccine associated Paralytic poliomyelitis: Indian Pediatr. 2001;38:1068-9.
15. Shah N. Indian Vi conjugate typhoid vaccine: Misleading claims. Indian Pediatr. 2010;47:447.
16. Singh MP. Fundamental Rights. The Constitution of India, 1st edition. New Delhi, Delhi: Law House; 1999. pp. 8-47.
17. Tiwari S, Tiwari K. Legal Issues in Immunization. In: Tiwari S, Baldwa M, Tiwari M, et al. (Eds). Textbook on Medicolegal Issues Related to Various Medical Specialties, 2nd edition. New Delhi: Jaypee Brothers Medical Publishers; 2019. pp. 461-9.
18. Tiwari S. Consumer Problems & the Pediatrician. In: Suraj G (Ed). Recent Advances in Pediatrics-19: Hot Topics. New Delhi: Jaypee Brothers Medical Publishers (P) Ltd.; 2010. pp. 72-84.
19. Tiwari S. Legal and Ethical issues in immunization. Indian J Pract Pediatr. 2021;23(1):48-52.
20. Tiwari S. Legal issues related to vaccinology today. In: Vashishta VM, Kalra A (Eds). IAP Textbook of Vaccines, 2nd edition. New Delhi: Jaypee Brothers Medical Publishers (P) Ltd.; 2020. pp. 810-8.
21. Tiwari S. Medical Ethics: Are we going in right direction? Mathur GP, Mathur S (Eds). Current Trend in Pediatrics, Volume 2, 1st edition. Delhi: Academa Publishers; 2006. pp. 67-71.
22. Varma S. (2012). Unfair practices: Pharma companies fined $13bn in 4 years. [online] Available from https://timesofindia.indiatimes.com/business/international-business/unfair-practices-pharma-companies-fined-13bn-in-4-years/articleshow/14972186.cms [Last accessed September, 2024].
23. Vashishtha VM. Status of immunization and need for intensification of routine immunization in India. Indian Pediatr. 2012;49:357-61.
24. World Health Organization. Rotavirus vaccine and intussusception: report from an expert consultation. Weekly Epidemiol Rec. 2011;86:317-24.
25. Yewale V, Choudhury P. Rota virus vaccine contamination with PCV 1. Indian Pediatr. 2010;47:589-91.

CHAPTER 38

Legal Issues in Junk Food

Ashish Jain, Neetu Jain

INTRODUCTION

Childhood is the most important period of growth and development of an individual. Healthy nutritional practices are of paramount importance at this time. Changing food habits and replacement of nutritious food with unhealthy junk food which is high in sugar, salt and fat content is leading to problems like childhood obesity, etc. Junk food consumption is increasing steeply, both in urban and rural areas. The ease of availability, taste, low cost for small packs, peer pressure and aggressive marketing strategies is making it popular with children and adolescents. As television and internet is reaching the remotest areas, so is junk food. Children watch television where fast food advertisements are rampant, leading to change in their food behavior. As a consequence, junk food is replacing traditional food items in daily life both because of convenience and taste. According to the National Institute of Nutrition (NIN) dietary guidelines, "the shift from traditional to 'modern' foods, changing cooking practices, increased intake of processed and ready-to-eat foods and intensive marketing of junk foods and 'health' beverages have affected people's perception of foods as well as their dietary behavior". Irrational preference for energy-dense foods and those with high sugar and salt content pose a serious health risk to the people, especially children. Moreover, children are unaware of effect of junk food on their growth and development and are unable to make educated choices.These practices have led to increasing number of overweight and obese people in the community. The consequent burdens of chronic noncommunicable diseases necessitate systematic nutrition and educational interventions on a massive scale.

The salt, sugar and fat content of the food items needs to be regulated. Junk food is not standardized in Indian regulations. This comes under category of foods which should declare their composition and comply under general regulation of Food Safety and Standards Act of India (FSSAI) **(Box 38.1)**. Regulations are needed on marketing and availability of junk food, especially where it can influence food choices of children. The society as a whole needs to understand the implications of junk food and associated legal issues.

WHAT IS JUNK FOOD?

There is broad concept of "Unsafe Foods" whose nature, substance or quality is affected so as to render it injurious to health. These also include those food items which are misbranded

Box 38.1: Food guidelines for schools in india (FSS ACT, 2006).

- Identify foods high in fat, salt, and sugar
- Restrict/limit availability of the following food items in schools and 50 meters nearby; chips, fried food, carbonated/noncarbonated sugar beverages, ready to eat noodles, pizzas, burgers, potato fries and confectionary items
- List food items needing regulation such as *samosa, chana bhatura*, etc.
- Implement a canteen policy based on color coding
- Green category (Healthy) foods-should constitute 80% of available foods
- Red category (unhealthy) foods-shouldn't be sold or served in schools

or promoted with false and misleading claims. Junk foods lie in the category of these unsafe foods. As per the NIN, *"Unhealthy (junk) foods are those containing little or no proteins, vitamins or minerals but are rich in salt, sugar, fats and are high in energy (calories)."* Globally, foods with similar attributes in different regions are also termed as foods "High in Fat, Salt and Sugar", (HFSS), "Foods of Minimal Nutritional Value" (FMNV) or "Energy-Dense Low-Nutrient Density Foods" or "Energy Dense and Nutrient Poor Foods for Children" (EDLNF or EDNPFC). Fast foods are rapidly prepared and quickly served in a packaged form. The terms junk and fast foods are interchangeably used frequently.

Examples of junk foods are fast foods (pizza, burger, noodles, pasta, chips, etc.), soft drink (coke, pepsi, etc.) and snacks (biscuits, chocolates, doughnuts, etc.).

Processed Foods

These are defined as "foods that are subjected to technological modifications either for preservation or for converting into ready to use/eat foods, eliminating laborious household procedures".

Why should Junk Food be Regulated?

As per WHO, there is a strong association between consumption of this food and non-communicable diseases (NCDs) like diabetes, hypertension and heart diseases and cancer. Junk food consumption is considered leading cause of childhood obesity which is one of the most critical public health problems especially among children and adolescents today. A recent report has suggested that the mothers who consumed junk food during pregnancy are more likely to have children who are more prone to obesity and other NCDs like diabetes and hypertension.

Despite, harmful effects of junk food, one can argue that people can make their own choices and there is no real need for legal regulation. This case scenario is same as what was presented by the tobacco lobby against legal regulation against cigarettes. Junk food marketing is primarily aimed at the population which is not equipped to make choices, the most important of them are children.

Children are not the best judges of their food choices. They have a limited understanding about the impact of food on their health and can easily be influenced especially through various modes of media. Broadly, they are not aware about the concept of balanced diet and what kind of food is to be consumed or avoided. They also lack the required know-how on diseases and their relation to diet. Despite this, they are being aggressively targeted by food marketing. They are one of the biggest viewer groups of television, and food advertisements constitute a major share of overall TV, radio and print advertisements across the world. Big food and drink companies are not only bombarding children with junk food advertising and sophisticated marketing techniques but also creating brand loyalty in children that they will carry into adulthood. Only 2% of a food company's budget goes into research and development against 50% into advertising. Also, today's children have more autonomy and they play a vital role in buying of any good or service in the market. "Pester Power" refers to children's ability to nag their parents into purchasing item they may not otherwise buy. Though we can educate children but it can be done to a limited extent only, hence, it is important to regulate marketing of junk food.

All the junk food companies target schools to promote their product which should be discouraged. School is a place to learn the right values and constructive behavior for a lifetime. Since food consumption at school is a significant part of the overall daily diet, schools should not allow canteens to promote food habits that not only negatively impact the health of children but also inculcate life time habit of junk food consumption.

Finally, the benefits of balanced, fresh and traditional food cannot be replaced. Junk food is not standardized in Indian regulations. Such products are only expected to declare their nutritive value, contents and comply under the general guidelines of "Food Safety and Standards Act."

What is being Done at International Level?

In 2004 Global Strategy of WHO on diet, physical activity and health stated that "food advertising messages that encourage unhealthy dietary practices should be discouraged and the government should develop a multisectoral approach to address any such issues."

Later in 2012–2013, the WHO provided a framework for implementing the set of recommendations on the marketing of food and nonalcoholic beverages to children, and also acknowledged that marketing of food and beverage products that are high in fat, sugar and salt to children is recognized as an important cause of child obesity and diet-related NCDs. Several countries have adopted one or more of the following three approaches for regulating the exposure and availability of junk food to children.

- Ban availability in schools
- Regulate advertisement and promotion
- Impose taxes
- High-profile campaigns, where celebrities shun endorsement of this food and push for healthier options.

Ban on Junk Food in Schools

Several countries across the world have begun to regulate availability of junk food over a few years. Specific legislations have been adopted that are aimed to promote health of school children, and provide healthy and nutritious food. Measures adopted include:

- Formulating nutrition standards and criteria to help decide on foods to be allowed or banned
- Keeping school canteens, kiosks, and vending machines under purview of the ban
- Replacements with healthier traditional foods at most times.

Some of the legislations are:
- *Canada*: "School Food and Beverage Policy, 2010" under the "Healthy Food for School Act, 2008"
- *Peru*: "Promoting Healthy Food for Children Act", 2013
- *UAE*: "Guide of Health and Nutritional Practices of School Canteen", 2011
- *United States*: "Smart Snacks in Schools", nutrition standards for all foods sold in schools under the "Healthy, Hunger-Free Kids Act, 2010"
- *England*: "Nutritional Standards and Requirements for School Food"(England) Regulations, 2007

Restriction on Junk Food Advertisements and Marketing

Numerous studies and scientific evidence across the world reflecting the extent of impact of food and nonalcoholic beverages on children through advertisements and promotion, suggest that advertisements directly influence the majority of the eating and drinking preferences of children. They are exposed to the pervasive marketing of unhealthy food via advertisements on television, internet, social media, viral marketing, and endorsement through cartoon characters and celebrities. About 40% of the children are only aware of the selling and persuasive intent of advertisements at the age of 11–12 years. Taste and healthiness are reported as the most important factors in snack food choices, but when faced with the actual food choice, children aged 5–12 years, predominantly choose unhealthy foods. Children aged 4–6 years prefer foods having popular cartoon characters on the packaging. Overweight children especially aged 4–8 years are more likely to recognize fast food restaurant logos than other food logos.

Taxing Junk Food

Several countries have imposed or proposed taxes on various junk foods in order to limit the overall consumption of foods that are high in fats, sugar including carbonated beverages, energy drinks, sugar sweetened/flavored beverages, packaged sweets, ice creams, jams, salty snacks, chocolates, and food flavorings, etc. This measure makes "price" a limiting factor in consumption and adds to "revenues" that would contribute to public health expenditure. Popularly, these taxes have been named as "chips tax", "fat tax", and "soda tax", etc.

Regulation of Marketing

The Dilemma: Self Regulation or Mandatory Government Regulations

There are contrasting views among industry experts on whether there should be self or government regulations in controlling unhealthy food practices.

Self Regulation

Large food companies participate in a variety of voluntary initiatives at global, regional and country levels like "The European Union (EU) Pledge" which was launched in 2007 by 11 leading food and beverage companies with an objective to change the way of advertising food and beverage over different forms of media (television, print, and internet) targeted at children. But these self regulatory initiatives have their own limitations and non, performance has raised doubts over its effectiveness. It was later observed that, in countries like Germany, Australia, Canada, and Spain, children's exposure to food commercials has largely remained unaffected. In the US, adolescent exposure to food advertisements increased by over 20% during 2004–2011. Companies have their own selection criteria about foods that are not to be advertised, moreover, the self-made rules are narrow and limited. Furthermore, these regulations are either erratically monitored or weakly enforced.

Mandatory Control

This is a strategy in which certain regulations are legally enforced upon food companies and they are bound to follow them. Considering the nonperformance and bias issues of the companies, only laws could make advertising company stick to the desired norms.

Labeling in Junk Food

The WHO says that, "Providing accurate, standardized and comprehensive information on the content of food items is conducive to consumers making healthy choices." Various labeling practices such as *"Nutrition facts" labeling, "Front-of-pack" labeling* and *"Menu" labeling* are considered as global best practices.

"Nutrition Facts" Labeling

"Nutrition Facts" labeling is practiced in countries like the US and is becoming popular in other parts of the world. It is aimed at enabling informed dietary decisions by the consumers. These labels must provide complete information on the nutrient content, depicting serving size and nutrient information per serving as percentage of the daily value. The presentation should be standardized to limit confusion, promote easy understanding and should be based on recognized scientific criteria.

"Front-of-Pack" Labeling

It is a figurative representation of key information on the front of the pack (FoP) and is a useful labeling tool that complements at the labeling at the back of pack. Several FoP labeling initiatives are being practiced across the world like:

The "Traffic Light" System Practiced in the UK

It has a mandatory nutrition declaration at back of pack. Color coding—Green, Amber and Red is an additional expression in line with EU FIC (food information to consumers).

The "Keyhole" Sign in Countries such as Denmark, Sweden and Norway

It is a positive label that suggests fulfilling a certain criteria on dietary fiber, salt, sugar, fat and saturated fats. It indicates a healthier option to consumers.

"Menu" Labeling

It is proposed by the US Food and Drug Administration (USFDA). It refers to listing of calorie content and nutrients such as sodium, added sugar, trans fat, saturated fat, and protein, etc., displayed on menus, menu boards (including drive through menu boards), food wrappers, vending machines and containers of fast food outlets and restaurant chains.

Nutrient Profiling Models to Categorize Food

As per the WHO, "Nutrient profiling is a science of classifying or ranking foods according to their nutritional composition for reasons relating to preventing disease and promoting health." It helps to assess the quality of food with reference to levels of nutrients such as fats, sugar, salt, vitamins, minerals and dietary fiber. Several countries have developed their own models.

Nutrient Profile Model (FSA-Ofcom Model) of the UK (Table 38.1)

It has been developed to introduce broadcasting restrictions on advertisements of junk foods and encourage promotion of healthier alternatives. The model uses a simple scoring system wherein points are allocated on the basis of nutrient content of 100 g of a food or drink. Points are awarded in 2 categories; "A" nutrients (energy, saturated fat, total sugar and sodium), and "C" nutrients (fruit, vegetables and nut content, fiber and protein). Final Nutrient Profile Score = Score for "A" nutrients–Score for "C" nutrients. Foods scoring 4 or more points and drinks scoring 1 or more points, are classified as "less healthy" and are subject to controls on the advertising of foods to children.

Legal Status in India

In India, there exist no specific guidelines or laws that deal with regulation of advertising and marketing of junk food. The FSSAI has laid down science based standards for manufacture, storage, supply and distribution of food. It has various sections which include restriction on advertisements (section 24) and penalty for misleading advertisements (section 53) among many others. There are few other acts such as Food Adulteration Act 1994 and Cable

Table 38.1: Scores depicting unhealthy junk foods (as laid by CSE, based on Nutrient Profiling Model, UK).

Food item	*Cut-off score*	*Score*
Lays Potato Chips	4	14
Haldiram Aloo Bhujia	4	18
Maggi Noodles	4	19
McAloo Tikki Burger	4	7
Cadbury Dairy Milk Chocolate	4	24
Coca Cola	1	2
Pepsi	1	2
Slice	1	3
Maaza	1	2

Television Networks Act, 1995. NGO Uday Foundation, filed a PIL in Delhi High Court in the year 2010, which sought for an immediate ban on junk food in schools and in their vicinity. In Sept. 2013, the High Court ordered the government to set up a committee to frame guidelines for junk food in India. This Committee included—Top Officials from Center for Science and Environment (CSE), NIN, All India Food Processors association, National Restaurant Association of India and medical professionals. On 16th March 2015, Delhi High court ordered strict implementation of new guidelines by government body **(Box 38.1)**. While approving the guidelines, the court gave Centre and FSSAI, 3 months' time to convert these into law and start enforcing them.

What is Needed?

India needs a suitable national policy for regulation of unsafe foods/junk food with a system to monitor and evaluate it periodically. Such a policy should be able to avoid potential conflict of interests. It should strengthen international cooperation to decrease the impact of cross-border marketing.

What Regulations can be Enforced by Court of Law?

In India, as with rest of the world, issues are similar, so we feel; the remedy should be on same lines. The laws should be stringent and there should be penalties for noncompliance with the laws. India has a diverse heritage of various foods and the calorie and nutrient content especially that of fats depends upon the cooking methods adopted. Most of the Indian fast foods are prepared by deep frying in fats especially saturated and trans-fats. In our country the regulations should not be limited to the fast food giants but the Indian street food should be regulated as well **(Table 38.2)**. This can be a mammoth task as these foods are not even standardized and need a comprehensive review.

There is a big issue with "exaggerated health claims" with food marketing in India. The food regulatory agency has indicted several household brands, including Britannia biscuits, Complan and Horlicks health drinks and Kellogg's breakfast cereals, for misleading claims about some of their food products amounting to "puffery" which means to make exaggerated claims about the product, which cannot be proved. Food companies should be punished for pushing unhealthy food if they are unable to substantiate their claims. In this regard several such food companies were taken to task by FSSAI.

In June 2016, the FSSAI banned the use of potassium bromated as an additive after a study by the Centre for Science and Environment (CSE) said its presence in bread products could

Table 38.2: Common and nonstandardized Junk foods.

Most common junk foods	***Nonstandardized junk foods***
Chips, fried packaged foods and similar packaged food items	*Samosa*
Carbonated beverages	*Chhole bhature*
Sugar sweetened noncarbonated beverages	*Bread pakora*
Instant noodles	*Tikki, Chaat*
Potato fries, burgers	*Pav bhaji*
Confectionery items such as chocolates, candies, and gums, etc.	

cause cancer. Though, the use of potassium iodate—also claimed to be carcinogenic by the CSE study, was referred to a scientific panel for further investigations.

A very important agenda in Indian context is availability of junk food in and around schools. Cafeterias at the schools offer sodas, cold drinks, chips, samosa and many other foods which can be classified among junk foods **(Table 38.2)**. This should be discouraged and healthy food choices should be promoted **(Box 38.2)**. As per laws, no fast food should be available in the schools and within 200 m radius of schools.

Central Board of Secondary Education (CBSE) in 2016 came out with circular for promotion of healthy food in CBSE affiliated schools. The consumption of junk food is known to cause many diseases including dyslipidemia, chronic inflammation, type 2 diabetes, hypertension, and hyperinsulinemia with increased risk of cardiovascular diseases in future. Schools should ensure that there is no HFSS foods (such as chips, fried foods, noodles, pizzas, burgers, carbonated beverages, potato fries and items like, chocolates, candies, bread pakora, samosas, etc.) available in and around 200 m of the school canteens.

Now, in 2015 CBSE's ***"sugar board"*** mandate, is a starting point for integrating nutrition education into curriculum amid growing dietary and lifestyle concerns including type 2 diabetes, childhood obesity, and related comorbidities. The boards aim to visually represent how much sugar is present in commonly consumed junk foods, snacks or drinks, comparing it with the recommended daily intake. Cases of obesity and diabetes are rising among students due to wrong food habits hence there is need to increase awareness among children and helping them make healthier food choices. As per this CBSE initiative schools would need to install Sugar Boards, which are visually interactive display boards installed in the campuses countrywide to make students aware of the unfavorable effects of excessive sugar consumption.

As in UK there should be laws to make nutrition food labeling mandatory in India. Though studies have shown mixed results of practice of food labeling on calorie intake and food behavior, but it definitely makes consumer aware of choices they are making. Labeling issues were highlighted by Centre for Science (CSE) study, 2012. Many of the food items tested claimed to be free of trans fats, but the study showed otherwise. Some brands did not mention the nutrition information for a serving size. The serving size was not standardized; it varied between brands and also from country to country. There was no mention of the amount the ingredients contributed to the RDA. Nonpackaged junk food items such as burgers, fries and pizzas had their nutritional value and content on their respective websites which is of little or no value. The nutritional attributes of these food chains mentioned on websites also varied between different country regions and within the same country also.

Box 38.2: Healthy menu options.

Suggested healthy menu options:

- Fruit *salad*, fruits, *paneer*/vegetable cutlets
- *Khandvi*
- *Poha*
- *Uthapam*
- *Upma*
- *Idlis*

One of the most important issues is regulation of food advertisements on television, print media and internet, etc. that lure children toward unhealthy food habit of consuming junk food. In India, media advertisement and publicity is under the control of Ministry of Information and Broadcasting. Media rules and regulations are set under Indian Cable Television Network Act 1994 and Advertising Standard Council of India (ASCI). There is an urgent need to formulate guidelines for regulation of quality of food products advertised on television. There should be guidelines banning advertisement that promotes unhealthy food behavior on channels frequently viewed by children. The timing of such advertisement should also be regulated so that no such advertisement is displayed at the peak hours, when children viewership is high. There should be agencies to monitor exaggerated claims and unscientific ads should be banned. The companies which violate these laws should be punished with heavy penalties and should be boycotted. Sportsman and celebrities should be taken to task for promotion of unhealthy foods as happened in a recent case of a celebrity who was served a notice for promoting a leading noodle brand. Keeping the prevailing scenarios in notice, on June 29th 2016, food regulator FSSAI joined hands with the Advertising Standard Council of India (ASCI), the self regulatory body for the advertising industry, to check the misleading campaigns for food and beverages.

Is Law the Only Answer?

Laws are made for various issues but most important is awareness among general public and participation of various sections of society to improve food habits among children and society at large. Health care professional should make people aware of healthy options and reinforce healthy food habits among children. Parents and community should not be impressed by misinformation and fads promoted by advertisements. Parents are instrumental in inculcating healthy food habits for life, they should be aware and motivated to do so. Media should be responsible enough to show only evidence based advertisements and those with exaggerated health claims should be rejected. Government should also take responsibility of making, monitoring and implementing stringent laws. Last but not least international agencies such as WHO and UN should actively work in this field to stop this epidemic of obesity and non-communicable diseases.

CONCLUSION

Eating junk food has become a part of our culture and life in past few years. Indian food with low nutritious value were always there but now other foods and beverages like pizza, burger, sodas and crisps are also part of routine diet. Children are lured by attractive marketing strategies and peer pressure. Consumption of diet high in saturated fats, sugar, salt and calories can lead to childhood obesity and cardiovascular complications later. High intake of junk food by children can be controlled by stringent laws against marketing and availability of these foods. Nutritional labeling can improve the quality of these foods and can give consumers insight into the content of such low nutritional value foods. Overall, we need strong legal guidelines, which should be as aggressive as those for tobacco industry. The government at all levels has an obligation to act, given the harmful effect of junk foods on the health of children.

BIBLIOGRAPHY

1. Anderson JW, Patterson K. Snack foods: comparing nutrition values of excellent choices and "junk foods". J Am Coll Nutr. 2005;24(3):155-6.
2. Campbell N, Duhaney T, Arango M, et al. Healthy food procurement policy: an important intervention to aid the reduction in chronic noncommunicable diseases. Can J Cardiol. 2014;30(11):1456-9.
3. Children 'pester' for advertised junk food. Community Pract. 2015;88(3):8.
4. Chopra M, Darnton-Hill I. Tobacco and obesity epidemics: not so different after all? BMJ. 2004;328(7455): 1558-60.
5. Evans CE, Greenwood DC, Thomas JD, et al. SMART lunch box intervention to improve the food and nutrient content of children's packed lunches: UK wide cluster randomized controlled trial. J Epidemiol Community Health. 2010;64(11):970-6.
6. Food Safety and Standards Rules. In: MOHFW 2011.
7. Franck C, Grandi SM, Eisenberg MJ. Taxing junk food to counter obesity. Am J Public Health. 2013;103(11): 1949-53.
8. Fung C, Kuhle S, Lu C, et al. From "best practice" to "next practice": the effectiveness of school-based health promotion in improving healthy eating and physical activity and preventing childhood obesity. Int J Behav Nutr Phys Act. 2012;9:27.
9. Garg A. Experts shy from ban on junk food. The Times of India. 2014.
10. Gracey M. Junk food or 'junk eating'? Nestle Nutr Workshop Ser Pediatr Program. 2005;56:143-50.
11. Graff S, Kunkel D, Mermin SE. Government can regulate food advertising to children because cognitive research shows that it is inherently misleading. Health Aff (Millwood). 2012;31(2):392-8.
12. Hammond D, Lillico HG, Vanderlee L, et al. The impact of nutrition labeling on menus: a naturalistic cohort study. Am J Health Behav. 2015;39(4):540-8.
13. Harper TA, Mooney G. Prevention before profits: a levy on food and alcohol advertising. Med J Aust. 2010;192(7):400-2.
14. Harrison K, Marske AL. Nutritional content of foods advertised during the television programs children watch most. Am J Public Health. 2005;95(9):1568-74.
15. Hawkes C. Regulating and litigating in the public interest: regulating food marketing to young people worldwide: trends and policy drivers. Am J Public Health. 2007;97(11):1962-73.
16. Jackson P, Romo MM, Castillo MA, et al. Junk food consumption and child nutrition. Nutritional anthropological analysis. Rev Med Chil. 2004;132(10):1235-42.
17. Jochelson K. Nanny or steward? The role of government in public health. Public Health. 2006;120(12): 1149-55.
18. Kaur M, A MH. Are we Aware of what we are, we are what we eat: An Epidemiological Survey. Int J Clin Pediatr Dent. 2008;1(1):13-6.
19. Kelly B, Hattersley L, King L, et al. Persuasive food marketing to children: use of cartoons and competitions in Australian commercial television advertisements. Health Promot Int. 2008;23(4):337-44.
20. Kerr MA, McCann MT, Livingstone MB. Food and the consumer: could labeling be the answer? Proc Nutr Soc. 2015;74(2):158-63.
21. Lloyd-Williams F, Bromley H, Orton L, et al. Smorgasbord or symphony? Assessing public health nutrition policies across 30 European countries using a novel framework. BMC Public Health. 2014;14:1195.
22. Malik VS, Popkin BM, Bray GA, et al. Sugar-sweetened beverages, obesity, type 2 diabetes mellitus, and cardiovascular disease risk. Circulation. 2010;121(11):1356-64.
23. McClure AC, Tanski SE, Gilbert-Diamond D, et al. Receptivity to television fast-food restaurant marketing and obesity among U.S. youth. Am J Prev Med. 2013;45(5):560-8.
24. Miller SA, Taveras EM, Rifas-Shiman SL, et al. Association between television viewing and poor diet quality in young children. Int J Pediatr Obes. 2008;3(3):168-76.
25. Misra A, Vikram NK, Sharma R, et al. High prevalence of obesity and associated risk factors in urban children in India and Pakistan highlights immediate need to initiate primary prevention program for diabetes and coronary heart disease in schools. Diabetes Res Clin Pract. 2006;71(1):101-2.
26. MOI and BI. The Cable Television Networks (Regulation) Act, 1995.
27. Nishida C, Uauy R, Kumanyika S, et al. The joint WHO/FAO expert consultation on diet, nutrition and the prevention of chronic diseases: process, product and policy implications. Public Health Nutr. 2004;7(1A): 245-50.

28. Popkin BM. The nutrition transition and obesity in the developing world. J Nutr. 2001;131(3):871S-3S.
29. Sacks G, Veerman JL, Moodie M, et al. 'Traffic-light' nutrition labeling and 'junk-food' tax: a modeled comparison of cost-effectiveness for obesity prevention. Int J Obes (Lond). 2011;35(7):1001-9.
30. Sreevatsava M, Narayan KM, Cunningham SA. Evidence for interventions to prevent and control obesity among children and adolescents: its applicability to India. Indian J Pediatr. 2013;80 (Suppl 1):S115-22.
31. Tandon PS, Wright J, Zhou C, et al. Nutrition menu labeling may lead to lower-calorie restaurant meal choices for children. Pediatrics. 2010;125(2):244-8.
32. The European Union Pledge: white paper. 2007.
33. The Food Safety and Standards Act, 2006.
34. Uribe R, Fuentes-Garcia A. The effects of TV unhealthy food brand placement on children. Its separate and joint effect with advertising. Appetite. 2015;91:165-72.
35. Vashishtha VM. Advertisement of food products for children: a tale of legality, ethics and indifference. Indian Pediatr. 2010;47(10):857-9.
36. Waxman A. Prevention of chronic diseases: WHO global strategy on diet, physical activity and health. Food Nutr Bull. 2003;24(3):281-4.
37. WHO. Guideline: Sugars Intake for Adults and Children. 2015.
38. Yamamoto JA, Yamamoto JB, Yamamoto BE, et al. Adolescent fast food and restaurant ordering behavior with and without calorie and fat content menu information. J Adolesc Health. 2005;37(5):397-402.

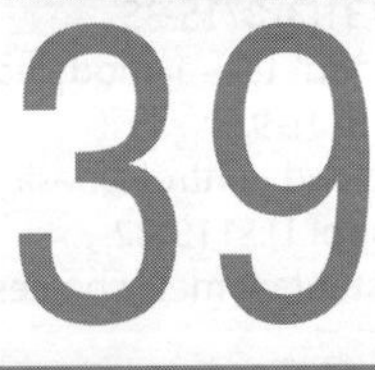

39

CHAPTER

Legal Issues in Unborn Fetus

Murli Janardan Sabath

INTRODUCTION

Human life begins in the mother's womb at the time of conception and progresses through a period of approximately 9 months till its delivery. A child, since its birth, attains access to all rights and privilege akin to any other person. However, it is still a matter of debate whether any legal rights exist for the life that begins in a mother's womb till it is unborn. The right to life under Article 21 of the Indian Constitution reads "*No person shall be deprived of his life or personal liberty except according to a procedure established by law*." Article 21 also casts an obligation on the state to preserve life. It is the obligation of those in charge of the community's health to protect life so that the innocent may be protected and the guilty may be punished. Questions such as "whether an unborn baby is considered a person according to the definition as per Article 21" and '"whether an unborn has similar rights as of a born child" keep creating debates; however, the unborn child is conferred with several rights such as the right to property under succession law, etc.

The strange uncertainty about legal acceptance of rights of an unborn fetus leaves several lacunae that may be exploited by unscrupulous people in committing crimes toward the unborn fetus. Action against pregnant women causing miscarriage forcibly or illegal abortion due to gender based reasons, etc may go unnoticed or unpunished, which need strict vigilance and prompt action. The unborn child deserves to be protected from harm and should have right to life at par with any other person.

DEFINITIONS

A fetus is that stage of a human being's life that begins at about ninth week of pregnancy and extends till about 38 weeks after fertilization. While it takes about 8–9 weeks for development of all organs of a child in the womb, the heart beat can be heard only between the second and third week of pregnancy.

As per *Surrogacy (Regulation) Act, 2021, "Foetus" means a human organism during the period of its development beginning on the fifty-seventh day following fertilisation or creation (excluding any time in which its development has been suspended) and ending at the birth."*

The fetus has also been described as *"...a living entity that comes into being as the result of the fertilization (in vivo or in vitro) of a human egg by a sperm and that develops in the uterus of a woman or that is physically separated from a woman's body, but is capable of surviving outside the uterus to some extent."*

GLOBAL PERSPECTIVE

The 1924 Geneva Declaration of the Rights of the Child recognized for the first time that special requirements of children need to be addressed with much care and concern. It was emphasized that there should not be any discrimination based on nationality, caste, or creed before or after birth of the child. The first draft of the International Covenant (1947) recognizes the concept of human rights protection for "*any person, from the moment of conception*" in the very first session. The fourth Geneva convention clearly accepts and considers the child before birth as a fundamental humanitarian duty. A similar protection was provided to the infant before birth and the infant after birth at the time of the universal declaration of 1948. The Geneva Protocol also raises its primary concern toward the unborn child, which states that a woman who is pregnant or whose children are of young age should not be awarded capital punishment, that is, death penalty. The UN Declaration of Rights of the Child (1959) stipulates in its principle 1 that "*Every child, without any exception whatsoever, shall be entitled to these rights, without distinction or discrimination.*"

INDIAN PERSPECTIVE

The unborn child exists physically in the mother's womb and under natural circumstances, it would be coming out of the womb of his or her mother eventually. Hence, it seems unreasonable to have doubts whether to consider an unborn child as a normal human being and grant him all fundamental rights which a normal person would deserve. Therefore, the law of our country should clearly emphasize that the fetus should be treated similar to a normal human being and it deserves every right that a normal human being deserves.

Based on this philosophy, till the year 1971, it was considered a criminal offence to undertake abortion in India under Section 312 of the Indian Penal Code (IPC). Permission to terminate pregnancy was allowed only in exceptional cases where there was any serious health risk to the life of the baby or the mother. It was only after 1971 that termination of pregnancy was legally permitted under provisions of the medical termination of pregnancy (MTP). Initially, it was granted until 20 weeks of pregnancy, which was later amended in 2020 and raised to 24 weeks.

Indian laws related to the rights of the fetus are surrounded by a typical uncertainty whether to consider the unborn fetus as living or not. The Article 21 of Indian Constitution states that "*No person shall be deprived of his life or personal liberty except according to a procedure established by law.*" But whether the term "*person*" applies to an unborn child too who can be provided with all rights similar to that of a normal person is still a matter of debate.

LEGAL PROTECTION OF THE UNBORN

The unborn fetus is vulnerable at every stage of development and requires constant precautions by the pregnant mother as well as the environment to ensure its smooth growth till the birth of a healthy living baby. Protection of the unborn child from illegal abortion has been monitored by law for a long time. The Hippocratic oath taken by doctors and practitioners since the 19th century prohibits any wrong treatment to their patients and dictates to never procure a woman to terminate a child in her womb. The medical practitioners have a duty not to engage themselves in any sort of illegal clinical practices such as sex determination of the unborn fetus, illegal abortions, or termination of pregnancy, etc. Any act that causes death of a quick, unborn child amounts to culpable homicide in the eyes of law. The existing provisions under Bharatiya Nyaya Sanhita 2023 penalizes any person causing miscarriage in a pregnant women without her consent.

As demonstrated by scientific research and medicine, life begins at origination. Though a child in its mother's womb may inherit the rights to property, but rights and privileges of an unborn child depends upon the fact whether he is born alive or not. The fundamental right to life under Article 21 of the Constitution confers a duty on all to preserve life of every person; that person can be an unborn person too.

While the MTP Act 1971 (duly amended) decriminalizes abortion in specific medical conditions, legislators still fear that liberalization of the law in such circumstances may result in killing of unborn babies, especially the girl child. This has led to enactment of stricter provisions under laws such as the Pre-Natal Diagnostic Techniques (PNDT) Act and empowers the government health departments for penal actions to defaulters. Legal aspects of viability state of fetus have become a critical point of concern especially for those involved in carrying out genetic studies and counseling.

The *International Convention on the Rights of the Child,* which is universally acceptable as the most authoritative standard setting instrument in the field, emphasizes that every child has right to life and survival, to a nationality, to an identity, and other rights similar to other individuals including health. However, the convention is unclear whether such rights also apply to the unborn.

MILESTONE JUDGMENTS

Fetal rights got its recognition following a landmark judgment in *Roe versus Wade.* In this 1973 abortion case, termination of pregnancy was requested on the basis of a sonographic diagnosis of fetal anomalies. The Court in its decision held that under the terms of the fourteenth amendment to the US Constitution, *a fetus is not a person.* This decision of the court was debated in various segments of the society. The State of Texas argued that "*the fetus is a 'person'* within the language and meaning of the Fourteenth Amendment." To which Justice Harry Blackmun responded, "*If this suggestion of personhood is established, the appellant's case, of course, collapses, for the fetus' right to life would then be guaranteed specifically by the Amendment.*" Justice Blackmun then came to the conclusion that "*the word 'person,' as used in the Fourteenth Amendment, does not include the unborn.*"

The Court finally held that while right to abortion in the first trimester in a pregnant woman has constitutional acceptance, she also has a right to terminate her pregnancy medically in the second trimester if situation so arise. However, the state may reserve that right if the procedure itself poses a serious health risk to the mother that is greater than the risk of carrying the fetus to term.

Dr Kenneth Edelin who underwent a trial in Boston was found guilty of manslaughter causing death of a "baby boy" following a hysterotomy. The prosecution kept on stressing on the gestational age of the fetus to prove its viability and made every attempt to bring out that the baby was "killed" between the 24th and 28th weeks of pregnancy. This raised the discussions on the concept of fetal viability.

Rights of Pregnant Women versus Rights of the Unborn: Some Important Judgments and Cases

The women's right to make reproductive choices as part of their right to "personal liberty" has been recognized by Court under Article 21 of the Indian Constitution in *Suchita Srivastava case*. This judgment is important because it accepts a women's right to decline participating in any sexual activity and allows her to choose between carrying her pregnancy till delivery, her choice for use of birth control measures, or seek abortion.

In "Z" versus State of Bihar, the Supreme Court held that denial for termination of unwanted pregnancy in a woman can cause "grave mental torture," which affects her dignity and self-respect. The court further emphasized that as per the Medical Termination of Pregnancy Act (1971) for an adult women not suffering from mental illness, only consent of the woman is required for abortion.

The Bombay High Court on its *Own Motion* versus *State of Maharashtra* recognized that forceful continuation of unwanted pregnancy can be deleterious to a woman's mental health. It further added that *"a person is vested with human rights only at birth; an unborn foetus is not an entity with human rights."*

The Supreme Court has also emphasized during deciding multiple cases such as *Meera Santosh Pal versus UOI, Sarmishtha Chakrabortty versus UOI,* and *Mrs X versus UOI* that a pregnant woman cannot be compelled to continue with a high-risk pregnancy; she has every right to preserve her life and protect herself from any harm to her physical or mental health.

In *Tapasya Umesh Pisal versus Union of India*, the Supreme Court took exception in granting permission to terminate a 25-week pregnancy on the ground of fetal impairment, which would require multiple corrective surgeries after birth and had a high risk of mortality and morbidity after birth. The Court referred to Section 3 (2) (b) (ii) of the MTP Act, which permits MTP up to 20 weeks and held that abortion may be permitted in the interest of justice in circumstances where there is a substantial risk to the child if born to *"suffer from such physical or mental abnormalities as to be seriously handicapped."*

Thus, majority of cases as above favor the concept of preserving a woman's life and mental well-being over the existence of unborn fetus whose viability remains uncertain.

Existing Laws Providing Rights to the Unborn

Despite the prevailing uncertainty, several provisions exist under various existing laws that acknowledge the existence and rights of an unborn fetus. Some of these are enumerated as follows:

- *Bharatiya Nyaya Sanhita (BNS), 2023. Section 92 of BNS states that "Whoever does any act under such circumstances, that if he thereby caused death he would be guilty of culpable homicide, and does by such act cause the death of a quick unborn child, shall be punished with imprisonment of either description for a term which may extend to ten years, and shall also be liable to fine." (This supersedes erstwhile Section 315 of Indian Penal Code, 1860)*
- *Transfer of Property Act, 1882*: Section 13 of the said Act provides that for the benefit of an unborn person a property can be transferred through a trust. The section states, *"...where, on a transfer of property, an interest therein is created for the benefit of a person not in existence at the date of the transfer, subject to a prior interest created by the same transfer, the interest created for the benefit of such person shall not take effect, unless it extends to the whole of the remaining interest of the transferor in the property."*

- *The Indian Succession Act, 1925*: Section 114 of the Act recognizes the prior interest to make an unborn child the owner of a corporeal or incorporeal property, however, holds that *no property will be deemed to be vested in the unborn child until he is born alive as per the Act.* The "Hindu Succession Act, 1956" under Section 20 acknowledges the right of the child in the womb in the same way as a born child with respect to inheritance of intestate of a deceased person.
- *Bhartiya Nagrik Suraksha Sanhita (BNSS), 2023. Section 456 of BNSS (erstwhile Section 416 of Criminal Procedure Code, 1973) state that "If a woman sentenced to death is found to be pregnant, the High Court shall commute the sentence to imprisonment for life."*

Fetal Rights Need to be Recognized

Society acknowledges existence of the unborn fetus, thus it seems logical for law making authorities to amplify under article 21 that an unborn child is entitled to receive the "Right to Life" irrespective of caste, creed, sex or nationality on the same grounds as any other living child. And why not? If a property can be transferred to a baby who is not yet born, then why not the fundamental Right to Life?

The preamble of Declaration on the Rights of the Child, includes that, "the child, by reason of his physical and mental immaturity, needs special safeguards and care, including appropriate legal protection, before as well as after birth," and thus indicates inclusion of protection of legal rights of the unborn as well. Miscarriage of a pregnant mother is also to be prevented under fetal rights.

With advancement of technology in medical profession, it is now possible to regard the fetus as an independent patient. Many legal experts recognize the need to clarify the legal status of the fetus. Some scholars even recommend to pass a model fetal rights act so that states are able to address the issue of fetal rights with a more coherent legislative approach.

Fetal viability has gained much importance with advent of the practice of gene studies. Genetic studies empower the professionals to make an informed decision regarding termination of pregnancy based on findings of such studies. However, it takes almost 21–40 days for the biochemical analysis results to be available. That means, a woman can take an informed decision for MTP only during 20th or 21st week of her pregnancy at the earliest. But at this stage, the fetus is already approaching "viability" and state may pose hinderance for nontherapeutic abortions.

Risks to an Unborn Child

Once conceived, the fetal growth and development depends upon several factors and requires due care and necessary preventive measures. The unborn may be exposed to the callousness or careless attitude of the parents that can endanger its life. Consumption by the pregnant woman of alcohol, drugs, smoking, etc., during the period of conception may have serious consequences causing grave danger such as retarded growth, deformities, or may even lead to miscarriage in certain cases.

By early 1990s, it was estimated that in the United States, about 375,000 children were born annually who exhibited effects of illegal drugs consumed by their mother during pregnancy. In some countries, women were held criminally liable on charges of using illegal drugs during pregnancy that had harmful effect of the fetus and in several cases, hefty penalty was sought by the prosecutors as a deterrent to such behavior by women against their fetus.

Another threat prevailing in Indian society pertains to the illegal practice of female feticide. The age old misbelief and misperception, which renders preference to a male child over a girl child, has increased the rate of termination of pregnancy once it was detected to be a female fetus. To combat such illegal practice, the "pre-conception and pre-natal diagnostic techniques act, 1994" was enacted and further amended in 2002 that forbids any unethical practices related to determination of sex of a child before delivery. Obstetric sonography has since become under scrutiny in the eyes of law and monitors all wrongful births and wrongful deaths.

Courts have held in several cases that no woman can be compelled ethically by any law or a person to carry on a pregnancy that she does not want. However, there has been several instances where fetus has progressed to viability during pregnancy, thus it is prudent to have a holistic view of the situation not only from the point of the woman but also from the well-being of the potential child.

CONCLUSION

The unborn baby starts the process of developing itself since the day of conception. It is high time the law recognizes legal status of the unborn baby and grants "Right to Life" similar to a normal person to them as well. Bharatiya Nyaya Sanhita 2023 (Sec 92) has established that causing death of a quick unborn child by any act amounts to culpable homicide. However adequate measures should be taken to ensure strict compliance of these legal provisions that protects the fetus during its development in a healthy environment without any threat to the life. Appropriate rules should be in place for strict legal action against those voluntarily causing harm to the fetus or those committing the heinous crime of female feticide. By adopting an integrated approach, the Government can enhance community awareness and strengthen the legislative framework to curb any unfair and unethical practices that harms the unborn fetus.

KEY LEARNING POINTS

- Unborn fetus has a physical existence in the mother's womb.
- Unborn fetus deserves equal recognition and fundamental rights similar to any other living human being.
- Any attempt to harm the existence of an unborn fetus amounts to criminal offence and should be strictly penalized by law.
- Unethical practices of sex determination leading to female feticide cases and illegal abortions need to be curbed with stringent actions against those involved.
- Law should be made simpler and clearer by defining the rights of an unborn fetus as integral to any other human being.

BIBLIOGRAPHY

1. Bharatiya Nyaya Sanhita, 2023.
2. Bhartiya Nagrik Suraksha Sanhita, 2023.
3. Chandra A, Mrinal S; Center for Reproductive Rights. Securing Reproductive Justice in India: A Casebook. Delhi: Centre for Constitutional Law, Policy and Governance, National Law University.
4. Glantz LH. The Legal Aspects of Fetal Viability. Boston: Centre for Law and Health Sciences, Boston University of Law.

5. Janoff AF. Rights of the pregnant child vs. rights of the unborn under the Convention on the Rights of the Child. Boston Univ Int Law J. 2004;22(1):163-88.
6. Kamale .VN Rights of unborn child and social state of antenatal care. New Indian J Pediatr. 2019;8(3).
7. Kuthe A, Kuthe D. Legal rights of the fetus. New Indian J Pediatr. 2019;8:3.
8. Macones AJ, Lev-Toaff AS, Macones GA, et al. Legal aspects of obstetric sonography. AJR Am J Roentgenol. 1989;153(6):1251-4.
9. Sandeep N. Rights and status of unborn. [Online] Available from https://www.legalserviceindia.com/legal/article-3345-rights-and-status-of-unborn.html [Last accessed May, 2024].
10. Sayi GR. Legal rights and status of a person, unborn child and environmental resources. [Online] Available from https://blog.ipleaders.in/legal-rights-status-person-unborn-child-environmental-resources/ [Last accessed May, 2024].
11. West's Encyclopedia of American Law. Fetal rights. [Online] Available from https://www.encyclopedia.com/law/encyclopedias-almanacs-transcripts-and-maps/fetal-rights [Last accessed May, 2024].
12. Yuvaraj R, Sneha J. A study on the legal status of the unborn child in India. Juscholars Journal. Volume1, Issue 2.

40

CHAPTER

The POCSO Act

Chandrika Rao

INTRODUCTION

Child sexual abuse (CSA) is a broad term used to describe sexual offenses against children (below age of 18). As per World Health Organization (WHO) definition, "all forms of physical and/or emotional ill-treatment, sexual abuse, neglect or negligent treatment or commercial or other exploitation, resulting in actual or potential harm to the child's health, survival, development, or dignity in the context of a relationship of responsibility, trust, or power."

Child sexual abuse is a complex event involving multifaceted factors based on the social interaction of the alleged child, the family, community, and societal factors. Studies have shown poor impact of future physical and mental health outcomes of CSA in India.

POCSO ACT, 2012

The POCSO (Protection of Children Against Sexual Offences) Act, 2012 is a law that has been provided to protect children from the offenses of sexual assault, sexual harassment and pornography, while ensuring that the interests of the child are safeguarded during all the stages of the judicial process. The Act came into force with effect from 14th November, 2012 followed by an amendment in 2019.

The Criminal Law (amendment) Act, 2013 amended the Indian Penal Code, the Code of Criminal Procedure, 1973, the Indian Evidence Act, 1972, and the Protection of Children from Sexual Offences Act, 2012. The Criminal Law (Amendment) Act 2013, also mentions punishment on stalking, disrobing, voyeurism, trafficking, and acid attack.

COMPONENTS OF THE POCSO ACT, 2012

The act protects children from sexual assault, sexual harassment, and pornography. It also lays down clear procedures for the medicolegal procedures, court trials, punishments with guidelines for all stakeholders such as the police, judiciary, and child protection committee to collaborate and give a combined response to protect the sexually abused child.

The POCSO act has classified sexual offences into categories, defined them and outlined punishments for all. It also lays down procedures for courts and legal authorities, and doctors to follow.

The Act has mandated compulsory reporting of sexual offences. Failure to do so attracts an imprisonment for a duration of 6 months and/or a fine. This casts a legal duty on every citizen, parent, neighbor, police, doctors, and any person who has knowledge about sexual abuse to a child, to report the offence.

Classification

According to the POCSO Act, 2012, sexual offences against children can be classified as the following:

- Penetrative sexual assault
- Aggravated penetrative sexual assault
- Sexual assault
- Aggravated sexual assault
- Sexual harassment

Children who reported an abusive experience usually faced more than one category of abuse; abuse in one category was significantly associated with abuse in other categories such as physical or emotional abuse. The Act recognizes almost every known form of sexual abuse against children including eve teasing, abetment to sexual offences and oral sex, insertion of object of any kind into vagina, anus or mouth and penile sex as punishable offences. Earlier acts such as digital penetration was not considered an offence under the IPC.

As per the POCSO Act, aggravated sexual assault occurs if the abused child is mentally ill or if the abuse is committed by a person in a position of trust or authority such as a family member, police officer, teacher, or doctor.

CHAPTER II: SEXUAL OFFENCES AGAINST CHILDREN

The POCSO Act prescribes severe punishment including a fine as per the level of offence. The punishment can extend up to a maximum term of rigorous imprisonment for life.

The definition and punishment for each of the sexual offences are described in **Tables 40.1 and 40.2.**

SALIENT FEATURES OF POCSO ACT, 2012

- *Burden of proof on the accused:* POCSO Act has placed the responsibility on the alleged accused to prove that he/she is innocent. According to Section 29 of the Act, the Special Court shall presume, that such person has committed or abetted or attempted to commit the offence, unless the contrary is proved. The law recognized that the child will not be able to describe the events properly and has lifted the pressure from the child to prove that the crime took place.
- *Gender neutral law:* POCSO Act is gender neutral and takes cognizance of all sexual crimes committed against both girls and boys under the age of 18 years. It has outlined punishment for perpetrators irrespective of age and gender. As cases from boys are largely under reported, there is a need to have strategies addressing both boys and girls.
- *Severe punishment when protectors are perpetrators:* These are included in the category of "aggravated" which has been described in the Act.

Table 40.1: Definition for each of the Protection of Children Against Sexual Offences (POCSO).

Sexual offence	*Definition*
Penetrative sexual assault	• Penetrates his penis to any extent, into the vagina, mouth, urethra, anus of a child or makes the child to do so with him or any other person • He inserts to any extent any object or part of the body, not being the penis into the vagina, mouth, urethra, or anus of a child or makes the child to do so with him or any other person • Manipulates any part of the body of the child so as to cause penetration into the vagina, urethra, mouth, anus, or any part of the body of the child or makes the child do so with him or any other person • He applies his mouth to the penis, vagina, urethra, or anus of the child or makes the child to do so to him or any other person
Aggravated penetrative sexual assault	• Whoever, being a police officer commits penetrative sexual assault on a child: ○ Within the limits of the police station or premises at which he is appointed ○ In the premises of any station house ○ In the course of his duties ○ Where he is known or identified as an officer • Whoever being a member of the armed forces or security forces commits penetrative sexual assault on a child: ○ Within the limits of the area where the person is deployed ○ In any area under the commands of forces ○ In the course of his duties ○ Where the person is said to be identified as a member of security or armed forces • Whoever being a public servant commits penetrative sexual assault • Whoever being on the management or staff of a hospital, whether government or private commits penetrative sexual assault • Whoever being on the management or staff of an educational or religious institution, commits penetrative sexual assault • Whoever commits gang penetrative sexual assault on a child
Sexual assault	Whoever with sexual intent touches the vagina, penis, anus, or breast of the child or makes the child do so to him or any other person, or does any other act with sexual intent which involves physical contact without penetration is said to commit sexual assault
Aggravated sexual assault	• Whoever, being a police officer commits sexual assault on a child: ○ Within the limits of the police station or premises at which he is appointed ○ In the premises of any station house ○ In the course of his duties ○ Where he is known or identified as an officer • Whoever being a member of the armed forces or security forces commits sexual assault on a child: ○ Within the limits of the area where the person is deployed ○ In any area under the commands of forces ○ In the course of his duties ○ Where the person is said to be identified as a member of security or armed forces

Continued

Continued

Sexual offence	***Definition***
	• Whoever being a public servant commits sexual assault • Whoever being on the management or staff of a hospital, whether government or private commits sexual assault • Whoever being on the management or staff of an educational or religious institution, commits sexual assault • Whoever commits gang sexual assault on a child
Sexual harassment	• A person is said to commit sexual harassment upon a child when such person with sexual intent: ○ Utters any word or makes any sound, gesture or exhibits any object or body part with the intention that such word or sound will be heard or such gesture or object or body part shall be seen by the child ○ Makes a child exhibit his body or any other body part so as to be seen by such a person or any other person ○ Shows any object to a child in any form or media for pornographic purposes ○ Repeatedly or constantly follows or watches or contacts a child either directly or through digital, electronic, or any other means ○ Entices a child for pornographic purpose or gives gratification

Table 40.2: Punishment for each of the Protection of Children Against Sexual Offences (POCSO).

Sexual offence	***Punishment***
Penetrative sexual assault	Imprisonment for a term which shall not be <7 years but may extend to imprisonment for life and shall also be liable to fine
Aggravated penetrative sexual assault	Imprisonment for a term which shall not be <10 years but may extend to imprisonment for life and shall also be liable to fine
Sexual assault	Imprisonment for a term which shall not be <3 years but may extend to 5 years and shall also be liable to fine
Aggravated sexual assault	Imprisonment for a term which shall not be <5 years but may extend to 7 years and shall also be liable to fine
Sexual harassment	Imprisonment for a term which may extend to 3 years and shall also be liable to fine

- *Child-friendly measures:* Child-friendly rooms, questioning techniques, provision of female doctors to examine female children, and child friendly procedures in court have been mentioned.
- *Support to the child and family:* The POCSO act has guided the legal authorities to support the family in the form of support person who is appointed from the government.
- *Every citizen is accountable toward child protection:* The Act has made it mandatory to report all such cases of sexual offences toward children to the police and has included punishment for failure to report or record a case also.

- *Confidentiality of the child:* The Act has stressed on maintaining confidentiality of child and family and applies to all stakeholders including Press too.

The main stakeholders in the Act:
- Police
- Courts
- Doctors, psychiatrists, and psychologists
- Counselors
- Institutions to provide a safe place for the children.

The following principles should be kept in mind while helping a family and the child:
- Right to life and survival
- The best interests of the child
- The right to be treated with dignity and compassion
- The right to be protected from discrimination
- The right to be informed
- The right to be heard
- The right to effective assistance
- The right to privacy
- The right to safety
- The right to compensation

The role of each stakeholder has been described as follows:
- *Police:* Police are the protectors of the child as per the Act. They have to ensure that the child is in a safe environment immediately, facilitate any emergency treatment, and ensure child friendly protocols during the investigative procedure.
  They have to inform the matter to Child Welfare Committee (CWC) within 24 hours of receiving the report. The CWC takes care of further hospitalization, shifting child to shelter home, providing an attender if necessary.
- *Medical professionals:* The Act has made detailed provisions for the medical examination, treatment, forensic evidence collection of the child to be carried out by a medical professional. The parent or another trusted person is allowed to accompany the child. A female child is examined by a female doctor. Consent of parent and assent in older children is necessary.

ROLE OF MEDICAL PROFESSIONALS AS PER THE POCSO ACT, 2012

The role of the doctor:
- Be aware of the processes involved
- Document details of history, examination in non-judgmental, and empathetic manner
- Examine the child in detail including forensic examination, evidence collection.
- Be able to do a psychological evaluation.
- Provide required treatment, pregnancy, and sexually transmitted diseases (STDs) prevention.
- Formulate a medical report with diagnosis.
- Testify in court when required.
- Be available for follow-up.

Differential diagnosis must be considered when a child has a complaint of:
- Vaginal discharge
- Abdominal pain or encopresis (soiling)
- Incidental findings such as enlarged hymenal ring

Das S et al. reported four cases to stress that CSA is not uncommon in India, and sexually transmitted infection (STI) in a child always means CSA. Their study showed that CSA is complicated by lower socioeconomic status, overcrowding, single mother, and the popular belief that sex with a child cures STD.

PROCEDURE FOR REPORTING CASES

Mandatory Reporting

The Act mandates that doctors must report to police (all acts of child abuse should be reported to the police). The medical establishment must make arrangements with the appropriate authorities (i.e., the police or the relevant person within his/her organization who will then contact the police). The Act has provided punishment for not reporting.

A sexual abuse report can include the following:
- Names, address
- Child's age
- Description of the child's injuries
- Identity of the person responsible for the abuse
- Doctor`s name and address

Why should Reporting be Done?

The alleged victim, the child may feel scared or ashamed due to sexual abuse. The family may have excuses not to report and may not support the child. The possible involvement of a parent, family member or friend, in the abuse makes it complex for the children to report sexual abuse. The POCSO act has, therefore, placed the responsibility to report not on the child but on a surrounding adult who may be in a better position to help.

Failure to Report

Failure to report the offence or who fails to record the offence are also prescribed punishment of fine or imprisonment up to 6 months or both as per the POCSO Act, 2012 under Section 21(1).

Reporting False Information

Making a false report, giving false information under sections 3, 5, 7, and 9 are also prescribed punishment up to 6 months imprisonment, fine or both under the POCSO Act, 2012, when such report is made other than in good faith.

If it has been made with the intention to humiliate, extort, threaten or defame the accused, the person giving false information shall be punished with imprisonment up to 6 months–1 year, fine or with both.

SPECIAL COURTS

The POCSO Act further makes provisions for Special Courts to hear child abuse cases. It has to follow child friendly mechanisms for reporting, evidence recording, investigations with a parent or other trusted person can be present at the time of testifying. It has also laid time limits for trial periods and ensures a speedy trial. The said Act stipulates that a case of child sexual abuse must be disposed of within 1 year from the date the offence is reported.

Child-friendly atmosphere includes trial in-camera to avoid re-victimization is given importance. The child cannot be repeatedly called to testify in court and can testify through video-link rather than in a courtroom. The identity of child should also be protected.

The compensation awarded by the special court to a sexually abused child, can be used for the child's medical treatment and rehabilitation **(Fig. 40.1)**.

The POCSO act further states that no hospital under the jurisdiction of the Indian Constitution can refuse to admit the victim of child sexual abuse for examination and treatment. This issue has been re-emphasized in Section 23 of the Criminal Law Amendment Act, which inserts Section 357C into the Code of Criminal Procedure, 1973. All hospitals should provide first-aid or medical treatment, free of cost and immediately to the victims of a sexual offence. Treatment to a rape victim cannot be refused by any public or private hospital as per the amended Act, Section 166B of Indian Penal Code 8.

POCSO ACT 2019 AMENDMENT BILL

According to the NCRB Report on Crimes against children, there was an increasing number of crimes against children despite a strong legal framework. Hence, POCSO Act was amended in November 2019 to make it more effective in dealing with cases of child sexual abuse.

The Amendment Act provided for more stringent punishments as increase in the imprisonment period and depending on the gravity of the offence, the court could impose death penalty on the perpetrator in extreme cases of aggravated penetrative sexual assault.

As stated in the POCSO Act 2019 Amendment:
"Whoever commits penetrative sexual assault on a child below sixteen years of age shall be punished with imprisonment for a term which shall not be less than twenty years, but which may extend to imprisonment for life, which shall mean imprisonment for the remainder of natural life of that person and shall also be liable to fine."

And punishment for *aggravated penetrative sexual assault* is mentioned in the Act as follows:
"Whoever commits aggravated penetrative sexual assault shall be punished with rigorous imprisonment for a term which shall not be less than twenty years, but which may extend to imprisonment for life, which shall mean imprisonment for the remainder of natural life of that person and shall also be liable to fine, or with death."

CHALLENGES AND CONTROVERSIES IN POCSO ACT

- *Consent:* This area involves a lot of confusion and controversies. In some cases, the family member or police officer insists on medical examination but the child/adolescent refuses to undergo medical examination, the POCSO Act has not given clear direction. Forceful

Recording a child's statement

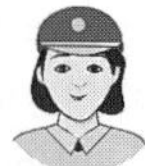

Statement should be recorded preferably by a woman police officer, not in uniform

It should be recorded at the child's home, or any place he/she finds comfortable

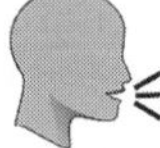

It should be recorded in the language of the child, as spoken by the child

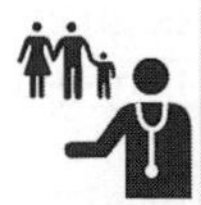

Statement should be recorded in presence of trusted adult and/or an expert, interpreter, translator or social worker

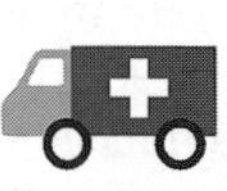

Medical examination within 24 hours in the presence of parent or trusted adult

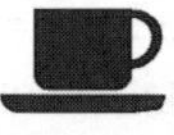

Take frequent breaks while the child narrates the incident. Don't rush the child while recording the statement

Audio or video recording devices should be used, if available

Police officer should read out loud the recorded statement to the child

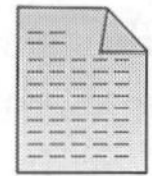

Child/parent must get a copy of the statement

Fig. 40.1: Recording a child's statement.

Source: nyaaya.in.

examination without the adolescent's consent becomes an offence and hence should not be done even if parents are insisting on it unless there is bleeding or it is a medical and surgical emergency. Consent should be taken from parent in a child (<12 years) and consent from both parent and the child in ages 12–18 years. However, emergency treatment can be initiated without getting into legality to protect the life of the child.

- *Medical examination:* The POCSO Act, Section 27(3) mandates that in case of a female child/adolescent victim, the medical examination should be done by a female doctor. On the other hand, the Criminal Law Amendment Act, Section 166A of Indian Penal Code mandates the Government medical officer on duty to examine the rape victim without fail. Issues arise when a female doctor is not available.
- *Treatment cost:* The law has said medical care to the survivors should be free. Medical establishments have on occasions provided costly care for a long time to children and care to prevent substandard medical treatment procedure just for the issue of cost should not arise.
- *Consented sexual intimacy:* Adolescents engage in mutual consent sexual act before age of 16 in many cases which is considered illegal under the POCSO Act 2012, irrespective of consent or marriage.
- The latest amendment of the Indian Penal Code concerning rape laws has fixed the age of consent for sex at 18 years. Hence, consensual sex with a child <18 years comes under POCSO act. Since the MTP (medical termination of pregnancy) cases (<18 years) now need to be reported, cases of girls not accessing medical care should not increase.
- *Training:* Examination of sexual assault child cases should be covered more in the undergraduate medical curriculum. Training of all physicians, nurses, and medical personnel in a child protective service, school and college teachers, judges, lawyers, police, and other legal agencies is necessary as per the POCSO Act, 2012. All the MBBS undergraduates and Indian medical graduates should be trained in conducting all child protective services for an alleged child abuse case including interview in a child-friendly manner, proper evaluation, regular and forensic evidence collection, investigations and should be knowledgeable in STDs and human immunodeficiency virus (HIV) prophylaxis, counseling, and regular follow-up. Research and monitoring are challenges and should be done on a larger scope.

- *Role of mental health professional:* Every child abuse case should ideally be evaluated by a psychiatrist or psychologist. Mental health professionals need to be recruited in follow-up care of the victim by providing individual counseling, family therapy, and rehabilitation.
- *Reporting:* It is difficult for the families to report as investigations may be intrusive. More friendly procedures need to be involved. In a study in India, 64% of respondents had an idea about an online complaint system for child abuse, and 70% were aware of the availability of a one-stop center at a respondent's hospital.

CONCLUSION

The POCSO Act, 2012 is a well-crafted legislation **(Flowchart 40.1)**. It has documented all forms of sexual abuse against children as punishable offence. A collaborative multi-agency team and multi-tier approach should be planned and accessible in all areas to deliver complete and comprehensive care in one center for children exposed to sexual abuse with child-friendly legal and medical practices.

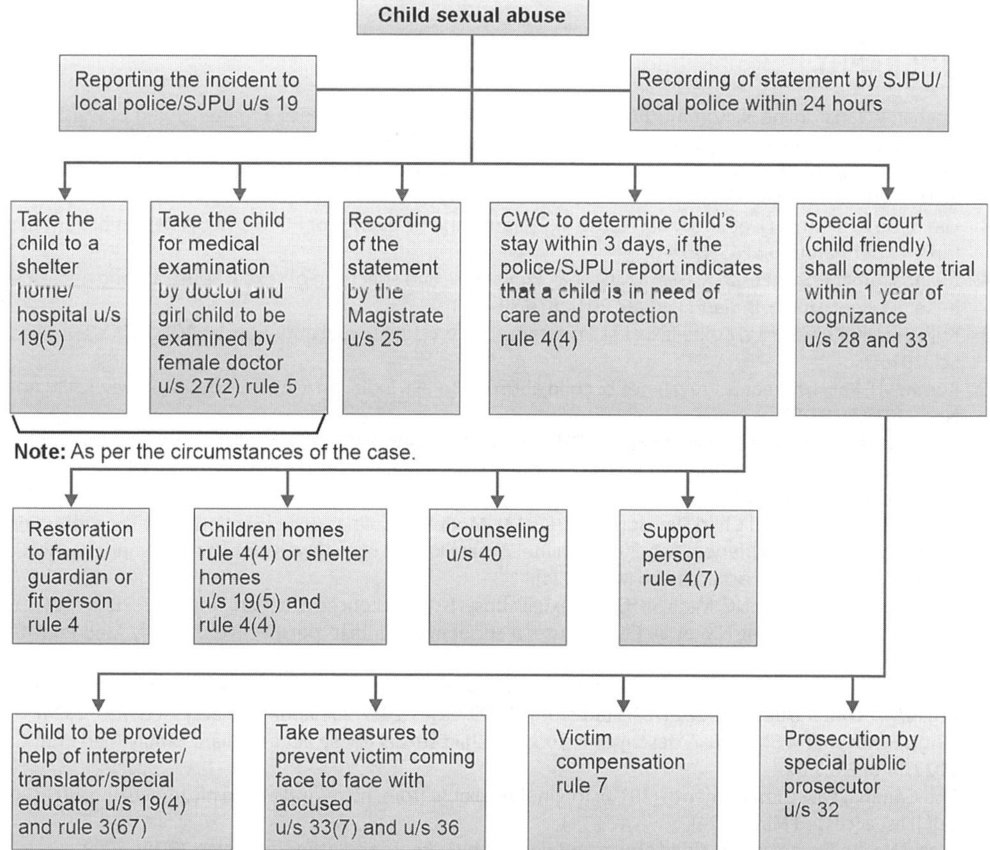

Flowchart 40.1: Processes under Protection of Children Against Sexual Offences (POCSO).
(CWC: child welfare committee; SJPU: special juvenile police unit; u/s: under section)

KEY LEARNING POINTS

- Child sexual abuse is when a person involves the child below the age of 18 years in sexual activities for his/her sexual gratification, commercial gain, or both.
- The POCSO Act, 2012 is a comprehensive law that provides for the protection of children from the offences of sexual assault, sexual harassment, and pornography, while safeguarding the interests of the child at every stage of the judicial process.
- The Act defines different forms of sexual abuse such as nonpenetrative, penetrative assault, sexual harassment, and pornography.
- The Act prescribes stringent punishment graded as per the gravity of the offence, with a maximum term of rigorous imprisonment for life, and fine. The POCSO Act ensures punishment for all perpetrators irrespective of age and gender.
- Role of medical professionals in the context of the POCSO Act, 2012 is well defined including mandatory reporting.
- The POCSO Act further makes provisions for avoiding re-victimization, child-friendly atmosphere through all stages of the judicial process and gives paramount importance to the principle of "best interest of the child."

BIBLIOGRAPHY

1. Anchan V, Janardhana N, Kommu JVS. POCSO act, 2012: Consensual sex as a matter of tug of war between developmental need and legal obligation for the adolescents in India. Indian J Psychol Med. 2021;43(2):158-62.
2. Choudhry V, Dayal R, Pillai D, et al. Child sexual abuse in India: A systematic review. PLoS One. 2018;13(10):e0205086.
3. Das S, De A, Sharma N, et al. Sexual Abuse in Children and Relevance of POCSO Act-A Report of Four Cases. Indian J Dermatol. 2020;65(1):74-6.
4. Krishnakumar P, Satheesan K, Geeta MG, et al. Prevalence and spectrum of sexual abuse among adolescents in Kerala, South India. Indian J Pediatr. 2014;81:770-4.
5. Kulkarni UK, Kulkarni KV, Kokre RN, et al, Forensic study on child sexual abuse under POCSO act. Eur J Pharm Sci. 2016:3:7.
6. Kumar MT, Kar N, Kumar S. Prevalence of child abuse in Kerala, India: An ICAST-CH based survey. Child Abuse Negl. 2019;89:87-98.
7. Ministry of Health and Family Welfare. (2014). Guidelines and Protocols. Medico-legal care for survivors/victims of sexual violence. [online] Available from https://main.mohfw.gov.in/sites/default/files/953522324.pdf [Last accessed May, 2024].
8. Ministry of Women and Child Development. (2013). Model Guidelines under Section 39 of The Protection of Children from Sexual Offences Act, 2012. [online] Available from https://wcd.nic.in/sites/default/files/POCSO-Model Guidelines.pdf [Last accessed May, 2024].
9. Moirangthem S, Kumar NC, Math SB. Child sexual abuse: Issues & concerns. Indian J Med Res. 2015;142(1):1-3.
10. Paul V, Rathaur VK, Bhat NK, et al. Child abuse: a social evil in Indian perspective. J Family Med Prim Care. 2021;10(1):110-5.
11. Satyarthi Childrens Foundation. (2021). Status of POCSO cases in India. [online] Available from https://satyarthi.org.in/wp-content/uploads/2021/03/Status-of-POCSO-Cases-2017-2019.pdf [Last accessed May, 2024].
12. Singh R, Koushal V, Bharti B. A descriptive study on child sexual abuse act in India. J Family Med Prim Care. 2022;11(6):2923-32.
13. The Criminal Law (Amendment). (2013). [online] Available from: http://indiacode.nic.in/acts-in-pdf/132013.pdf [Last accessed May, 2024].
14. World Health Organization. Child abuse and neglect by parents and other caregivers (PDF). 2002.

CHAPTER 41

The IMS Act

Preeti Srivastava, Tapas Sarangi, Kumar Diwakar

INTRODUCTION

World Health Organization (WHO), Indian Academy of Pediatrics (IAP) as well as Infant and Young Child Feeding (IYCF) recommend initiating breastfeeding within an hour of birth, preferably within 30 minutes. They also recommend exclusive breastfeeding for the first 6 months and continued breastfeeding until 24 months of age. It is well established that early initiation of breastfeeding as well as exclusive breastfeeding for the first 6 months of life significantly reduces neonatal mortality by 20% and under-five mortality by 13%. However, it is astounding to note that only 38% of infants under 6 months are exclusively breastfed despite the strong evidence of the protective role of breastfeeding against infection-related neonatal and infant mortality. As per the data of the Indian Rapid Survey 2013–2014, exclusive breastfeeding was seen in 64.9% Indian population as compared to the world average of 38%. Several factors cause suboptimal breastfeeding like lack of awareness in mothers regarding advantages of breastfeeding, socioeconomic factors, mother's education level, support system for mothers at home and workplace to facilitate breastfeeding, easy availability of infant milk substitutes (IMS), which involves less effort, and lack of motivation in mothers to breastfeed.

In 1992, infant milk substitute, feeding bottles and infant food act was adopted in India to provide regulation for production, supply, and distribution of IMS, feeding bottles, and infant foods with an aim to protect, promote, and support breastfeeding as well as ensure proper use of infant foods. "Infant milk substitute" means any food being marketed or otherwise represented as a partial or total replacement for mother's milk (for infants up to the age of 2 years). It is important to regulate IMS as it helps to create an environment conducive to promoting breastfeeding. It also prevents inappropriate marketing of food products that compete with breastfeeding and are very often responsible for interfering with breastfeeding, and protects newborns from unethical marketing practices.

The IMS Act was further strengthened in 2003 after making amendments. The Act has incorporated all essential components of the all essential components of WHA code were incorporated in the act; however, the greatest challenge is the implementation of the Act.

BACKGROUND OF IMS ACT

The 34th session of the World Health Assembly (WHA) adopted the International Code of Marketing of Breast-milk Substitutes in 1981 through a WHA resolution as a minimum requirement to protect and promote appropriate infant and young child feeding. The Code represents an expression of the collective will of governments to ensure the protection and promotion of optimal feeding for infants and young children. The Code provides detailed guidelines regarding the following:

- Information and education on infant feeding
- Promotion of breast-milk substitutes and associated products to the public and mothers
- Promotion of breast-milk substitutes and associated products to healthcare workers, hospitals, and other healthcare settings
- Quality of breast-milk substitutes and related products as well as their process of labeling
- Implementation and monitoring of compliance to the Code.

Subsequent years have witnessed several clarifications to the Code. The salient points in the latest clarification, published in 2016 as WHA 69.9, outlines that:

- "Follow-up formula" and "growing-up milk" should not be promoted as they lie within the scope of the Code.
- Complementary foods should clearly display, in their messages, that breastfeeding should be continued till 2 years, and complementary food should not be started before 6 months of age.
- Labeling and designing of breast-milk substitutes should be distinct and separate from products other than breast-milk substitutes to prevent cross-promotion.
- Companies selling breast milk substitutes and infant food should not make any donations to healthcare systems, health workers, or professional associations, as it represents a conflict of interest and should be strongly prohibited.
- It is recommended to the companies selling foods for infants and young children to not provide sponsorship for scientific meetings of health professionals.

OBJECTIVES OF IMS ACT

The objectives of the IMS Act are as follows:

- Facilitate and support breastfeeding.
- Prohibit any kind of promotion of IMSs.
- Create awareness in pregnant and lactating mothers about the importance of breastfeeding and IMS Act.
- Take measures to curtail the use of IMS and infant foods.
- Impose restrictions on marketing and promotional activities of companies manufacturing baby food.
- Clearly define roles and responsibilities of healthcare workers and healthcare institutions.
- Ensure appropriate use of breast-milk substitutes in relevant situations.

ACCEPTABLE CRITERIA FOR USING ALTERNATE FEEDS

There are certain unavoidable situations where the infant is unable to receive breastfeeding and is dependent on formula feeds. A majority of them are, however, temporary scenarios like very sick mother (or suffering from serious psychiatric illness), relocating mother, rejection of infant by mother, or infant dependent on artificial feed. But situations like a deceased mother or human immunodeficiency virus (HIV) positive mother, who chooses to use breast-milk substitute, are examples of justified use of formula feeds.

KEY PROVISION OF IMS ACT

Key provisions of IMS Act include the following:

- Undue commercialization of infant milk substitute is strictly banned, and therefore zero tolerance for any promotion
- No provision for free samples
- No free or subsidized supply of IMS or educational material related to these products to be given to any person.
    - In May 1986, Governments at the WHA urged a ban on donated supplies of baby milk (WHA 39.28).
    - WHO/United Nations Children's Fund (UNICEF) Baby-friendly Hospital Initiative (BFHI) pledged to achieve a target of ending free supplies in all countries.
    - It is believed that a hospital cannot be baby-friendly if it receives free supplies of breast milk substitutes.
- Labels on all IMS, feeding bottles, and infant food should clearly mention that "Breastfeeding is the BEST" in English as well as in the local language. There should be no display of pictures of women, infant, or phrases on the labels, which are designed to promote the sales of these products.
- The Act provides clear guidelines for advertisements and educational materials, whether audio or video, related to pre and postnatal care/infant feeding.
- Posters are strictly prohibited.
- The Act does not permit any kind of financial assistance.
- The Act clearly states that no commissions should be given to any salespersons or employees.

IMS Act bans the following:

- Advertisements to promote IMS
- Distribution of gifts and free samples
- Donation of products, educational material, or equipment
- Labels displaying pictures of mothers, baby, etc.
- Incorrect or incomplete information through educational material or advertisements
- Providing payments or sponsorships to healthcare workers and their associations
- Providing commission to salespersons or employees to increase sales

IMS Act violations (whether intentional or unintentional) are supposed to occur if anyone:

- Promotes any food under any label for kids up to 2 years old
- Encourages consumption of "infant food" prior to the age of 6 months
- Advertising on any platform, including radio, television, newspapers, magazines, journals, short message service (SMS), e-mails, pamphlets, etc.
- Distributes infant food, feeding bottles, and milk substitute products, or samples thereof, to anyone
- Provides any kind of incentives, including rebates, free gifts, or other benefits, to anyone who uses or purchases infant formula, feeding bottles, or baby food
- If anyone provides mothers, families, and other groups with information and educational materials pertaining to the promotion of IMS, feeding bottles, and infant foods. If the educational material contains the information laid down by IMS Act, 2003, clause 7, they may distribute it to health professionals including doctors, nurses, and others. Only true information should be used in educational materials; no company-sponsored products should be mentioned.

- Displays the tins, cartons, or accompanying brochures for these items with cartoons, phrases, or other images featuring mothers or babies or any other similar images
- Exhibits placards or posters promoting IMS, feeding bottles or infant foods in a hospital, nursing home, chemist shop, etc.
- Offers financial incentives or gifts to health professionals or their family members with the intention of promoting the use of IMS, feeding bottles, or infant foods
- Shows mothers or any members of her family how to feed these products; however, a doctor can show the mother how to accomplish this
- Provides financial incentives to medical professionals, nurses, or organizations such as IAP, Indian Medical Association (IMA), National Neonatology Forum (NNF), etc., such as funding for the organization of seminars, meetings, conferences, contests, fees for educational courses, or sponsorship of projects, research program, or tours
- Sets employee commission based on the overall volume of these products sold

Penalties stipulated for violating the IMS Act:
- *Imprisonment:* 6 months to 3 years
- *Fine:* ₹2,000–5,000

Violation of IMS Act can be reported to:
- Breastfeeding promotion network of India (BPNI)
- Association of Consumer Action on Safety and Health (ACASH)
- Indian Council for Child Welfare (ICCW)
- Central Social Welfare Board (CSWB)

CONCLUSION

The act was passed by the government. However, nothing is turning out the way it was envisioned. Manufacturers frequently use legal justifications or lacunas to their advantage to thwart the spirit of the law. After a law is enacted, the Government's and policymakers' work is not accomplished. To put the act's policies and provisions into effect, they should act with strength and determination. We have a right to information about the IMS Act. The Human Resource Development Department, Women and Child Development Department, and Health Ministry should start actively promoting and reinforcing breastfeeding on television and radio. Even a decade after this Act's enactment, only about 61.7% of doctors, 28.1% of nurses, and 25.6% of chemists are aware of its provisions, according to a BPNI Delhi study (personal communication). It is now necessary for us to actively promote this Act so that more medical professionals and other healthcare professionals are aware of it. The mother and her family should receive health education about the benefits of breastfeeding and the negatives of IMS and infant food. Workshops on human lactation management and the BFHI movement could support this education. One of the well-liked initiatives to accomplish this is the BFHI. The Baby-Friendly Medical Store Initiative (BFSI) should now be planned for. We shouldn't allow the Act to degenerate into a mere "toothless paper tiger" as responsible citizens. As a result, we must become activists who can assist our peers in comprehending the objective and spirit of the Act. There ought to be "zero tolerance" for Act violations. All of us who are working to improve the health of children must make a commitment to safeguard, aid, and promote breastfeeding.

KEY LEARNING POINTS

- Only two-thirds of infants younger than 6 months are breastfed exclusively, even though there is ample evidence to support breastfeeding's numerous benefits, including a decreased likelihood of neonatal and infant death.
- To regulate the manufacturing, supply, and distribution of IMS, feeding bottles, and infant foods, the Indian Parliament passed the Infant Milk Substitutes, Feeding Bottles, and Infant Foods Act in 1992 and was further strengthened in 2003 after making amendments.
- The act's aim is to safeguard the use of infant food and to protect, support, and promote breastfeeding.
- IMS means any food being marketed or otherwise represented as a partial or total replacement for mother's milk for infant up to the age of 2 years.
- IMS act also specifies acceptable criteria for using alternate feeds in certain unavoidable circumstances.
- The IMS Act prohibits the use of advertisements, the provision of gifts and free samples, the dissemination of false or misleading information through educational materials or advertisements, providing payments or sponsorships to healthcare professionals and their associations, and the payment of commission to salesperson or employees in order to increase sales.
- IMS Act violations (whether deliberate or inadvertent) are punishable by imprisonment for up to 3 years but not less than 6 months and a fine of between ₹2,000 and 5,000.

BIBLIOGRAPHY

1. Hoche S, Meshesha B, Wakgari N. Sub-optimal breastfeeding and its associated factors in rural communities of Hula district, Southern Ethiopia: A cross-sectional study. Ethiop J Health Sci. 2018;28(1):49-62.
2. India Code. 2024. The Infant Milk Substitutes, Feeding Bottles and Infant Foods (Regulation of Production, Supply and Distribution) Act, 1992 as Amended in 2003 (IMS Act). [online] Available from https://www.indiacode.nic.in/handle/123456789/1958?view_type=browse#:~:text=An%20Act%20to%20provide%20for,connected%20therewith%20or%20incidental%20thereto. [Last accessed May, 2024].
3. Jones G, Steketee RW, Black RE, et al.; Bellagio Child Survival Study Group. How many child deaths can we prevent this year? Lancet. 2003;362:65-71.
4. Ministry of Women and Child Development, UNICEF. (2014). Rapid Survey On Children (RSOC) 2013-14. [online] Available from http://wcd.nic.ic/acts/rapid-survey-children-rsoc-2013-14 [Last accessed May, 2024].
5. Phukan D, Ranjan M, Dwivedi LK. Impact of timing of breastfeeding initiation on neonatal mortality in India. Int Breastfeed J. 2018;13.
6. Sankar MJ, Sinha B, Chowdhury R, et al. Optimal breastfeeding practices and infant and child mortality: A systematic review and meta-analysis. Acta Paediatr. 2015;104(467):3-13.
7. Tiwari SK, Chaturvedi P. The IMS Act 1992: Need for more amendments and publicity. Indian Pediatr. 2003;40(8):743-6.
8. UNICEF, World Health Organization. (2009). Acceptable medical reasons for use of breast milk. substitutes. [online] Available from https://www.who.int/nutrition/publications/infantfeeding/WHO_NMH_NHD_09.01/en/ [Last accessed May, 2024].
9. World Health Assembly (WHA). 2016. Ending inappropriate promotion of foods for infants and young children. [online] Available from http://apps.who.int/gb/ebwha/pdf_files/WHA69/A69_R9-en.pdf [Last available May, 2024].
10. World Health Organization. Baby-Friendly Hospital Initiative: Revised, Updated and Expanded for Integrated Care. Geneva: World Health Organization; 2009. [online] Available from https://www.ncbi.nlm.nih.gov/books/NBK153486/ [Last accessed May, 2024].
11. World Health Organization (WHO) Secretariat. (2010). Early Initiation of breastfeeding: the key to survival and beyond. [online] Available from http://new.paho.org/hq/dmdocuments/2010/Eight%20Pager%20English%20FINAL.pdf [Last accessed May, 2024].
12. World Health Organization. (1981). International Code of Marketing of Breastmilk Substitutes. [online] Available from www.who.int/nutrition/publications/code_english.pdf [Last accessed May, 2024].

CHAPTER

Telemedicine and Electronic Consultations

Brij Bhushan Sahni, Mahesh Baldwa

INTRODUCTION

The World Health Organization defines telemedicine as, "The delivery of healthcare services, where distance is a critical factor, by all healthcare professionals using information and communication technologies for the exchange of valid information for diagnosis, treatment, and prevention of disease and injuries, research and evaluation, and for the continuing education of healthcare providers, all in the interests of advancing the health of individuals and their communities."

TELEMEDICINE PRACTICE GUIDELINES APPROVED BY THE NATIONAL MEDICAL COMMISSION

Enabling registered medical practitioners to provide healthcare using telemedicine [This constitutes Appendix 5 of the Indian Medical Council (Professional Conduct, Etiquette and Ethics Regulation, 2002)], gazetted on 25-03-2020.

The name of Government of India's free telemedicine service is eSanjeevani.

The National Telemedicine Service, "eSanjeevani," a digital health initiative of the ministry supports two types of teleconsultation services: Doctor–doctor (eSanjeevani) and patient–doctor [eSanjeevani outpatient department (OPD)] teleconsultations.

LEGAL ISSUES

The issues being debated pertain to professional liability, credentialing, confidentiality and reimbursement, development of standards and telecommunications and infrastructure. Legal conundrums may arise with respect to data protection, product liabilities and standards, freedom of information, personal and organizational responsibility, what bodies are responsible for legal guidance, cross-border transmission, teleconsultation equipment, and so on.

LEGAL RISKS OF DISCLOSURE OF CONFIDENTIAL RECORDS

The legal risks relating to the disclosure of inaccurate or confidential medical information are significant. Such disclosure may result in defamation claims by the patient whose record is disclosed. This becomes more pertinent in an era when the media is more interested in sensationalism of news than pragmatism. Therefore, patients' consent to disclosure of information is a very important part of the agreement between the doctor or his institution and the patient.

Potential privacy and security issues that create heightened compliance challenges in telemedicine, according to Quashie and Lerman, include: Data management. Sharing data management responsibilities with other providers. Privacy and security risks during telemedicine encounters, "Responsibilities for securing and managing the electronic health information generated through telemedicine encounters must therefore be clearly defined."

TELEMEDICINE IN THE NEXT MILLENNIUM

It is here and now a swiftly growing trend. Traditionally, healthcare has taken into account social, cultural, ethnic beliefs, education, socioeconomic group, geographical location, and age assuming that the healer and the healed hail from the same region. Access to telemedicine has brought new dimensions to healthcare. The practice of telemedicine—through access to tertiary level specialist healthcare, even transmission of digitized data, audio, video, and images—is getting popular all over the world. It provides hitherto unavailable specialized advice in geographically remotest areas without displacement of the patient, physician, or the equipment.

It is not only cost-effective to the patient but cost beneficial to the society also.

It will be appropriate to get to know the meanings of terms used in e-medicine to enable us to understand the legal issues which can arise.

Telemedicine would also be governed by the Information Technology Act, 2000. In the absence of any central or overarching legislations providing for registration or licenses for practicing telemedicine in India, state-specific laws governing the practice of "medicine" generally have to be considered.

TELEMEDICINE

- *Is telemedicine routinely allowed by law?*
  No, it was allowed for coronavirus disease 2019 (COVID-19) pandemic. It was allowed to cover emergency COVID-19 situations for the time being. There are contradictory messages from decided cases on telemedicine where the Supreme Court two-judge bench says no prescription should ordinarily be given without actual examination. The tendency to give prescription over the telephone, except in an acute emergency, should be avoided. This is according to 2009 Martin F D'Souza vs. Mohd Ishfaq, (SC) 2009 AIR (SC) 2049, which says precautions which doctor/hospitals/nursing homes should take: (b) No prescription should ordinarily be given without actual examination. The tendency to give prescription over the telephone, except in an acute emergency, should be avoided.
- *Teleconsultation not allowed*—according to 2018, Bombay High Court (HC) says emergency telephonic advice not allowed in case of *Deepa Sanjeev Pawaskar vs. State of Maharashtra, (Bombay) 2018(3) Crimes 576* where patient Dnyanada discharged after lower segment cesarean section (LSCS). A day later, patient readmitted in emergency was being treated by two nurses who were administering medicines on the telephonic instructions of the

doctor. The condition of the patient deteriorated. Some other doctor attended belatedly. Patient died. Criminal case filed based on expert medical opinion. Anticipatory bail application rejected.

- *Teleconsultation was allowed in COVID-19*. Now recently in 2020, Delhi HC allows treating non-COVID illnesses by telemedicine in *Yash Aggarwal vs. Union of India (Delhi)(DB) 17.04.2020*, where it said that a citizen-friendly web-based teleconsultation has also been launched, where patients can have a safe and structured video-based clinical consultation with the doctor while remaining in the confines of home. HC said cancer or chronic kidney diseases, etc. are not being treated is incorrect.
- *Government of India portal on e-Health and Telemedicine*—Ministry of Health and Family Welfare (MoHFW) has undertaken various initiatives using Information and Communication Technologies (ICT) for improving efficiency and effectiveness of the public healthcare system.

  E-Hospital:
  - *Website*: https://dashboard.ehospital.gov.in/dashboard-testing2/
  - *Website*: https://ehospital.nic.in/ehospitalsso/

  National Telemedicine Network (NTN): *WB has its own website.*

  Telemedicine services to the remote areas by upgrading existing Government Healthcare Facilities [medical college (MC), district hospital (DH), subdistrict hospital (SDH), primary health center (PHC), and community health center (CHC)] in states.

  In the first phase of the NTN project, it is proposed to connect 500 PHC/CHC/SDH at remote/rural locations with 100 DH and 50 MC. So far, financial aid has been provided to seven states. This is because 70% rural and 90% secondary and tertiary care in cities.
- *Telemedicine guideline in COVID-19*:

  The National Medical Commission (NMC)—approved medical council published 48 pages guidelines on telemedicine prescription of medicines guidelines during COVID-19. The salient points are:

  List-0: Over-the-counter medicines
  List-A: Video conferencing first consultation
  List-B: Follow-up consultations
  Prohibited list: Psychotropic drugs
- *Telemedicine consent, documentation, and consultation digital recording in prescribed format*—but it is nearly the same as we routinely use name, gender, age, address, history, diagnosis and treatment, and signature.
  - One can consult on audio calls for old, known patients, where consent is not needed—WhatsApp (WA) call with consent sent on WA and e-mail from patient party Zoom, Google Meet, and WA video with consent—if need to be record the consultation. Send prescription via email, preferably on letter head.
  - Telemedicine and consent according to 2008-3JJ

    Real consent in writing Samira Kohli vs. Doctor Prabha Manchanda
    Part 1: Name, address, mobile, and e-mail
    Part 2: Patient signature, write proper prescription with history, investigation, advise, or treatment given
    Part 3: Disclose benefit, >10% risks, complications, and alternatives
    Part 4: Doctor's name, registration number, and signature

Telemedicine consent: Patient has to sign and send by email or WA or suitable app or alternatively record telemedicine consultation. Witness is needed if sent by e-mail/WA along with ID by Aadhar/PAN card, etc.

- *Always remember*:
    - Always avoid off-label use, higher and longer duration use, and use of banned drug.
    - Remember 2013—the Supreme Court three-judge bench—steroids in higher dose for longer duration used, highest claim to the tune of more than 11 crores.
    - Also remember 2009—the Supreme Court two-judge bench *Martin D' Souza vs. Md Ishfaq*. Supreme Court 2009—amikacin 500 mg twice a day to chronic renal failure (CRF) patients for *Klebsiella*. More than 21 days result in deafness.
    - Also remember *Vijaya Laxmi vs. Dr Krishna Kumar*, the Supreme Court 2006 claimed 2.84 crores for alleged nimesulide use which is a banned drug.
- *Documentation in telemedicine*:
    - Preserve all documents such as consent, written documented advices, and digital recordings.
      Record teleconsultation because patients and doctors shall forget, but medical documents and records will always remember. Medical records are nonrebuttable evidence in court of law.
    - Remember:
        - *No records*: No defense
        - *Poor records*: Poor defense
        - *Good records*: Good defense

      In a Supreme Court two-judge bench 2019 decision on maintenance of records in *Federation of Obstetrics and Gynecological Societies of India vs. Union of India, (2019) 6 SCC 283*, ratio decidendi reason for a judge's decision in a case, while obiter dicta-persuasive precedent. Considering the nature of services rendered by medical professionals, proper maintenance of records is an integral part of the medical services.
    - *Use good or capital handwriting—2020 HC*: Doctors shall write name of drugs in good or capital handwriting in *Krishna Mandal vs. State of Odisha, BLAPL 3541/2020*, which says doctors shall write name of drugs in good or capital handwriting, avoid illegible scrawls that leaves room for ambiguity.
- *Records preservation in telemedicine*:
    - Legally for 3 years only
    - Income tax 6 years but not part of medical records
    - Xerox to be given to the patient if demanded within 72 hours
    - Record digitally all teleconsultations, keep consent, and prescriptions saved

LAWS AND LEGAL ISSUES IN HEALTHCARE INFORMATION TECHNOLOGY

The Information Technology Act, 2000, Data Protection Rules, 2011, and Intermediaries Guidelines, 2011 codified law-governing regular exchange of information and personal data regarding health issues and advisory thereon among patient and the service provider; protecting personal data is of prime concern as per law.

The Central Drug Standards Control Organisation (CDSCO) is the prime regulatory authority which regulates the provisions of "The Drugs and Cosmetics Act, 1940 and Rules thereof." Further, the practice of medicine is regulated by the Medical Council of India. In addition, the protection in terms of intellectual property is regulated under the Office of the Controller General of Patents, Designs and Trade Marks (CGPTDM), and copyright is governed by the Copyright Office, both under the Department for Promotion of Industry and Internal Trade (DPIIT). In addition, the Indian Council of Medical Research (ICMR) has been instrumental in encouraging research for implementing the National Digital Health Blueprint (NDHB) by MoHFW.

The legal and regulatory framework is usually governed by the following relevant acts:

- The Information Technology Act, 2000, the Information Technology (reasonable security practices and procedures and sensitive personal data or information) Rules, 2011, and the Information Technology Rules, 2011
- Other Service Providers Regulations under the New Telecom Policy, 1999
- The Drugs and Cosmetics Act, 1940 and Drugs and Cosmetics Rules, 1945
- NMC approved the Indian Medical Council Act, 1956 and the Indian Medical Council (Professional conduct, Etiquette and Ethics) Regulations, 2002
- The Drugs and Magic Remedies Act, 1954 and Drugs and Magic Remedies Rules, 1955
- Unsolicited Commercial Communications Regulations, 2007 and Telecom Commercial Communication Customer Preference Regulations, 2010
- The Clinical Establishments Act, 2010
- Personal Data Protection Bill, 2019 was introduced in Lok Sabha, on 11 December 2019. The said Bill seeks to provide for the protection of individuals' personal data and establishes a Data Protection Authority for the same. However, in the absence of any strict adherence to these, no standards have yet been set to mandate the implementation of data protection and security till date.

INFORMATION TECHNOLOGY IN HEALTHCARE SCHEMES

National Level

The healthcare sector is important in India and various healthcare schemes are currently in force which can be broadly classified under Central Sector Schemes, Centrally Sponsored Schemes, and State Schemes. At national level, the MoHFW is the supreme body.

Various schemes such as Pradhan Mantri Swasthya Suraksha Yojana; the National AIDS and STD Control Program; Family Welfare Schemes; the National Pharmacovigilance Program; National Organ Transplant Program; Impacting Research Innovation and Technology (IMPRINT) Scheme; and Swachhta Action Plan (SAP) are covered under Central Sector Schemes. In addition, various programs such as the National Health Mission (NHM), National Rural Health Mission (NRHM), and National Urban Health Mission (NUHM) are centrally sponsored schemes which are representing various other subschemes.

State Level

Further, at state level, this organization is under the Department of Health and Family Welfare of each state which is headed by a minister and has a secretariat under the charge of the Secretary or Commissioner (Health and Family Welfare) belonging to the cadre of the Indian Administrative Service (IAS).

Regional and Zonal Setup

In addition, at regional level, each regional and zonal setup covers three to five districts and acts under authority delegated by the State Directorate of Health Services; at district-level, the structure of health services is a middle-level management organization that provides a link between the state and the regional structures on one side, and the PHCs and subcenters on the other. Furthermore, at community level, one CHC has been established which provides basic specialty services in general medicine, pediatrics, surgery, obstetrics, and gynecology.

Key ongoing initiatives in digital health being implemented by MoHFW include Reproductive Child Healthcare (RCH); Integrated Disease Surveillance Program (IDSP); Integrated Health Information System (IHIP); e-Hospital, e-Shushrut, Electronic Vaccine Intelligence Network (eVIN); Central Government Health Scheme (CGHS); Integrated Health Information Platform (IHIP); National Health Portal (NHP); National Identification Number (NIN); Online Registration System (ORS); Mera Aspatal (Patient Feedback System); Health Management Information System (HMIS); and National Medical College Network (NMCN). These initiatives are operational at a significantly mature level and continuously generate an enormous amount of data in the health sector for providing benefits to the public. Since health is a state subject, states are supported under the NHM for associated services such as Telemedicine, Tele-Radiology, Tele-Oncology, Tele-Ophthalmology, and Hospital Information System (HIS).

FUTURE DIGITAL HEALTH TECHNOLOGIES

- *Telemedicine/virtual care*: NMC has provided guidelines—48 pages on Telemedicine Practice Guidelines enabling registered medical practitioners to provide healthcare using telemedicine.
- *Robotics*:
  - Energy storage
  - Ethics and security
- *Wearables*:
  - Cost of device
  - Battery life
  - Safety, security, and privacy
- *Virtual assistants (e.g., Alexa)*:
  - Lack of accuracy
  - Lack of analytical interpretation
- *Mobile applications*:
  - Competitive market
  - Promotion and marketing
- *Software as a medical device*:
  - Software development lifecycle
  - Product safety and security
  - Data collection and privacy
- *Artificial intelligence (AI)-as-a-Service*:
  - Reliance
  - Transparency and governance
  - Long-term cost

- *Internet of Things (IoT) and connected devices*:
    - Compatibility of operating systems
    - Identification and authentication of devices and technologies
    - Integration of IoT products and platforms
    - Connectivity
    - Data analytics, security, and privacy
    - Consumer awareness
- *Three-dimensional (3D) printing/bioprinting*:
    - Piracy
    - Misinterpretation of results
- *Natural language processing*:
    - Understanding of natural language
    - Reasoning about multiple documents
    - Identification of data and evaluation of problem

Clauses of Secrecy and Privacy of Health Data

The primary contractual consideration to ensure secrecy and privacy for the various stages from collecting database to use the same would be to enter into nondisclosure data and confidentiality of patients in agreements with other healthcare employees and other healthcare influencers involved providing remedies due to breach of predefined contractual conditions such as consent, permissions, etc. The key issues in sharing personal data are primarily, but not limited to, transparency and control of data collection and exchange; security and privacy during transition; and information sharing, trust, responsibility, and accountability.

POSTCOVID-19 PHYSICIAN'S LIFE NOW

One day, the COVID-19 pandemic will no longer be a global healthcare crisis. However, it will significantly change both the way medical practices operate and clinicians practice medicine.

Problems to Tackle

The year 2020 has been a remarkably challenging period for the healthcare industry, with intense pressure on physicians during the COVID-19 pandemic. A small number of physicians running small private practices around the country have reported steep declines in revenues and drops were so significant that some of them have closed their clinic or hospital, especially senior general practitioners. Though most doctors have learned to cope with new safety protocols, much of the healthcare industry has absorbed the financial impact of reduced elective procedures and patient volumes. It was an opportunity for those providers on the frontlines of acute care who have worked tirelessly, helping patients in need, risking their health in the process of treating the COVID-19 patients. For many physician practices, changes presumed to be temporary just a few months ago may in fact become part of more permanent changes to their practice structure. We anticipate there will be changes in the way doctors practice post-COVID-19, citing likely trends such as fewer in-person patient visits and fewer visits from medical sales representatives. It is also increasingly likely that what doctors will return with "new normal" in medical practice many ways.

Opportunities to Grasp for Future

- *We have to redefine patient access and treatment options in the following ways*:
    - Telemedicine is quick and significant shift in response to the pandemic will result in an increased demand for telemedicine services post-COVID-19. This will continue to promote social distancing and avoid risk; many providers are relying more heavily on telemedicine to deliver services to their patients.
    - A shift in the point-of-care shall shift. The importance of digital health solutions was made clear during these challenging times. They are ready-made options to bring healthcare to patients rather than the other way round. Telemedicine's use has skyrocketed.
    - All the training in the world would not help Indian patients if they do not feel comfortable using the digital technology or do not have access to telemedicine. It could be a huge stumbling block for geriatricians and elderly patients. In India, telemedicine coverage includes services delivered by audio-only telephone calls also, which likely would help patients who lack Wi-Fi and a computer.
- *Sustainable medical care and living healthy solutions*: If this pandemic taught us anything, it is that our life (as it used to be) is not sustainable for our planet. We all had to experiment with digital solutions, be it virtual meetings for work, digital education for students, or virtual events instead of in-person conferences. These proved not only to be effective but also an environmentally friendly way to operate in a connected world. We are not saying everything is going digital, but it makes sense to make digital anything that is not more efficient in real life, if possible. Telemedicine and digital health technology already show their aptitude to make this a possibility. They just need to be adopted on a large scale.
- *We have to sensitize regulatory agencies and insurance providers and make them perceive new opportunities by*:
    - To support adaptation and adoption to telemedicine by providing additional coverage and expanded flexibility to telemedicine technology, since it is operating from distant sites and may not be in territorial jurisdiction of patient.
    - Telemedicine-benefitted patients are to experience ease of access healthcare that eliminates transportation logistics, virus exposure concerns, and long waits. As the pandemic plays out, societal habits and norms shall be shifting for telemedicine, and the impacts of these changes will likely permeate into healthcare practices across a range of specialties. In terms of the practice environment, the COVID-19 pandemic appears to have accelerated the use of telemedicine.
    - Physicians associate the trend of reduced in-person visits as opportunity and the emergence of telemedicine and the convenience it provides to patients; some further note that patients may delay nonessential treatment or visits in-person.
- *Physician's inclination to use established therapies*: Healthcare providers have opportunity to shift toward more established therapies and generic drugs, potentially making it easier for them to manage adverse events or titrate therapies.
- *Opportunities to avoid in-person meeting of sales representatives and reliance on review articles published in peer-reviewed journals*:
    - Physicians can expect to use sales representatives and in-person meetings less often as sources of medical information.
    - Physicians are expected to read review articles published in peer-reviewed journals and websites to gather new information that can help them in practice. This shift in

channels provides an opportunity for other pharmaceutical industry professionals aiming to communicate with physicians to optimize their approach for physician convenience and comprehension.

- *Opportunities to avoid in-person examination of patient, but if they come then observe certain rules of hygiene*: The COVID-19 pandemic has forced doctors to take the waiting patients, as physicians quickly see as many patients with masks as they can by maintaining social distancing and by observing certain other rules of hygiene.
- *Opportunities toward maintenance of medical records by more use of electronic medical records (EMR)*: Post-COVID-19 pandemic, we will take a historic stride toward most promising way of maintaining medical records by electronic health records, which we never realized that they are more efficient, convenient, and affordable in healthcare system.
- *Opportunities due to patient's trust diminished in treatment in globalized foreign treatment*: In the prepandemic globalized world, patients enjoyed a certain level of trust mostly took for granted to go abroad for treatment. Patients could travel almost without limitations, meet foreign doctors without restrictions, and order foreign products worldwide. Patients will not be able to travel that freely or enjoy the supply chains of medicines from the world so easily. Patients will think twice before going somewhere or to take treatment abroad. The pandemic is already exacerbating signs of social anxiety and agoraphobia among patients. Regaining trust will take time and these trends will take place over months.
- *Opportunities to upgrade governmental medical services*: The overburdened government hospitals need an upgrade on every level from their infrastructures to their processes. These will be needed to ensure a safe environment for the healthcare personnel and patients, as well to better cope with any emergency situations. We can expect to see many governments put more focus on healthcare.
- *Opportunities to inculcate brand-new good hygiene habits in patients*: Awareness for personal and public hygiene measures saw a surge thanks to the contagion. Health authorities are advocating for regular hand washing with soap for at least 20 seconds. Social distancing measures are in place. People are getting used to wearing facemasks which is leading to overall better hygiene. We might see people wearing masks wherever they go and unintentionally be more cautious when visiting elderly people. We should never shake hands again.
- *Opportunities to use AI as a necessary tool in medical practice*: We have stressed the need to implement AI in the healthcare setting for years, but the novel corona virus' damage highlighted this need even more. We saw how an AI platform assisted in sending out the first alerts of the outbreak. Algorithms are used to help screen for those potentially affected. AI can help hospitals manage their resources. These developments go on to show that AI will help us better prepare for the next public health crisis. These algorithms are not solutions in themselves but rather tools aiding professionals to perfect their craft.
- *Opportunities for surgical branches post-COVID rebound of patient overload may occur*: We have to understand increase in patient volumes once elective procedures can be performed again, there will be increased competition to capture the backlogged demand.
- *Opportunities to do multitasking by paramedical and nonmedical support staff*: Medical practices have historically maintained by putting paramedical and nonmedical staff to work for healthcare practitioner. Now, few staff members may fill multiple roles, particularly between front office and back office functions to maintain cash flow. There is increased adoption of computer technology to get payments from patients and maintain electronic records.

Changes to Absorb

- *How the pandemic could influence the next generation of healthcare professionals*: Being a physician has always been considered a noble and honorable profession, but ever since COVID-19, physicians, along with the nurses and other healthcare professionals working on the front lines, have become bona fide heroes. The public now sees these courageous men and women risking their lives for others (sometimes without the protective equipment they need) while isolating themselves from their own families to do so. But with this adulation has come an enormous cost. More than hundreds of doctors and nurses across the world have died from the novel coronavirus. Such grim numbers have shocked both the public and those already in or considering a career in healthcare. Yes, these careers involve hardwork, life or death levels of responsibility, and many stressful situations.
- *Acute care hospitals and health systems*: The market is gradually gaining greater visibility on the financial and operational impact of the pandemic to hospitals and health systems. This will continue in post-COVID era.
- *Ambulatory surgery centers*: Due to their substantial focus on emergency care, post-COVID-19 surgery center industry was near complete standstill. Now, they will pick up.
- *Long-term behavioral health*: Those who did not show signs of depression, anxiety, or substance abuse may be at a heightened risk of developing tendencies in post-COVID-19 environment.
- *Hospital dialysis to home dialysis*: Dialysis clinics, which provide life-saving services to patients, have remained open during COVID-19, as they cannot defer or cease treatments without considerable risk to the patients they serve. There is reason to expect these standard treatment protocols will trend to home dialysis over the short term and potentially continue in the long term.
- *Imaging in medicine*: The COVID-19 pandemic has caused many imaging centers to have a material decrease in scan volume due to a reduction in elective scans. Now, they will pick up.
- *Importance of digital health solutions*: Audio and video teleconsultation, audio and video telediagnosis, electronic maintenance of health records, and use of AI in diagnosis and treatment of patients.
- *More use of electronic gadgets for measuring*:
  - Digital temperature
  - Digital pulse
  - Digital oxygen saturation (SpO_2)
  - Digital blood pressure
  - Digital blood sugar
  - Heart rate
  - Tele-electrocardiogram (ECG)
  - Tele-otoscope
  - Telefundoscopy

GOVERNMENT UPDATE ON TELEMEDICINE

Dr RS Sharma, Chief Executive Officer, National Health Authority, said that with the tectonic shift seen in the uptake of digital in the COVID-19 pandemic, there could not have been a more opportune time for Ayushman Bharat Digital Mission (ABDM) to come into being. While teleconsultations have been talked about for the past decade, this tectonic shift caused the emergence of telemedicine for consultations and outpatient departments (OPDs) in an unparallel manner. There is evidence from the success of the eSanjeevani app which has facilitated over five million teleconsultations till date which now sees 40,000 teleconsultations per day. ABDM will help create a superhighway to seamlessly connect all stakeholders of the healthcare ecosystem digitally. However, to redefine access to digital health and reinvent service delivery, we need a strong collaboration between public and private health programs. In ABDM, open design, inclusivity, and security are at its core. ABDM will be scalable and provide a cohesive ecosystem for private sector innovation. Further, with all health records linked under health ID, the patients will be able to access their health history anytime and anywhere without worrying of losing their health records.

CONCLUSION

Post-COVID-19 pandemic will change global healthcare practices and significantly change both the way medical practices shall operate. Clinicians shall rely on digital and virtual examination and consultation rather than "in-person" service. This will improve efficiency by use of digital gadgets and AI, save time of doctor and patient, and increase safety of both doctor and patient. New era shall be full of opportunities and challenges both for patients and doctors to change for better.

KEY LEARNING POINTS

- Currently, telemedicine is available for legally and ideally OPD patients and not for in-patient department (IPD).
- Legally, currently, telemedicine availability for Indian interstate practice is in gray area and not allowed for foreign countries.
- Digitalization of medicine is available now in form of electronic medical record, keeping with hard copies of consent in PDF format.
- It remains to be seen whether clinicians shall rely on digital and virtual examination and consultation rather than "in-person" service.
- Digitalization of medicine will improve efficiency by use of digital gadgets, AI, save time of doctor and patient, increase safety and satisfaction of both doctor and patient.
- We shall see new era shall be full of opportunities and challenges both for patients and doctors to change for better, but hope legal luminaries will not oppose it.

BIBLIOGRAPHY

1. Appendix 5 of the Indian Medical Council (Professional Conduct, Etiquette and Ethics Regulation, 2002). https://www.maharashtramedicalcouncil.in/Files/Notifications_26032020_MCI%20Notification%20Regarding%20TELEMEDICINE.pdf
2. Baldwa M, Baldwa V, Padvi N, et al. Legal Issues in Critical Care. India: CBS Publishers & Distributors Pvt Ltd; 2022.
3. Baldwa M, Baldwa V, Padvi N, et al. Legal Issues in Medical Practice. India: CBS Publishers & Distributors Pvt Ltd; 2018.

4. Deepa Sanjeev Pawaskar vs. State of Maharashtra, (Bombay) 2018(3) Crimes 576, https://indiankanoon.org/doc/160266477/
5. Federation of Obstetrics & Gynecological Societies of India v/s Union of India, (2019) 6 SCC 283, https://indiankanoon.org/doc/123238150/
6. Increasingly Popular, Telemedicine Faces Legal Hurdles-Allen Smith
7. Krishna Mandal v/s State of Odisha, BLAPL 3541/2020, https://indiankanoon.org/doc/5796405/
8. Legal position of telemedicine, 2014.
9. Ministry of Health and Family Welfare. National Telemedicine Service: Bridging the Digital Health Divide.
10. Mohd. Ishfaq, (SC) 2009 AIR (SC) 2049, https://indiankanoon.org/doc/1092676/
11. Samira Kohli vs Doctor Prabha Manchanda, https://indiankanoon.org/doc/438423/
12. Solimini R, Busardò FP, Gibelli F, Sirignano A, Ricci G. Ethical and Legal Challenges of Telemedicine in the Era of the COVID-19 Pandemic. Medicina (Kaunas). 2021;57(12):1314.
13. Telemedicine in India—A Legal Perspective. 2002;12:185-8.
14. Vijaya Laxmi v/s Dr Krishna Kumar. https://www.casemine.com/judgement/in/5609067ee4b014971116463a
15. Yash Aggarwal v. Union of India (Delhi)(DB) 17.04.2020. https://indiankanoon.org/doc/43780306/

43

CHAPTER

Legal Issues in Medical Education

CM Chhajer, Satish Tiwari

INTRODUCTION

It has now been accepted that there is "holistic or spiritual component" in the health of an individual. It includes integrity, ethics, purpose in life, and commitment to some higher being. The recent industrialization, commercialization, and globalization have their effects on medical education also. The technical and scientific developments have resulted in many positive changes. But at the same time, it has some negative changes as well as ill effects. There is maldistribution of rural-urban healthcare providers, decrease in moral values, corporate culture in healthcare services, and of course decreasing standard and commercialization of medical education.

PRIVATIZATION OF MEDICAL EDUCATION

The mushrooming of private medical colleges and deemed universities has added fuel to the fire. Inconsistencies in the cases of many deemed universities is too evident to be overlooked. The myth that private institutions have better facilities has also been disproved. They often use their clout to flout norms and unfairly profit from the business of higher education. These private medical schools are run by managing committees which are under the influence of politically heavyweight personalities. These politicians form the backbone of these institutions whose aim is only to mint money at any cost. Unfortunately, ethical considerations are often of least importance in such institutions. You can not only buy an undergraduate seat but also a postgraduate degree. The medical education has been made a commodity for the rich. The private managements are not only fooling the students and their parents but also the government, judiciary, and regulatory bodies.

NATIONAL MEDICAL COMMISSION

The National Medical Commission (NMC) formed in 2019 [replaces the erstwhile Medical Council of India (MCI)] now regulates the standard of medical education in India. But the present observation suggests that the commission has been unable to solve the issues in which the MCI had badly failed. Though it is too early to come to a conclusion, it is felt that nothing much has changed.

According to chapter 1.4.2, physicians shall display as suffix to their names only recognized medical degrees or such certificates/diplomas and memberships/honors which confer professional knowledge or recognizes any exemplary qualification/achievements. This regulation is very ambiguous because the word "or" for the certificates/diplomas, honors, etc., does not apply to MCI-recognized achievements only. Similarly, according to chapter 7.20, a physician shall not claim to be a specialist unless he has a special qualification in that branch. Here again, the regulations are ambiguous regarding whether the qualifications should be MCI recognized or any qualifications. The effect of these ambiguous regulations or guidelines is that there are many organizations, institutes, or bodies who are running unrecognized courses and cheating the students, parents, people, and the communities. The State Medical Councils which were formed to look in the matters of state-wise registration of medical graduates are recognizing such (MCI unrecognized) qualifications for practicing in a particular state only. This is not only creating a confusion in the minds of medical graduates, but it also raises the very vital issue regarding the powers of the various councils as far as regulation of medical education is concerned. There is need to tackle this paradox since the NMC (MCI) is the highest body as far as regulation of medical education is concerned. Hence, if the NMC does not recognize a particular course or qualification, the various State Medical Councils cannot over rule these NMC guidelines and recognize these courses in their respective states. If a proper decision is not taken on this issue, it will create a chaos in the future because in India, we have more than 28 states and each and every state can frame its own guidelines and regulations for medical education in its respective states. So, there has to be a highest regulatory body whose decision shall prevail in case any controversy or ambiguity arises.

ROLE OF REGULATORY BODIES

As discussed earlier, the regulatory bodies such as medical and dental commissions or councils have been formed with the aim of regulating the medical education and practice of medicine in different systems. Various private medical colleges mushroomed all over India defying all the prescribed NMC/MCI norms. Many institutions are conferring unrecognized degrees, diplomas, certificates, etc., and thus cheating the highest regulatory body of India. Cheating of regulatory bodies has become a norm rather than exception. The unethical practice is ignored and guilty doctors remain undetected and unpunished by otherwise highly qualified, resourceful, and powerful medical bodies.

PRESENT SCENARIO

The medical education system has totally failed on cost-effective and input-output analysis. These industries can produce only commercially sound but morally weak graduates. They will produce doctors for the classes and not for the masses. Our health system needs "*barefoot doctors*" (as experimented in China) who will serve the masses and not the classes. The emphasis is changing from healthcare for the people to healthcare by the people.

The teaching faculties in private institutions are mostly part-time, "*daily-wage earners,*" fixed salaried, "transient teachers," or the so-called "ghost faculties" are substandard and frustrated individuals willing to "sort things out" as per the need of the management. Most of the teachers in clinical specialties who have well-established private practices hardly find time to teach. Serious teaching and research have been affected badly. The few who are enthusiastic are disheartened by uncongenial atmosphere. Associated with this, the commercialization of medical education has further deteriorated the already "rotten system." Money can buy marks and merit but not the sincerity and morality. The important issue is whether the higher education shall be the right of a citizen? Should government nationalize and act as a watch guard in controlling the corruption and financial mismanagement in running the private institutions of "political heavyweights?"

Are we going to produce ethically and morally motivated graduates from these "money-spinning educational factories?" The long felt need is that the government should enact a legislation to provide equal opportunities for higher/professional education to the poorest of the poor citizens.

Regretting that some "privilege remains unchanged" even after 68 years of independence, the Supreme Court stated that national interest requires doing away with all forms of reservation in institutions of higher education and urged the center to take effective steps "objectively." A bench of Justice noted that despite several reminders to the central and state governments to make merit the primary criteria for superspecialty courses, the ground reality remains that reservation often holds sway over merit. While dealing with the issue of reservation in superspecialty courses in medical institutions, the court had said "there should really be no reservation" since it is in the general interest for improving the standard of higher education, and thereby improving the quality of available medical services to the people of India. It also referred to a body of judgments asking government authorities to abstain from relaxing the eligibility criteria based on various kinds of reservation since it would defeat the very object of imparting the best possible training to selected meritorious candidates.

CROSS PATHY VERSUS INTEGRATION

The cross pathy is one of the highly debated hot issues at present. Many state governments are allowing AYUSH (Ayurveda, Yoga and naturopathy,. Unani, Siddha, and Homoeopathy) doctors to practice modern medicine in their states. The Medical Universities have also asked for Ayurvedic and homeopathic outpatient departments (OPDs) in the medical colleges. The NMC has made it compulsory for every medical college to have a "Department of Integrative Medicine Research" to promote integration of modern medicine with homoeopathy and Indian systems of medicine such as Ayurveda. The central government is also promoting AYUSH by having a separate department or ministry for them. The modern medicine doctors see this "mixopathy" as unlawful, harmful to the society as the AYUSH doctors are "half baked" and not adequately trained in medicines used in allopathy. The Indian Medical Association wanted the Government to rethink regarding integration of different systems of medicine. They are protesting this at various levels, while the authorities say that as modern medicine doctors are not giving their services in rural areas, the only option with government is to allow modern medicine practice through AYUSH doctors. The *SC in Civil Appeal Nos. 8553-8557 of 2014, State of Gujarat vs. Dr PA Bhatt* (decided on April 26, 2023) held that we have no doubt that every alternative system of medicine may have its pride of place in history. But today, the practitioners of indigenous systems of medicine do not perform complicated surgical operations. A study of Ayurveda does not authorize them to perform these surgeries. Therefore, even while recognizing the importance of Ayurveda doctors and the need to promote alternative/indigenous systems of medicine, we cannot be oblivious of the fact that both categories of doctors are certainly not performing equal work to be entitled to equal pay.

One of the suggestions on the issue is to integrate the different systems and have a common undergraduate degree. On the matter of interaction of allopathy and alternative medicine, the Group of ministers has pointed out that the "prejudice of AYUSH being a nonscientific field can be overcome by integrating it in the MBBS curriculum." This means that the undergraduate Ayurvedic and homeopathic courses shall be scrapped or abolished. At undergraduate level, there should be only MBBS or BBMS (bachelor of basic medical sciences) where students shall be taught about some of the common medicines from allopathy, Ayurvedic, homeopathy, etc. The New Educational Policy (NEP) 2020 that has been approved by the cabinet calls for a healthcare education system that must be integrative.

The specialization in Ayurvedic and homeopathy shall be during postgraduation, i.e., there should be MD and MS in Ayurveda, homeopathy, etc., as we have in pediatrics, medicine, surgery, orthopedics, etc., for modern medicine. The undergraduates can practice all the system of medicine, but those who are MD Ayurveda or homeopathy shall practice only their specialty. In the present scenario, this seems to be one of the most practical solutions for the present controversy regarding mixopathy, cross pathy, or integration of medical sciences.

TIME FOR "GURUKUL MEDICAL EDUCATION"

The big multispecialty or corporate hospitals exist in splendid isolation in the community, acquiring the euphemism "an ivory tower of diseases." There is no doubt that we have to accept the development and advances in medical sciences so as to improve the health and quality of the life of an individual and the nation. Medicine will continue to evolve so long as man's quest for better health continues. But the important issue that arises is that should we continue with commercialization of medical education? or should we go back to simplified and basic methods of teaching medical sciences? Should there be centralization of medical education and that too in the hands of capitalist or the process should be decentralized in the benefit of common layman in the community. This is the time to review our errors and accomplishments. Can this be included in "Millennium Development Goals?" The Government of India along with NMC is planning to start medical colleges to educate rural students and deploy them there to provide basic healthcare to villagers. Many villagers rely on indigenous systems of medicine. The doctors taught in villages or small towns (Taluka places) might prefer to work in that area following the footsteps of their "*Guru*." Thus, it can solve the problem of maldistribution of doctors in remote areas. This means that technical advances in health services are not going to fulfill the dreams of Indian population as well. We are going to provide services to classes at the expense of masses. This trend cannot be cost-effective in developing countries such as India. What we need is healthcare for the people that too preferably by the people. This can be achieved only if we have more healthcare personnel (including qualified medical graduates) catering to the needs of community including rural community.

There are many good academicians who are engaged in stand-alone clinics, hospitals, or private practice. Because of their busy schedule, they are unable to keep pace with technical advances in medical sciences. Teaching liabilities may encourage them to update their knowledge by reading and attending continuing medical education (CME), workshops, panel discussions, etc. There is no paucity of good, morally strong medical teachers (Gurus) even in present era. In fact, the postgraduate medical education is completed under a guide (Guru).

Then what is the harm if undergraduate candidates are also taught by the Guru? Why should we not allow them to select the *"Shishya"* from the community and train them for this noble profession? Can Indian method of Gurukul teaching solve this problem of commercialization? The graduates taught in Gurukul can be examined, evaluated by an authorized agency (as we are doing for undergraduate students from overseas or foreign universities), and subsequently trained for latest advances in medical sciences at specialty hospitals (government or corporate) with minimum expenses and as per the need. In this manner, there are more chances of producing morally strong and educationally qualified graduates. Thus, we can achieve the concept of "healthcare for the people and by the people."

CONCLUSION

The stakeholders seem to be confused regarding the status of medical education in our country. The medical education needs to be reenvisioned so that the duration and structure matches the role requirements of the graduates. Our health education system must be integrative so that the basic understanding of modern medicine as well as AYUSH with emphasis on community medicine and preventive healthcare. There is need to restructure the medical education. Competency-based medical education (CBME) developed by the NMC can be one step in this direction.

KEY LEARNING POINTS

- In ancient India, there were many health consultants or experts. The Lord Dhanvantari is known as God of health.
- In modern era, the corporate culture has destroyed the basic healthcare concept.
- There is need to integrate various systems practiced in our country.
- We need to discuss the various options available to improve the healthcare facilities.
- Gurukul medical education can be another option to prevent the commercialization.
- Let us work together to create health workers for the people by the people.

BIBLIOGRAPHY

1. Chattopadhyay S. (2023). Govt needs to rethink the strategy of mixopathy: IMA President Dr Sharad Kumar Agarwal. [online] Available from https://medicaldialogues.in/news/health/govt-needs-to-rethink-the-strategy-of-mixopathy-ima-president-dr-sharad-kumar-agarwal-105148 [Last accessed September, 2024].
2. Chhajer C, Tiwari S. Legal issues in medical education. In: Tiwari S, Baldwa M, Tiwari M, et al. (Eds). Textbook on Medicolegal Issues Related to Various Medical Specialties, 2nd edition. New Delhi: Jaypee Brothers Medical Publishers (P) Ltd.; 2019. pp. 485-8.
3. Garima. (2020). Group of Ministers on health call for shorter MBBS duration, integration with PG medical courses: Report. [online] Available from https://medicaldialogues.in/news/education/group-of-ministers-on-health-call-for-shorter-mbbs-duration-integration-with-pg-medical-courses-report-72273 [Last accessed September, 2024].
4. Jayanth AS. (2022). NMC bats for integration of modern medicine with Ayush. [online] Available from https://www.thehindu.com/news/national/kerala/nmc-bats-for-integration-of-modern-medicine-with-ayush/article65918077.ece [Last accessed September, 2024].

5. National Medical Commission (Indian Medical Council). (2002). Code of Medical Ethics Regulations, 2002. [online] Available from https://www.nmc.org.in/rules-regulations/code-of-medical-ethics-regulations-2002/ [Last accessed September, 2024].
6. Park K (Ed). Health care of the community. Park's Textbook of Preventive and Social Medicine, 25th edition. Jabalpur: Banarsidas Bhanot Publisher; 2019. pp. 950-81.
7. Singhania MA. (2015). Supreme Court has directed institutions to scrap quota for specialty medical courses. [online] Available from https://medicaldialogues.in/supreme-court-asks-govt-to-scrap-quotas-in-super-speciality-medical-courses?infinitescroll=1 [Last accessed September, 2024].
8. Singhania MA. (2020). New Education Policy calls for Integration of Allopathy, AYUSH system of medicine. [online] Available from https://medicaldialogues.in/news/health/government-policies/new-education-policy-calls-for-integration-of-allopathy-ayush-systems-of-medicine-68177 [Last accessed September, 2024].
9. The Times of India. Deemed below par: Editorial. Nagpur: The Times of India; January 21, 2010. p. 10 (Col. 1-2).
10. The Times of India. MCI plans 300 rural Medical colleges. Nagpur: The Times of India; February 7, 2010. p. 11 (Col. 5-6).
11. Tiwari SK. Medical ethics: Are we going in right direction? In: Mathur GP, Mathur Sarla (Eds). Current Trends in Pediatrics, Volume 2, 1st edition. Delhi: M/s Academa Publishers; 2006. pp. 67-71.

44

CHAPTER

Medical Tourism

Mukul Tiwari, Abhyuday Tiwari

INTRODUCTION

Medical tourism can be defined as "traveling by patients to another country or another region in the same country, to get treatments, which may come at a lower but in some cases, at a higher cost, and may or may not be available in their home town/country, without legal hindrances, the kind of medical procedures and innovative treatments they desire."

There is opportunity for the medical tourist to enjoy tourism and the holiday in the country they visit. In this way, he is having extra benefit. Medical tourism includes three basic components, namely hospital services, hotels, and travel/leisure. There are immense economic growth and infrastructure development opportunities for countries which have attractive policies and correct marketing strategies.

The global medical tourism market size is projected to grow from $24.14 billion in 2023 to $93.38 billion by 2030, at a compounded annual growth rate (CAGR) of 21.3% over the forecast period. Its growth prediction is impressive and may even surpass the expectation. The reasons for such exponential growth are progress in healthcare technology, increasing tendency and will to travel, increasing prosperity, and increasing need for specialized treatments. The most sought-after medical tourism destinations in the world are: Thailand, India, South America, Singapore, Hong Kong, Hungary, Malaysia, and recently the Middle Eastern countries.

HOW MEDICAL TOURISM EVOLVED?

Medical tourism is not a new trend. Since the dawn of civilization, human beings have visited other locations to get treatment for their ailments. The Egyptians and the Greek in the ancient times visited different Mediterranean places for purification and spiritual treatment. Earliest documented instances of medical tourism are probably of the Greek pilgrims who visited Epidaurus, a place in the Sardonic Gulf, known as sanctuary of Asclepius, the healing god.

Since the 1500s, India became a known destination for teaching yoga as well as offer Ayurveda treatment to patients worldwide. Roman and British patients visited hot springs for health rejuvenation and healing. 18th century onward, Europeans visited medical spas in Germany, seeking relief from grievous and disabling ailments such as tuberculosis, liver diseases, and gout. In Europe, the affluent and capable have traditionally visited health spas to "take the waters" for curing ailments.

In the 20th century, patients began traveling in search of alternative forms of treatment, for example, Hoxsey Clinic, Tijuana, Mexico; Bumrungrad International Hospital and Bangkok International Hospital, Asia. In the 21st century, the United States (US) began to promote internationally its centers of excellence, for example, University of Pittsburgh Transplant Center, Mayo Clinic, Cleveland Clinic, and MD Anderson Cancer Center.

In recent times, even less developed countries have raised their level of expertise and facilities for cutting-edge treatments relative to that of the developed countries. These nations have come up with feasible policies and strategies to encourage medical tourism.

TYPES OF MEDICAL TOURISM

Medical tourism has evolved over the decades into many subspecialties. One subspecialty is health/recuperative tourism, i.e., travel to a recuperative climate with natural therapeutic resources. The health tourism business provides mainly yoga, massages, traditional Ayurveda medicine, and spa resorts. This type of tourism does not involve high technology but needs a good infrastructure.

Fertility tourism is another branch of medical tourism gaining popularity. The main causes behind the growth in fertility tourism are strict legal codes in the native place of the patient which makes it a cumbersome process for them. Another reason is lower cost in the less developed countries. In vitro fertilization (IVF) and donor insemination are the main treatments offered. For example, before 2016, couples from the People's Republic of China visited fertility clinics outside the country to bypass the government ruling of one-child policy. Numerous nations have no policy on the number of embryos transfer. India used to be is one of the top centers for surrogacy because of economy of the treatments. Indian infertility clinics are at par with those in the western world because of improved technology and infrastructure. After 2016, surrogacy laws in India have made it difficult for foreign couples to obtain surrogacy treatments in India.

There are other countries where surrogacy is legal, for example, Russia, Ukraine, and Georgia. Russian legislations have made Russia an attractive destination for "reproductive tourists" (couples seeking babies). In Russia, many clinics and facilities offer oocyte donation as well as surrogacy services for couples with advanced age and single marital status for both men and women. In Russia, commercial surrogacy is legal. The US is an attractive destination for couples seeking green card through surrogate mothers. Surrogacy laws vary worldwide and also in a single country from state to state. In the US, it is allowed in some states but banned in others. In India, Canada, and the United Kingdom (UK), only altruistic surrogacy is allowed. In Georgia, meanwhile as in Ukraine and Russia, both forms are legal.

Euthanasia tourism is also in practice. It is not a major branch of medical tourism. A few countries provide this service, namely Switzerland, Netherlands, etc. Lots of regulations exist to avail of the facilities.

INDIA'S MEDICAL TOURISM

Medical tourism is one of the fastest growing sectors in India. In 2022, medical tourism market was approximately US $6 billion. Approximately, two million patients visit India every year for medical, wellness, and IVF treatments. The industry is expected to reach $13 billion by 2026, backed by the government's Heal in India initiative. Ministry of tourism (MOT) has built

National Strategy and Roadmap for Medical and Wellness Tourism in 2022. Corona caused a severe decline (>40% in 2021), but medical tourism bounced back to precorona level in 2022 and is now expected to meet its precorona predictions. According to some estimates, India is now second biggest tourist destination after Thailand, while other reports say it is one of the top five medical tourism destinations. In India, Gurugram is the biggest center, followed by Chennai.

In 2019, the Indian government waved off necessity for foreigners to arrange medical visa to receive medical treatment. These initiatives will go a long way in helping India boost tourism market. India has 40 hospitals accredited by the US Joint Commission. As the treatment costs in the developed world increase out of the affordability limits, more and more westerners are likely to choose cheaper destinations.

India is also quite popular with African patients seeking overseas treatments. The main treatments for which tourists come to India are alternative medicine, bone marrow and organ transplants, cardiac bypass, eye surgery, hip replacement, dental treatments, fertility treatments, oncology problems, etc. The Government has also started various initiatives that can be of great push to help international patients get the right kind of treatment at affordable prices.

Medical tourism in India is a major revenue source. According to the medical tourism index, a bypass surgery in India costs roughly US $10,000 as opposed to US $113,000 in the US. According to the medical tourism resource guide, a heart valve replacement costs about $15,000 in India, versus $150,000 in the US; Chennai is drawing highest numbers with 45% of patients from abroad and 30–40% domestic.

Ministry of Tourism, India might expand its market development assistance (MDA) scheme so that it can develop the Joint Commission International (JCI) and National Accreditation Board of Hospitals (NABH) certified hospitals. An official announcement is likely soon.

Advantages of India as a medical tourism hub is familiarity with English language, new state of the art technologies, and an increasing compliance to international quality standards. A big hurdle in the growth of the industry is poor infrastructure of the country and widespread poverty, but hopefully things will improve in future. Recently, it was calculated that the medical packages in India were costing only a fifth of what was being charged in the US or Britain.

India gets a sizable patient flow from neighboring countries which have less developed healthcare, such as Bangladesh, Pakistan, Myanmar, and central Asian countries. Patients also come from African countries and the Middle East. The country is also becoming popular with even Americans, Canadians, and Europeans for cost reasons.

RISKS AND HURDLES IN MEDICAL TOURISM

Medical tourism carries the following risks:

- Communication is a major issue. In destination country, because of language barriers, the visitor and care givers may not be able to communicate effectively, leading to errors and misunderstanding.
- In some south eastern countries such as India, Malaysia, or even Thailand, the patients might get exposed to microbial agents and infections which are absent in their country and what if they do not possess the required immunity to combat them, for example, gastrointestinal diseases—amoebic dysentery, typhoid, paratyphoid, hepatitis A, mosquito-transmitted diseases, tuberculosis, and influenza. Such infections, if contracted by tourists, can complicate the prognosis of the disease for which they are being treated. Therefore, healthcare professionals must be utmost careful in diagnosing such infections.

- Another note of concern is that the medical tourists are also at risk of acquiring blood-borne infection because of poor blood collection, screening, and storage facilities. Patients visiting for organ transplantations are especially at higher risk for contracting severe infections and facing the complications.
- Another point of concern is that medical tourists may carry the infection to their home countries. A notable example to be remembered is the New Delhi metallo-beta-lactamase 1 (NDM-1) fiasco where the patients took the strain back to their native countries.
- The care and quality of the treatment as well as postoperative care might be different between the destination country and the developed world; even in the same country, there may be differences between the hospitals and may be different from European or US standards. In 2004, the World Health Organization (WHO) launched the World Alliance for Patient Safety, acknowledging that there are differences in healthcare provider standards around the world. The main function of this body is to help hospitals and governments around the world set up patient safety policies and practices which help in providing safe and high standard medical care.
- After a treatment or postoperatively, patients have to travel home on long-distance flights with decreased mobility and cramped seating, which can be harmful and cause life-threatening situations such as deep-vein thrombosis or pulmonary embolism. This phenomenon is also known as "economy class syndrome."
- In destination country, the quality of medicines may be poor or counterfeit, especially where corruption is more prevalent and government regulations are weak.
- For patients who go back early to their home countries, posttreatment complications are a problem. In research on Omani patients, it was found that at least 15% patients who took treatment abroad faced complications after treatment; British Association of Plastic Reconstructive and Aesthetic Surgery also conducted a survey and found that 37% of members had patients who had complications from medical tourism.

LEGAL ISSUES IN MEDICAL TOURISM

- In many countries, there are inadequate policies to deal fairly with and address dissatisfied patients' complaints. Medical tourism is still a new field and there are many issues not addressed properly.
- In many developing countries, there is limited and uncertain litigation cover, which accounts for slow growth of medical tourism there. Although some countries which are attractive medical tourism destinations provide legal remedies for medical malpractice, such remedies may not be adequate to cover all the issues of the medical tourist. In case of problems, patients may not be covered sufficiently by personal insurance or may not be able to find compensation by malpractice lawsuits.
- In some places, even hospitals and/or doctors may not have sufficient indemnity cover/insurance cover by insurance companies to pay the financial damages awarded by the court. Things are changing and newer insurance policies are available which protect the patient even in such circumstances.
- Coming to another set of issues, there was an allegation of illegal purchase of organs and tissues for transplantation in countries such as India and China (before the rules became stricter in 2007). If a racket is apprehended by police, what outcome the patient has to face in such cases is another question. Is there any liability of the patient?

ETHICAL ISSUES IN MEDICAL TOURISM

- Medical tourism creates some ethical issues. There are worries that medical tourism, which is afforded by mostly rich people, will lead to a divide between haves and have-nots. For example, in Thailand, in 2008, it was observed that doctors had become so preoccupied with foreigners that Thai patients were being neglected. Same issue stands true for India. Is the rise in medical tourism good for poor Indians who are not deriving any benefit from it? In India, where hundreds of patients die from preventable illnesses, should the government focus on medical tourism by making medical tourist-friendly policies and help private hospitals that cater mainly to the demands of the affluent people? A concept of cosmopolitan nationalism must guide solutions to these dilemmas. According to this view, medical tourism in India can only be ethically justified if basic hygiene and health is improved and provided to all.
- A clear-cut example of "rich favoritism" is a leading hospital in New Delhi. The land (15 acres) was donated by the Government of Delhi and the hospital was built in 1996. Construction of the hospital was assisted by the Government funds and equity capital was also contributed by the Delhi Government, which also provided tax and duty waivers on import of equipment. All of this assistance was offered with the agreement that the hospital would reserve one third of its beds for the treatment of poor patients at no cost. In 1999–2000, only 2% patients in this hospital were treated free and most of these were relatives of staff, bureaucrats, and politicians.
- Centers which deal with stem cell treatments have a dubious reputation for misinformation, lack of scientific rationale, and profiteering. It is need of the hour to put a break on technologies which are sprouting but are more of unproven claims and are costly. There is also need to differentiate between a proper medical innovation and self-claimed innovations.
- Presently, proper legal frameworks for medical tourism do not exist. There are differences in regulations in different countries. In some countries, the legal cover is insufficient, although awareness is increasing. Ironically, the countries which have weak legal covers are also attracting a good number of medical tourists, whereas countries such as the USA, which have a good legal framework and policies in place, have not attracted much medical tourism because of increased legal liability and policy.
- In reproductive tourism which involves abortions/IVF and also in euthanasia tourism, lots of ethical issues are involved. In reproductive tourism, people travel to another destination to benefit from a service which is not available in home country due to legal reasons or because it is much costlier. There may be ethical objections regarding abortions and decisions surrounding IVF. Same is true for euthanasia tourism.
- Consumer's rights are important issues in reproductive and euthanasia tourism. Consumers have a right to seek treatment in alternative locations if their countries are not friendly or unreasonable and a different country has more policies which serve their rights. This is more relevant for procedures such as abortions, IVF, as well as euthanasia.
- There were reports of illegal selling of organs and tissues in countries such as China and India (before the rules became stricter in India) for transplantation.

INTERNATIONAL HEALTHCARE ACCREDITATIONS

Good standards are important in health care. In medical tourism, international healthcare accreditation, evidence-based medicine, and quality assurance, there are many parallel issues.

Most reputed accreditations worldwide include the JCI in the USA. They inspect and impart the accreditation to medical tourism facilities worldwide. They are the biggest guiding source for Americans seeking treatment internationally. Coming to the UK and Hong Kong, the Trent International Accreditation Scheme is underway.

There are variations in quality, cost, size, intent, intensity and intensity of marketing in different international healthcare accreditation schemes. Their costing to the hospitals and healthcare institutions is also variable from institution to institution.

Many hospitals world over try to acquire international accreditations, JCI for the US patients, and Trent for British and European patients.

There are other organizations in this field as follows:
- The Society for International Healthcare Accreditation (SOFIHA)
- HealthCare Tourism International is a US-based nonprofit organization (NPO). It looks after accreditation of health institutions for nonclinical aspects such as business practices, language issues, and unethical advertising
- The International Medical Travel Association (IMTA, based in Singapore)
- The United Kingdom Accreditation Forum (UKAF)
- *Medical Tourism Association*: Another NPO which inspects the quality and pricing

CONCLUSION

Medical tourism is an enormous developing market globally. India has turned out as one of the most favorable destinations for global medical tourists. It has a great chance at becoming the top leader in the field because of many advantages it offers. However, lack of international accreditations, poor infrastructure, and ill-defined legalities are still major hurdles toward achieving this goal. Development of litigation policies and a proper framework is the need of the hour to prevent disputes, conflicts, and legal battles.

KEY LEARNING POINTS

- Global medical tourism is a sizable and fast-growing market.
- It is estimated to be US $24.14 billion in 2023, of which India alone has a share of US $6 billion.
- Majority of tourism is for transplantations, surgeries, fertility, and oncology treatments.
- Legal framework and policies are still not well-developed in many places.
- Misinformation, language barrier, and shady practices are still major hurdles to be overcome.
- India has to prepare itself for the opportunity and challenges medical tourism offers.

BIBLIOGRAPHY

1. Adeoye AO. Assessing the associated medical, legal, and social issues in medical tourism and its implications for Nigeria. Pan Afr Med J. 2023;45:145.
2. Agnihotri A. (2022). Medical Tourism in India: Top destinations, scenarios and all you need to know. [online] Available from https://www.hindustantimes.com/lifestyle/travel/medical-tourism-in-india-top-destinations-scenarios-and-all-you-need-to-know [Last accessed September, 2024].

3. Crooks VA, Turner L, Cohen IG, et al. Ethical and legal implications of the risks of medical tourism for patients: a qualitative study of Canadian health and safety representatives' perspectives. BMJ Open. 2013;3(2):e002302.
4. Meštrović T. (2023). Medical Tourism History. [online] Available from https://www.news-medical.net/health/Medical-Tourism-History.aspx [Last accessed September, 2024].
5. Mishra V, Sharma MG. Framework for Promotion of Medical Tourism: A Case of India. JGBC. 2021;16(Suppl 1): 103-11.
6. Scrivens E. International trends in accreditation. Int J Health Plann Manage. 1995;10(3):165-81.
7. Singh H. (2022). India eyes to be a huge medical tourism hub in coming years. [online] Available from https://timesofindia.indiatimes.com/blogs/voices/india-eyes-to-be-a-huge-medical-tourism-hub-in-coming-years [Last accessed September, 2024].

45 CHAPTER Surrogate Motherhood

Gita Guin, Deepshikha Sahu

INTRODUCTION

The word "surrogate" originated from the Latin "subrogare" which means "appointed to act in place of". Surrogacy is the process of giving birth as a surrogate mother or of arranging such a birth. Surrogacy is an arrangement often supported by a legal agreement, whereby a woman agrees to deliver/labor on behalf of another couple or person, who will become the child's parent after birth. Surrogacy may be of different types like natural (traditional/straight) or gestational.

DIFFERENT TYPES OF SURROGACY

Different types of surrogacy include:

- *Natural (traditional/straight) surrogacy*: The surrogate is pregnant with her own biological child, but this child was conceived with the intention to repudiate the child to the biological father and possibly his spouse or partner, and thus the child that results is genetically related to the surrogate mother. The child could be conceived via numerous methods like sexual intercourse, home artificial insemination using fresh or frozen sperm, or impregnated via intrauterine insemination (IUI), or intracervical insemination (ICI) which is performed at a fertility clinic. Sperm from the male partner of the "commissioning couple" may be used, or alternatively, sperm from a sperm donor can be used. Donor sperm will, for example, be used if the "commissioning couple" are both females or if the child is commissioned by a single woman.
- *In gestational (host) surrogacy*: The surrogate is only a carrier and is not genetically or biologically related to the child. After birth, the surrogate hands over the child to the biological mother and/or father to raise, or to the adoptive parent(s) (in which case, the embryo would have been a donated embryo). The surrogate mother may be called a gestational carrier.
- *Commercial surrogacy*: This is a form of surrogacy in which a gestational carrier is hired/paid a said or agreed amount by the couple who couldn't become pregnant due to various issues. This procedure is legal in several countries including India. Commercial surrogacy is also known as "wombs for rent", "outsourced pregnancies", or "baby farms".
- *Altruistic surrogacy*: It is a situation where the surrogate receives no financial reward for her pregnancy or the relinquishment of the child (although usually all expenses related to the

pregnancy and birth are paid by the intended parents such as medical expenses, maternity clothing, accommodation, diet, and other related expenses).

The intended parents/commissioning couple may enter into a surrogacy arrangement because of:

- *Infertility*: Female infertility, or other medical issues which may make the pregnancy or delivery risky.
- *High-risk pregnancy*: The intended mother could also be fertile and healthy but due to some high-risk factors or medical conditions either could not carry the pregnancy or complications to may occur during labor.
- *Same-sex couple*: Surrogacy can help same-sex couples realize their dream of having their own child, which is otherwise not possible for them to have a child of their own by natural way.
- *Single parent*: For those who want to fulfill their desire to have a child without a partner, surrogacy is a ray of hope.

Surrogates may be relatives, friends, or strangers. There are agencies running who basically make a match of intended couple with the surrogates; through monetary benefits and legal agreements, they carry out the same.

Since a gestational carrier is exposed to potential obstetric complications, careful screening is needed to assure the good health of the mother as well as the baby born through surrogacy. In compensated surrogacies, the remuneration to the surrogate varies anything between a few thousand to over a lakh rupees depending on the bargaining process, conditions and need of both parties (surrogate mother and intended parents), as also the literacy and poverty of the surrogate.

Surrogacy is a complicated and varied issue involving many individuals whose beliefs, expectations, and interests are not always aligned. The primary individuals are:

- Intended parents
- Surrogate
- Fertility specialists
- Lawyers
- Surrogacy agencies

World over, in whichever country surrogacy is allowed, the primary condition is that at least one of the intended parents must be biologically related. Thus, a scenario where either of the intended parents is not biologically related is not allowed.

The extreme social stigma associated with childlessness in India, availability of good medical infrastructure at a relatively low cost as compared to Western world, together with easy availability of potential surrogates have made surrogacy a million-dollar industry in India. It has become a hub for foreigners due to the low cost and ease of availability of women as surrogates. Though the expenses of surrogacy in India are about a third of that it would cost in the United Kingdom, the exact economy of surrogacy in the country is a mere guess due to the immense potential of such medical establishments to generate huge unaccounted money. Some of the couples pay around ₹35–40 lakh for a child through surrogacy; a study backed by the United Nations in July 2012 estimated the business at more than $400 million a year with over 3,000 fertility clinics across India, and both the numbers presumably must be growing.

Surrogacy laws vary from country to country and sometimes within the different provinces of the same nation (e.g., in the United States of America, surrogacy is legal in Florida, California,

Pennsylvania, and Delaware but not in New York). Commercial surrogacy has been legal in India since 2002, but now after so many years finally "Surrogacy Act 2021" has been commenced to regulate this havoc of the surrogacy market. Previously, when the law was not made, we had seen a lot of cases needing to be dealt in the court of law; one of them is mentioned as follows: "In Baby Manji Yamada vs. Union of India (2008)", wherein baby Manji was born through a surrogate mother to Japanese biological parents, the apex court paved the way for the framing of appropriate guidelines. A Japanese couple chose a surrogate in Anand, Gujarat. However, due to matrimonial discord, the couple separated before the birth of the baby, and the baby's custody was subsequently handed over to her grandmother. This petition which was filed by M/s Satya, stated to be an NGO, as a public interest litigation was dismissed by the Honorable Supreme Court, and the petitioner was directed to the National and State Commissions for Protection of Child Rights and Children's Court which was required to formulate suitable guidelines.

The Ministry of Law and Justice (Legislative department) has made recently the Surrogacy (Regulation) Act, 2021—an act to constitute the National Assisted Reproductive Technology and Surrogacy Board, State Assisted Reproductive Technology and Surrogacy Boards, and for appointment of appropriate authorities for regulation of practice and process of surrogacy has been enacted by the parliament.

1. *On and from the date of commencement of this Act*:
   (i) All surrogacy clinics need to be registered and verified by the local and national governing bodies before conducting or associating with the surrogacy procedures.
   (ii) Any gynecologist or any registered medical practitioner cannot undertake or employ any person or conduct or promote or avail commercial surrogacy in any form. They have to conduct any such procedures in registered surrogacy clinics.
   (iii) No person can promote or advertise with the aim to induce a person or force or commercialize a person for going into surrogacy or to become surrogate for any benefits.
2. *According to the Act*:
   (i) No place including a surrogacy clinic shall be used or cause to be used by any person for conducting surrogacy or surrogacy procedures, except for the purposes specified in clause clause (ii) of above mentioned and after satisfying all the conditions specified in clause (iii) of above mentioned point.
   (ii) No surrogacy or surrogacy procedures shall be conducted, undertaken, performed or availed of, except for the following purposes, namely:
      (a) Couple who intend to become parents via surrogacy should be Indian or if not, they should at least get a certificate through the board bearing the reason and permission for getting a surrogate
      (b) When it is only for altruistic surrogacy purposes
      (c) When it is not for commercial purposes or for commercialization of surrogacy or surrogacy procedures
      (d) When it is not for producing children for sale, prostitution or any other form of exploitation
      (e) Any other condition or disease as may be specified by regulations made by the Board
   (iii) No surrogacy or surrogacy procedures shall be conducted, undertaken, performed or initiated, unless the Director or in charge of the surrogacy clinic and the person

qualified to do so are satisfied, for reasons to be recorded in writing, that the following conditions have been fulfilled, namely:

(a) The intending couple should provide an appropriate certificate defining the medical indication for which they need gestational surrogacy from a district medical board and also insurance coverage for the surrogate in case of any complications occur during the course of pregnancy and delivery of approximately 36 months.
An order concerning the parentage and custody of the child to be born through surrogacy has been passed by a court of the Magistrate.

(b) The surrogate mother has to obtain a fitness certificate in order to become a gestational surrogate; namely, she should be between the ages of 25 and 35 years, married, and have a child of her own. She should be explained regarding the procedures to be performed on her and the risks associated. Women should be herself willing to become a surrogate but not due to force or pressure. She can become a surrogate only once in her lifetime and need to obtain a medical and psychological fitness certificate before commencing procedure.

(c) Indenting couple also need to produce some documents and certificates clarifying that they are married and have no surviving children. They should be between the ages of 23 and 50 years in case of females and between 26 and 55 years in case of males on the day of certification.

3. No person including a relative or husband of a surrogate mother or intending couple or intending woman shall seek or encourage to conduct any surrogacy or surrogacy procedures on her except for the causes that are previously mentioned.
4. The surrogacy procedure needs to be explained in local language with proper written consents to be obtained before commencing the procedure. The surrogate mother shall have the option to withdraw her consent before the commencement of the procedure.
5. The intending couple or intending woman shall not abandon the child, born out of a surrogacy procedure, whether within India or outside, for any reason whatsoever, including but not restricted to, any genetic defect, birth defect, any other medical condition, the defects developing subsequently, sex of the child, or conception of more than one baby and the like.
6. A child born out of surrogacy procedure, shall be deemed to be a biological child of the intending couple or intending woman and the said child shall be entitled to all the rights and privileges available to a natural child under any law for time being in force.
7. It has to be earlier prescribed the number of embryos that are being implanted in the womb of surrogate.
8. No person, organization, surrogacy clinic, laboratory, or clinical establishment of any kind shall force the surrogate mother to abort at any stage of surrogacy except in such conditions as may be prescribed.

RULES FOR THE ESTABLISHMENT OF SURROGACY CLINICS

The rules for the establishment of surrogacy clinics under the Surrogacy (Regulation) Act, 2021 are as follows:

- The surrogacy clinics need to be duly registered under the appropriate authority. No person shall establish any surrogacy clinic for undertaking such procedure before being registered.

- Proper application to be filed to the local authorities and procedures to be conducted after the appropriate authority is satisfied that such clinic is in right position to provide facilities and maintain standards needed.
- The appropriate authority shall after holding an inquiry and after satisfying itself that the applicant has complied with all the requirements of this Act and the rules and regulations made thereunder, grant a certificate of registration to the surrogacy clinic, within a period of 90 days from the date of application received by it, in such form, on payment of such fees and in such manner, as may be prescribed.
- Registration of the clinic is to be provided after proper inquiry and giving the opportunity to the applicant to explain all the issues raised by the authority.
- Every certificate of registration shall be valid for a period of 3 years and shall be renewed in such manner and on payment of such fees as may be prescribed.
- The certificate of registration shall be displayed by the surrogacy clinic at an appropriate place.
- The appropriate authority can issue a notice to the clinic for cancellation of the registration or file a complaint in case of noncompliance with the rules. If after hearing to the surrogacy clinic they find a breach of the provisions of the Act or rules or the regulations, they may take any specified actions including suspension of the registration.
- Any intending couple or the surrogacy clinic after receiving a rejection of application can reapply within 30 days with appropriate reasons and certificates to the following:
    - The State Government, where the appeal is against the order of the appropriate authority of a State;
    - The Central Government, where the appeal is against the order of the appropriate authority of a Union territory, in such manner as may be prescribed.
- There shall be an established Registry to be called the National Assisted Reproductive Technology and Surrogacy Registry for the purposes of registration of surrogacy clinics under this Act.

OFFENSES AND PENALTIES

Offenses and penalties include:

- No commercial advertisement, or any information on social media related to the procedures or services to be published by any individual or an organized group. No brokers or rackets are to be run under any clinic or by any organizations to bribe or forcefully make surrogates to enter in this vicious cycle. The child born out of surrogacy cannot be disowned, abandoned, or exploited in any form. If any form of selling, purchasing, or trading of human embryos were found, strict actions to be taken; this could even be cancellation of license and judicial custody.
- If above-mentioned points were not followed by any person, he/she shall be an offense punishable with imprisonment for a term which may extend to 10 years and with a fine, which may extend to ₹10 lakh rupees.
- For the purposes of this section, the expression "advertisement" includes any notice, circular, label, wrapper, or any other document including advertisement through internet or any other media, in electronic or print form, and also includes any visible representation made by means of any hoarding, wall-painting, and signal (light, sound, smoke, or gas).
- Powers of appropriate authorities; assigned by the state government (local).

PROHIBITION OF COMMERCIAL SURROGACY

- Any medical professional including gynecologists, embryologists, microbiologists, or any person who owns a surrogacy clinic found doing any misconduct shall be punishable under this Act for the imprisonment of term up to 5 years even including a fine which may extend to ₹10 lakh.
- In case of subsequent or continuation of the offense mentioned in the above point, the name of the registered medical practitioner shall be reported by the appropriate authority to the State Medical Council concerned for taking necessary action including suspension of registration for a period of 5 years.
- Any intending couple or intending woman or any person who seeks the aid of any surrogacy clinic, laboratory, or of a registered medical practitioner, gynecologist, pediatrician, embryologist, or any other person for not following the altruistic surrogacy or for conducting surrogacy procedures for commercial purposes shall be punishable with imprisonment for a term which may extend to 5 years and with fine which may extend to ₹5 lakh for the first offense, and for any subsequent offenses with imprisonment which may extend to 10 years and with fine which may extend to ₹10 lakh.
- Whoever contravenes any of the provisions of this Act, rules, or regulations made thereunder for which no penalty has been provided in this Act, shall be punishable with imprisonment for a term which may extend to 3 years and with a fine, which may extend to ₹5 lakh rupees, and in the case of continuing contravention with an additional fine, which may extend to ₹10 thousand for every day during which such contravention continues after conviction for the first such contravention.
- No court shall take cognizance of any offense punishable under this Act except on a complaint in writing made by:
    - The appropriate authority concerned, or any officer, or an agency authorized on this behalf by the Central Government or the State Government, as the case may be, or the appropriate authority assigned by the state government (local).
    - A person, including a social organization, who has given notice of not less than 15 days in the manner prescribed, to the appropriate authority, of the alleged offense, and of his/her intention to make a complaint to the court.

  No court inferior to that of a Metropolitan Magistrate or a Judicial Magistrate of the first class shall try any offense punishable under this Act.

The Surrogacy (Regulation) Act, 2021 largely supports surrogacy in India and attempts to initiate a legitimate way of operating surrogacy clinics in Indian conditions. While it remains wanting in many areas, it is a great step forward. The exploitation of women through surrogacy is a matter of immense concern. The Law Commission has strongly recommended against commercial surrogacy. But in a country where a woman hardly has a say in matters as personal and relevant as contraception and abortion, to even assume that she has willingly consented to surrogacy and has therefore given herself to all the social, emotional, and physical trauma associated with pregnancy for someone she may meet only a few times without any material gains is a preposterous presumption. What is more important is probably to follow the Surrogacy Act strictly and take actions against those who misuse surrogacy for commercialization. Israel is the first country in the world to implement a form of state-controlled surrogacy in which each and every contract must be approved directly by the state in accordance with the "Embryo Carrying Agreements Law". Ironically such state scrutiny has only resulted in Israeli intended parents turning to India for easy surrogacy laws. This in itself makes a case for the legislation of surrogacy in India. Government and nongovernmental organizations (NGOs) must have an active and well-defined role in monitoring the in vitro fertilization (IVF) and surrogacy clinics.

There is no doubt that the parliament will enact a law so as to weed out the dubious practitioners. However, the view of many is that in a country that is struggling to provide a caring home to its abandoned and orphaned children due to very rigid laws of adoption, there is a greater need to promote adoption rather than letting its poor and vulnerable women be exploited for their reproductive potentials by those who can afford IVF and surrogacy. Such an attitude only promotes the patriarchal notion of "own child as the true heir" and is a rather feudal concept.

Fertility tourism or reproductive tourism involves patients traveling to another country for fertility treatment to bypass legal prohibitions, nonavailability of procedures, or its high cost in the home country. A complex situation is thus created involving the laws of both lands. The intended parents must precisely be sure about the surrogacy law in their country. It is essential to have a thorough interaction with a legal attorney in order to safeguard against exigencies. Countries like Japan, Netherlands, Belgium, Hungary, Canada, and France prohibit commercial surrogacy. The United States of America (USA) confers American citizenship on all children born in the US through surrogacy irrespective of the nationality of the intended parents. The issue of Indian citizenship was addressed in Jan Balaz vs. Union of India.

In Jan Balaz vs. Union of India, the Gujarat High Court conferred Indian citizenship on two twin babies fathered through compensated surrogacy by a German national in Anand district. The court observed: "We are primarily concerned with the rights of two newborn, innocent babies, much more than the rights of the biological parents, surrogate mother, or the donor of the ova. Emotional and legal relationship of the babies with the surrogate mother and the donor of the ova is also of vital importance." The court considered the surrogacy laws of countries like Ukraine, Japan, and the United States.

Because India does not offer dual citizenship, the children will have to convert to overseas citizenship of India if they also hold non-Indian citizenship. We have an example of this as follows:

- Balaz, the petitioner, submitted before the Supreme Court that he shall be submitting his passports before the Indian Consulate in Berlin. He also agreed that an NGO in Germany shall respond back to India on the status of the children and their welfare. The Union of India responded that India shall make all attempts to have the children sent to Germany. German authorities have also agreed to reconsider the case if approached by the Indian authorities. In May 2010, the Balaz twins were provided the exit and entry documents that allowed them to leave India for Germany. The parents agreed to adopt them in Germany according to German rules.

Needless to say that the law will not support sex-selective surrogacy but whether simply laying the law will be effective given that despite having strict laws banning preimplantation (a lawful option in the USA) and postimplantation sex selection, the child sex ratio in the country is shamefully skewed. Surrogacy has only added an extra tool to the mal intentions of both unscrupulous doctors and affording parents whose arguments may be, "if I am spending as much for surrogacy, why not spend a little more and beget a son." After all, it will not only remove the stigma associated with childlessness but will also restore the honor of the entire family.

Some infertility clinics require that the surrogates stay in hostels during the entire period of gestation under the supervision of doctors so that their health needs are well addressed. It is often alleged that such pregnant women are only allowed very infrequent interactions with their near ones. Such young women will usually have their own children left behind in the care of husbands and in-laws, often in conditions of deprivation. Honest social organizations will need to be roped in to monitor the homes of surrogates so that it will not become another legal formality that can be easily bypassed with the money power of assisted reproductive technology (ART) clinics.

CONCLUSION

Surrogacy has been a way of our culture since ancient times where a king or even a commoner would have sex with another woman to beget offspring to be reared by the couple who were either childless or had no son. It is no doubt a blessing in some situations, for example, same-sex marriages, which are not presently legal in India. But it definitely has put abeyance on adoption by childless couples who can afford the costs of surrogacy. It is set to widen the gap between "our own child" and "our adopted child". The debate on the ethics and legalities of surrogacy will be unending until the enactment of laws, the constitution of appropriate monitoring authorities, and above all revisiting one's own conscience to decide, to what extent can one stretch righteousness and where should wrong begin.

KEY LEARNING POINTS

- Surrogacy is an arrangement often supported by a legal agreement, the intended parents/ commissioning couple may enter into a surrogacy arrangement.
- Careful screening is needed to assure the good health of the mother as well as the baby born.
- The primary condition is that at least one of the intended parents must be biologically related.
- Surrogacy laws vary from country to country and sometimes within the different provinces of the same nation.
- The surrogacy clinics need to be duly registered under the appropriate authority.
- The Act largely supports surrogacy in India and attempts to initiate a legitimate way of operating surrogacy clinics.
- Fertility tourism or reproductive tourism involves patients traveling to another country for fertility treatment to bypass legal prohibitions.

BIBLIOGRAPHY

1. Casemine. (2009). Jan Balaz(S) v. Anand Municipality & 6 (S). [online] Available from https://www.casemine.com/judgement/in/56b48efa607dba348fff6a16 [Last accessed July, 2014].
2. India Code. (2021). The Surrogacy (regulation) Act. 2021 (The Gazette of India). [online] Available from https://www.indiacode.nic.in/bitstream/123456789/17046/1/A2021-47.pdf [Last accessed July, 2024].
3. Lok Sabha Secretariat. (2021). Legislative note. The Surrogacy (Regulation) Bill 2019. [online] Available from https://loksabhadocs.nic.in/Refinput/New_Reference_Notes/English/29012021_103307_102120474.pdf [Last accessed July, 2024].
4. Surrogacy Law in India . [online] Available from https://www.indiacode.nic.in.
5. Surrogacy motherhood: History and concept. [online] Available from https://www.britannica.com; https://dl1.cuni.cz (univerzita karlova).
6. Surrogacy in India: Current Perspectives. [online] Available from https://www.medicalsciencejournal.com.

46

CHAPTER

Legal Issues for Doctors in Government Service

Piyali Bhattacharya

INTRODUCTION

Medical practice is an ethical and legal minefield. It is a combination of medical and legal knowledge that can help us manage these dilemmas in an effective way! The two main legal issues faced by doctors in government services are:

1. Handling medicolegal cases (MLC), especially Protection of Children from Sexual Offences (POCSO)
2. Postmortem in suspected cases of foul play

HANDLING MEDICOLEGAL CASES

Medicolegal cases are an integral part of medical practice that is frequently encountered by medical officers (MO). Proper handling and accurate documentation of these cases is of importance to avoid any legal complication. The decision to label a case as MLC should be based on sound professional judgment, after detailed history taking and thorough clinical examination. A MLC is defined as "any case of injury or ailment where the attending doctor after history taking and clinical examination considers that investigations by law enforcement agencies are warranted to ascertain circumstances and fix responsibility regarding the said injury or ailment according to the law."

Medical institutions are usually apprehensive in dealing with a MLC as it implies a lot of disputes, unwanted burden, rough-speaking police officials, inordinate hours in the court, unrelenting defense counsels, etc. With improper understanding about implications of the cases, they invite mistakes and deliberation, which may land them in trouble.

The medical professionals need not have only scientific knowledge and technical skill but also awareness about the relevant laws of the land. A physician should know the provision of state acts such as the Pharmacy Act, Drug and Cosmetics Act, Narcotics Drugs and Psychotropic Substance Act, Medical Termination of Pregnancy Act, Mental Health Act, Transplantation of Human Organ Act, Environmental Protection Act, Pre-Conception and Pre-Natal Diagnostic Techniques (PCPNDT) Act, Biomedical Waste Rules, POCSO, National Medical Commission (NMC) Regulations 2023, and Right to the Information Act, 2005. Members of the medical profession are liable to be called upon to give medicolegal assistance in varied circumstances and situations by police and law.

List of Medicolegal Cases

- Assault and battery, including domestic violence and child abuse
- Accidents such as road traffic accidents (RTA), industrial accidents, etc.
- Cases of trauma with suspicion of foul play
- Electrical injuries, chemical injuries, burns, and scalds
- Poisoning, alcohol, drug overdose, drug abuse, etc.
- Undiagnosed coma
- Sexual offences
- Criminal abortions
- Attempted suicide
- Case of asphyxia as a result of strangulation, hanging, drowning, suffocation, etc.
- Death in the operation theater
- Unnatural deaths, custodial deaths
- Death due to snake bite or animal bite
- Fire arm injury
- Brought dead to the emergency/or deaths occurring without a diagnosis within 24 hours of hospitalization

In the casualty, while attending to an emergency, the doctor should understand that his first priority is to save the life of the patient. He should do everything possible to resuscitate the patient and ensure that he is out of danger. All legal formalities stand suspended till this is achieved. This has been clearly exemplified by the Honorable Supreme Court of India in Parmanand Katara vs. Union of India. Every doctor is bound to provide medical aid to the victims irrespective of the cause of injury; he cannot take any excuse of allowing law to take its course. In the same case, the Medical Council of India (MCI) filed an affidavit stating that "the MCI expects that all registered medical practitioners must attend to the sick and the injured immediately and it is the duty of the practitioner to make immediate and timely care available to every injured, whether he is injured in an accident or otherwise...Life of a person is far more important than the legal formalities."

Again, in Pattipati Venkaiah vs. State of Approaches, the Honorable High Court of Andhra Pradesh decreed that doctor's duty is to attend to the injuries of the person produced before him. His primary effort should be to save the life and then inform the police/document clearly all the injuries observed in MLC. This means that the duty of the doctor to provide medical aid, even in MLCs, has been extended to private doctors also.

General Guidelines for Dealing with Medicolegal Case

In an emergency, resuscitation and stabilization will be carried out first and medicolegal formalities may be completed subsequently. The consent for treatment is implied in all emergencies. All cases of trauma will be labeled as MLCs, if there is a suspicion of foul play, even if the incident is not of recent origin. All emergency rooms and hospitals will maintain a MLC register and the MLC will be initiated and documented in the register. Personal particulars, identification marks, and finger prints of the individual will be noted. Particulars of the person accompanying will also be noted.

During examination, a male/female attendant should be present for a male patient and a female for a female patient. Otherwise the doctor may be charged with indecent assault under

Section 354 of Indian Penal Code (IPC) and the punishment may be imprisonment up to 2 years and/or fine.

Medicolegal documents should be prepared with utmost care, giving all necessary details, preferably written and avoiding overwriting. If any overwriting or correction is made, it should be authenticated with full signature and stamp of MO. Abbreviations should be avoided.

The medical superintendent (MS) or equivalent person has to be informed as and when a MLC is registered or admitted. Particulars of the registered/admitted patient should be mentioned in the emergency report book along with a short summary of the case.

Next of kin should be informed if the address is available.

Police information: Every big hospital usually has a police post near the casualty or has a police official posted there for this purpose. Police should also be informed regarding the discharge/death of the said patient in the casualty/any other department of the hospital.

Under Section 39 of Criminal Procedure Code (CrPC), the doctor attending the MLC is legally bound to inform the police. Failure to report may invite prosecution under Sections 176 and/or 202 of IPC. The verbal communication should invariably be followed by communication in writing.

According to the Honorable Supreme Court, whenever any MLC comes to the hospital, the MO on duty should inform the duty constable, giving the name, age, sex, and the place of occurrence of the incident and should start the treatment. It should be the duty of the said constable to inform the nearest concerned police station or higher police functionaries for further action.

Triaging, preliminary treatment, and safe transfer of a MLC from one facility to another should be not delayed because of the medicolegal nature of the case.

In cases with injury to bones/joints, any opinion on severity of injuries should be given after the X-ray reports are received.

Seal, label, and hand over all collected samples/specimens to the investigating officer. Medicolegal documents are confidential records and must be stored in safe custody to avoid any tampering. Case sheets, X-rays, investigation reports, and all documents pertaining to the MLC should be preserved meticulously in the medical record section (indefinitely) and handed over only to the police investigating officer/court or such concerned authority as and when required.

Dying declaration: A magistrate must be intimated in cases where the patient wishes to make a dying declaration. In case the MO feels that he might not be able to reach in time, the MO may record the dying declaration himself in presence of two independent witnesses. Dying declaration should have the signatures of the doctor, the patient, and the two witnesses. The MO is also required to certify the person making the dying declaration is in a sound state of mind at the time of making the declaration.

In case of controversy between the medicolegal report given by the hospital and the police investigation thereafter, a certificate from the investigating officer along with a copy of the Panchnama has to be kept in record whenever the body is returned to the hospital.

Precautions to be Taken in Medicolegal Cases

- Two identification marks with other available particulars of the patient and particulars of the person accompanying have to be recorded.

- The doctor should never rely on memory while writing reports or during recording of evidence in a court.
- It is wise to discuss pros and cons in complicated cases with seniors and colleagues.
- Cause of death should be stated as "Exact cause is to be ascertained by postmortem examination" in the death certificate.
- The civil police should be informed and the MLC body be handed over to them (not to the relatives of the dead person). The police, after the medicolegal formalities are authorized, has to hand over the body to the relatives.
- A MLC should be reported by the first healthcare-receiving establishment. The hospital to which he is transferred can also initiate the report when a patient has been transferred before initiation of a report. Comprehensive medical records mentioning whether medicolegal formalities have been initiated should be mentioned by the first-receiving doctor in the transfer notes.

Preservation of Medicolegal Evidence

All evidences must be identified, sealed, labeled properly, and kept in safe custody. They should be handed over to the investigating officer for forensic examination and production as evidence in a court. The loss/destruction of evidence after collection is punishable offence under Section 201 of IPC.

In *case of injury*—the following articles should be preserved in sealed envelopes:
- Clothing worn by the patient showing evidence of injury, for example, torn clothes, bullet holes, cuts, blood stains, etc.
- Encircle and number each piece of evidence like multiple tears, cuts, or holes in the clothes, with matching description in the MLC report and case sheet.
- Bullets recovered from a body should be marked by etching an initial or a mark on the bottom before preservation.
- All evidence collected should be mentioned in a document.

Suspected poisoning—preserve and forward the following articles for forensic examination:
- Vomitus/soiled clothing/gastric contents
- Blood, urine, or any other body fluid depending on the poison ingested

Burns and carbon monoxide poisoning—preserve the following articles:
- Articles soiled with inflammable substances such as burnt pieces of clothing, scalp hair, etc. in sealed envelopes
- Blood (and not serum) for carbon monoxide levels

In *sexual offences*—preserve:
- Clothing worn by the patient and showing evidence of blood stains or seminal stains and stains of mud, tears/cuts, etc. in sealed envelopes
- Vaginal swab preferably from posterior fornix/anal swab

Guidelines for Attending Alleged Victim of Sexual Offence

- *Initiate a case sheet*: Note personal particulars along with date and the time of reporting and fill the MLC register at emergency room. At least two identification marks of the victim will be mentioned in the case sheet as well as in MLC register.

- Admit the alleged victim if the condition is serious.
- Inform the Senior registrar/MS of the hospital.
- Inform civil police telephonically, followed by information in writing. The police report can be made in the name of the victim or as an unknown case if name is not known. Care must be taken to preserve the confidentiality from others not related with the case. Police will either register a case under the relevant section of the IPC or take the victim and the accused for medical examination at an authorized hospital for medicolegal workup.
- Consent of the victim must be obtained before starting the examination. The steps of examination and their purpose should be explained in a language he/she understands. The examination is to be carried out in the presence of a female attendant in case the abused person is a female. All injuries present on the body will be recorded. Line diagrams depicting the front and back of the body may be used for a better description of location of the injuries. If the clothes are the same as those worn during the occurrence of alleged offence, they should be carefully examined for the presence of blood, seminal stains, mud, etc. If there are any marks of suspicious stains, the clothes should be preserved with a view to forwarding them to the Chemical Examiner of Forensic Science Laboratory (FSL). If there are foreign hairs, fibers, debris under the nails, etc., they must be carefully preserved and sent to experts of FSL for comparison with those found on the accused.
- If the victim reports herself directly to the hospital after the alleged crime, the police will be called to the hospital instead of sending her to the police station.

Precautions in Case of Sexual Offence

- A duplicate copy of the case sheet and medicolegal report shall be preserved for future reference.
- If an accused in the case of sexual offence is brought for examination in police custody, consent is not required.
- In cases of alleged sodomy, all injuries shall be recorded.
- Neither victim nor accused in cases of sexual offences should be permitted to wash or take a bath till the examination is completed. Care must be taken to preserve the vaginal/anal swab for forensic examination.
- Collected samples may be handed over to the police for forensic examination.

MISCELLANEOUS ISSUES

Medicolegal Aspects of Poisoning

Administration of any substance with the intention of causing hurt or death is punishable as per Indian law. Offences related to handling and administration of poisonous substances fall under Sections 284, 299, 300, 304A, 324, 326, and 328 of IPC [286, 100, 101, 106, 118(1), 118, 123 of BNS].

Guidelines in Case of Poisoning

When poisoning is suspected, a case sheet with personal particulars of victim, date, and time of reporting has to be initiated. The particulars of the person accompanying must always be noted. The patient will be admitted if condition is serious. Thereafter, a MLC will be initiated by filling the MLC register and the civil police be informed. The victim must be protected from further exposure of poisoning; however, no clothing should be discarded, as they might be useful for chemical analysis.

If the MO conceals the information, he/she is liable to be prosecuted under Section 202 of IPC, but if he/she gives false information, he/she is liable to be charged with the offence of giving false information under Section 193 of IPC.

Noncompliance is punishable under Section 201of IPC. If it is proved that the doctor did it with the intention of protecting the accused. However, if the doctor is sure that the patient is suffering from suicidal poisoning, he is not bound to inform the police.

The registrar/MS of the hospital will also be informed. The treating doctor/authorized nursing staff will only be permitted to administer food and medicines to the patient. A careful history is to be elicited, including relationship of food or medicine taken and the toxic manifestations. All signs and symptoms are to be noted carefully. The vomitus, urine, feces, stomach wash, and sample of food or medicine taken should be preserved in a sterile bottle. Any suspicious bottle or utensil seen near the victim and the clothes and bed clothes used last by the victim must be preserved for chemical analysis.

Suitable preservatives may be used for these purposes depending upon the nature of the sample. The name and concentration of preservative used should invariably be mentioned in the label and/or accompanying documents. It is advisable to take the second opinion and advice of a senior colleague in all matters regarding diagnosis and treatment. Use of poison information services may also be made. If there is any indication of danger to the general public, for example, food poisoning from a hotel, the public health authorities must be notified so that suitable remedial measures are taken.

Where required, a magistrate should be called to take down the dying declaration.

Precautions to be Taken in Cases of Poisoning

- Always initiate emergency medical treatment. Consult and discuss with senior colleagues.
- While issuing a medical certificate, write "Cause of death to be ascertained after chemical analyses."
- Always preserve samples of medicolegal importance and hand over to the police for forensic examination.
- Obtain and preserve a receipt from the police for all samples which have been handed over by you.

CONCLUSION

Doctor should be aware about laws in relation to medical practices (legal obligation), for example, IPC Sections 118, 176, 177, 182, 191, 192, 193, 194, 195, 197, 201, 203, 204, and 312–316 (58, 211, 212, 217, 227, 228, 229, 230, 231, 234, 238, 240, 241, 88–92 of BNS).

Medical ethics and acts related to medical practice should be emphasized in postgraduate curriculum and examinations.

Periodical continuing medical education (CME)/reorientation programs involving forensic medicine should be made compulsory for all doctors.

KEY LEARNING POINTS

- Doctor should know that on the slightest doubt, he should send police information (section 39 of CrPC).
- He should carefully examine and treat the patient and record date, time, place, brought by whom, and examination findings.
- At least two identification marks of the victim will be mentioned in the case sheet as well as in MLC register.
- However, the MO should initiate emergency medical treatment if patient is very sick. Consultation and discussion with senior colleagues can be helpful.
- Inform civil police telephonically followed by information in writing.
- Consent of the victim must be obtained before starting the examination.
- Always preserve samples of medicolegal importance and hand over to the police for forensic examination.
- Obtain and preserve a receipt from the police for all samples which have been handed over by you.
- A duplicate copy of the case sheet and medicolegal report shall be preserved for future reference.
- While issuing a certificate write "cause of death to be ascertained after chemical analysis/after postmortem."
- He should record dying deposition/declaration if there is imminent danger of death. He should not issue death certificates if death occurred in suspicious circumstances and recommend postmortem examination for cause of death and police should be informed.

BIBLIOGRAPHY

1. Dogra TD, Rudra A. Lyon's Medical Jurisprudence & Toxicology, 11th edition. Delhi: Delhi Law House; 2005. p. 367.
2. Jayapalan VK. Practical Medico-Legal Manual, 1st edition. India: Indian Academy of Forensic Medicine; 1988. p. 26.
3. Parmananda Katara vs. Union of India. AIR 1986 SC 2039.
4. Pattipati Venkaiah vs. State of Andhra Pradesh. 1985(2) Crimes 746 at p. 749.

47

CHAPTER

Role of Government

Sudhir Mishra

INTRODUCTION

Traditionally, a doctor-patient relationship has been that of mutual trust and respect. This relationship has taken a beating with the increasing commercialization of medical practice. Increasing lawsuits have led to higher insurance premiums for doctors. This is then transferred to patients directly by increasing the cost of care and indirectly by adopting defensive medical practice. The increasing cost of medical care in turn brings discomfort and distrust among the patients leading to increased chances of legal conflict between the two. It is evident from the fact that most legal cases have been against big hospitals, doctors working in corporate hospitals, or doctors with steep fee structures. This vicious cycle needs to be broken. The Government has a responsibility in this respect.

The Government can act in many ways: Strengthening the medical infrastructure of the country, strengthening regulatory bodies like National Medical Council/Universities, providing improved facilities at Government-run educational institutions, making laws for continuously upgrading knowledge of medical practitioners, implementing laws that exist against fake/poor-quality drug manufacturers, review the laws against counterfeit or spurious drugs, vaccines, irrational combinations specially in formulations used for children and ensuring the availability of quality instruments, clearly defining medical negligence, providing definitive guidelines for execution of these laws by enforcement agencies, making laws that will reduce the gains of lawyers involved in frivolous lawsuits, building provisions for compensation to aggrieved doctor or hospital in case a suit is found frivolous, and fixing upper limits for compensation depending on extent of damage where courts find doctors, hospitals, or both negligent or lacking in services. Rules can be framed for insurance companies to calculate realistic premiums for doctors. In addition, laws to deal with cases of physical assault on medical service providers including nurses and other workers in hospitals or the destruction of property of medical establishments like hospitals, nursing homes, clinics, laboratories, etc., are required. Some states have passed the "Medical Protection Act" by this name or slightly different names. However, it needs to be passed by all states or preferably by the Central Government, so that it is effective across the country.

STRENGTHENING MEDICAL INFRASTRUCTURE OF THE COUNTRY

Though there is some improvement in the Government Health system, especially in larger cities, it remains poor in most backward states and rural areas. Poor infrastructure in the Government sector has led to the proliferation of different types of private healthcare centers. These include corporate hospitals with excellent medical infrastructure and private nursing homes, many of whom do not have even one trained nurse, some of them do not have a doctor available round the clock on nursing home premises but claim to provide round-the-clock services and laboratories run by technicians. Whereas many such "hospitals" provide some healthcare in rural areas where none exists, most of these do not provide the kind of care they promise or do not fulfill the kind of expectation they raise. This mismatch of expectations and service delivery is the key factor in creating a feeling of being cheated or not provided with what was promised. This leads to frustration and legal action or sometimes even direct action leading to loss of property or life or both. It is estimated that India falls short of 1.4 million doctors and 2.8 million nurses as per the World Health Organization (WHO) norms for developing countries. The Government has to play a key role in establishing, promoting, subsidizing, or financing quality healthcare services. There has been some improvement in the number of medical institutions in countries. However, nursing and paramedical services still need many more institutions. In addition, the availability and quality of faculty members in many such institutions are suspicious and lead to poor outcome in the quality of new doctors. The National Exit Examination proposed and likely to be implemented may help to some extent. However, this examination being in objective type pattern cannot assess the knowledge, skills, or ability of doctors to provide quality service. On the other hand, students will start preparing for the objective-type examination from the final year or even earlier. This can lead to compromised clinical learning.

As of May 2025, the Indian government's approach to promoting generic medicines involves a combination of regulatory mandates, public health initiatives, and evolving state-level policies. This policy aims at providing cheaper medicines to general public thereby reducing the cost of healthcare. An overview of the current landscape is presented below.

NATIONAL POLICIES ON GENERIC MEDICINES

Prescription guidelines: The Indian Medical Council (Professional Conduct, Etiquette and Ethics) Regulations, 2002, stipulate that physicians should prescribe drugs using their generic names legibly and preferably in capital letters. This aims to encourage the use of cost-effective generic alternatives.

National Medical Commission (NMC) directive: In 2023, the NMC issued regulations mandating that all doctors prescribe only generic medicines. Non-compliance could lead to penalties, including suspension of medical licenses. However, due to concerns raised by medical associations about drug quality and implementation challenges, this mandate was put on hold.

Public health facilities: Under the National Health Mission (NHM), the government supports the provision of essential generic drugs free of cost in public health facilities. This initiative includes strengthening procurement systems, quality assurance, and supply chain management.

PRADHAN MANTRI BHARTIYA JANAUSHADHI PARIYOJANA (PMBJP)

Overview: Launched in 2008 and rebranded in 2016, PMBJP aims to provide quality generic medicines at affordable prices through dedicated outlets known as Pradhan Mantri Bhartiya Janaushadhi Kendras (PMBJKs). These medicines are priced 50–90% lower than their branded counterparts.

Quality assurance: Medicines under PMBJP are procured from WHO-GMP certified suppliers and tested in NABL-accredited laboratories to ensure quality and efficacy.

Some states have adopted the scheme well whereas other states like Karnataka have abandoned it after initially adopting, in favor of free drugs through its own hospital and health centers. However, even in the system adopted, Procurement Strategy for hospitals has remained focused on procuring affordable generic medicines via the Karnataka State Medical Supplies Corporation from the Bureau of Pharma Public Sector Undertakings of India (BPPI). The move has not remained uncontroversial as the efficacy of hospital systems remains suboptimal. The decision faced criticism from various quarters, including opposition parties and PMBJK owners, who argued that it undermines access to affordable medicines and affects the livelihoods of pharmacy entrepreneurs.

REGULATORY OVERSIGHT AND CHALLENGES

Quality concerns: Despite efforts to promote generic medicines, challenges persist regarding the uniform quality of these drugs. Some healthcare professionals express skepticism about the efficacy of generics, citing inconsistent quality control across manufacturers.

Regulatory bodies: The Central Drugs Standard Control Organization (CDSCO) is responsible for the approval and regulation of generic medicines in India, ensuring their safety, efficacy, and quality.

STRENGTHENING REGULATORY BODIES

Regulatory bodies exist but are not able to control malpractice. The National Medical Commission has replaced the Medical Council of India, which is the body that recognizes medical institutions. The state of medical institutions in the country and standards of education have declined. Such organizations need to play a decisive role in ensuring that the condition of our institutions improves and the institutions are able to provide for adequate training to doctors and set an example for doctor–patient relationship that is fiduciary in nature. National Medical Commission (or such other organizations) may be given the responsibility of overseeing the functioning of corporate hospitals, especially its social responsibility aspect. They should have quasi-judicial authority to force adequate corrective action or take punitive action against the erring organizations or individual doctors. Faith in these organizations will prompt the medical malpractice cases to go to them for quicker solutions and less damage (reputation, mental or economic) to the doctors. This will improve societal satisfaction as well.

A lot of fake medical practitioners or "quacks" often called registered medical practitioners (RMPs) are practicing medicine in this country. In the case *(Dr) Baleshwar Prasad versus Firtu Das*, the District, State, and later National Commission unanimously observed that the doctor has produced a certificate issued by the Council of RMP Bihar, but the validity of the certificate itself is doubtful. He cannot be allowed to practice and should shut down his dispensary.

PROVIDING BETTER FACILITIES AT GOVERNMENT EDUCATIONAL INSTITUTIONS

Improved facilities at free (or subsidized) government organizations will attract patients who are unable to pay the huge bills of private or corporate organizations. Often it is the anger arising out of a disproportionate bill (to paying capabilities) that culminates in unrealistic expectations on the part of patients. Unmet expectations then drive them to seek redressal from other sources including judiciary. Availability of good services including some tertiary care services at government institutions will certainly avoid this situation. In this respect, Ayushman Bharat seems to have helped but needs strengthening.

LAWS TO UPGRADE THE KNOWLEDGE OF MEDICAL PRACTITIONERS

Upgrading knowledge is an integral part of medical practice. New evidence makes old practices irrelevant sometimes even proving them to be dangerous. For example, in the past, steroids were used in the treatment of hypoxic-ischemic encephalopathy (HIE) as a matter of routine. Current evidence suggests that there is no role of steroids in the management of HIE. On the other hand, steroids were considered a last resort or even denounced in the management of asthma but have become the treatment of choice, by inhaled route. Not adopting a new concept where it has become the accepted standard of care or continuing to use old obsolete treatment modalities can lead to a legal problem if the aggrieved party approaches court. The role of continuing education is clear. Some countries have made it mandatory to accrue some points on medical education for continued suitability for practicing in those parts of the world. One can see the phrase, "continuing medical education (CME) credit available till this date" in Medscape articles. It is desirable to adopt some such strategies for our country as well. Technology is of great help in this regard and online submission of answers to questionnaires can easily be adopted as a mechanism of continued education. In case of default, one has to forego the right to practice or appear in a refresher crash course on payment, which may be organized either by accrediting bodies or by professional associations or academies like The Indian Academy of Pediatrics for Pediatricians.

It is proved that this gives doctors enough reasons to be alert to the changing scenario in the medical world, and consequently adopt better care strategies for their patients.

FAKE OR POOR-QUALITY DRUGS

Fake or poor-quality drugs are known to be rampant in our country. Using these drugs does not give an appropriate response to patients and can result in life-threatening situations. If the drug was provided by the doctor or hospital, the doctor may be considered at fault. Counterfeit artesunate causing havoc in Southeast Asia is well documented. Doctors have no method to find/check the quality of the drug. Technology can be of help again in this respect. An identification method can be adopted that will ensure the traceability of the medicine to the right source. If it is found that the medicine cannot be traced to the lawful manufacturer, the retailer should discard it. In this situation, the liability to ensure that the retailer is selling the right product will rest with him. This will ensure that the end users get the right medicine. In addition, more stringent laws to punish those involved in fake drug rackets are required. The Government of India set up a committee called the Mashelkar Committee in January 2003 to comprehensively look into the regulatory infrastructure. The committee was asked to study the extent and problem of substandard or spurious drugs in the country. The Committee was asked to suggest methods for implementation of the recommended measures, so that this problem can be completely removed from India. The committee found that there is no mention of spurious drugs in the Indian Penal Code (IPC). The punishments for offenses are in consonance with the Drugs and Cosmetics Act 1940 (D&CA) and Rules. The offenses are bailable. This Committee has recommended that the offenses be made nonbailable, cognizable, and prosecution may be initiated by an officer of the rank of a sub-inspector (at present it is not less than an inspector). This Committee also recommended death penalty as the maximum punishment for spurious drugs [like in Vietnam and some middle-east countries including the United Arab Emirates (UAE), Kuwait, Oman, Qatar, and Bahrain].

Summary of important recommendations of this Committee are as follows:

- Recommend a new structure for the drug regulatory system in the country including the setting up of a National Drug Authority.
- Recommend measures to strengthen the drug regulatory infrastructure in the Centre and States. The proposed authority should have ten divisions within it. These include:
  i. Division for Regulatory Affairs and Enforcement
  ii. Division for New Drugs and Clinical Trials
  iii. Division for Biological and Biotechnology Products
  iv. Division for Pharmacovigilance
  v. Division for Medical Devices and Diagnostics
  vi. Division for Imports
  vii. Division for Organizational Services
  viii. Division for Training and Empowerment
  ix. Division for Quality Control Affairs
  x. Division for Legal and Consumer Affairs

There are detailed recommendations in relation to other related issues including:

- *Other related drug regulatory issues*:
  - Health food/dietary supplements/therapeutic foods
  - Indian systems of medicine (ISM), herbal products, and drugs of natural origin
  - Over-the-counter (OTC) drugs
  - Medical devices and diagnostics
  - Drug development including clinical research
  - Storage and distribution
- Evaluate the extent of spurious and substandard drugs and recommend measures required to deal with the problem.

The gist of the recommendations to tackle the spurious drugs problem is as follows:

- Creation of effective interaction between the stakeholders, i.e., industry and regulators, industry and consumers, trade and regulators, and medical professionals and regulators
- Creation of intelligence cum legal cells in State and Central offices
- Discouragement of the proliferation of drug distribution outlets
- Making changes in the law to provide enhanced penalties, making the offenses cognizable and nonbailable in the light of similar provisions in the Narcotic Drugs and Psychotropic Substances Act
- Designation of special courts for trial of the cases of spurious drugs
- Preparation of dossiers of suspected dealers and manufacturers
- Provision of secret funds and incentives to informers
- Creating effective networking system between States
- Checking on drug supplies to practitioners who buy and supply drugs to their patients

- Creation by the industry of its counterfeit drug strategies, better surveillance, and efficient complaint handling system
- Creation of a better surveillance system by the trade association on defaulting members and to take strict action against them
- Creation of better awareness amongst consumers

More specifically to prevent the sale of spurious drugs, the following recommendations were made:

- The penalty for the sale and manufacture of spurious drugs that cause grievous hurt or death should be enhanced from life imprisonment to death. Even the penalty for manufacture and sale of spurious drugs that do not cause grievous hurt or death should also be made more severe.
- The offenses related to spurious drugs should be made cognizable and nonbailable. The bail, if considered by the court should be granted only after 3 months.
- The penalty for not disclosing the source of purchase of drugs by a dealer should be made stringent.
- A provision should be included in the D&CA to enable the Central and State Governments to designate special courts for speedy trial of spurious drug cases.
- A provision for compounding of offenses should be included in the D&CA.
- Under the D&CA, besides the drug inspectors, police should also be authorized to file prosecution for offenses related to spurious drugs.

The Committee also recommended measures to be adopted by other stakeholders like the pharmaceuticals, pharma trade associations, consumers, and other professional associations.

In addition to these recommendations, the Central Government should take proper measures to prevent cross-border infiltration of counterfeit medicines. Training programs for the pharmacists on detection of counterfeit drugs should be conducted at regular intervals. Reorientation courses including introduction to newer technology and methods in the detection of counterfeit medicines should be organized through the professional bodies of the pharmacists. The Government should ensure that medicines made for export are regulated and controlled according to standard quality. A quick response (QR) code as a ready source of the drug from the actual manufacturer may be made mandatory for quick identification of the source of medicine. End users will also be able to identify and will be assured of using the original drug.

In addition to fake drugs, irrational combinations of drugs are rampant and they come out of approval from respective bodies of Central or State Governments. In 2003, it was estimated that there were 70 irrational fixed-dose combinations (with 1,000 brands) in the market. This number has swelled many folds over the years and is harmful to the patients. It is the utmost responsibility of the governments that these combinations are removed and fresh irrational combinations do not appear in the market.

GUIDELINES FOR LAW ENFORCEMENT AGENCIES

Administrative officers, especially police officers, are the executive arm of the Government for implementation of the laws enacted by the lawmakers or the precedents or directives set out by the courts, especially the Hon'ble Supreme Court. Medical practitioners face the maximum problems at this stage as it may even go to the arrest and imprisonment till the court orders. This may be because of ignorance about the sections or clauses the offense belongs to. **Sections**

106(1) and 106(2) of BNS exemplify this best. The basic difference between the two sections is that **Section 106(1)** deals with death caused intentionally, which is a non-bailable offense, as against **Section 106(2)** that deals with acts not done with the intention to cause death. The offense in this section is bailable. It will make a big difference to the medical service providers if Section 106(1) is applied in place of **Section 106(2)**. Even the Hon'ble Supreme Court in the case Dr *Jacob Mathew vs. State of Punjab* has given its guidance: "A doctor may be arrested only if the investigating officer believes that she/he would not be available for prosecution unless arrested." Corresponding sections in IPC were 304 and 304A.

The police officer needs to be apprised of the clauses concerning medical negligence and should be held accountable for the same. Provision for refresher courses in law should be available for police officers. The Government is responsible for making these provisions. It is also incumbent on the Government to hold guilty police officers responsible and take corrective actions for the same.

REDUCE THE GAINS OF LAWYERS INVOLVED IN FRIVOLOUS LAWSUITS

Lawsuits are a phenomenon originating in the West. It is, therefore, good to follow the natural course of development as in the West. We should not wait for adverse natural developments to take place and then correct them. Frivolous lawsuits are common in the West. Since Act 13 came into being, in the state of Pennsylvania alone, over a period of 30 months, 5,600 doctors were sued. What was more surprising was of the 5,600 cases that the medical board looked at, it went through 3,600 cases, reviewed and analyzed them, and found that in only four of them, it was necessary to go ahead with the legal suit as required in Act 13. It is obvious that there were so many frivolous lawsuits. This is happening with the active connivance of lawyers or attorneys who are looking for quick financial gains. In many situations, insurance companies do not want to go through the full trial and settle it out of court, which encourages the lawyers to "search and create" more cases of negligence.

A register for the effect of the involvement of lawyers in frivolous medical negligence suits may be maintained. Repeated inclusion of a lawyer's name should automatically result in forfeiting the license to practice (at least criminal law).

If India encounters a similar situation, there will be millions of cases. We need to build the safety net against such a situation now. This can be done in many ways. One of them is to reduce the gains for lawyers from the suits. Many times, it is found that lawyers take up these cases on a "fraction of the gain" basis. Fixing the highest limits for the lawyer's fee in malpractice suits, and fixing the highest limits for compensation for nonfinancial loss such as pain or mental trauma can reduce the gains for the lawyer and is likely to reduce such cases.

BUILT-IN PROVISIONS FOR COMPENSATION FOR AGGRIEVED DOCTOR(S) OR HOSPITAL

There should be an in-built provision for compensating the doctor and hospital in case a lawsuit against the doctor fails. It should be in proportion to the claim of the plaintiff. The more is the compensation claimed, the higher could be the damages in the event of loss. This will not only reduce the number of cases but will also lead to more realistic claims from doctors or insurance companies. This can be in addition to the present compensation which generally involves the cost incurred in fighting the case for doctors.

FORMULATE A COMMON LAW WITH MEDICAL NEGLIGENCE IN FOCUS

The doctors can be prosecuted in the civil courts, under the Consumer Protection Act (CPA) 2019 or criminal negligence under section 106(1) and 106(2) (IPC Section 304A or erroneously under 304). They are also being prosecuted under BNS section 123 [IPC Section 336 (rash or negligent act endangering human life)], BNS section 124(1) (IPC Section 337) (causing hurt to any person by doing any rash or negligent act as would endanger human life) or BNS section 124(2) [Section 338 of the IPC (causing grievous hurt to any person by doing any rash or negligent act so as to endanger human life)]. None of these acts were primarily formulated with medical negligence in mind. Hence, they are subject to interpretation by the public, police, lawyers, and courts of law. It would be a great service to humanity in general and the medical profession in particular, if the provisions of all these acts can be redefined with the perspective of medical negligence and a law is created for the purpose with clear guidance for criminal or civil prosecution. It should also incorporate the sections that often come to the defense of the doctors. Doctors may use BNS section 14 and 27 (Sections 80 and 88 of the IPC) for their defense. BNS Section 14 deals with accidents in doing a lawful act. It states that nothing is an offense that is done by accident or misfortune and without any criminal intention or knowledge, in the doing of a lawful act in a lawful manner by lawful means, with proper care and caution. BNS section 27 (IPC Section 88) protects a person against accidental injuries caused during an act in good faith, for the other's benefit, even if there is a risk. The patient may have given consent explicitly or implicitly, or may not be in a position to give consent.

The court has also directed the Central Government to frame guidelines to save doctors from unnecessary harassment and undue pressure in performing their duties. It ruled that until the Government framed such guidelines, the following guidelines would prevail:

- A private complaint of rashness or negligence against a doctor may not be entertained without prima facie evidence in the form of a credible opinion of another competent doctor supporting the charge. In addition, the investigating officer should give an independent opinion, preferably of a Government doctor. Finally, a doctor may be arrested only if the investigating officer believes that (s)he would not be available for prosecution unless arrested.

PROVISION OF LONG-TERM INSURANCE AGAINST MEDICAL MALPRACTICE SUITS

At present insurance companies provide insurance against medical malpractice suits on a yearly basis. Usually, a surcharge is added if you happen to get a case against you (which is why you take the policy in the first place). The law should be enacted to convert it to a life insurance kind of fixed premium-based insurance. Just like the detection of a disease does not lead to the addition of a surcharge in life insurance premiums, it should not be the case in insurance against medical malpractice premiums. This will go a long way to protect doctors from the repeated surcharge from insurance companies in the event of a suit. It will benefit society by not increasing the cost of insurance that is passed on to the patients. It will also discourage insurance companies from making out-of-court settlements, which is seen to contribute to an increasing number of cases, in search of easy money.

THE LAW AGAINST PHYSICAL ASSAULT ON PERSONS/MEDICAL ESTABLISHMENTS

Growing incidents of physical assault on doctors and other service providers in hospital or nursing home settings have led to frequent disruption of services to the poor and needy. In response to an attack on doctors at Niloufer and Government Maternity Hospital and subsequent strike by the doctors, the Andhra Pradesh Government promulgated an ordinance on 18 December, 2007. This ordinance seeks to prohibit violence against medicare service persons and damage to property in medicare service institutions and for matters connected therewith and incidental thereto. It states that medicare service persons in relation to medicare service institutions shall include: (a) RMPs working in medicare institutions (including those having provisional registration), (b) registered nurses, (c) medical students, (d) nursing students, and (e) paramedical workers employed and working in medicare service institutions. It further states that any act of violence against medicare service persons or damage to the property in a medicare service institution is hereby prohibited.

Subsequently, medical protection acts have been enacted in many states. However, their implementation remains poor and so far there is no known conviction in the act. Still, the state governments that do not have a medical protection act should bring it at the earliest possible.

Any offender who commits any act in contravention of Section 3 shall be punished with imprisonment for 3 years and with a fine, which may extend up to ₹50,000. Any offence committed under Section 3 shall be cognizable and nonbailable. In addition to the punishment specified in Section 4, the offender shall be liable to a penalty of twice the amount of the purchase price of medical equipment damaged and loss caused to the property as determined by the court trying the offender. If the offender has not paid the penal amount under subsection (1), the said sum shall be recovered under the provisions of the Andhra Pradesh Recovery Act, 1864 as if it were an arrears of land revenue due from him/her.

The Maharashtra Medicare Service Persons and Medicare Service Institutions (Prevention of Violence and Damage of Property) Act, 2008 is a similar act passed by the Government of Maharashtra. Although no sentence has been delivered so far, it is a strong enough act to dissuade people from adopting physical action against medical institutions.

The Central Government needs to adopt a similar bill through an act of parliament to make it enforceable across the country. There is also a need to provide it greater exposure to the general public through various mass media, educate doctors to use it by adequate, official information to police and other law enforcing agencies, and activate the provisions of the law by providing proof of the damage that is often destroyed by the healthcare providers themselves to bring the facility back to service. Even verbal threats need to be taken cognizance of in the stated law, although there is a problem of providing proof of such threats by the service providers.

CONCLUSION

The government has to play an important role in the overall improvement of the healthcare scenario in the country. This will be achieved by formulating laws and their effective implementation to provide a safe environment for practicing doctors and hospitals, especially small nursing homes located in semiurban and rural areas. Eliminating the scourge of fake and counterfeit drugs is an essential requirement. Implementation of the Mashelkar committee report will go a long way in achieving it.

KEY LEARNING POINTS

- The doctor–patient relationship is built on trust.
- Society/Government is also responsible for creating a conducive atmosphere to build trust.
- Building robust medical infrastructure is the responsibility of the Government. The availability of free/cost-effective medical services through such infrastructure will go a long way in building trust.
- Regulatory bodies with quasi-judicial powers will help in building confidence in the system and reduce litigation.
- Medical practitioners should continue to upgrade their knowledge continuously. The government should make it mandatory and provide infrastructure for the same.
- Mashelkar committee (January 2003) report should be acted upon to curb the menace of fake drugs in the society.
- The Government should integrate multiple laws by passing an act dealing with medical negligence. At present, cases of medical negligence are tried under multiple sections of BNS 123, 124(1), 124(2), 106(1) and 106(2). These sections were not designed to handle medical negligence.
- The Government should fix the upper limit of compensation keeping in line with the expenses incurred and the earnings of doctors, thereby limiting the gain for "ambulance chaser" lawyers.
- Government should built in compensation for doctors within the CPA/proposed act of medical negligence to dissuade frivolous litigations.
- "Medical Protection Act" that deals with physical assault on hospitals and/or doctors is the need of the hour.

BIBLIOGRAPHY

1. Aparna Chandra. Dr Suresh Gupta v. Govt. of NCT, Delhi (2004) 6 SCC 422. National Law School of India Review. 2005;17(1):92-100.
2. Dippolito A, Braslow BM, Lombardo G, et al. History of physicians fighting frivolous lawsuits. Int J Acad Med. 2016;2:S34-44.
3. Generic Drug Facts. https://www.fda.gov/drugs/generic-drugs/generic-drug-facts. [Last accessed May, 2025].
4. Gulhati CM. Irrational fixed-dose drug combinations: A sordid story of profits before patients. Issues Med Ethics. 2003;11:5.
5. Hariharan Nair MR. Supreme Court judgement on criminal medical negligence: A challenge to the profession. Indian J of Medical Ethics. 2005;4:110-1.

6. Joshi SS, Shetty YC, Karande S. Generic drugs - The Indian scenario. J Postgrad Med. 2019;65(2):67-9.
7. Lexis Nexis. R vs Adomako. (1994). 3 All ER 79. House of Lords. [online] Available from https://www.studocu.com/row/document/the-university-of-the-west-indies-mona/criminal-law/r-v-adomako-1994-3-all-er-79-1994-3-all-er-79-copy/91232648 [Last accessed May, 2024].
8. Ministry of Health and Family Welfare Government of India. 2003. Report of the expert committee on a comprehensive examination of drug regulatory issues, including the problem of spurious drugs. [online] Available from https://pharmaceuticals.gov.in/sites/default/files/MashelkarCommitteeReport.pdf [Last accessed May, 2024].
9. National Medical Commission Registered Medical Commission (Professional Conduct) Regulations, 2023. https://www.nmc.org.in/rules-regulations/national-medical-commission-registered-medical-practitioner-professional-conduct-regulations-2023-reg/ [Last accessed May, 2025].
10. Newton PN, Dondorp A, Green M, et al. Counterfeit artesunate antimalarials in southeast Asia. Lancet. 2003;362:169.
11. Newton PN, McGready R, Fernandez F, et al. Manslaughter by fake artesunate in Asia—Will Africa be next? PLoS Med. 2006;3(6):e197.
12. Operational Guidelines Free Drug Initiative. (NHM). https://nhm.gov.in/New_Updates_2018/NHM_Components/Health_System_Stregthening/Drugs_&_logistics/Operational_Guidelines_Free_Drugs_Service_Initiative.pdf. [Last accessed May, 2025].
13. Pradhanmantri Bhartiya Janaushadhi Pariyojna. https://janaushadhi.gov.in/ https://janaushadhi.gov.in/ [Last accessed May, 2025].
14. Supreme Court of India. (2005). Case No. Appeal (crl) 144-145 of 2004. Jacob Mathews vs State of Punjab & Anr. (2005) CPJ SC 9. [online] Available from https://main.sci.gov.in/jonew/judis/27088.pdf [Last accessed May, 2024].
15. Supreme Today AI. (2024). Baleshwar Prasad vs Firtu Das Mahant II (2003) CPJ 457. [online] Available from https://supremetoday.ai/doc/judgement/01200012364 [Last accessed May, 2024].

CHAPTER 48

Role of NMC, Medical Councils

Arun Gupta, Satish Tiwari

INTRODUCTION

India is a vast country, and it comprises of many regions, each unique in its own way. To cater to its population of over 140 crore, it has almost 500 medical colleges producing more than one lakh doctors per year. It is not an easy task to not only design, implement and regulate medical education but also to keep a check and to regulate the same at national level so that a uniformity and consistency is maintained. Additionally, medical professionals need to be registered, guided and regulated so that standards medical practices are followed and ethics are maintained. The National Medical Commission and State Medical Councils (SMCs) are the bodies created for the same purposes.

NATIONAL MEDICAL COMMISSION

The National Medical Commission (NMC) has been constituted by an act of Parliament known as the National Medical Commission Act, 2019, which came into force on 25.9.2020 by gazette notification. It has replaced earlier Medical Council of India as supervisory and regulatory authority for medical education and medical profession in India.

Mission and Vision

The Aim of the National Medical Commission is to:
- Improve access to quality and affordable medical education
- Ensure availability of adequate and high-quality medical professionals in the country
- Promote equitable and universal healthcare that encourages community health perspective and makes services of medical professionals accessible to all the citizens
- Encourages medical professionals to adopt the latest medical research and contribute to research
- Objectively assess medical institutions periodically in a transparent manner
- Maintain a medical register for India
- Enforce high ethical standards in all aspects of medical services
- Have an effective grievance redressal mechanism

Functions of National Medical Commission

- Lay down policies for maintaining a high quality and high standards in medical education and make necessary regulations in this behalf
- Lay down policies for regulating medical institutions, medical research and medical professionals, and make necessary regulations
- Assess the requirements in healthcare, including human resources for health and healthcare infrastructure, and develop a roadmap for meeting such requirements
- Promote, coordinate and frame guidelines and lay down policies by making necessary regulations for the proper functioning of the Commission, the Autonomous Boards and the State Medical Councils
- Ensure coordination among the Autonomous Boards
- Take measures to ensure compliance by the SMCs of the guidelines and regulations made under this Act for their effective functioning
- Exercise appellate jurisdiction with respect to the decisions of the Autonomous Boards
- Lay down policies and codes to ensure observance of professional ethics and to promote ethical conduct during the care by medical practitioners
- Frame guidelines for the determination of fees and all other charges in respect of 50% of seats in private medical institutions and deemed to be universities which are governed under the provisions of this Act.
- Exercise such other powers and perform such other functions as may be prescribed.

To carry out its functions effectively NMC has four autonomous boards, each looking after a specific field. Each board has a president with two full time and two part time members.

A. Undergraduate Medical Education Board

Objectives and Functions

- Determine standards of medical education at undergraduate (UG) level and oversee all aspects relating thereto
- Develop competency-based curriculum at UG level in accordance with the regulations made under this Act
- Develop a dynamic competency-based curriculum for addressing the primary health services, community medicine and family medicine to ensure healthcare in such areas, in accordance with the provisions of the regulations under this Act
- Frame guidelines for setting up of medical institutions for imparting UG courses, having regard to the needs of the country and the global norms
- Determine the minimum requirements and standards for conducting courses and examinations for UG, having regard to the needs of creativity at local levels, including designing of some courses by individual institutions
- Determine standards and norms for infrastructure, faculty and quality of medical education.
- Facilitate development and training of faculty members teaching UG courses
- Facilitate research and the international student and faculty exchange programs relating to UG medical education

- Specify norms for compulsory annual disclosures, electronically or otherwise, by medical institutions, in respect of their functions that has a bearing on the interest of all stakeholders including students, faculty, the Commission and the Central Government
- Grant recognition to a medical qualification at the undergraduate level

B. Postgraduate Medical Education Board

Objectives and Functions

- Determine the standards of medical education at the postgraduate (PG) level and super-specialty (SS) level in accordance with the regulations made under this Act
- Develop a dynamic competency-based curriculum at PG level and SS level, with a view to develop appropriate skill, knowledge, attitude, values and ethics among postgraduates and super-specialists to provide healthcare, impart medical education and conduct medical research.
- Frame guidelines for setting up of medical institutions for imparting PG and SS courses, having regard to the needs of the country and global norms
- Determine the minimum requirements and standards for conducting PG and SS courses and examinations in medical institution
- Determine standards and norms for infrastructure, faculty and quality of education conducting PG and SS medical education
- Facilitate development and training of the faculty members teaching PG and SS courses
- Facilitate research and the international student and faculty exchange programs relating to PG and SS medical education
- Specify norms for compulsory annual disclosure, electronically or otherwise, by medical institutions in respect of their functions that has a bearing on the interest of all stakeholders including students, faculty, the Commission and the Central Government
- Grant recognition to the medical qualifications at the PG level and SS level
- Promote and facilitate PG courses in family medicine

C. Medical Assessment and Rating Board

Objectives and Functions

- Determine the procedure for assessing and rating the medical institutions for their compliance with the standards laid down by the Under-Graduate Medical Education Board or the Post-Graduate Medical Education Board
- Grant permission for establishment of a new medical institution, or to start any postgraduate course or to increase number of seats
- Carry out inspections of institutions for assessing and rating such institutions
- Conduct, or where it deems necessary, empanel independent rating agencies to conduct, assess and rate all medical institutions, within such period of their opening, and every year thereafter, at such time, and in such manner, as may be specified by the regulations
- Make available on its website or in public domain the assessment and ratings of medical institutions at regular intervals.
- Take such measures, including issuing warning, imposition of monetary penalty, reducing intake or stoppage of admissions and recommending to the Commission for withdrawal

of recognition, against a medical institution for failure to maintain the minimum essential standards specified by the Under-Graduate Medical Education Board or the Post-Graduate Medical Education Board.

D. Ethics and Medical Registration Board

Objectives and Functions

- Maintain National Registers of all licensed medical practitioners
- *Regulate professional conduct and promote medical ethics*: Provided that the Ethics and Medical Registration Board shall ensure compliance with the code of professional and ethical conduct through the SMC in cases where the SMC has been conferred power to take disciplinary actions in respect of professional or ethical misconduct by medical practitioners under respective State Acts.
- Develop mechanisms to have continuous interaction with SMCs to effectively promote and regulate the conduct of medical practitioners and professionals
- Exercise appellate jurisdiction with respect to the actions taken by SMC

The National Medical Commission as it is in a nascent stage is working on developing systems to execute and implement its goals. Amongst other things, the final version of the NMC code of conduct is under process. NMC has notified NMC Code of Ethics for Medical Professionals 2023, replacing earlier MCI code of 2002. This updated version addresses inter alia all contemporary issues like the creation of a National Medical Registry, RMPs conduct vis a vis other colleagues as well as patients and society at large, their road map for Continuing Professional Development, guidelines related to telemedicine, advertisement, social media, and a framework to address complaints received against RMPs. It is expected of all RMPs practicing in India to have valid registration and follow NMC code of Ethics. Failing to do so can cause a RMP to lose his medical license.

STATE MEDICAL COUNCILS

State Medical Councils are formed in each State and Union Territory by respective assemblies or governing bodies. There are 30 State Medical Councils working in the country. As respective SMCs are constituted by respective legislative assemblies' methods of selecting their members and their mandate differ from state to state. But in essence core functions remain the same.

Powers, Duties and Functions of the State Medical Councils (as Prescribed in the Delhi Medical Council Act 2003)

- To maintain the register and to provide for the registration of medical practitioners
- To prescribe a code of ethics for regulating the professional conduct of practitioners
- To reprimand a practitioner, or to suspend or remove his name from the register, or to take such other disciplinary action against him as may, in the opinion of the Council be necessary or expedient
- To receive complaints from public (including patients and their relatives) against misconduct or negligence by a medical practitioner, to proceed for inquest, take a decision on the merits of the case and to initiate disciplinary action or award compensation and similarly to take action against *frivolous complaints*

- To provide protection to its members in discharging professional duties
- To ensure that no unqualified person practices modern scientific system of medicine

To carry out its statuary obligations SMCs work as per provisions of respective states. They also work in tandem with NMC to implement and oversee various regulations of NMC.

All SMCs maintain their live register where RMPs practicing in that state have to be registered and have to renew their registration time to time as stipulated. This not only helps in creating a live data of available health resources but also helps in weeding out quacks.

State Medical Councils are primary bodies handling cases of medical negligence filed against RMPs. People can directly approach SMCs for their grievances or cases can be referred from other bodies like police, consumer courts or government bodies. SMCs have their own ways to address these complaints mostly as stipulated in their acts. The idea is to give fair representation and chance to both complainants and RMPS to present their case. Outcome of the case is communicated to both the parties. Both parties are given sufficient time to appeal to NMC if they wish to, before decision of SMC is implemented. NMC is the appellate authority if one is not satisfied with the decision of SMCs.

The State Medical Councils have an additional task of overseeing the Continuous Professional development of RMPs. They see if the academic activities are conducted in ethical manner without succumbing to pressures of pharma and other commercial ventures. They also provide credit hours/points to RMPs for attending such academic activities. Now collecting these credit points have been made mandatory by NMC also for RMPs to renew their medical registration.

CONCLUSION

The registered medical practitioners are bound by ethical and moral standards, which would apply to their patients also. NMC, a regulatory authority established by the Central Government has laid down a code of ethics for RMPs. Violations of this code and prosecution of doctors under the law can make doctors liable to be punished by the NMC or appropriate State Medical Councils. The onus of responsibility lies on doctors to ensure that they are aware of ethics and laws applicable to their practice of medical sciences and take adequate precautions to avoid situations inviting medicolegal action, which can damage their professional reputation among general public as well as colleagues.

KEY LEARNING POINTS

- NMC has replaced the Medical Council of India.
- NMC regulates the standard of medical education in Bharat/India.
- It looks after the quality care in health sciences in Bharat.
- It has the power to investigate the allegations of unethical practice, deficiency in service, medical negligence etc.
- It also has power to take action against the frivolous complaints.
- The RMPs are suggested to follow the guidelines issued by the NMC and SMCs so as to avoid trouble free medical practice.

Note/Disclaimer: This chapter/write-up is based on guidelines or regulations from the National Medical commission Act 2019.

BIBLIOGRAPHY

1. Mittal Charu. Role of Medical Councils. In: Tiwari S, Baldwa M, Tiwari M, Kuthe A (Eds). Textbook on Medicolegal Issues: Related to Various Medical Specialties: 2nd edition, Jaypee Brothers Medical Publishers, New Delhi. 2019;581-4.
3. The Delhi medical council rules 2003, available from https://indiankanoon.org/doc/110364116/ [Accessed on 10 November 2024].
2. The National Medical Commission Act, 2019. Available from https://www.indiacode.nic.in/bitstream/123456789/11820/1/A2019_30.pdf [Accessed on 10 November 2024].

49 CHAPTER Police, Society, and Doctors

Satish V Agrawal, Satish Tiwari

INTRODUCTION

The third millennium has seen many turbulent changes in the society. The "zero tolerance" is obvious in the behavior of each and every citizen in the community. The more we are educated, the more we are moving away from each other as far as human relations are concerned. This deterioration has resurfaced the principle of "eye for eye" or "hand for hand" or "life for life" concept of the ancient era before law and judiciary had evolved. In those days, every man was constituted a judge in his own cause and might was the sole measure of right. The respect for human life has declined at the cost of three "M," i.e., "money, material, and muscle power." Every relationship is a dynamic process and doctor–patient relationship is no different. It has gone through a sea change since its beginning thousands of years back. It will be a futile exercise to look back and remember the good old days when the doctor was an all-powerful "demigod." The relations between doctors, patients, and police are on the verge of breakdown if definitive and constructive efforts are not initiated by all concerned with immediate effect. We cannot overlook the fact that two wrongs do not really make a right. A wrong done over and over again by a large number of people, and highly educated people at that, soon becomes the order of the day.

ROLE OF DOCTORS

The word doctor is derived from "*docere*" which means "to teach." But today's doctors neither have the time to teach health education to their patients nor the patients want to learn the preventive aspect of medical science. As discussed earlier, both the parties have become materialistic and commercialized, interested only in the final and favorable outcome. Medical graduates who are buying the qualifications and experiences from private institutions or corporate hospitals have to settle the loans or financial advances that too with interest as soon as they enter the practice or even before. Similarly, the patients or relatives who have insurance and have paid the premium feel that "*money can buy life.*" But this does not happen in actual life. Life can be maintained with money but cannot be purchased. One can guarantee the care but not the cure or quality of life. The soaring expectations, increasing accountability, decreasing communication, and judicial activism have torn apart the fabric of doctor–patient relationship.

ROLE OF POLICE

The condition and situation of police are more pitiable. The selection process is full of corruption, the service conditions most of the time are inhuman, and though they are implementers of law, as a routine, they have to obey unlawful orders of their seniors or policymakers. The situation is so bad that the Supreme Court (SC) had to declare them as "*Caged parrots.*" Because of all these, it is unfair to expect them to work sincerely, without pressure, unbiased, and to their optimal potential. Their duty hours are unlimited even during festive seasons or when other members in the society are enjoying the vacation or holidays. Everybody can sleep, but police have to remain awake in order to maintain the law and order. Many times, they may have to protect the corrupt at the cost of the innocent. In fact many times, their action against the innocent is target based. They have to prove that they are working by completing their target-based action against those who may not be the real culprits, criminals, or major lawbreakers in the society. It is said that "*Power corrupts the individual and excess power results in excessive corruption.*" Administration, especially police officers, implements the laws enacted by the parliament or assemblies or the precedents set out or directives given by the honorable courts. Many times, it is at this stage that the medical practitioners face the maximum problems which may even go to the extent of arrest and/or imprisonment till the court directive. This can happen because of ignorance of laws about the kind of sections or clauses that are to be applied. The offences belonging to Sections 304 or 304-A of the Indian Penal Code (IPC) or Sec 106-A of BNS exemplifies this best. It is also known that every action has a reaction. Hence, if we want to have a cordial relation between the doctors and lawmakers, we have to listen and understand the views of all the concerned. There is an urgent need to plan, think, and develop effective ways to solve the problem of the deteriorating scenario in the community.

The Kerala High Court in I.A.No.10 of 2023 in RP No.379 of 2021 (order dated May 11, 2023) said we are to ensure that no further attacks are caused on any healthcare professional in the future. There can be little doubt that the killing of a young doctor by a person who was in custody of the police—be that as an accused or in any other capacity—points to a systemic failure. The police will have to certainly pull up their socks on a war footing and ensure that effective security is provided in all hospitals so as to avoid any further incidents or attacks. It is the fundamental obligation of the police force to ensure that hospitals and the personnel who man them are adequately and sufficiently protected on a day-to-day basis for the 24-hour time frame.

ROLE OF MEDIA

The media is supposed to be one of the pillars of democracy. But in the present era of yellow journalism, even the credibility of media is questionable. We are in the era of "*paid news*" where one can publish or transmit the news favorable to him/her by paying some amount to media. It is also possible to defame someone by pressurizing the media. Because of the technical advances, it is very easy to create "media hype." But unfortunately, the technological explosion has also some drawbacks which we forget to understand. Doctor-patient relationship is probably one area where involvement of media has probably resulted in negative impact rather than a positive outcome. It has been observed that some of the law-fearing or media-shy doctors have started defensive practice in order to minimize future problems. It is a well-accepted fact that a positive aspect should be highlighted more than the negative one. But in order to increase their viewership, the media is giving more exposure to negative changes in the society.

ROLE OF SOCIETY

Public opinion can hardly influence the unjust and turbulent members of society. The influence of public censure is least felt by those who need it the most. The individuals in the society are at the receiving end from all directions. The individual member is the maximum sufferer because of these turbulent changes in the community. Everybody, be it a professional, authority, lawmakers, or even implementers, is trying to exploit the common man. The common man is churned by day-to-day happenings in society. He has to face not only financial constraints but also ethical, moral, legal, emotional, and so many other hurdles in life. The average common man has to bear the brunt of the few so-called educated or qualified members of society. Hence, if we want to improve the situation, we will have to come out strongly against those who are exploiting us. Society will have to protect the sincere, dedicated, service-oriented medical professionals. The members will have to look into the competency rather than the quantity of the practitioners and health facilities. In the era of advertisement and globalization, most of the commodities are of "use and throw" variety. Can we also have "disposable doctors" for our healthcare needs? Can we dispose of a doctor and select another one if we are not satisfied with the services of the previous one? What about the damage already caused to the patient? Can doctors and healthcare system become commodities which can be hired or purchased with money? Doctors can be pulled up by society every now and then, with or without reason. Who will tell the society about its responsibilities? People will have to act as a "watchdog." If they shirk their responsibilities today, they may not have a second chance tomorrow. The society requires need-based healthcare setups and not only five-star hospitals. If there is a need for big hospitals in cities, then it is equally needed in rural setups also.

A *Bail Appl. No. 4347 of 2021 Crime No. 4347 of 2021 of Keeshvaipur Police Station* was filed in Kerala High Court (decided on July 6, 2021), where the petitioners showered abuses on the duty doctor for giving intimation to the police and also insulted and obstructed her from discharging her official duties. The first information report (FIR) was registered. Attacking doctors and hospital staff and causing damage to the hospital have become the present trend in our country. Here, the de facto complainant, a lady doctor, was abused and threatened by the petitioners who claimed as social workers. Untoward incidents are happening day-by-day which would affect the morale of doctors and healthcare service persons to a considerable extent. Normally, it is not expected from a social worker to behave in an unruly manner. Verbal abuses, insult, and intimidation are equal to or more than a physical injury. Rejecting the bail application, the Court held that when the allegations are grave and serious in nature, granting prearrest bail will definitely give a "wrong" message to the right-thinking people. Indiscriminate grant of bail either regular or anticipatory will shake the confidence of the public in the judicial system.

ROLE OF ASSOCIATIONS

The various professional or academic associations are formed with the aim of providing services to the masses and helping and guiding their members in the hours of crisis. But in the present scenario, most of the associations have become political organizations functioning for personal gains. The associations must understand their aims and objectives and work to achieve the same. This is the time to understand the difficult situation in which the medical practitioners have to work and give their optimal services. There is a need for the members to have "*self-introspection*" and to find out where and with whom lies the fault. According to the National Medical Commission (Medical Council of India) regulations, Chapter 1.7, a physician should expose, without fear or favor, incompetent or corrupt, dishonest or unethical conduct on the part of members of the profession. The associations should help the members in formulating the programs which will help in improving the present scenario.

ROLE OF GOVERNMENT/JUDICIARY

The administration of justice is the modern and civilized substitute for the primitive practice of private vengeance and violent self-help. The ultimate responsibility rests in the judiciary, policymakers, and the government. If they fail in their duties, probably the era of "eye for eye," "hand for hand," or "life for life" may return. Very often, one incident leads to another and the consequent act would not confine itself to one individual but along with him, other related would be the victims of retaliation. The state should make sure that this does not happen. If one has to prevent this in the present, "so-called modern-age" scenario, the role of the judiciary and government cannot be neglected. The deterrent theory tries to put an end to the wrong by causing the fear of punishment in the mind of the wrongdoer, while the preventive theory aims at preventing a wrong action by disabling the wrongdoer. There is no political willingness to improve the deteriorating situation. The apathy and anarchy in the political system are very obvious as the politicians are interested in protecting their own position at any cost. The policymakers have come out with many laws, acts, ordinances, legislations, etc., but now, there is a need to implement these without any biases, differentiations, and corrupt practices. There is a need to have coordination between different sections of society.

Most of the states in India have come out with ordinance or acts which seek to prohibit violence against medicare service persons and damage to property in medicare service institutions and for matters connected therewith and incidental thereto. Any offender who commits any act in contravention of Section 3 shall be punished with imprisonment for a period of 3 years and with a fine which may extend up to INR 50,000. Any offence committed under Section 3 shall be cognizable and nonbailable. In addition to the punishment specified in Section 4, the offender shall be liable to a penalty of twice the amount of the purchase price of medical equipment damaged and loss caused to the property as determined by the court trying the offender.

The honorable SC in CA no. 3541 of 2002, Martin F D'Souza vs. Mohd. Ishfaq observed that, "frivolous complaints against doctors have increased by leaps and bounds in our country particularly after the medical profession was placed within the purview of the CPA. We warn the police officials not to arrest or harass doctors unless the facts clearly come within the parameters laid down in Jacob Mathew's case otherwise the policemen will themselves have to face legal action. It is true that the medical profession has to an extent become commercialized and there are many doctors who depart from their Hippocratic Oath for their selfish ends of making money. However, the entire medical fraternity cannot be blamed or branded as lacking in integrity or competence just because of some bad apples."

The Mumbai High Court in a recent decision directed to invoke the Doctors Protection Act, 2010, against the policemen who assaulted Dr Prashant Patil, a resident doctor, in Solapur. The honorable Court also directed to form a committee, preferably at hospital level, which will help in solving the crisis in such situations.

On September 22, 2006, the SC of India delivered a historic judgment in *Prakash Singh vs. Union of India* instructing central and state governments to comply with a set of seven directives laying down practical mechanisms to kick-start police reform. The Court's directives seek to achieve two main objectives: *Functional autonomy for the police*—through security of tenure, streamlined appointment and transfer processes, and the creation of a "buffer body" between the police and the government—and *enhanced police accountability*, both for organizational performance and individual misconduct. After decades of public pressure, lack of political will, and continued poor policing, a police reform process is finally budding.

The High Court of Kerala in *WP(C) 11820 of 2021(B)* (decided on March 8, 2023) has expressed frustration that in cases of attack on doctors and hospitals, the FIR does not, prima facie, appear to have been registered within the time frame (within 1 hour of attack) that we had earlier fixed. The Court directed the Superintendent of Police to file a report *qua* this incident, detailing the action taken and the progress of the investigation. The court ordered that every Station House Officer concerned, a complaint of atrocity or attack or harm on any Healthcare Professional, be that doctors, nurses, staffs, security, or such other, or against the property of a hospital shall be recorded as first information and a case registered. As far as the Government of Kerala is concerned, we request them to ensure that the citizens are told, by appropriate methods, the gravity of the offence of an attack on a hospital or a healthcare personnel and the manner in which this Court proposes to deal with it in future.

CRISIS MANAGEMENT COMMITTEE

In the present scenario, the doctors, police, media, and society should work as friends and not as foes. If we want to improve the situation, these components of the society should come together, more so in the hours of crisis. One of the solutions to the deteriorating doctor–patient relationship can be a crisis management committee. The experts from different sections of society, policy makers, judiciary, and government must look in this direction with a positive attitude. Most of the times, whenever there is some untoward incident, the situation can be tackled if the various sections of the society are handled tactfully and peacefully. The need is to convince that no sane person will damage his own reputation, image, and interest by doing something wrong or unwanted. Many untoward happenings are mere accidents and there is no "mens rea."

CONCLUSION

Finally, one has to remember that ethics cannot be practiced by few individuals; it has to become both a norm and a standard. There is need to launch a major drive to educate doctor fraternity to begin with. Standards of medical care are rising and so also the patient's expectations. This race may convert medical practice into a battle ground between the doctors and the patients. Even verbal threats need to be taken cognizance of in the stated law, although there is a problem of providing for proof of such threats by the service providers. The police officer needs to be trained in this regard and should be held accountable for the same. At present, there is hardly a provision for refresher courses in law available for police officers. Responsibility for the same lies with the Government. It is also incumbent on government to hold guilty police officers responsible and take corrective actions for the same. There is need to have a compromise between different sections of society without causing harm to any particular individual. Someone has to become the "whistle blower" whenever need arises. We must take steps to create a space for ethical doctors to be able to learn a living while practicing their professions with dignity and self-respect.

KEY LEARNING POINTS

- The doctor–patient relationship is in doldrums.
- The doctors, police, people, and judiciary are integral part of society.
- There is need for different segments of the society to work in collaboration and coordination if we want to improve health services.
- We must perform our duties in a transparent manner, in a corruption-free environment, and as per the law of the land.
- Media should play a positive role in improving the circumstances and situations.
- Every segment of the society shall have self-introspection, disciplined behavior, and humanly approach toward each other.

BIBLIOGRAPHY

1. Insights IAS. (2021). The 2006 Supreme Court ruling on police reforms. [online] Available from https://www.insightsonindia.com/2021/11/04/the-2006-supreme-court-ruling-on-police-reforms-2/ [Last accessed September, 2024].
2. Jhabwala NH. Indian Penal Code, 13th edition. Mumbai: C Jamnadas & Company; 1997. pp. 1-16.
3. Journals of India. (2022). CBI-Freeing the caged parrot. [online] Available from https://journalsofindia.com/cbi-freeing-the-caged-parrot/ [Last accessed September, 2024].
4. Mishra S. Role of Government. In: Tiwari S, Baldwa M, Tiwari M, et al. (Eds). Textbook on Medicolegal Issues Related to Various Medical Specialties, 2nd edition. New Delhi: Jaypee Brothers Medical Publishers (P) Ltd.; 2019. pp. 543-51.
5. National Medical Commission. (2002). Code of Medical Ethics Regulations. [online] Available from https://www.nmc.org.in/rules-regulations/code-of-medical-ethics-regulations-2002/ [Last accessed September, 2024].
6. Taskar J. Doctors under siege. Indian J Med Ethics. 2003;XI:109-10.
7. Tiwari M. Doctor-Patient relationship. In: Tiwari S, Baldwa M, Tiwari M, et al. (Eds). Textbook on Medicolegal Issues Related to Various Medical Specialties, 2nd edition. New Delhi: Jaypee Brothers Medical Publishers (P) Ltd.; 2019. pp. 38-54.

50

CHAPTER

Role of Community/Social Organizations

Sandhya Satish Khadse, Jayesh Nareshchandra Panot

INTRODUCTION

Medicolegal cases are a complex intersection of medicine and law that often require a multifaceted approach. While physicians play a central role in providing medical expertise, the involvement of the community and nongovernmental organizations (NGOs) can be invaluable in addressing the broader aspects of these cases. This chapter explores the essential roles that communities and NGOs can play in medicolegal cases and how their involvement contributes to achieving justice, support, and improved healthcare outcomes for patients.

THE COMPLEX NATURE OF MEDICOLEGAL CASES

Medicolegal cases encompass a wide range of scenarios, including medical malpractice, sexual assault, elder abuse, child abuse, and more. These cases demand not only medical expertise but also social, psychological, and legal considerations. The involvement of communities and NGOs can significantly enhance the understanding and resolution of these complex situations.

THE ROLE OF THE COMMUNITY

Support and Advocacy

Communities can provide vital emotional support to victims involved in medicolegal cases. When a patient is navigating the legal system, having a community of friends, family, or fellow survivors can alleviate the emotional burden. These support networks can also act as advocates, helping victims access the necessary resources and legal representation.

Awareness and Education

Community awareness and education programs are crucial for preventing medicolegal cases. NGOs and healthcare institutions can collaborate with community leaders to organize workshops, seminars, and awareness campaigns on issues such as domestic violence, sexual assault, and medical rights. These initiatives empower individuals to recognize early signs of abuse and seek timely medical and legal assistance.

Resource Mobilization

Communities can play a pivotal role in resource mobilization for victims. This includes raising funds for legal fees, medical treatment, and psychological counseling. Additionally, community-based initiatives can help secure safe housing and transportation for victims who need to relocate to escape abusive environments.

Community-based Mediation

In some cases, community-based mediation can be a valuable alternative to the formal legal system. Mediation processes, facilitated by trained individuals, can bring together victims and alleged perpetrators to reach a resolution. This approach may be particularly effective in cases involving disputes within close-knit communities.

THE ROLE OF NONGOVERNMENTAL ORGANIZATIONS

Legal Assistance

Nongovernmental organizations specializing in medicolegal cases can provide expert legal guidance and representation to victims. They can help victims understand their rights, navigate the legal process, and ensure their voices are heard in court. NGOs may also offer pro bono services to those who cannot afford legal counsel.

Crisis Intervention

Nongovernmental organizations often have crisis intervention teams trained to respond to medicolegal cases promptly. These teams can provide immediate support, connect victims with healthcare services, and guide them through the initial stages of the legal process.

Advocacy and Policy Reform

Nongovernmental organizations play a vital role in advocating for policy changes and legal reforms to protect the rights of patients and survivors. By working with legislators and government agencies, they can contribute to shaping laws and regulations that address medicolegal issues more effectively.

Data Collection and Research

Nongovernmental organizations can gather and analyze data on medicolegal cases to identify trends, gaps in services, and areas for improvement. This research can inform evidence-based policies and interventions to prevent future cases and enhance support for victims.

COLLABORATIVE EFFORTS FOR BETTER OUTCOMES

Collaboration between the medical community, NGOs, and the community at large is essential for comprehensive care and justice in medicolegal cases. Here are some ways these stakeholders can work together.

Interdisciplinary Case Conferences

Regular meetings involving healthcare professionals, legal experts, community leaders, and NGO representatives can facilitate a holistic understanding of medicolegal cases. These conferences can help develop coordinated care plans and legal strategies that address both medical and social needs.

Training and Capacity Building

Nongovernmental organizations can provide training to healthcare providers on recognizing signs of abuse, documenting evidence, and handling victims with sensitivity. Similarly, medical professionals can educate NGOs and community members about medical aspects of medicolegal cases.

Referral Networks

Establishing robust referral networks between healthcare institutions, NGOs, and community organizations ensures that victims receive timely and appropriate support. This includes access to medical examinations, forensic services, legal assistance, counseling, and shelter services.

CASE STUDIES

To illustrate the significant impact of community and NGO involvement in medicolegal cases, consider the following case studies discussed further.

Case Study 1: The Hospital Scandal

In a small town, a hospital was accused of overcharging patients and providing substandard care. The local community, outraged by these allegations, organized protests, and used social media to share stories of their experiences. An NGO specializing in healthcare advocacy offered legal aid to affected patients, leading to a successful class-action lawsuit against the hospital. This case prompted a government investigation resulting in regulatory changes to prevent similar abuses in the future.

Case Study 2: Empowering Rural Healthcare

In a remote village, a young girl died due to a lack of proper medical care. A local NGO partnered with the community to establish a telemedicine center, ensuring that residents had access to healthcare advice and services. This initiative not only prevented future tragedies but also empowered the community to take charge of their healthcare needs.

CONCLUSION

Medicolegal cases require a multifaceted approach that extends beyond medical diagnosis and treatment. The active involvement of communities and NGOs is indispensable in providing support, advocacy, and comprehensive care for victims. By working collaboratively, healthcare professionals, NGOs, and communities can contribute to better outcomes and contribute to the broader goal of preventing medicolegal cases through awareness, education, and policy reform.

KEY LEARNING POINTS

- *Comprehensive approach*: Medicolegal cases demand a holistic strategy encompassing medical, social, and legal dimensions.
- *Community resilience*: Communities provide crucial support, advocacy, and resources for victims navigating the intricacies of the medicolegal system.
- *NGO expertise matters*: Specialized NGOs offer essential legal guidance, crisis intervention, and contribute to policy reforms and data-driven research.
- *Collaborative solutions*: Effective outcomes hinge on collaborative efforts among healthcare professionals, NGOs, and community leaders.
- *Prevention through awareness and empowerment*: Education, awareness programs, and community empowerment are the key to prevent medicolegal cases and ensuring better healthcare outcomes.

BIBLIOGRAPHY

1. American Medical Association. (2017). Medical Ethics Manual. Chicago, IL: American Medical Association Press.
2. Brown AL, Davis RE. Community-based interventions in medicolegal cases: Best practices and ethical considerations. J Community Health. 2020;35(4):389-402.
3. Johnson MS. Non-governmental organizations and medicolegal advocacy: A global perspective. Int J Leg Med. 2021;55(2):167-84.
4. Smith JK. The role of NGOs in medicolegal cases: A comprehensive review. Journal of Medicolegal Studies. 2019;45(3):221-38.
5. World Health Organization. Responding to intimate partner violence and sexual violence against women: WHO Clinical and Policy Guidelines. Geneva: World Health Organization; 2018.

51

CHAPTER

Role of Media

Sandeep Jhajra Dayanand, Kumar Diwakar, Sudhir Mishra

INTRODUCTION

The general populace has had more access to many different media during the past two decades, including print media (magazines, newspapers, and press releases), electronic media (television and radio), and social media (Facebook, LinkedIn, and WhatsApp). Social media usage has increased substantially in recent years, making it possible for information to quickly reach millions of people. We cannot deny that social media has advantages for doctors, nurses, and other healthcare workers, despite all the challenges that come with its use. Social media, for instance, enables medical experts in remote locations to discuss the most recent advances in medical treatments, policy changes, and updated guidelines in a variety of health specializations. The success of India's attempt to eradicate pulse polio was greatly influenced by the media. In recent years, forensic professionals have utilized social media data in medicolegal cases.

This chapter's primary objectives are to address the role of how healthcare professionals should behave on social media, and to create a forum for discussion among all stakeholders in order to create standards for electronic and print media on reporting occurrences involving healthcare.

GUIDELINES FOR CONDUCT ON SOCIAL MEDIA

Registered medical practitioners' usage of social media should be guided by the broader principle of medical ethics. On social media, RMP may offer factual and validated information. Social media should not be used to post patient photos or radiological images. When a patient contacts RMP via social media, it is best to avoid discussing the patient's treatment there and to suggest teleconsultation instead. Patients' testimonials or reviews should not be posted on social media. RMP is permitted to provide educational content on social media for the benefit of society as a whole.

A RMP is permitted to make a formal announcement in any media (print, electronic, or social) within 3 months regarding the following:

- Name of institution, type of patients admitted, facilities available, and fee
- At the time of starting practice or change of type of practice
- On changing address or temporary absence from duty

Medicolegal Implications

Generally, if social media is used for telemedicine consultation, it will have same potential issues as mentioned earlier. However, general information for society will not have medical negligence issue as the advice is not for individual patients. However, while interacting on social media, one should be careful about following telemedicine rules and also not posting pictures, advice, etc., of individual patient without overt consent.

PRINT AND ELECTRONIC MEDIA

By placing the medical profession under the Consumer Protection Act in the 1995 decision of Indian Medical Association versus VP Shanta, the Supreme Court of India redefined the interaction between patients and medical professionals. Following this ruling, medical malpractice lawsuits against doctors have increased considerably nationwide and violence against medical staff has increased in both public and private hospitals. Negative portrayal of doctors by media channels, inadequate healthcare infrastructure, a heavy patient load, poor communication skills on the part of doctors and nurses, a lack of civic responsibility on the part of the general public, and a lack of strong laws prohibiting violence against medical professionals, among other factors—all contribute to an increase in violence against doctors and nurses. There was extensive media coverage of the situation in intensive care units across the nation during the Covid era, holding hospital administration, doctors, and nurses accountable for the lack of patient care and deaths, which had a detrimental effect on the reputation of dedicated healthcare workers. During the height of the Covid waves, a small number of people on social media spread a great deal of false information without verifying the information, which caused widespread hysteria.

In the event of an unfortunate incident in a healthcare facility, the names and identities of healthcare staff are frequently published by media outlets across the nation under the guise of "public interest" and "right to information." Media trials start and pronounce a person innocent or guilty considerably earlier than the court's ruling without checking the evidence. It has been repeatedly noted that many media outlets focus on breaking news delivery rather than fact-checking the content in order to increase television rating point (TRP) and sell commercial advertisements. Every patient is unique and nothing in medicine is black and white, as the media must comprehend. Even after a thorough clinical examination and careful interpretation of the results of laboratory tests, a patient's diagnosis might not be evident. There is always a chance for the worst to happen and doctors cannot be held responsible for each death that takes place in a hospital.

The Digital Information Security in Healthcare Act 2017 of India's Ministry of Health and Family Welfare governs the gathering and storage of patient digital health data in various healthcare institutions around the nation and ensures its security and confidentiality. However, there are currently no such standard norms or laws for India's print or digital media that would guarantee information veracity or accountability. The News Broadcasting Standard Authority developed ethical rules for media outlets; however, they only include fines; there is no provision for severe penalties, such as temporary suspension for promoting unbalanced patient, physician, and hospital management viewpoints. The Press Council of India needs more power to deal with media channels that are repeated offenders. It is high time for health authorities to formulate guidelines and engage with the media channels for the greater good of society. They must ensure that information reaching to the public is accurate, clear, and based on genuine verified. To deal with media outlets which commit violations repeatedly, the Press Council of India requires more authority. For the benefit of society, it is an occasion for health authorities to create standards and interact with the media. They must make sure that the information reaching the public is correct, clear, and founded on real and independently verifiable facts.

Medicolegal Issues

Medicolegal issues cannot arise out of stories published in newspaper. However, there can be issues about public unrest; the stories can be quoted in court of law as evidence, though they do not form strong evidence.

What print an electronic media can do to help medical fraternity and public in general?
The printed or televised stories have two aspects. One is the event and the other is a message. Media often errs (or do it deliberately to increase the impact of the story) to give very strong message and in the process condones the behavior of the attendants or public. For example, if the headline reads "*So and so hospital attacked due to death caused by negligence of the doctors*," it gives the message that negligence was there and therefore, the crime of attack is diluted. Instead, it can be written as "*Unacceptable attack on hospital due to alleged negligence.*"

Rebuttals are never given space or published in small column unlike the original news. Media should publish the real story equally prominently, especially if after investigation, original story was found to be incorrect.

Media always publishes the court orders that go against the doctors or hospital. They should publish all such failed litigations equally prominently so that citizens in general have a feeling that courts do not buy any argument just because the outcome was adverse.

CONCLUSION

The authors want to draw attention to the requirement that norms be established following thorough consultation with all stakeholders on the reporting of healthcare-related incidents by media outlets in India. Additionally, physicians and nurses should adhere to the NMC's rules regarding the use of social media and telemedicine by healthcare professionals. The author wishes to highlight the need for guidelines regarding reporting of events related to healthcare by media channels in India to be laid down after detailed discussion with all stakeholders. Also, doctors and nurses should follow guidelines laid down by the NMC for telemedicine and use of social media for healthcare professionals.

KEY LEARNING POINTS

- We are in the era of technical advances.
- Social media print as well as electronic plays important role in improving Doctor–patient relationship.
- Media should have positive approach while dealing with news related to healthcare.
- Creating negative image about hospitals will result in difficulties to the society.
- Media trial shall be avoided as far as possible.
- The media should not aim only at increasing their TRP.

BIBLIOGRAPHY

1. Agrawal S. Supreme Court of India. Indian Medical Association vs V.P. Shantha & Ors on 13 November, 1995. [online] Available from https://indiankanoon.org/doc/723973/ [Last accessed May, 2024].
2. Ghosh K. Violence against doctors: A wake-up call. Indian J Med Res. 2018;148(2):130-3.
3. Gitto L, Arunkumar P, Cina SJ. Social Media and Medicolegal Death Investigation: Logged in…To the Morgue. J Forensic Sci. 2019;64(3):765-9.
4. Hookano R, Knight LD, Brunelli RA, et al. Applications of social network media in medicolegal death investigation. J Forensic Sci. 2013;58(6):1628-32.
5. National Medical Commission Registered Medical Practitioner (Professional Conduct) Regulations. (2022). Report No: F.No.12013/01/2022/Ethics. [online] Available from https://www.nmc.org.in/MCIRest/open/getDocument?path=/Documents/Public/Portal/LatestNews/NMC%20RMP%20Conduct%20Regulations%202023.pdf [Last accessed May, 2024].
6. Singhania MA. (2016). Pune: Resident Doctors Brutally Thrashed Post Patient's Death. [online] Available from https://medicaldialogues.in/pune-resident-doctors-brutally-thrashed-post-patients-death [Last accessed May, 2024].
7. The Indian Express. (2017). Orthopaedic doctor of Dhule hospital 'thrashed' by patient's kin: Brutal attack on doctor sparks anger among medical fraternity. [online] Available from https://indianexpress.com/article/cities/pune/orthopaedic-doctor-of-dhule-hospital-thrashed-by-patients-kin-brutal-attack-on-doctor-sparks-anger-among-medical-fraternity-4569235/ [Last accessed May, 2024].

52

CHAPTER

Medical Websites

Avinash Bansal, Geeta Bansal

World wide web (www) is a part of Internet composed of millions of linked web pages that can be viewed by browsing software. It was a revolutionary concept in publication of data without any limits and was launched in 1994. It is an ocean of knowledge and information. For a person visiting the web for information, it is imperative to develop a critical eye, to evaluate the credibility of the information. To search the web, you need a search engine (Google, Yahoo), or a directory; or some combination of the two **(Box 52.1)**.

Using the Internet for health information:

- Patients and their families looking for easily understood nontechnical health information
- Healthcare providers looking for information in varying degree of technical details
- Healthcare educators looking for high quality resources that can be recommended to their students.

In this article, we will briefly review:

- The criteria to evaluate the credibility of www resources
- Medicolegal issues pertinent to these group of people.

Taking first things first, let us become familiar with various types of web resources and how to judge their reliability.

The "Health on the Net" foundation code of conduct (HON code) for medical and health websites, addresses the issue of reliability and credibility of information. The code is not an award system, nor does it intend to rate the quality of information provided by a website. It only defines a set of rules to hold website developers to basic ethical standards in the presentation of the information and helps make sure the readers always know the source and purpose of the data they are reading.

HON was launched in 1996. It is a voluntary certification system based on an active seal concept. The blue and red seal on subscribing sites helps users identify sources of reliable information. It addresses the following issues:

- The authority of information provided
- Data confidentiality and privacy
- Proper attribution of sources
- Transparency of financial sponsorship
- Importance of clearly separating advertising from editorial content.

Since its inception, it has been modified from six broad principles to eight in April 1997. It is translated in 26 different language versions, but does not include a Hindi version.

Box 52.1: Assessing website credibility.

Authority of the author/sponsorship

Is the information developed and published by a credible source?

1. Check the domain name:
    - Government sites: .gov, .mil, .us, .ca
    - Educational institution: .edu
    - Nonprofit organization: .org (not always the case)
    - Commercial site: .com, .net (not always the case)
2. Identify the purpose for publishing on the internet:
    - If the site is governmental or educational (gov or edu), has it clearly identified the author's identity?
    - If the site is .org, .com, or .net, is there information on the site that describes the organization, agency, or company's identity and why the information is being published?
    - If the site is .org, .com, or.net, find out if the organization, agency or the company is being sponsored by other reputable organizations.
    - Is the purpose of the site is to generate revenue in some way?
3. Check for tilde ~ in the URL:
    - A tilde ~ in the URL indicates that this information was published by an individual and may not reflect the originating domain
4. Determine who authored this information:
    - Is the author stated with his/her e-mail address?
    - What qualification does this author have for publishing this information?

Testing the Validity of the Contents

Is the content rich and valid for this research?

1. Determine if the content is fact or opinion:
    - Does the content cite other resources that were used when creating this information?
    - Does the content have limited advertising and does the domain clearly state the reasons for presenting this information?
    - Does this resource include the name of the institution or organization hosting or funding this information?
2. Check how current is the information:
    - Does it state when this resource was created?
    - Does it state when this resource was last updated?
    - Do all the links still work?
3. Consider how rich is the information:
    - How does the resource compare with other similar resources on the internet?

Websites and webmasters who have a clear motive should apply for HON code certification. If one wishes to make a comment on issue of credibility and reliability one can e-mail at Honcode@healthonnet.org. There are now over 2,800 websites which are certified by HON code. For more information, readers can visit the HON code website www.hon.ch. One can also look for urac seal of credibility (www.urac.org).

Coming to the second issue; medicolegal aspects involved with internet medical practice and medical education. Till date you do not require a license to "broadcast" on internet. This is a venue for limitless open communication and unlike radio, newsprint and television, remains largely unregulated.

Problems with Regulation of Internet

- It has no national and cultural boundaries.
- It is growing at a bewildering speed.
- No physical recording like newsprint or radio. It is highly volatile; here today gone tomorrow.
- Internet community itself has a record of stiff resistance to attempted government regulation.
- Legislative bodies seem unable, if not unwilling, to tame the global medium in a timely manner.
- International nature and freedom of speech/freedom of choice issues prevent imposition of restrictions.

Medicolegal Issues in Use of the Web

Medical websites which only provide health information are over 1,400 as per data of study for G-8 group of countries and they are being added at an annual rate of 21%. It is easy to regulate drugs and medical devices but none of this is directly applicable to the information on net. The net is a source of valuable information but at the same time life-threatening, incorrect, misleading, and outdated information is available in plenty.

Incorrect, fraudulent information regarding diagnosis and treatment, prospects of miracle cure may all harm the patient. Who is responsible?

- E-mails, issues of privacy, security and confidentiality in relation to medical information
- Telemedicine: Issues of licensing and jurisdiction.

A regulatory body by the American Federal Trade Commission is targeting false and unsubstantiated health claims on the net through "Operation Cure. All", a law enforcement and consumer education corporation. Their website (www.ftc/bcp.) helps consumers to recognize health fraud. It also provides guidance for business on how to ethically market health products. Medicolegal authority and financial resources are limited to deal effectively with the problem. To help consumers we have anti-quacking websites. The most popular is www.quackwatch.com It is operated by a retired psychiatrist Dr Stephen Barrett. Another one is US National council against health fraud (www.ncahf.org). A wider organization is anti-quackery webring (http://g.webring.com/hub). These sites fill the medicolegal void against websites.

There are sites in USA which provide the patient, physician profile information including malpractice claim data (www.doc/info.org, www.vahealthprovider.com). Questionable doctor site (www.questionabledoctors.org) contains data on disciplinary action taken for medical incompetence, misprescribing drugs, sexual misconduct, criminal conviction, ethical lapses and other offences.

The medical groups are helpful for support but the flip side is that the information is anecdotal and distributed by people who are not fully knowledgeable. Problem of miracle cure for chronic diseases is a matter of concern. No medicolegal help is available. The only resource is education concerning the negative consequence of taking unproven treatment.

Use of e-mail in health care raises issues related to privacy, security and confidentiality in relation to medical information. The American medical informatics organization (www.amia.org) has published guidelines for e-mail communication and for administrative and medicolegal aspects of e-mail.

What happens if the information is incorrect? If e-mail is intercepted containing confidential parent information. What are the liability issues? Legal liability issues also figure prominently in any discussion of inaccurate and potentially harmful medical information. Jurisdiction becomes irrelevant given the international nature of the world wide web.

Questions arise as to who is responsible if unverified and ultimately harmful information is distributed by a discussion group. Is the person volunteering that information liable? Or is it always expressed in caveat emptor? What onus is there on individuals who use this content? What responsibility do website and usenet administrator bear? In case of international communication in whose legal jurisdiction would liability proceedings take place? Should liability claims apply only to peer reviewed or organization certified sites?

There are number of websites which collect patient data for purpose of research, pre/post marketing survey, or for their database. This information is confidential and any divulgence without consent of the patient is illegal and comes under Law of Torts. It also comes under purview of Health Information Portability and Accountability Act (HIPAA) in USA. It is one of the most powerful and robust protection for medical information.

To control information on net or have legislation is not only extremely difficult but also exorbitant in terms of cost and labor. Therefore, a voluntary control and accreditation is recommended to ensure quality of data on the website. The following strategy may help:

- Self regulation by the website owner; use of kite mark or use mark grading
- Use of downstream or upstream filters depending on the qualification and profession of the users
- Accreditation seal from various voluntary organizations, for example:
  - Health on the Net Foundation (honcode), *www.hon.ch*
  - Internet Health Coalition, *www.healthcoalition.com*
  - American Medical Association, *www.ama.assn.org*
  - Health Internet Ethics, *www.hiethics.com*
- Sites which are not accredidated may be ignored by search engines and browsers.

A health site is liable for litigation under consumer protection act and civil court:

- If it charges a fee for its service and the information causes health injury to the person
- Breaks its own code of privacy
- Provides e-consultation and dispensing
- Advertisements which are illegal under the law of the state, e.g. advertisement of breast milk substitute is illegal under the "Infant Milk Substitute, Feeding Bottle and Infant Food Regulation Act, 2003 in India".

The wonder world of websites is here to stay. We only need to ensure the quality and genuineness of the data. It will be of immense use for the medical profession and the consumer alike.

"Internet is the spring of knowledge". Let us drink deep of touch note the spring for its shallow draughts and after and drinking largely sobers us again.

Some credible health sites, which may be recommended to parents:

- **4 R Kids Sake:** *http://www.1 to 9 months.com.* A nonprofit organization whose mission is to protect our children from preventable injuries and death, through awareness, education, legislation and prevention.
- **American Association of Pediatrics:** *http://www.aap.org/advocacy/mediamatters.htm.* National public education campaign of the American Academy of Pediatrics. To help

pediatricians, parents and children become more aware of the influence that media have on child and adolescent health.

- **Facts of Life:** *http://www.unicef.org/ffl.* UNICEF presents practical, effective and low cost ways to protect children's life and health. Includes child development and early learning, nutrition and growth, immunization, hygiene, and injury prevention.
- **FDA Kids:** *http://www.fda.gov/oc/opacom/kids/default.htm.* Food and Drug Administration provides medicine cabinet information, vaccination facts and other health concerns about children.
- **Focus on Kids' Health:** *http://www.medicinenet.com/healthy_kids/focus.htm.* Complete listing of all health information about kids and teens, including acne, AIDS awareness, allergies and asthma, attention deficit disorders and dyslexia.
- **Healthy Child Online:** *http://www.healthychild.com.* Children's health information and parenting resources in a searchable library of articles and links covering vaccinations, ear infections, childhood illnesses, ADHD and various other child health conditions, diseases and concerns.
- **India Parenting Guide to Childrens' Health:** *http://www.indiaparenting.com/babyhealth.* Part of parenting portal with information on childhood illnesses, diseases, medical conditions like measles. Also first aid for fever, colds, cuts, burns.
- **Kids' Health Info for Parents:**
  - *www.kidshealth.org*
  - *www.teenshealth.org.* Both these sites provide information on child health, parenting, etc.
  - *www.generalpediatrics.com.* Provides information on common child and teen illnesses in alphabetical order A to Z.
  - *www.cdc.gov.vaccines.* Facts sheets on common conditions are available for browsing or downloading. Prepared and updated by the Royal Children's Hospital, Melbourne, Victoria, and Australia.
- **Poison Prevention Tips:** *www.cincinnatichildrens.org.* The Cincinnati Drug and Poison Information Center offers safety tips to prevent poisoning in children and pets.
- **Immunization Websites:**
  - *www.immunize.org* website of vaccine alliance organization. (Provides vaccine information in many languages including Hindi)
  - *https://acvip.org.* The immunization website of Indian Academy of Pediatrics. It gives latest information on vaccination schedule and different vaccines
  - *www.who.int/topics/vaccines/en* (website of WHO)
  - *www.rch.org.au* (website of Royal college of pediatrics Australia)
- **Medicolegal Websites for Doctors:**
  - *www.medicolegalupdate.org*
  - *www.legalserviceindia.com*
  - *www.aclm.org*
  - *www.racgp.org.au*
  - *www.issuesinmedicalethics.org*
  - *www.mlcd.in*

53

CHAPTER

Professional Indemnity

Ruchita Shukla, Satish Tiwari

INTRODUCTION

The beginning of the third millennium has brought us at the doorstep of information and technology era. Things are different today. The market economy had swallowed us. The age-old doctor–patient relationship is no exception to these negative changes in the society. The enactment of Consumer Protection Act in 1986 and subsequently in 2019 and its application to medical practitioners has added fuel to the fire. The process of liberalization and globalization has resulted in mushrooming of many insurance and risk management companies with different products and schemes.

DEFINITIONS

Indemnity means "to make good the loss sustained by the insurer." The doctor's indemnity policy provides insurance protection to the doctors against their legal liability to pay damages arising out of their negligence in the performance of professional duties. The insured includes the policyholder and his qualified assistants or employees named in the proposal.

The "*retroactive date*" means the first incepted date of policy, which is renewed without any break. The "*policy period*" means the hours shown in the schedule and terminating at midnight on the expiry date.

TYPES

The different types of professional indemnity or hospital insurance policies are:

- *Doctor's indemnity policy*: For individual doctors as per their field of practice
- *Doctor's composite package policy*: These policies also cover loss or damage to the property as the case may be.
- *Doctor's protection shield*: Includes protection from various hazards to which doctors are exposed, such as buildings, computers, other appliances, and electronic equipment.
- *Doctors' and medical establishment policy*: These policies include nursing homes, hospitals, or medical establishments.

According to the rate per mille or limit ratio, it can be:
- *Any one year limit (AOY)*: For the act of negligence committed in that year (single act arising out of all acts)
- *Any one act limit (AOA)*: In the ratio of 1:1, 1:2, 1:4, etc., where the compensation limit will be divided into the number of acts of negligence committed in that year as per the option given at the time of selecting the policy.

CRITERIA/REQUIREMENTS

- The individual must be a registered medical practitioner.
- The act should occur during the period of insurance (commencing from retroactive date), resulting in a claim made in writing against the insured.
- The medical establishments shall be registered with competent authority as per the local regulations or should have minimum facilities as per the requirements of insurers.
- There should not be any misrepresentation, wrong description, or nondisclosure of any material information.

PREMIUM RATE

The premium rate depends on the specialization (physician, surgeon, super specialists, etc.) and the nature of services provided by the insured and the number of qualified assistants, nurses, nature of equipment, etc. If the doctors wish to cover unqualified staff working with them, an additional premium is required. It also depends on the limit ratio opted, i.e., AOA to AOY and the type of policy opted. It also depends on different aspects to be covered as per the protection shield.

LEGAL ASSISTANCE AND BENEFIT SCHEME

These schemes are launched by various academic organizations for *assisting their members* by:
- Providing *medicolegal guidance* in hours of crisis—a subject experts committee is formed which guides members in hours of crisis.
- *Expert opinion* is provided if there is case in court.
- A *crisis management committee* support may be made available at the city/district/state levels. (It can be city/district/state branch of that association).
- *Financial assistance* as per the terms of agreement.

SCOPE

It applies to claims arising out of bodily injury, illness, and/or death of any patient caused by or alleged to have caused by an error, an act of omission, or an act of commission during the professional service/duty. The other policies cover loss or damages to property, building, equipment, etc. One must inform the insurance company when you shift your nursing home or consulting room. Disclose your attachments with other hospitals or nursing homes otherwise company may refuse to take liability arising in those places.

EXCEPTIONS/EXCLUSIONS

- Any act committed in violation of any law/ordinance
- Services rendered while under the influence of any intoxicants or narcotics
- The third party public liability, such as accidents/injury in hospitals
- Claims arising out of "cosmesis," such as plastic surgery, cosmetic surgery, hair transplants, etc.
- Claims arising from any conditions related/associated with human immunodeficiency virus/acquired immunodeficiency syndrome (HIV/AIDS)
- It does not cover liability arising out of deliberate, willful, or intentional noncompliance of any statutory provisions.
- It does not cover liabilities arising out of personal injuries, such as libel, slander, or any other form of defamation.
- Company may not be liable if the doctor practices in specialty other than the mentioned in the application form.
- The policies do not cover the liabilities caused by radiations or radioactive substances.
- Experimental treatments are excluded.

ADVANTAGES

- With the prior permission of insurance company, the legal expenses incurred by the insured for defending the case are also payable.
- The insurer is bound to pay as per the coverage if those parties were liable to pay at the end. The nonjoining of insurance company could not vitiate the trial; this was held in *S Panchori versus Dr K Pandey I (1999) CPJ 332.*
- The Company will always have the right to take over the conduct of the defense of any proceedings filed against the insured before the medical councils or any other criminal proceedings against the doctor connected with his professional capacity.

LIMITATIONS

- No liability for any claim prior to the retroactive date specified in the policy
- The insurers may arrive at *compromised settlement* without the legal establishment of negligence in a court of law, as it is cheaper, simpler, and of least resistance to them rather than fighting out the case.
- It has been observed that if the patient or their advocate knew that the doctors are insured, there are more chances of negligence suits.
- The employees shall take all reasonable precautions to prevent all accidents and shall comply with all statutory or other regulations.
- After the amendment of Consumer Protection Act in 2019, the limits of compensation at District, State, and National levels have been enormously increased. The companies may be hesitant in indemnifying such a big amount or give only part payments, especially if there are suits pending against the doctors.
- The Company is not liable for the promise or payment made or given by the doctor for compromise without taking the insurance company in confidence.

OUT-OF-COURT SETTLEMENT

The litigations in the courts can continue for years or decades. Hence, some of the companies or the practitioners are of the opinion that "out-of-court settlement" is a better option than prolonged judicial procedures. Sometimes, if there is obvious negligence, then many companies may opt for such proposal so as to avoid prolonged litigation with unfavorable outcome and exorbitant compensations. Some of our colleagues also feel that such settlement is better than long-drawn battle in the court rooms. Hence, such proposal can be accepted after following various procedures for out-of-court settlements as per the legal provisions in presence of various stakeholders and appropriate authorities.

NO-FAULT INSURANCE

Many medicolegal consultants are now suggesting that there should be provisions for "no-fault insurance." The details of these are discussed in Chapter 54.

WHICH SCHEME ONE SHOULD OPT?

Many of us believe that we should go for indemnity from government companies. Still many prefer private companies or risk management–service contract companies. There are distinct advantages of adopting the schemes from academic associations. It is better if we take the decision based on our previous experiences, experiences of our colleagues, and the reliability of services by various companies.

PROCEDURE

In the event of any notice from advocates or courts received by the insured doctor regarding compensation, it should be immediately forwarded to the policy issuing office with details and should cooperate with insurance company for defending the case on behalf of the insured.

Doctors are very soft target for any financial institution. The role of insurance companies may not be controversial or questionable, but one must be alert and involve them whenever there is a medicolegal difficulty. The professional indemnity may not protect from legal problems, but it may turn out to be a protector for financial losses. Thus, it gives mental peace over and above financial relief. While signing a contract for professional indemnity, hospital insurance, or risk management, one must read in between the lines. It is necessary that the system should be doctor- and patient-friendly and not insurance company-friendly. The *Supreme Court of India, in Civil Appeal No. 6224 of 2013* (decided in April, 2023), Nagarmal Modi Sewa Sadan versus Prem Prakash Rajagaria has observed, clarified, and directed that it is the insurance company which would have to reimburse the compensation to the extent of the liability under the policy as against the said respondents.

The insurance or risk management companies are coming with newer and newer policies for attracting the beneficiaries. It is desirable for a doctor or hospital to have adequate insurance in present era. The doctor's indemnity policy provides insurance protection to the doctors against their legal liability to pay damages arising out of their negligence in the performance of professional duties. In *M/s Sheth M L Vaduwala Eye Hospital versus Oriental Insurance Company Limited CA 7611-34/2021* (decided in December, 2021), the honorable Supreme Court has held that hospital cannot claim protection under insurance obtained by the doctors against claims of medical negligence. In this case, a cataract eye camp was conducted without following the aseptic precautions. The individual doctors had indemnity, but hospital did not. The Oriental Insurance Company Limited refused to pay the compensation as the indemnity policies were obtained by individual doctors and not by the hospital.

CONCLUSION

In this era of consumerism, the cases of medical negligence are increasing by leaps and bounds. Many of us believe that health is not a commodity which can be purchased with money and hence, patient is not a consumer. But the judiciary, people, and policymakers think differently. The patients or relatives are approaching the courts even for minor faults and alleged deficiency in service. In such situations, professional indemnity provides financial security if court sanctions compensation against the hospitals or doctors. If we have insurance for our vehicles, buildings, instruments, etc., we should not hesitate for adequate amount of indemnity including indemnity for unqualified staff from a reliable company.

KEY LEARNING POINTS

- Medical services are included under the Consumer Protection Act 2019.
- There is no capping on the extent of compensation that can be sanctioned against hospitals or doctors.
- Unfortunately, the compensation amounts are increasing day by day.
- The best way to protect the financial liability is professional indemnity.
- We should have adequate indemnity as per the type of services, place of practice, specialization, and jurisdiction of courts.

BIBLIOGRAPHY

1. Joshi MK. A-Z of Medical Law 2000, 1st edition. Ahmedabad; 2000. pp. 289-92.
2. Shah RM (Ed). General Insurance Ready Reckoner, 23rd edition. Baroda: New India Assurance Co Ltd; 2005. pp. 149-61.
3. Tiwari S, Baldwa M. What is medical negligence. In: Baldwa M, Tiwari S, Tiwari M, et al. (Eds). Legal Problems in Day-to-Day Pediatrics Practice, 2nd edition. Hyderabad: Paras Publishing; 2010. pp. 14-39.
4. Tiwari SK, Baldwa M. Medical negligence. In: Gupte S (Ed). Recent Advances in Pediatrics (volume 14). New Delhi: Jaypee Brothers Medical Publishers (P) Ltd.; 2004. pp. 311-29.
5. Tiwari SK. Be safe from the clutches of Law. J Indian Med Legal Ethics Assoc. 2022;10(3):70-2.

54

CHAPTER

No-fault Insurance

Mahesh Baldwa, Amit Padvi, Namita Padvi

"No-fault" insurance pays immediately so it is patient friendly and so also doctor friendly! We cannot watch family lose everything after death of earning member. Hence, this insurance.

INTRODUCTION

The reach of masses to allopathic medical and surgical treatment is increasing with so many government schemes such as Ayushman Bharat, Rashtriya Swasthya Bima Yojana (RSBY), and below poverty line (BPL)-related health insurance schemes. Naturally, India with 1.3 billion population shall have more number of medical accidents and mishaps causing complications needing costly treatment. Rarely, some treatments may lead to fatalities and debilitating injuries to patients with comorbidities. India has already overburdened judiciary. This may become one more source of a litigation explosion to already strained judicial machinery.

How common is the situation in practice?

In healthcare system, deaths are common. Intensive care unit (ICU) in healthcare is extremely expensive. So, a death in ICU and healthcare becomes litigation prone. This leads to practice of defensive medicine. Doctors cannot give their 100% potential to patient being under fear of litigation. This is written with an aim to pave way to make a new statute, law, or legislate "no-fault" medical compensation law and indemnity insurance to cover for medical negligence, mishap, and accident under law of tort. This will pave way for healthcare practice of vigilant, vigorous practice of medicine to save lives of critically ill till last ditch effort. Patients will receive full potential of healthcare team.

What will be the immediate steps if the patient is brought to you?

No-fault insurance will restrain doctors from practicing defensive medicine. They will be able to give 100% of their potential to sick and serious. No doctor shall refuse any patient for fear of litigation. Patient shall receive all the treatment which scientifically and medically patient deserves. The goals of medicine, as laid down in the Hippocratic Oath, are founded on profound moral–ethical principles, which require healthcare providers to be committed to the mitigation of suffering, to uphold the primacy of life, and to recognize their corresponding obligations.

What are the legal provisions in that particular situation for patients/doctors?

The leading case on this matter is Parmanand Katara vs. Union of India and several other cases decided on this basis, the three judge bench of Supreme Court (SC) noted in writ filed by a public-spirited person in response to a news report of a scooterist who was knocked down by a car and died due to lack of medical treatment. Following the accident, the scooterist was taken to the nearest hospital but was turned away and sent to another hospital 20 km away, which was authorized to handle medicolegal cases. The scooterist died while he was being transported to the other hospital. Doctor is looked upon by common man as the only hope when a person is hanging between life and death, but they avoid their duty to help a person when he is facing death when they know that it is a medicolegal case. Though a physician is not bound to treat each and every one asking his services except in emergencies for the sake of humanity and the noble traditions of the profession, he should be ever ready to respond to the calls of the sick and the injured. Doctors cannot choose a patient who comes in emergency.

What will be the subsequent steps in management of such cases?

On such occasions, medical profession is approached and if he finds that whatever assistance he could give is not sufficient really to save the life of the person but some better assistance is necessary, it is also the duty of the man in the medical profession so approached to render all the help which he could and also see that the person reaches the proper expert as early as possible. "Preservation of/saving life" and "duty of care" are established as absolute, nonnegotiable, supreme constitutional obligations of the medical profession and the State. The doctors shall inform police and law enforcing authorities as required after giving first aid.

- Preservation of human life is of paramount importance.
- Every doctor, at a government hospital or otherwise, has the professional obligation to extend his/her services to protect life.
- There should be no doubt that the effort to save the person should receive top priority. This applies not only to the legal profession but also to the police and other citizens who are part of the matter.

What are the laws applicable in these situations?

The Indian Penal Code of 1860, The *Code* of *Criminal Procedure* of 1973, Indian Evidence Act of 1872, Law of Limitation of 1963, Consumer Protection Act of 2019, Civil Procedure Code of 1908, *Permanent Lok Adalat*, organized under Section 22B of The *Legal Services Authorities Act* of 1987, National Medical Commission Act of 2019, and similar laws comprise an unending maze of law. Punishment in India starts the moment a law is put in motion against doctor and it goes on and on. The judicial process itself is a punishment. At present, the SC has 193 working days annually, high courts have 210 days, and trial courts have 245 days a year. As per another expert's calculation, if no new actions are filed, 324 years would be needed to clear the dockets at current speed the courts are working. Law Minister Ravi Shankar Prasad in a written reply said 43.55 lakh cases are pending in the high court and out of these, 18.75 lakh relate to civil matters and 12.15 lakh are criminal cases. As on June 1, 2019, pending cases in the SC were 58,669. Roughly, three crore cases in all courts in India are pending.

What are the legal provisions in world?

In the world, most countries have same legal provisions as India with faster judicial clearance of cases. This is because India has 1.3 billion population with more than three crore cases still pending to be heard. Only two countries have "no-fault" systems. Sweden and New Zealand are maintaining "no-fault" systems. In New Zealand, there is no medical malpractice system but rather a publicly funded accident compensation scheme that bars suing for compensatory damages and separate medical professional accountability processes.

DIFFICULTY IN INTRODUCING REFORMS LIKE NO-FAULT

It must be considered that there is nothing more difficult to carry out, nor more doubtful of success, nor more dangerous to handle, than to initiate a new order of things. Any kind of reform has enemies in all those who profit by the old order system and only lukewarm defenders in all those who would profit by the new order.

No-fault Professional Indemnity

In its strictest form, the term no-fault provides for the payment for patients' party for economic losses by producing medical bills incurred to treat complications and lump sum immediate monetary compensation for disability, death arising out of professional medical treatment or surgery, and restrict the right to sue doctors. Because high-threshold no-fault systems restrict litigation, they tend to reduce costs and delays in paying claims.

By paving way for no-fault professional indemnity, one does not depend upon broad judicial interpretation of medical negligence substituted many a times as res ipsa loquitur for a complication or disability, death arising out of medical accident or mishap in treatment or surgery are done away so also lengthy, unending, seemingly speculative, frustrating court proceedings to all litigants. No-fault indemnity insurance eliminates the incentive to inflate claims.

ARE THERE INADEQUACIES OR PARADOXES IN EXISTING LAWS?

Main Shortcoming of Existing Law

The deficiencies in current tort law concerning medical negligence litigation have been examined, highlighting the need for its revision to benefit patients. This revision aims to foster transparency among medical professionals in reporting errors, mishaps, and accidents, enabling future corrective actions and learning from mistakes. Under the current system, trial under law of tort related to medical negligence is deterrent to reporting errors, mishaps, and accidents. It also promotes blame game and shame. The day litigation starts, doctors feel heat of punishment, which may or may not happen. Medical professionals laugh at colleagues who are caught in litigation but wish that this should not happen to them during their practice. Apart from financial and time-consuming repercussion of litigation, litigations are emotionally and psychologically exhausting. The judicial discretion keeps stifling the standard of care from case to case basis and its application and final outcome. It appears that one is speculating rather than litigating.

The Law of Tort is Failing

Despite favorable results predicted from application of a tort system to the commission of wrongful conduct, fissures have appeared in the tort system, prompting criticism of the system and arguments for various systemic changes and tort alternatives. "The law is failing. It is incomplete as a compensation device, terribly wasteful of legal and other resources, doubtful as a promoter of safety, the probable cause of significant socially and economically undesirable conduct, and generally unsuccessful as a mechanism for doing justice between injurers and victims." In spite of the growing list of its actual and perceived shortcomings, the current tort system has survived, only because no "sensible alternative" to the fault system has been presented and accepted.

STUDIES ON RESULTS OF DOCTOR–PATIENT LITIGATION

From India

One study from India revealed that it is easier to prove allegations of medical negligence against Surgery and Allied Specialty as compared to Medicine and Allied Specialty. Chances of proof of allegations of medical negligence against Diagnostic Specialty (Radiology, Pathology, Biochemistry, etc.) are highest at 50% cases, followed by Surgery and Allied Specialty with 34.48%, Dentistry with 25%, and the least chances of proof in Medicine and Allied Specialty with only 18.18%.

From the United States of America

When a case is dismissed, the road is typically long for both doctors and the patients suing. How long malpractice claims take to resolve or what proportion of them actually end in a payment to patients is studied. For this study, they looked at more than 10,000 malpractice claims against the United States' (US) doctors closed between 2002 and 2005. They found that of all claims, about 55% percent resulted in an actual lawsuit. Of those litigated claims, more than half were dismissed by the court. And out of the rest, most were resolved before a verdict; less than 5% ended up being decided by a trial verdict. When there was a verdict, it went in favor of the doctor 80% of the time.

For doctors, the outcomes of claims varied by specialty—e.g., internists were among the most likely to have cases against them dismissed in court. Pathologists and pediatricians were least likely—about 36% of cases against pathologists and a little over 40% against pediatricians were dismissed. Pathologists study laboratory test samples and are key in diagnosing diseases. If they seem to have missed something, there is going to be more scrutiny. The same may be true in cases against pediatricians because a child is involved.

Why are litigations tiring both for patients and doctors?

In a study on malpractice claims against the US doctors, it was found that these claims are often dismissed and when they go to trial, the verdict is usually in the doctor's favor. "Most claims go in favor of the physician and they take a long time to resolve." What is killing was the length of time the cases took to resolve even when they were dismissed. "It is hard on everyone—patient as well as doctors." On average, lawsuits dismissed against doctors in court took more than 20 months and some resolved out of the court before a verdict took over 28 months. Cases that went all the way to a trial verdict typically lasted a few years—39 months, on average, when it went in favor of the doctor and close to 44 months when the patient won.

Capping the compensation is not a solution if state has to pay for healthcare costs in the United States of America (USA).

President Bush had strongly advocated for the imposition of a $250,000 cap on noneconomic damages and an undisclosed cap on punitive damages for all cases of medical malpractice. He claims these measures would "curtail frivolous lawsuits, decrease insurance costs, and ultimately lead to lower healthcare costs and better care for patients." The President had directed much of his criticism at trial lawyers for their alleged pursuit of "frivolous" claims that drive up the federal government's healthcare costs by 28 billion dollars a year and clog up the courts to the detriment of more deserving litigants.

Litigations between doctor and patients based on law of tort as basis of medical negligence are:
- Long drawn out in time frame, even in consumer courts both for patients as well as doctors
- Costliest even in consumer courts both for patients as well as doctors
- It appears as if instead of litigation, they are in speculation.

Usual difficulties for patient party:
- Finding a qualified medical malpractice lawyer
- Convincing the judges that the doctor was negligent at admission stage of case
- Proving the doctor's negligence
- Complicated medical evidence
- Necessity of medical experts
- High cost of litigation

Usual difficulties for doctors:
- Disruption and distress of a trial to a doctor's practice and family life
- Paucity of time
- Monetarily and psychologically expensive
- Long-term stress due to psychic burden takes its toll in physical health
- Not able to understand shifting, stifling, wobbling, and variable legal algorithm and paradigm
- Real consent and medical records are impeached. Tacit consent has no place.
- The average litigation goes on from 3 to 5 years or more.
- Emotionally, it is consuming and exhausting.
- The allegations made are intensely personal and derogatory.
- Winning is better than losing because it just looks a pyrrhic victory even after win.
- All this may force them to settle out of court.

PROPOSAL OF "NO-FAULT" MEDICAL COMPENSATION LAW

It is always patients who suffer death, disability, and disfigurement due to alleged medical negligence. Though all death, disability, and disfigurement are not due to alleged medical negligence, most of the times, it is patients who suffer from preventable medical error may not indulge in litigation. Patient party suffers in silence. Hence, for all who receive medical treatment, whether they allege death, disability, or disfigurement due to medical treatment or not, should receive "no-fault" claim from insurance companies. This is a social benefit which they can choose, relinquishing tort remedy under alleged medical negligence law. This will also lead to proactive reporting and learning from committed error committed by doctors. "No-fault" medical compensation law should be promulgated to replace medical negligence under law of tort.

Identification of Medical Error and Accidents

In 2016, medical errors are found to be underrecognized cause of death. 10% of all the USA deaths are now due to medical error. Medical error is the third highest cause of death in the

USA. "To err is human" and so are medical errors. According to the Centers for Disease Control and Prevention (CDC), in 2013, 611,105 people died of heart disease, 584,881 died of cancer, and 149,205 died of chronic respiratory disease—the top three causes of death in the USA. The newly calculated figure for medical errors puts this cause of death behind cancer but ahead of the respiratory disease.

Insurance is a Win–Win Strategy for both Patients and Doctors

Universal insurance coverage of patient and doctors.

Insurance coverage for patient in form of Mediclaim, RSBY, Ayushman Bharat, and indemnity insurance for medical professional is becoming common in healthcare system in India. Ayushman Bharat is National Health Protection Scheme, which will cover over 10 crore poor and vulnerable families (~50 crore beneficiaries), providing coverage up to INR 5 lakh per family per year for secondary and tertiary care hospitalization. Ayushman Bharat—National Health Protection Mission will subsume the ongoing centrally sponsored schemes, RSBY and the Senior Citizen Health Insurance Scheme (SCHIS).

TORT-BASED MEDICAL NEGLIGENCE LITIGATIONS

Complex and Intricate Nature of Medical Science

Medical science has always been complex and is ill understood by common people. Hence, an illusory standard was created for medical profession. The illusory standard for conduct for physician was never defined. Initially, illusory standard was self-regulated in the form of medical ethics. Later, legal illusory standard was created. Legal standard was couched in negative words, meaning what physician ought not to do. Violation of legal standard was labeled as negligence. Legal standard kept on changing. The legal standard was tested on the basis of reasonability, responsibility, duty of care, proximity, and what not. The degree of standard also varied from situation to situation, physician to physician, geographical area, social values, economic conditions, and also from judge to judge.

What was always medical accident or mishap is mislabeled legally as negligence?
Tort law, a fundamental building block of every legal system, features prominently in mass culture and political debates, which was never codified, leaving room for judicial discretion. Law of tort is not simply a collection of legal rules and procedures set out by legal judicial pronouncements, based on set of cultural responses to avert risks, injury, assignment of responsibility, compensation, valuation, and obligation.

Medical Accidents versus Medical Negligence

There is a thin dividing line between medical accidents and medical negligence. In common parlance, "accident" means an event that occurs without one's sight or expectation and in the same way, law also adopts it. The word "accident" means occurring by mere chance. Accidents occur as unintentional, unexpected acts. Sometimes, further spontaneous downhill bad events continue to occur without any further acts or omissions, leading to additional damages.

Shift of Focus from Causation to Fault in Medical Negligence

Lately, in cases of negligence, court instead of focusing on causation, began to see occurrence of fault as most important factor for tortuous actions. With this shift in focus, it became less necessary to restrict actions to categories, where fault has set to have occurred because of falling short of prevailing professional standard.

Prevailing Standard of "Duty of Care"—a Nebulous Concept

The law of negligence requires professional people to conduct themselves in a manner that conforms to certain prevailing standards of conduct, which is also known as duty of care in conduct.

Before 1932, there was no such thing as a "tort of negligence." In 1932, Donoghue vs. Stevenson, Lord Buckmaster dissented saying, where will negligence end? Where does liability end? Expanding ambit of negligence like this could result in unlimited liability that would impede the progression.

"Use of Ordinary Care" with Respect to Medical Profession

Lack of precise legal definition "use of ordinary care" is fraught with subjective terminology as reasonability, rationality, and responsibility. The standards of care are nebulous, keep changing, and drifting with scientific technological advances with respect to time, place, and person.

Legal Uncertainty in Describing Precisely What "Negligence" is

The uncertainty in definition of negligence existed since its emergence. The development of law of negligence in the last 150 years provides a good illustration of adventurous nature of judicial discretion and adventurism. Therefore, interpretation of phrase "use of ordinary care" is left to judicial discretion which keeps changing. Medical practitioners who were duly qualified and licensed to practice by medical council also had to take test of "use of ordinary care" as per the interpretation of judiciary. Never medical profession was allowed to set a standard for themselves. Medical ethics have as such no legal force and are applied selectively when required.

Earlier, medical negligence judgments were related to conduct of medical care. Now, it got extended to medical opinions, medical interpretation of clinical judgment, and interpretation of blood and imaging reports. Not only that, it also extended Bolam rule to medical opinion, advice, and judgment also. All these years, Indian judiciary adhered to Bolam rule, encompassing defect and deficiency in conduct of medical care only with respect to treatment. Suddenly, it extended the rule to medical opinions and interpretation, complication, unexpected abnormal anatomy, and physiology of patient, causing mishaps and accidents. The "eggshell rule" blasted. The domain of consent meant what is written on consent form is real consent, leaving tacit consent gasping. Samira Kohli's judgment underlines "real consent." Anything beyond even for benefit of patient if not life-saving is not allowed. The matter related to diligent conduct of medical care is extending and widening scope. Scope is so wide that judiciary is expecting what cannot be contemplated by ordinary intelligence, interpretation, and judgment of practitioner in treating the patient. The judicial interpretation finds faults in conduct with respect to delay in diagnosis, delay in investigating, misinterpreting reports, misdiagnosis, and wrong diagnosis, which as a matter of fact is largely based on opinion of an average practitioner. The death, disability, and expenditure incurred by patient party creates a bias in favor of patient party, forcing judiciary judge the case much above the standards of average practitioner. Medical documents and records, if kept, were on several occasions considered tampered, manipulated, inadequate, meaningless. It also opened floodgates for what precautions were not taken from hindsight knowledge. Issue of hindsight knowledge is not easy. If not kept, they meant no defense. Medical records related to retinopathy of prematurity (ROP) show judicial discretion in V Krishnakumar vs. State of Tamil Nadu, saying "hastily written general warning." Court said, "We are not prepared to infer from 'Informed about alarms signs' that the parents were cautioned about ROP in this case." "A rule of happening of complication less than 10% with respect to what?" is applied. Court also said, "We are thus satisfied that we are not looking at the 1996 accident with 2007 spectacles."

It may not be hindsight knowledge in western countries and All India Institute of Medical Sciences (AIIMS) in Delhi, but its percolation and translation to practical knowledge and application as routine practice for average practitioner in rest of India is. During the litigation, the stands taken by doctors undergo legal posturing to meet legal requirement as per advice of lawyers. This legal advice of stifling, posturing by doctors to explain medical records create further weakness and medical records become foes.

So what is the point in contesting alleged medical negligence and speculating a win?

The "eggshell skull" rule: The term "eggshell skull" rule originated in the Dulieu vs. White & Sons (1901) judgment, in which the following pithy statement can be found, "If a man is negligently run over or otherwise negligently injured in his body, it is no answer to the sufferer's claim for damages that he would have suffered less injury, or no injury at all, if he had not had an unusually thin skull or an unusually weak heart." In Smith vs. Leech Brain & Co (1962), a widow claimed against her dead husband's employer (defendant) that their negligence led to a burn on her dead husband's lip, "leading to stem-cell transformation to carcinoma." The court ruled that it was unnecessary either to show that death by cancer was foreseeable or that an ordinary person would not have died from the injury. It was determined using the "eggshell rule" that the defendant was liable because the defendant must take the patient, victim, or plaintiff as the defendant finds him/her. The "eggshell rule" has important medicolegal ramifications, as clinicians cannot use a particular patient's specific predispositions to pathology and disease as legal excuses to diminish culpability.

■ Standard of Care and Uncertainty of Opinion

If the defendant is found to have a duty of care, what is the reasonable standard of care and was it breached is decided by judiciary. Usually, what is the standard is matter of law, but interpretation is left to judiciary. But was the standard breached? is a matter of fact, which again is left to discretion of judiciary.

■ Medical Accidents were Dubbed as Alleged Negligence

Medical accidents and mishaps are tried as alleged negligence all these years. What were accidents ab initio are for all these years labeled as acts of negligence. Medicine is a highly regulated profession. At every stage, there is competitive examination. After passing final examination, one has to obtain license to practice. All practitioners have to conduct themselves within four corners of medical ethics. With so much of tight regulation, the chances for medical professionals not to conduct as per standards sounds impossible. So now, whatever mishap causes death, disability, or huge expenses in an attempt to save life is alleged and dubbed as negligence.

Why I say medical mishaps cause death, disability, or huge expenses in an attempt to save life are nothing but accidents for following reasons:

"NO-FAULT" MEDICAL ACCIDENT CLAIMS TRIBUNAL: BANE OR BOON?

Doctors should stay warned of the challenges facing the healthcare profession in keeping pace with the information age. Medicine has always been quick to adopt and adapt new technologies and many advances in care have been due to utilizing advances made in other branches of science. Traditional boundaries between private and professional life are becoming blurred and the potential for members to inadvertently fall into medicolegal traps is increasing. Delivering high-quality communications with patients when something has gone wrong which is accidental be communicated in skillful manner to patient party. The objective of effective open communication when an error or accident happens if not reported and kept wrapped under the carpet is meaningless. There is a risk in such kind of legislation by creating a "tick-box" mentality, which does not support the intensely sensitive, personalized, and patient-centered conversations. You can have the best individuals with the best intentions, but in the wrong environment, they can succumb to what is the norm of wrapping under carpet—the truth about medical accident. Because there is no legislation which will compensate medical accidents; hence, it is dubbed as medical negligence to get the compensation.

Establishing a medical accident claims tribunal would not only enable patients to report serious injuries or deaths resulting from medical accidents, errors, mishaps, and complications but also facilitate learning from near misses transparently. This approach would enhance patient safety without attributing blame, fostering a win-win situation for doctors, hospitals, and patients. Medical accident claims would promptly compensate victims of all medical accidents. Compulsory insurance for doctors and hospitals, akin to the Motor Vehicle Act and Workmen Compensation Act, would also be mandated.

No-fault New Zealand in 1992: The 1992 reforms—compensable medical injury was defined as "medical misadventure," which was either "medical mishap" (a rare and severe adverse event) or "medical error" (in effect negligence). The 1992 reforms (unfairly) restricted access to compensation for those suffering medical injury as opposed to general injury. The restrictive definition also increased the possibility of litigation from those not covered under the scheme. Thus, in 1992, reforms introduced fault (medical error) into the otherwise no-fault scheme but obliged to report all findings of medical error to the Medical Council; the compensation claims process could result in discipline for doctors. This made some doctors (and patients) unwilling to participate in the compensation claims process. It also led some doctors to contest findings of medical error, further restricting and/or delaying access to compensation for injured patients.

No-fault New Zealand in 2005: Prior to 2005, patients could obtain compensation for medical injury under the scheme by proving "medical error." Medical error in effect amounted to negligence and as all findings of error were reported to the Medical Council, it could result in punishment for doctors. Fear of being labeled negligent and punished made some doctors reluctant to participate in the compensation claims process and also possibly drove to defensive practice and overdiagnosis.

Swedish no-fault system of 1975—Patient Compensation Insurance (PCI): The PCI was established in 1975 by voluntary contract between the county councils and a consortium of insurers in order to preempt the threat of statutory expansion of tort liability, possibly to a form of strict liability. Private practitioners entered into similar contracts and a voluntary contractual Pharmaceutical Insurance (PI) was established in 1978. The motivating political concern was lack of patient access to tort compensation—only about 10 patients per year received compensation for medical malpractice.

■ Why Medical No-fault Insurance?

New Zealand is small in population and state can compensate victims, but India has about one sixth of world population. Hence, medical no-fault insurance is more suited to India. This is to provide money to cover to victims of medical mishaps as back up concept of legislating "no-fault" medical accident tribunal. Legal rule is that every individual undergoing treatment is responsible for own injuries suffered in while taking medical treatment and same be termed as an accident, regardless of who is at fault. Its objective is to reduce the number of medical negligence litigation-related damage claims and universal coverage of medical professionals with indemnity insurance coverage. This will also weed out unqualified medical practitioners who because of their inability to take professional indemnity insurance will be exposed. No medical professional in country should be allowed to practice without professional indemnity insurance.

NO-FAULT

A kind of medical indemnity insurance that provides that each driver must collect the allowable amount of money from his or her own insurance carrier subsequent to a medical accident, mishap, or negligence regardless of who was at fault.

What is medical no-fault insurance?

In its broadest sense, no-fault insurance is any type of insurance contract under which insured are indemnified for losses by their own insurance company, regardless of fault in the incident, medical negligence, mishap, or accident generating losses. A policyholder (and his/her patients) are not only reimbursed by the policyholder's own insurance company without proof of fault but also restricted in the right to seek recovery through the civil justice system for losses.

What does no-fault mean?

A no-fault medical indemnity insurance system, such as patient compensation, works by paying claims regardless of who is to blame for an alleged medical negligence, mishap, or accident. This means that the insurance company pays patient compensation benefits no matter who is found to be at fault for the alleged medical negligence, mishap, or accident that resulted in the patient injuries during treatment. This provides an important layer of protection for patient who does not need to go through the additional burden of proving their case before receiving benefits from court of law or tribunal.

Description of No-fault Systems

No-fault systems generally exempt individuals from the usual liability for causing body injury. The insurance covers bodily injury of the patient party caused by medical negligence, mishap, or accident regardless of who is liable under ordinary common law tort and rules. No-fault insurance has the goal of lowering premium costs by avoiding expensive litigation over the causes of medical negligence, mishap, or accident while providing quick payments for injuries or loss to patients. Further, no-fault systems often grant "set" or "fixed" compensation for certain injuries regardless of the unique aspects of the injury or the individual injured.

Fault versus No-fault

This operates on a no-fault system, which means that it does not matter who is to blame for an alleged medical negligence, mishap, or accident. Either way, the injured patient is paid out to insurance cover with respect to medical expenses, expenses for extended treatment, disability, disfigurement, death, and also lost wages.

Fault-based claims find out who is to blame, which is crucial for receiving compensation. Patient parties involved in an alleged medical negligence, mishap, or accident must prove the fault of an opposing party (medical practitioner and team) before any compensation payments will be made. The benefit of no-fault systems is that claims can be processed much quicker given that there is no burden of proof or lengthy dispute over who bares blame. This helps victims receive money sooner and with much less hassle.

"No-fault" medical accident tribunal shall draw and be similar in provisions of "no-fault" law existing even today.

Existing "No-fault" Laws

Motor vehicle accident claims tribunals: They work on similar principles, rules, and regulations. Motor vehicle accident claims tribunals are operative on the basis of "no-fault" systems with usually a fixed schedule for compensation for various injuries.

Railway accident claims tribunal: It is operative on the basis of "no-fault" systems with usually a fixed schedule for compensation for various injuries.

Workers' compensation tribunals: Workers' compensation is a system of compensation which allows employees who are injured at work to obtain payment for lost wages, medical costs, and occupational rehabilitation expenses without regard to their personal negligence or fault.

Divorce law: The term no-fault is also used colloquially in reference to a type of divorce in which a marriage can be dissolved on the basis of irretrievable breakdown or irreconcilable differences, without a requirement that either party proves that the spouse was guilty of any misconduct causing the end of the marriage.

Proponents of No-fault Insurance

Proponents of no-fault insurance argue that medical negligence, mishap, or accident are inevitable and that at-fault medical practitioners are not necessarily at higher risk and should not necessarily be punished; moreover, they note that the presence of liability insurance insulates reckless or negligent medical professionals from financial disincentives of litigation and also protect injured patients. This will promote universal insurance among medical professionals. As such medical mishap and accidents dubbed as medical negligence are getting higher and higher in number; hence, no-fault systems may make more sense.

Replacing Tort of Medical Negligence with No-fault Legislations

The number of medical accidents, mishaps, and alleged negligence causing fatalities and debilitating injuries have become the source of a litigation explosion that was straining and in some areas like consumer courts, it is overwhelmingly the judicial machinery. Much legal thinking in academia is required to be devoted to the question of whether the tort system should be replaced with another method of allocating risks of loss from medical accidents, mishaps, and alleged negligence.

Traditional Tort Liability versus No-fault Liability

A "traditional tort" liability system for medical negligence for recovery is governed by principles of provable negligence.

It is obvious that costs for no-fault systems will be higher, which in turn shall escalate premium for indemnity insurance for particular specialty of medical professionals.

In the case of economic (medical and wage loss) damages, most no-fault systems permit injured parties to seek recovery only for damages that are not covered by available Mediclaim insurance benefits. In the case of noneconomic (pain and suffering) damages, most no-fault systems permit injured patients to seek compensation only in cases of exceptionally "serious" injury.

Extent of Coverage Under No-fault Systems

Medical no-fault systems focus solely on issues of compensation for bodily injury to patient arising out of medical treatment but could be extended to if medical professional additional premiums for alleged medical mishap, accident, or negligence that damages patient then patient may recover compensation for medical treatment along with excess medical expenses for treating medical complications if any.

The amount of damages to be paid by the insurance company is limited to actual medical and rehabilitation expenses, lost wages, and necessary expenses with a low maximum and for a limited period. In addition, an injured person can sue the negligent medical professional for medical costs above the amount of the insurance, pain, and suffering if the injuries required medical treatment or resulted in permanent injury, broken bones or disfigurement, or wrongful death.

Economics of Fault versus No-fault System

Just as the test of fault against standards of reasonable care was becoming confused with standards of near perfection, so did the final result depend too often upon the fortuitous assessment of the evidence or the fortuitous skill of lawyer. All seemed not only expensive but wasteful to the point of extravagance, as was demonstrated so clearly by the high proportion of funds which never reached the injured persons in respect of whom they had been collected. And there was the affliction of protracted delays in judicial system. More victims are paid, they do not have to prove fault from which massive savings result, and overall, everyone is better off. It is true that claims that every individual victim will be financially better off cannot be convincingly made. However, judged in the broad spectrum, the reforms provide a better set of arrangements than tort.

"No-fault" medical accident claims tribunal needs to be backed up by universal indemnity insurance.

All registered medical practitioners are insured with indemnity insurance. The benefits of no-fault include rapid payment of all medical expenses in most cases, elimination of lawsuits except in cases involving lesser injuries, very serious injury or death, and elimination of extensive and costly investigation, proof of negligence, and medical reports and depositions. Insurance companies and some court reform advocates who believe "no-fault" alleviates a clogging of the courts favor it.

How Does No-fault Work in the Patient Compensation Context?

Patient compensation benefits can still be claimed, regardless of whether the accident was caused by faulty equipment, following of incorrect instructions by a subordinate medical staff, the negligence of a third-party, or the carelessness of the employee under medical professionals himself.

Insurance companies' need for indemnity allows us to provide "no-fault" which is the most flexible and adaptive support provided to doctor members, especially during times of rapid change happening in medicolegal spheres where all complications, errors, and mishaps are being bundled as negligence, deficiency of service, or unfair trade practice which neither helps doctors nor patients who keep litigating in courts to prove complications, errors, and mishaps dubbed as negligence, deficiency of service, or unfair trade practice.

We hope all the stakeholders shall pave way for legislative "medical accident claims tribunal" for better "patient–doctor relationship" and "stress-free," "nondefensive" medical practice.

Compulsory No-fault Insurance

In fact, the registration for medical practice is given when doctor opts for "no-fault" insurance policy.

Future is no-fault compensation system if humanity wants to get rid of defensive medicine. A no-fault compensation system would address many of the injustices of our current malpractice system. It could offer an antidote to the poisonous specter of lawsuits that haunts hospital wards and harms the doctor–patient relationship. If done effectively, it could offer a path forward that is more dignified for the patients who suffer from medical errors and more navigable for the doctors who mean well.

CONCLUSION AND SUGGESTIONS

The limitations of the current tort law concerning medical negligence litigation have been examined, highlighting the need for its revision in favor of patients. This revision aims to encourage medical professionals to adopt transparency in reporting errors, mishaps, and accidents, facilitating future corrective measures and learning opportunities from mistakes. Current litigations related to medical negligence have financial and time-consuming repercussions; they are emotionally and psychologically exhausting.

Establishing a medical accident claims tribunal would not only enable patients affected by serious injuries or deaths due to medical accidents, errors, mishaps, and complications to report their cases, but also create opportunities to learn from near misses openly and transparently. This approach aims to enhance patient safety by fostering a culture where errors are acknowledged without obfuscation, benefiting both doctors and hospitals. Such measures would facilitate a balanced approach that compensates victims promptly for all medical accidents. Additionally, mandating compulsory insurance for all doctors and hospitals, akin to the Motor Vehicle Act and Workmen Compensation Act, would be essential steps in ensuring comprehensive coverage and protection.

Implementation of a comprehensive New Zealand-style no-fault system of compensation is far from becoming a reality in India and other countries. However, small expressions of interest may proliferate in the stasis of the current tort system in which doctors are increasingly choosing to change professions in the midst of their careers rather than face the uncertainty of potential painful lawsuits and the decreasing profitability of their profession based on skyrocketing overhead costs, which in India with Ayushman Bharat shall be borne by government only. Medicine as a profession shall not be opted by young and intelligent. The trend is bad for future of medicine.

KEY LEARNING POINTS

- No-fault does not play blame game, shame punish game.
- The victim who suffers damage or death is immediately paid compensation.
- Doctors are shown the root of the failure whether it is lack of knowledge, lack of skills, lack of experience, or lack of infrastructure and accordingly takes corrective measures; thus, doctors learn from it to fortify knowledge, skill, and experience and for improvement of infrastructure.
- Compensation is done by insurance company.
- Tort jurisdiction is excluded if opted for no-fault.

BIBLIOGRAPHY

1. Aironline. AIR 1989 Supreme Court 2039 ::(1990) 1 ACC 3.
2. Aironline. AIR 2015 Supreme Court 2836 ::2015 AIR SCW 4283. June, 2024.
3. Bal BS. An introduction to medical malpractice in the United States. Clin Orthop Relat Res. 2009;467(2):339-47.
4. Baldwa M, Baldwa V, Padvi N, et al. (Eds). Legislating "No-fault" Medical Compensation Law to Replace Medical Negligence Under Law of Tort. Legal Issues in Medical Practice. Delhi, India: CBS Publishers & Distributors Pvt Ltd; 2019. p. 715.
5. Bismark M, Paterson R. No-Fault Compensation in New Zealand: Harmonizing Injury Compensation, Provider Accountability, and Patient Safety. Health Aff (Millwood). 2006;25(1):278-83.
6. Bogdan J. (2011). Medical Malpractice in Sweden and New Zealand: Should Their Systems be Replicated Here? Available from https://www.centerjd.org/system/files/WP_SwedenNZ_F.pdf [Last accessed June, 2024].

7. Brennan TA, Studdert DM. (2001). No-Fault Compensation for Medical Injuries: The Prospect for Error Prevention. JAMA. 2001;286(2):217-23.
8. CNN.com/Inside Politics. (2003). Bush outlines medical liability reform. [online] Available from http://edition.cnn.com/2003/ALLPOLITICS/01/16/bush.malpractice/ [Last accessed June, 2024].
9. Danzon PM. The Swedish Patient Compensation System: Myths and Realities. Int Rev Law Econ. 1994;14:453-66.
10. Donoghue v Stevenson [1932] UKHL 100. [online] Available from https://lawteacher.net/cases/donoghue-v-stevenson.php [Last accessed June, 2024].
11. Johansson H. The Swedish system for compensation of patient injuries. Ups J Med Sci. 2010;115(2):88-90.
12. Harleston J. (2003). No-fault medical liability compensation system. [online] Available from https://www.cga.ct.gov/2003/olrdata/ins/rpt/2003-R-0386.htm [Last accessed June, 2024].
13. India Today. PIL: Why does Supreme Court work for only 193 days in entire year? [online] Available from https://www.indiatoday.in/mail-today/story/pil-why-does-supreme-court-work-for-only-193-days-in-entire-year-1241141-2018-05-25 [Last accessed June, 2024].
14. India.gov.in. Ayushman Bharat is National Health Protection Scheme. [online] Available from https://www.india.gov.in/spotlight/ayushman-bharat-national-health-protection-mission [Last accessed June, 2024].
15. Krishna Kumar Vs. State of Tamil Nadu. [online] Available from https://www.casemine.com/search/in/ [Last accessed June, 2024].
16. Machiavelli N. The Prince (1532). London, United Kingdom: Penguin Books; 1995.
17. Norton A. (2012). Docs win most malpractice suits, but road is long. [online] Available from https://www.reuters.com/article/us-docs-win-most idUSBRE84M11N20120523 [Last accessed June, 2024].
18. Rasheed J. A Study of Medical Negligence Cases decided by the District Consumer Courts of Delhi. J Indian Acad Forensic Med. 2015;37(1):50-5.
19. RCEM Learning. Understanding Clinical Error. [online] Available from https://www.rcemlearning.org/modules/an-introduction-to-human-factors-and-patient-safety/lessons/section-1-clinical-error/topic/understanding-clinical-error/ [Last accessed June, 2024].
20. Sternberg S. (2016). Medical Errors are Third Leading Cause of Death in the US [online] Available from https://www.usnews.com/news/articles/2016-05-03/medical-errors-are-third-leading-cause-of-death-in-the-us [Last accessed June, 2024].
21. Wallis K. New Zealand's 2005 'no-fault' compensation reforms and medical professional accountability for harm. NZ Med J. 2013;126(1371):33-44.
22. Wikipedia, the free encyclopedia. Hippocratic Oath. [online] Available from https://en.wikipedia.org/wiki/Hippocratic_Oath [Last accessed June, 2024].

Clinical Establishment Act

Kumar Diwakar, Tulsi Prasad, Bhupendra Kumar Gupta

INTRODUCTION

The Clinical Establishment Act was passed by parliament of India on 17th August 2010. The Clinical Establishment Act aims to register and regulate clinical establishment based on minimum standards to improve the quality of public healthcare in the country.

OBJECTIVES

- Make a digital registry of clinical institutions at District, State, and National level
- The registration of such establishment will prevent quackery by unqualified or unregistered practitioners
- The quality care improvement through standardized facilities with minimum standard services for different categories of establishments except teaching hospitals, and to ensure compliance of standard management guidelines, stabilization patients in emergency, display of charges or rates, and document maintenance, etc.

PRESENT STATUS OF SERVICES AND INFRASTRUCTURE IN INDIA

In India healthcare suffers from under regulation, poor quality of treatment, quackery, and high cost. Therefore, it is important to have minimum standards in both Private and Public Sectors. High cost in the Private Sector raises the issue of affordability and equity. Quality depends on factor such as personal competency, adherence to protocols, standard guidelines and availability of infrastructure ensured in accredited hospital but remain suspect in non-accredited hospital (**Table 55.1**).

SALIENT FEATURES OF CE ACT 10 AND CE RULES 12

Definition: Clinical Establishment

A hospital, nursing home, dispensary, maternity home, clinic, sanatorium or an institution that offers services, facilities requiring investigations, treatment, diagnosis, or care for illness, deformity, injury, abnormality or pregnancy in any system of medicine established, maintained, or administered by any individual or group of persons, whether incorporated or not.

Table 55.1: The summary of health regulations in states/UTs.

Group 1	The states in which CEA 2010 has become applicable are Himachal Pradesh, Arunachal Pradesh, Mizoram, and Sikkim because of their prior resolution passed in assembly
Group 2	CEA 2010 has become applicable by their adoption in state assemblies: Bihar, Assam, Jharkhand, Uttarakhand, Uttar Pradesh, and Rajasthan
Group 3	States/UTs which have their own Act. They may repeal their own Act before adopting the CEA 2010: Maharashtra, West Bengal, Andhra Pradesh, Odisha, Manipur, Delhi, Madhya Pradesh, Nagaland, and Punjab.
Group 4	Other states which had enacted their own Acts: Haryana, Chhattisgarh, J&K, Tamil Nadu, Meghalaya, and Tripura. (Only Chhattisgarh and Tripura implemented the Act)
Group 5	The states which have not adopted CEA 2010 nor have their own Act been: Gujarat, Kerala, and Goa

A place an independent entity or an establishment referred as in sub-clause (i), for the diagnosis or treatment pathological, genetic, radiological, bacteriological, chemical, biological investigations or any other services of laboratory or medical equipment, are carried on, administered or maintained by an individual or group of persons, whether incorporated or not, and includes an establishment owned, controlled or managed by:
- Government department
- A public or private trust
- A corporation/society registered under any Provincial or State Act
- By a local authority
- An individual doctor

Coverage: All clinical establishments—including diagnostic centers and single doctor clinics, across all recognized systems of medicine in both private and public sector (except Armed Forces establishments).

Date of commencement of the Act: The Act shall come into force in a State, or a State adopts the Act by resolution to this effect in the state legislatures.

The various systems of medicine recognized under the Act are:
- *Modern medicine*: Medical and dental
- *AYUSH*: Homoeopathy, Unani, Siddha, Ayurvedic, Naturopathy, Yoga, and Sowa Rigpa (Sowa Rigpa was recognized by the Ministry of AYUSH after passing of clinical establishments bill)

Registry: The digital registry of CEA at District, State and, National level.
- *Standard application form*: Application may be made in person, by post or online through website.
- *Registration is mandatory*: Within 1 year from commencement of Act, each and every existing clinical establishment shall apply for registration and new establishments, i.e., which come into existence after commencement of Act shall apply for registration within 6 months.

The Act provides for two types of registration:
Provisional registration: No enquiry is to be done prior to grant of certificate of provisional registration, which is granted for one year at a time.

PERMANENT REGISTRATION

- Permanent registration is to be considered after notification of minimum standards.
- Clinical facilities must meet minimum standards before being approved for permanent enrollment.
- Temporary registration is not renewed after 2 years from the minimum standard notification date for existing clinics and 6 months after the minimum standard notification date for new clinics (effective after the minimum standard notification date). Permanent registrations are issued for 5 years at a time.

Conditions each clinical facility must meet to receive registration (permanent) and renewal:

- Minimum standards for services and facilities
- Minimum requirements for personnel
- Providing and maintaining reports and records
- Each clinical facility shall provide care "within the limits of personnel and facilities available" to stabilize the emergency medical condition of persons admitted or brought to the clinical facility
- *Details of charges and available services must be prominently displayed in the local language and English*:
    - Clinical facility charges for procedures and services within limits set by the central government from time to time in consultation with the State Government.
    - Clinical facilities must adhere to standard practice guidelines that may be issued by central/state governments.
    - Each clinical facility must maintain information and statistics in accordance with all applicable laws and regulations.
- *Registration, renewal and appeal fees*:
    - As specified by the relevant State/UT Administration in Section 54
    - State/UT may charge fees by category.
    - Fees may increase if you do not request an extension by the deadline.
    - State/Utah may charge a fee for filing an appeal with the State Legislature/Utah.
- *Registration renewal application deadline*:
    - 30 days before certificate expiration for temporary registration
    - 6 months before certificate expiration for permanent registration
- *Cancellation of registration provided by clinical institutions after registration*:
    - For non-compliance with the conditions of registration
    - A clinical establishment management officer has been convicted of committing a crime under this law.
    - In case of imminent danger to the health and safety of patients, the authorities may immediately suspend the activities of a medical institution after its abolition.
- *Penalties under the Act* **(Table 55.2)**:
    - No imprisonment under this Act
    - Monetary penalties: Rupees 10,000–500,000; depends on size, category, type and local conditions

Table 55.2: Penalties under Clinical Establishment Act.

Offence	*Penalty in Rupees up to*		
	First offence	*Second offence*	*Subsequent offence*
Running establishment without proper registration	50,000	200,000	500,000
Contravention of other provisions	10,000	50,000	500,000
Whoever knowingly serves in any unregistered establishment	25,000		
Minor deficiencies not posing imminent danger	10,000		

BENEFITS OF ACT

Comprehensive registry of establishments and systematic collection of various information:
- Policy formulation
- Better surveillance, response and management of outbreak and public health emergencies
- Engagement with private providers
- Clinical establishments with categories which makes it feasible to prescribe uniform standards for particular category
- *Transparency*:
  - Process of registration, data in public domain
  - Details of facilities, charges, to be prominently displayed at a conspicuous place in the establishment
- Multistakeholder participation in institutional mechanisms (National and State councils, District Registration Authority—consensus-based decisions)

Effective regulation of providers leads to:
- Improved quality of health care based on standard protocols
- Increased patient confidence
- Improved brand value of establishments
- *Deterrent against quackery*: Registration is allowed only for clinical establishments belonging to recognized systems of medicine
- Better management of emergency conditions
- Better maintenance of reports and records

Opposition to the Clinical Establishments (Registration and Regulation) ACT, 2010 by IMA

The Indian Medical Association (IMA) leadership had articulated reasons for its opposition.
- Doctors are already regulated by laws like the Pre-natal Diagnostic Techniques Act, Biomedical waste laws and the Consumer Protection Act and this bill would give regulators excessive authority and prevent doctor from protecting themselves against accusations.
- This measure will lead to the end of licensing and the practice of family doctors providing affordable healthcare.
- "Regulation and licensing" will exacerbate the tendency of young medical graduates to avoid family practice and work in specialty hospitals.

- The stringent requirements that must be contained in the law for the minimum required number of trained paramedical personnel cannot be met due to the widespread shortage of trained paramedics even in government agencies. Also, this will increase the cost of treatment, which can increase many times over

CONCLUSION

If the Clinical Establishment Act is taken and implemented in the right spirit it will be a boon for public and overall progress of our nation. The Clinical Establishment Act aimed to bridge the gap between private and public healthcare services in India by providing for a standard minimum to be followed by all medical establishment as well as regulating the quality of services availed through urban and rural area alike.

KEY LEARNING POINTS

- Clinical Establishment Act ensures digital registry of clinical establishment at National, State, and District level
- It prevents quackery by unqualified person by introducing registration system.
- It helps in improving quality care through standardization by prescribing the minimum standard of facilities and services.

BIBLIOGRAPHY

1. Clinical Establishments (Registration and Regulation) Act, 2010, Act No. 23 of 2010. Available from: https://clinicalestablishments.gov.in/WriteReadData/2591.pdf
2. Phadke A. The Indian Medical Association and the Clinical Establishment Act, 2010: irrational opposition to regulation. Indian J Med Ethics. 2010;7(4):229-32.

56

CHAPTER

Are Doctors Greedy and Money Sharks?

Mahesh Baldwa, Amit Padvi, Namita Padvi

"Sharks eat humans and doctors save human lives."

INTRODUCTION

The medicine practice is capable of mitigating illness by rendering state-of-art service through diligent medical care with due care and caution by doctors. The previous warm and good relations between doctor and patient have changed due to the corporate culture coming to run medical profession, culminating in heavy commercialization of so-called noble profession. This phenomenon is not in synchrony with the Hippocratic Oath. Quick and up-to-date daily advances in medical science and related technology are proving to be tools for the doctors shaping the better diagnosis and treatment of the sick and serious patients. Advancements are responsible for misuse too and have become tools for the commercial misuse and exploitation of the gullible patients by hospitals run by corporate sector. Large corporate hospitals that render service are now recognized by patients and no patient knows treating doctors in these hospitals. The elite hospitals providing facilities akin to a 5-star hotel treat the patients as ATM machines and work in league with insurance companies to make a mockery of the Hippocratic Oath. Only a portion of hospital costs are covered directly by patients. The majority of expenses are paid for by the Government in public hospitals and private health insurers in private hospitals.

They are not making as much money as you think!

DOCTORS START EARNING AFTER AGE OF 35 YEARS

Doctors put in so many years in study, so they start earning late in life. Unlike most high-end professionals, doctors begin making money only after the age of 35 years. By then they have bank debts because of expensive and specialized education. Some continue to fight debt further into their life by buying big houses and cars out of social pressure. So, the debt trap glitters more than the glamorous life of a doctor's practice.

SOLO DOCTOR'S PRACTICE

The difficulties of running a successful business overwhelm doctors who begin a solo practice. They are treated unfairly for several years after they join a group practice before they are made partners. They receive a salary when they work for a hospital, but they are subject to strict management and only receive 5% of the entire income generated by the facility.

MEDICAL DOCTORS ARE NOT AT ALL GOOD AT RUNNING HOSPITAL BUSINESS

As doctors most of them do not run profitable medical ventures. In reality, many doctors give up medical practice completely because slowly and steadily making a living in medical practice is not enough. In the United States of America (USA), about 40% of medical doctors feel stressed and wish to leave clinical practice during their next 5 years.

NORMAL BILL OF A CORPORATE PRIVATE HOSPITAL

Corporate private hospitals hand over an exorbitant bill that needs to be analyzed for expenses as to what goods/services go for what amount? If one goes to the depth of corporate private hospital bills then it will show the details about doctor's fees. One will wonder that the treating doctors get peanuts out of the huge bill of a corporate private hospital.

ARE DOCTORS MONEY SHARKS?

Corporate hospitals are owned by nondoctor businesspersons. They are opened to earn money, they provide excellent service, like star-rated hotels, and charge accordingly. It is not the qualified doctors who take your money but corporate private hospitals are money sharks and they exist with the sole purpose of emptying your pockets. Only around 4% of a corporate private hospital's total profit goes into the bank account of a caregiver doctor. So technically, it is about 4% of huge hospital bill raised by corporate that is going to the treating doctor's bank account. When it comes to blaming doctors, they are labeled as money sharks for none of their "faults".

WHY ARE THE DOCTORS OF CORPORATE PRIVATE HOSPITALS SO EXPENSIVE?

What do you think why patients are made to pay so much? A corporate hospital bill includes various charges, e.g., bed charges, nursing charges, junior doctors charges, oxygen charges, ventilation charges, intensive care unit (ICU) charges, medication charges, equipment charges, operation theater charges, and other myriads of charges. So virtually, nothing except the treating consultant doctor's visit fee that goes to the bank account of the doctor. Occasionally, the procedure performance charges or surgical charges go to the treating doctor's bank account. Still while blaming the huge bill, the treating doctors are labeled as money sharks. There is none of their "fault" in corporate billing. All fees and charges are determined by the hospital administration unilaterally. Doctors get paid for the piece of work they do. This is less than employed doctors.

Corporate private hospitals are run like by any business ventures, often under the leadership and patronage of politicians who have links with various big corporates. So, corporations and insurance companies decide and determine from where sick and serious patients will seek medical services treatment. The corporate insurance companies, third-party administrator

(TPA), and corporate hospitals rule the medical services. They decide whom to employ and give appointment letters among the leading practicing doctors. It is surprising that treating doctors get insignificant, notional portion of income from the hospitalization of patients, the laboratory tests ordered, procedures conducted, operations performed, and the medicines and drugs prescribed by them. Because practice is individualized, there are no checks and balances. Professional body fee schedules are overcome by itemizing; For example, a case of appendicitis can be billed for multiple items: One fee for laparoscopy, another for removal of appendix, another for suturing abdomen, another for wound care, and so on. There are clever accountants to advise them along the way for a fee.

ANALYSIS BY ANALYZING BY WAY OF EXAMPLES

Let us see a clear image with an example. A cardiac stenting operation that is free at any government hospital costs roughly ₹1.5 lakhs at a corporate private hospital.

A similar picture can be found in the antibiotic scene. The general public is not expected to be aware of such confidential matters. Zuventus Pharma charges ₹1,271 for a common antibiotic used in ICUs, while Cipla charges ₹2,140 for the same medication. The government is well aware of the situation, but why does it never look into such discrepancies? It is easy to utilize populist methods and threaten the doctors in the forefront. The Government avoids confrontation with corporate private hospitals owned by industrialists and the multinational companies (MNCs) and never ever takes them to task.

For example, a three-way stopcock (bivalve, by Romsoms) used in intravenous infusion that hospitals purchased for ₹5.77 was sold to patients for ₹106, resulting in a 1,737% profit for hospitals.

Similarly, a syringe without a needle (Lifelong Meditech Ltd) purchased by the hospital for ₹15.29 was sold to patients for ₹200, resulting in a profit margin of 1,208%. The investigation reveals that hospitals, rather than medicine and equipment producers and distributors, are the most profiting.

"The total cost on scheduled medicines used in the treatment is only 4.10% as compared to 25.67% on non-scheduled formulations," the study noted. As per the study, "It is amply clear that for claiming higher margins, doctors-hospitals preferred prescribing and dispensing non-scheduled branded medicines instead of scheduled medicines." According to the study, "new drugs" and "fixed-dose combinations" introduced by manufacturers to escape price restriction have become the preferred option for the manufacturing and medical communities, so undermining the intent of classifying drugs as essential. What nobody realizes is that the biggest money maker in hospital segment is actually the Government, with zero investment and zero risk. The goods and services tax (GST) is virtually free income to the Government.

ACCOUNTABILITY, AUTONOMY, ETHICS OF INDIVIDUAL DOCTOR, AND CORPORATE ECONOMICS

Corporate economics wants individual doctors to meet quarterly revenue target so as to meet return on investment (ROI) on corporate investment. Usually, quarterly revenue targets are difficult to meet by individual doctors. Even if an individual doctor wants to meet, he/she will have to do unethical things to the patient. Even accountability and autonomy of individual doctors are also at stake. The main thing is to meet 100% of the quarterly revenue target for 5% of the total revenue share.

Let's take one example, a corporate hospital gives quarterly target of 1 crore for revenue to a neurosurgeon. Now, the neurosurgeon is under pressure. This may lead to losing personal and professional autonomy in the first place. Secondly, in order to meet the revenue target, he/she may indulge in unethical advice of tests, imaging studies, and extra surgery. So, accountability to patients gets eclipsed.

DOCTORS ARE UNDERPAID IN INDIA

Actually, the problem is increasing with each passing year due to numerous reasons:

- Health is never a priority in India, be it in Government policies or to people. So, people will never be ready to spend money on doctor's fees; instead, they will spend on festivals and entertainment resources.
- There is increasing saturation for doctors in cities. So, freshers and new doctors are struggling to earn enough.
- Government hospitals offer good enough salaries but not excellent
- Established doctors are also struggling since they do not want to invest in ultramodern facilities.
- Finally, doctors join corporate hospitals where they are paid decently, but just 5% of the total revenue of the hospital is earned by them, and with each quarter their target for generating hospital revenue gets escalated.

WELFARE STATE FUNCTION AND GOVERNMENT HOSPITALS

The government operates government hospitals as per the Constitution of India, as a welfare state.

But whose welfare it is? When those with substantial political ties, high-ranking government employees, and their families spend days on end in very important person (VIP) cabins, intensive coronary care unit (ICCU)/high-dependency units (HDU)/cardiac care unit (CCU) beds, the phrase "welfare state" loses all meaning. Doctors are frequently criticized for preferring to work in private business settings due to their desire for high salaries. Given the kind of living a doctor enjoys at a government facility, this is not surprising. Let us look at and emphasize a few points regarding government doctors:

- Doctors perform tasks like giving injections and analyzing test results, for which they are paid peanuts.
- A junior doctor is permitted to sleep on mattresses with bed bugs; the lack of access to even hygienic restrooms can be a serious issue for female doctors.
- During the scorching summer months, a doctor working in an outpatient department of a government hospital is required to visit at least 80 patients each day, occasionally while using a broken fan.

Primary healthcare center (PHC) in rural areas have no water supply, intermittent electric supply, and are full of dirt. They are mosquito-infested and unclean toilets and bathrooms attached to quarters are provided. Even municipal and government hospitals of tier one and tier two cities provide similar resident doctors quarters with 10 by 10 feet room being occupied by two to three doctors.

MEDIA MENACE

Whatever antiphysician fuel the news outlets have been feeding you, there is one thing you must grasp. Authorities tell and threaten the poor doctor that it is critical that they focus solely on one thing: the patient's recovery. And the doctor is so bound and permitted to undertake this task at any cost. Doctors take the Hippocratic Oath at an early age, which directs them to prioritize a sick patient above everything else. In their right mind, no doctor would ever do anything to add to a patient's pain.

MEDICAL LAW

Medical legislation is changing dramatically. The evolution of professional misconduct and negligence law is far from adequate. The laws are insufficient and do not cover the complete scope of medical malpractice. Medical malpractice lawsuits can be reduced or prevented by taking steps to keep patients satisfied, adhering to policies and procedures, providing patient-centered care, and learning how to defend against malpractice judgments. In today's litigious environment, having adequate professional liability insurance is a must.

NOBEL PROFESSION

Because of the nature and importance of their work, as well as the devotion and sacrifice required by the profession, medical practitioners have enjoyed a high level of respect in society. For good reason, the profession is generally associated with a sense of nobleness.

CONCLUSION

Doctors are not money sharks, but it is the corporate hospitals that charge so much and pay hardly 4–5% of whole bill to the doctors, shifting the fault to poor doctors. But after all, the medical profession needs to be treated with dignity. The current system forces medical practitioners to be too defensive, ordering unnecessary tests and investigations that only add to the cost of therapy. The inclusion of health services in the Consumer Protection Act did not benefit society, but rather increased confusion and mistrust in the doctor–patient relationship. To prevent future deterioration of the medical profession, health services should be excluded from the scope of this Act. To restore the glory of this wonderful profession, the National Medical Commission must undertake changes.

KEY LEARNING POINTS

- The medicine practice is capable of mitigating illness by rendering state-of-art service through diligent medical care with due care and caution by doctors.
- The elite hospitals providing facilities akin to a 5-star hotel treat the patients as ATM machines and work in league with insurance companies to make a mockery of the Hippocratic Oath.
- Hospitals' expenses are only partly paid for directly by the patient. The majority of expenses are paid for by the Government in public hospitals and private health insurers in private hospitals.
- Doctors start earning after the age of 35 years.
- Solo doctors have difficulties in running a successful business.
- Corporate hospitals are owned by nondoctor businesspersons.
- Corporate hospitals give doctors a salary of less than 5% of revenue generated. Main thing is to meet 100% of quarterly revenue target of corporate hospitals to get 5% of the total revenue share.
- When it comes to blaming doctors, they are labeled as money sharks for none of their "faults".
- Medical professionals take the Hippocratic Oath at a young age, which commands doctors to put the needs of a sick patient before everything else.
- Medical legislation is changing dramatically. The evolution of professional misconduct and negligence law is far from adequate. The laws are insufficient and do not cover the complete scope of medical malpractice.

BIBLIOGRAPHY

1. Sumi Sukanya Dutta. (2018). The New Indian Express. How private hospitals make 1,700 per cent profit. [online] Available from https://www.newindianexpress.com/nation/2018/feb/20/how-private-hospitals-make-1700-per-cent-profit-1776300.html [Last accessed May, 2024].

CHAPTER 57

Consumer Protection Act

Neeraj Nagpal

INTRODUCTION

The first consumer organization was born in Denmark in 1947 and then in Great Britain in 1953. The World Consumer Rights Day is observed every year on March 15th. It was on this day that the President of the United States of America (USA) John F Kennedy had asked the US Congress to give its approval to the Consumer Bill of Rights. The rights mentioned in the document were: (1) Right to choice; (2) right to information; (3) right to safety; and (4) right to be heard. The right to consumer education was later added by President Gerald R Ford. The United Nations Guidelines for Consumer Protection were adopted by consensus in a resolution 39/248 on April 16th,1985, in the General Assembly, authorizing the Secretary General of the United Nations to persuade member countries to adopt these guidelines through changes in policy or law.

These guidelines outlined what the governments needed to do to promote consumer protection and constituted of the following:

(i) Physical safety of consumer
(ii) Protection and promotion of their economic interest
(iii) Safety and quality standards of consumer goods and services
(iv) Distribution facilities for consumer goods and services
(v) Measures ensuring that consumers are able to obtain redress
(vi) Certain measures specifically related to different areas like food, water and pharmaceuticals, etc.
(vii) Program to provide information and education to consumer

THE ACT

With these international events in mind, the Indian Parliament had enacted the Consumer Protection Act (CPA), 1986. The objective of the Act as stated was "to provide for better protection of the interests of consumers." The intention was to provide a speedy and inexpensive remedy to the consumer. The CPA of 1986 was supposed to be a benevolent social legislation intended to protect the consumers from exploitation. Unfortunately, as time has passed, neither is the process speedy nor is it inexpensive and benevolent.

DOCTORS AND CONSUMER PROTECTION ACT OF 1986

In the initial years after 1986 enactment of CPA, there was confusion regarding inclusion of healthcare within the definition of "services" as defined in Section 2(1)(o) of the CPA of 1986. Karnataka High Court in Dr AS Chandra vs. Union of India 1992 held that services rendered by doctors, nursing homes, and private hospitals must be construed as service for the purpose of the Act. In Dr CS Subramanian vs. Kumarasamy 1994, the honorable Madras High Court took the opposite view. Meanwhile, the National Consumer Redressal Commission decided that activity of providing medical services for payment falls within the scope of "service" as defined in the Act, but Government hospital services did not. The question whether the service rendered at a hospital/nursing home can be regarded as "service" under Section 2(1)(o) of the 1986 Act was finally decided by the honorable Supreme Court (SC) in the case of Indian Medical Association vs. VP Shantha and Ors 1995. The conclusions drawn in this judgment were:

(1) Service rendered to a patient by a medical practitioner would fall within the ambit of "service" as defined in Section 2(1)(o) of the Act.
(2) The fact that medical practitioners are subject to the disciplinary control of the Medical Council of India would not exclude the services rendered by them from the ambit of the Act.
(3) The honorable court held that relationship between a patient and the medical practitioner was not that of master and servant and hence, the services rendered by a medical practitioner could not be regarded as services rendered under a "contract of personal service." A doctor's services were held to be rendered under a "contract for personal services" and so is not covered by exclusionary clause within the definition of "service" contained in Section 2(1)(o) of the Act.
(4) The expression "contract of personal service" cannot be confined to contracts for employment of domestic servants only and would include the employment of a medical officer for the purpose of rendering medical service to the employer. This service under the contract of employment would be outside the purview of "service" as defined in Section 2(1)(o) of the Act.
(5) Service rendered free of charge where such services are rendered free of charge to everybody, would not be "service" as defined in the Act. The payment of a token amount for registration purpose only at the hospital/nursing home would not alter the position.
(7) Service rendered at a nongovernment hospital/nursing home where charges are required to be paid by the persons availing such services falls within the purview of the expression "service" as defined in the Act.
(10) Service rendered at a government or a charitable hospital where some persons paid for services and others were treated free of charge would also fall within the ambit the Act, irrespective of the fact that the service is rendered free of charge. Free service would also be "service" and the recipient a "consumer" under the Act.
(12) If the person availing the service has taken an insurance policy for medical care or where employer bears cost of treatment where the charges for medical treatment are borne by the insurance company or the employer, such service would fall within the ambit of "service" as defined in the Act.

AMENDMENTS

The Government made numerous amendments to the CPA 1986 starting from 1991, 1993, and then 2002. In the amendments, among other things, pecuniary jurisdiction of District

Commissions and State Commissions was enhanced and another important issue addressed was the one where death of complainant or opposite party would not abate the suit. However, these amendments still did not address the booming e-commerce industry and modern methods of providing goods and services such as online sales, teleshopping, direct selling, and multilevel marketing in addition to the traditional methods. The Government over the next decade or so instead of bringing another amendment decided to enact an altogether new Act.

The New Act

Keeping in view the 1995 judgment of the honorable SC, the draft Consumer Protection Bill 2018 placed before the parliament had included healthcare within the definition of "services" mentioned in it, but this Bill was stalled in Rajya Sabha due to objection by certain members regarding this inclusion of healthcare. This lead to the bill being lapsed. In the next session, when the bill was again introduced and passed, this time the parliament had by an act of commission, consciously dropped Healthcare from the list of services mentioned in definition of services in the CPA 2019.

Legislative intent had been clearly stated on the floors of both Houses of the Parliament, through multiple and extensively elaborate statements of the honorable Minister of Consumer Affairs, Food and Public Distribution, Late Shree Ram Vilas Paswan ji, that Healthcare has been deliberately kept out of the new CPA 2019, clearly citing the reasons for the same with examples. The parliament was aware of the IMA vs. VP Shantha and Ors judgment of 1995 which included doctors within the definition of service providers under the CPA 1986. Despite being so aware and despite including healthcare within Section 2(42) of Consumer Protection Bill 2018, the word "healthcare" was deliberately and consciously dropped, effectively going against the 1995 judgment of the SC.

If the intention of the Parliament was to follow the order of the SC given in IMA vs. VP Shantha and Ors' case in 1995, then they would have added the same in the Act and not consciously dropped it as decided in Vishakha vs. State of Rajasthan. Definition of sexual harassment given by the SC was later on added in the Act by the Parliament. Similarly, in Sowmithri Vishnu vs. Union of India (UOI)—Adultery Section—497 of Indian Penal Code (IPC) was declared unconstitutional and the SC asked the Parliament to legislate on the matter. This clearly indicates that the parliamentary intent of not including medical services was reflected in the final CPA 2019. Unfortunately, the Parliament did not notify specific exclusion of healthcare as was required under the CPA 2019. This appeared to be an oversight and led to unnecessary confusion.

Multiple public interest litigations (PILs) were filed in various high courts and SC to remove healthcare within purview of the CPA 2019, but all were rejected summarily. The two cases filed in Bombay High Court and the SC by Medicos Legal Action Group (MLAG) had only taken up the issue of parliamentary intent as the plea for exclusion of healthcare from within purview of the CPA 2019. Though MLAG lost the judicial campaign, the view, that maintaining status quo with healthcare remaining within the purview of the CPA 2019 is against the interest of consumers and doctors, as well as the nation, is gaining ground.

The CPA introduced nearly three decades ago has been used to prosecute medical professionals for errors causing damage to patients under their care. This legislative and judicial conversion of doctors into traders resulted in cases of alleged medical negligence being filed in courts and what was a trickle in 1990s has turned into a deluge in the past few years. Each and every negative or suboptimal outcome or known complication of medical treatment is now perceived as negligence. This has caused doctors to start practice of defensive medicine and what could be treated clinically is now first investigated and what could be managed at home is now treated in intensive care units (ICUs). Doctors who used to take on challenging cases with a firm hand and a strong heart now treat only low-risk patients and refer others to higher institutions. Doctors who are senior and experienced do not consider taking the risk worthwhile and the younger generation of doctors is not as experienced at least partly due to lacunae in medical education and training due to recent changes. Younger doctors are also leaving the profession or the country demoralized with the situation.

ACCOUNTABILITY WITHIN AND SELF-REGULATION OR PROSECUTION AS PER COMMON LAW

The consumer courts are neither equipped nor is the summary nature of the process suited to adjudicate complicated issues related to medical treatment. The argument that medical negligence cases should not be decided by nonmedical courts was dismissed by the honorable SC in IMA vs. VP Shantha and Ors in 1995. The SC in this judgment however had made it clear that only outright cases of medical negligence like amputation of wrong limb, leaving swab or clamp in body, and giving wrong anesthetic gases would be covered under CPA. Cases which required evidence of experts were not to be covered under CPA. What is standard medical practice in other hospitals or by other average surgeons was also held not to be negligence.

However, as we see it today, dose of medicine, wrong diagnosis, method of treatment, conservative vs. radical surgery, extension of surgical procedure depending on intraoperative findings, all have been adjudicated by consumer courts with the help of expert evidence even via video conferencing. Dragging doctors to consumer fora with increasing frequency is a trend with disturbing consequences. That medical professionals need to be held accountable for their actions is not in dispute. It is how they should be held accountable which is the matter of debate. The process under CPA is summary in nature and this is flawed and urgent remedial measures need to be made, failing which private healthcare establishments which provide a bulk of healthcare needs of the country will become slowly extinct. India spends <1.5% of its gross domestic product on healthcare and the public healthcare system simply cannot provide the necessary services to the teeming population. Government does not have the resources, inclination, or manpower to provide universal state-sponsored healthcare.

RESTITUTIO IN INTEGRUM

The quantum of compensation being awarded by consumer courts in India today in cases of medical negligence is bordering on absurd with serious implications for medical profession and patients alike. Medical professionals as mentioned earlier have now started practicing defensive medicine. While taking medical decisions, doctors have to contend with an additional factor of what the courts' view will be. The hand that holds the scalpel has become shaky. The sword of compensation claims of exorbitant amounts sufficient to exhaust a doctor's lifetime (and maybe next seven lives) earnings is now hanging over every doctor's head.

Since there are no free lunches in this world, for every patient who claims compensation in crores, millions of other patients will pay their doctors to cover for such eventualities.

What is absurd is the fact that any amount of compensation can be demanded from medical professionals as there is no cap on this amount and what was unthinkable a decade ago is being awarded today and exponential increase in this amount is expected few years down the line.

Since compensation awarded is based on earning capacity of the victim, a rich industrialist could be awarded 100s of crores as per CPA. Here, the penalty is not commensurate with the crime, whereas natural justice demands that for any crime, the punishment has to be proportionate. Human life cannot be valued differently. So, a common bile duct (CBD) injury during laparoscopic cholecystectomy will be awarded different penalty against the same surgeon and the same hospital depending on earning capacity of the patient.

Unlimited compensation claims and differential awards are unjustified because doctors do not charge fee for their services based on the earning capacity of the patient and hence commensurate with the risk (of higher compensation) that they undertake. If a patient's earning capacity is the criterion for computation of compensation award, then the fee for services should be linked to the earning capacity of the patient (hence the risk undertaken). On the contrary, under the Clinical Establishment Act as well as National Medical Commission Act and Regulations, doctors have to display their uniform rates clearly and government has the power to decide the rates being charged by doctors.

CONFRONTATION OF MEDICINE AND LAW

If the corona pandemic has taught us anything, it has exposed that India is a resource-poor country and in a critical situation, doctors frequently have to decide who the limited resources should be given to. Medical equipment such as ventilators, oxygen cylinders, and ICU beds were all in short supply and it is common to see many patients being ventilated on a trolley by their relatives using ambu bag while waiting for a ventilator/ICU bed. If two patients needed a ventilator in a hospital and only one was available, what was the doctor supposed to do. If one patient was a high net worth individual and his death could result in an astronomical compensation award, then the doctor would obviously choose him over a poor patient keeping the risk of exorbitant compensation in mind. Is the doctor supposed to restrict the use of medical resources to cater to the rich and hence bring a bias into treatment decisions because of the concept of *Restitutio in integrum* in law. This is a frightening but real prospect not faced earlier by medical men. *Are medical treatment and resources in India going to be the prerogative of the rich? This discrimination against poor patients is violative of Articles 14 and 21 of the Indian Constitution as well as medical ethics.*

MOTOR ACCIDENT CLAIM TRIBUNAL AND CONSUMER PROTECTION ACT

During treatment of a fatal disease, treatment given may lead to death earlier than the disease itself would have caused it. But this is the cornerstone of medicine. While handling an aneurysm, it may burst causing bleeding to prevent which surgery was being done in the first place. By this argument, no neurosurgeon should operate a head injury, no malignancy should be operated, no pancreatic abscess drained, or even an angioplasty performed because in doing so, death may occur. Despite actions of doctors being done in good faith, unforeseen and adverse outcomes are now on the basis of *res ipsa loquitur* condemned as negligence and sometimes even criminal prosecution of the doctor being done. The courts have already upheld that *mens rea* is not necessary in cases of medical negligence and gross negligence in performance of his duty by a doctor is sufficient. How is this comparable with killing or maiming normal healthy individuals either intentionally or contributing to it by negligence of a drunk driver of motor vehicle?

MEDICAL PRACTICE IN INDIA

Medical profession in India is unique from other professions as well as from medical profession as practiced in the western world. Medical professionals should not have been compared with other service providers as defined in CPA, keeping in view the adverse environment that doctors in India work in to provide healthcare which has now been declared a fundamental right of all citizens by a catena of SC judgments. The term services in the definition of CPA should have distinguished between routine services, essential services, and services which fulfill fundamental rights of citizens. Providers of services which are the fundamental right of all citizens should not have been shackled and deprived of their professional autonomy and forever under threat of litigation, leaving them with shaking hands and a sword hanging over their heads. As practiced in India, it is nothing short of miracle that healthcare indices have improved to a great extent and thanks to the dedication, work ethics, and empathy of doctors, we have cure rates similar to most developed countries for most of the diseases, increased life expectancy, and decreased maternal mortality. Because of the sheer volumes and variety of patients that Indian doctors have to deal with, they have far more experience than some of the foreign dignitaries who come to give lectures in conferences.

This is despite the fact that Indian doctors have to battle with quackery which is mostly condoned if not promoted by their Government. Myths, superstitions, and misconceptions are deep-rooted in Indian psyche. Working in such adverse environment would be impossible for the foreign and nonresident Indian (NRI) doctors who are invited to various conferences to deliver lectures and demonstrate procedures. Despite this, to try to impose compensations against doctors as applicable in USA to India is nothing short of absurd. If we want ideal medical treatment, then it can only be provided in ideal treatment environment.

CONSUMER PROTECTION ACT 2019

The recently notified Consumer Protection Amendment Act 2019 does not have any ceiling on the quantum of compensation which can be asked for in a District Commission. This has increased the apprehension of doctors regarding the increasing number and substantial increase in quantum of compensation being demanded by those who allege negligence. The increase in pecuniary jurisdiction of various commissions along with removal of penalty for frivolous complaints is expected to increase litigation against doctors manifold. Since patients who have paid up to INR 50 lakhs can now file complaint in the District Commission (irrespective of how much they have asked for in compensation); nearly all cases of alleged medical negligence are now expected to be filed in District Commissions and the introduction of the Section 41 (CPA 2019) requiring 50% of compensation awarded to be deposited before going for appeal will also ensure that cases will no longer be taken up for appeal, especially since the indemnity insurers refuse to make any interim payments. Since the 50% of penalty awarded is to be deposited before appeal, it is assumed that complainant if he loses the case will not have to deposit 50% of amount claimed if he or she decides to go in appeal. This is an indirect endorsement of inherent desire of consumer courts to award compensation to complainant irrespective of any finding of negligence. Also, since judgments of State Consumer Courts, National Commission, High Courts, and SC are reported, they remain in public domain, likely to be examined and academically discussed. The District Commission judgments were not reported and hence, all judgments in cases of medical negligence will henceforth tend to be arbitrary and without any fear of accountability, thus denying justice to medical professionals.

THE SERVANT

As mentioned earlier the VP Shantha judgment, while including the medical services within the purview of the CPA 1986, had considered the issue of "contract of personal service" vs. the "Contract for Personal Services" while expanding the definition of services. As decided in the judgment, "contract for services" implied a contract where one party undertakes to render services, for example, professional or technical services to another, but he is not subject to detailed direction and control but instead exercises professional autonomy using his technical knowledge and skill at his discretion. However, a "contract of service" implies relationship of master and servant and involves an obligation to obey orders in the work to be performed and as to its mode and manner of performance. The honorable court had held however that there can be a contract of personal service if there is relationship of master and servant even between the person availing his services and the doctor.

In 2008, however, the Samira Kohli vs. Dr Prabha Manchanda judgment also from the SC by honorable Justice *BN Agrawal, Justice PP Naolekar, and Justice RV Raveendran* stated clearly that during a surgery, while patient is under anesthesia, if an additional procedure is required, the doctor cannot do anything more than what the patient has given consent for. They said that it may be that the required additional procedure may be beneficial and may be in the interest of the patient and it may also be that postponement of the additional procedure (say removal of an organ) may require another surgery with its additional risks and costs, still doctors cannot proceed on their own. It was decided that even though additional removal of the affected organ during the initial diagnostic or exploratory surgery would save the patient from the pain and cost of a second operation, a doctor cannot do anything more than what has been asked of him by the patient. The court held as irrelevant any objections as to the impracticality or inconvenience caused by such decision not to proceed. "What is relevant and of importance is the inviolable nature of the patient's right in regard to his body and his right to decide whether he should undergo the particular treatment or surgery or not." Therefore, unless the unauthorized additional or further procedure is necessary in order to save the life of the patient and it would be unreasonable (as contrasted from being merely inconvenient) to delay the further procedure until the patient regains consciousness and takes a decision, a doctor cannot perform such procedure without the consent of the patient.

This obviously now means that as a doctor, he is now subject to detailed direction and control and cannot exercise his own professional or technical skill and use his own knowledge and discretion (thus making him a servant?) but has to do what is directed by the patient (master?). *Since "Contract of personal service" was excluded in definition of "services" in the CPA 1986 and also in the CPA 2019 would not doctors be excluded now since they are subject to detailed direction and control by his master/patient and also cannot exercise professional or technical skill or use his own knowledge and discretion.*

ACCOUNTABILITY OR SELECTIVE ACCOUNTABILITY

There is no denying of the need for all service providers to be accountable. However, though 40% of qualified doctors of modern scientific medicine in India today are facing at least one allegation of negligence in courts, the cases against professionals other than doctors are next to nil. The honorable SC has granted stay on the decision of National Consumer Disputes Redressal Commission (NCDRC) which had said that advocates are also covered within purview of the CPA 1986. This stay was granted in 2009 and it was only in 2024, in judgment DK Gandhi v. Bar of Indian Lawyers, that the Supreme Court finally gave its decision and held that advocates will not be covered within purview of CPA 2019. This concept of selective accountability applied against medical professionals has created a feeling of alienation among them and has left them with a feeling of persecution.

MULTIPLICITY OF JURISDICTION

Currently, doctors who are accused of medical negligence are being prosecuted by different courts, commissions, boards, and quasi-judicial fora. This leads to three to four different places where a doctor keeps running on different dates trying to defend a single case of alleged medical negligence, each moving at a different pace. Also, sometimes when a medical board has been formed, the doctor appears before this said medical board in addition. The legal process before three to five different courts, fora, boards, and commissions is more severe punishment for a practicing doctor than a 2-month imprisonment or suspension of registration.

The CPA 1986 in Section 3 and CPA 2019 in Section 100 state very clearly that provisions of the law shall be in addition to and not in derogation of other laws for the time being in force. This provides for prosecution of doctors under multiple laws in addition to CPA simultaneously. It has been argued that the current system where a doctor is held accountable in multiple courts, boards, and commissions simultaneously on same facts against complainants is undesirable.

SOLUTION

Ideal situation would however be (as is being followed in certain countries) that the indemnity insurance premium of doctors and hospitals should be uniform (such as motor vehicle insurance) based on their specialization for unlimited compensation. After this, any compensation awarded should be paid by insurer as a no-fault compensation without naming and shaming the doctor concerned.

Medicos Legal Action Group had suggested a special act be formulated and had shared it as a representation with the government. Under this act, doctors will remain accountable, consumer will get a reasonable compensation for his loss, and regulatory authorities retain the powers to temporarily or permanently remove the name of a registered medical practitioner from the state medical register.

The suggested "Medical Injury Compensation Bill" would encompass all aspects of alleged simple and gross medical negligence, professional misconduct, impropriety, and other legal issues related to the practice of medical profession.

Salient features of the bill suggested could be as follows:

- It should cover all aspects of compensation and punishment in cases of medical error and injury thereof exclusively.
- It should cover criminal negligence as defined in Jacob Mathew vs. State of Punjab and Martin F Dsouza vs. Mohd Ishfaq judgments by giving powers of Judicial Magistrate First Class to the Tribunal/Commission or Fora formed under this Act.
- It should override all other laws currently in place being a Special Act concerned with a specific problem. Multiple avenues of litigation should be barred. All litigation regarding alleged medical negligence should be under this Act.
- Introduce a cap on maximum compensation which can be awarded in case of medical error and injury thereof. This could be based on the fee charged for treatment. Consequent loss of earning of an individual should be compensated through life and other health Insurances which all individuals should take. Earning capacity of individual should be delinked from compensation awards since fee paid is not linked to earning capacity. A person whose life is worth 10 crores should anyway be having life insurance to the tune of 10 crores and hence, accidental (may be medical accident) death would anyway recompense the nominee for the financial loss.
- It should provide mechanism for independent medical opinion taken from experts working in similar establishments. An expert from a tertiary care institute may view events differently from an average practicing doctor in a similar area of work. Negligence has been defined now as doing something which an average practicing doctor would not do or not doing something which an average practicing doctor would do.
- The commission should comprise at least one MBBS doctor preferably who also has done LLB or may have been practicing in the region for >20 years outside tertiary institutes, one doctor of the specialty to which the case belongs besides a president who may be a judicial officer.
- It should provide mechanism of penalizing complainants for frivolous complaint. The penalty so imposed should be linked to the compensation asked for and not a ridiculously low figure. It should be sufficient to act as a deterrent for the mischievous.
- It should provide for provision to *ab initio* dismiss a complaint of alleged medical negligence by patient or relatives if they have indulged in violence at the medical establishment. This may be difficult for legal pundits to accept. The alternative is that it is likely that those who indulged in violence would also not have cooperated with doctors during treatment and are hence guilty of contributory negligence. Their conduct of violence would have caused other patients to be denied proper care which may even cause death of these other patients who are not involved in the incident of violence otherwise. The perpetrators should be saddled with 50% of whatever compensation is awarded and the total amount be deposited in poor patient fund of nearest government hospital. Under no circumstances should those who indulge in violence against doctors be beneficiaries of any compensation awarded.
- The commission under the Act should have powers to take action against perpetrators of violence against hospitals and doctors; the provisions could be similar to the Epidemic Diseases Amendment Act 2020.
- Mechanism for rates of medical treatment charges commensurate with earning capacity of patient should be made and any negligence thereafter should be compensated based on declared income and rates charged.

- The State Medical Council on application made by the complainant after decision of the District Commission under the Medical Injury Compensation Act would thereafter decide regarding any action for misconduct based on decision of the District Commission after giving opportunity to the doctor to defend himself.
- The decisions of all commissions formed under this Bill should be reported in law journals and online search engines.

It is necessary that all doctors and medical organizations to kindly initiate a discussion on this bill so that a consensus may be generated.

BIBLIOGRAPHY

1. Bandhua Mukti Morcha v. Union of India & Ors. (1997) 10 SCC 549.
2. Constitution of India as on 1st May, 2024; https://cdnbbsr.s3waas.gov.in/s380537a945c7aaa788ccfcdf1b99b5d8f/uploads/2024/07/20240716890312078.pdf; June 3, 2025.
3. Consumer Education and Resource Centre Vs Union of India 1995 AIR 922, 1995 SCC (3) 42.
4. "Cosmopolitan Hospital and Anr vs Vasantha P Nair"; [I (1992) CPJ 302 (NC)].
5. "Dr A S Chandra vs Union of India"; [1 Andh LT 713 DB].
6. "Dr C S Subramanian vs Kumarasamy"; [1996 86 CompCas 747 Mad].
7. Dr Vijil & Ors vs Ambujakshi T P WP (C) 970/2022 Kerala High Court.
8. F. Silva, A. Cavaliere, "I diritti dei consumatori e l'efficienza economica, in "La tutela del consumatore tra mercato e regolamentazione", a cura di F. Silva, Roma, 1996, p.12.
9. Giannotti v. Beleza Hair Salon, Inc., 296 Ga. App. 636, 642 (2009).
10. http://164.100.47.5/newsite/debatenew/newshow.aspx; Aug 6, 2019.
11. http://loksabhaph.nic.in/Debates/Result17.aspx?dbsl=1114; pg 89-90; July 30, 2019.
12. "Indian Medical Association vs. V P Shantha and Ors"; [1996 AIR 550].
13. "Jacob Mathew vs. State of Punjab and Another", [(2005) 6 SSC 1].
14. Kennedy, John F. (March 15, 1962). "John F. Kennedy: Special Message to the Congress on Protecting the Consumer Interest". presidency.ucsb.edu.
15. Kirloskar Brothers Ltd v. Emplyees' State Insurance Corpn (1996) 1 SCR 884.
16. "Martin F.D'Souza vs. Mohd. Ishfaq", [1(2009) CPJ 32(SC)].
17. Medicos Legal Action Group vs Union of India 2021 Bombay High Court PIL No 58 of 2021.
18. Medicos Legal Action Group vs Union of India SC 2022 SLP (C) No 19374/2021.
19. Nagpal N, Are large compensation payouts for negligence good for medicine in India? BMJ 2014; 349:g5229; https://www.bmj.com/content/349/bmj.g5229/rr/763402.
20. Paschim Banga Khet Mazdoor Samity vs. State of West Bengal 1996, SCC (4) 37.
21. Pradeep Arora vs Union of India SC 2022 Diary No 2562 /2022).
22. R v. Woolin [1998] UKHL 28; 1 AC 82.
23. "Samira Kohli vs. Dr. Prabha Manchanda", [(2008) 2 SCC 1].
24. Sexual Harassment of Women at Workplace (Prevention, Prohibition and Redressal) Act, 2013; URL: https://www.indiacode.nic.in/bitstream/123456789/2104/1/A2013-14.pdf; June 3, 2025.
25. "Sowmitri Vishnu v. Union of India", [1985 Supp SCC 137].
26. State of Punjab and Others vs. Mohinder Singh Chawala , JT 1997 (1) SC 416.
27. The Consumer Protection (Amendment) Act, 1991 (34 of 1991) (w.r.e.f. 15-6-1991); URL: https://www.indiacode.nic.in/repealedfileopen?rfilename=A1991-34.pdf.; Date Accessed on June 03, 2025.
28. The Consumer Protection (Amendment) Act, 1993 (50 of 1993) (w.r.e.f. 18-6-1993); URL: https://www.indiacode.nic.in/repealedfileopen?rfilename=A1993-50.pdf; Date accessed on June 03, 2025.
29. The Consumer Protection (Amendment) Act, 2002 (62 of 2002) (w.r.e.f. 15-3-2003); URL: https://www.indiacode.nic.in/repealedfileopen?rfilename=A2002-62.pdf; Date accessed on June 3, 2025.
30. The Consumer Protection Act 1986; URL: https://www.indiacode.nic.in/bitstream/123456789/6922/1/consumer_protection_act_1986.pdf; Date accessed on June 03, 2025.
31. The Consumer Protection Act 2019; URL: https://ncdrc.nic.in/bare_acts/CPA2019.pdf; June 3, 2025.

32. The Consumer Protection Bill, 2018; URL: https://prsindia.org/billtrack/the-consumer-protection-bill-2018; Date accessed on June 3, 2025.
33. Venkatchalam vs Ajitkumar C Shah (2011) 9 SCC 707 https://indiankanoon.org/doc/1399474/.
34. Vincent Panikulangara vs. Union of India, SC [1987] 2 SCC 165.
35. "Vishakha & Ors. vs. State of Rajasthan & Ors.", AIR 1997 Supreme Court 3011, [(1997) 6 SCC 241].

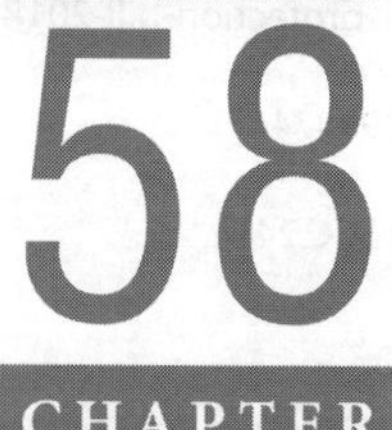

58 Advertising by Professionals

CHAPTER

Ashok Banga

INTRODUCTION

Any business or enterprise needs advertising to let the public know about its presence and the services offered. For one-upmanship, businesses advertise their products in a way to show that they are the best in the world. Similar trend may start or has already started among medical professionals as the competition hots up. In this era, simply saying no to advertisement by one prominent section of the society seems controversial if not unjustified. Once freely allowed to advertise, individual doctors and smaller groups will not be able to compete with the corporate hospitals. There can never be a level playing field. To limit this trend of advertising, the National Medical Commission (NMC) has laid down certain guiding principles and limiting points through regulations. Advertising by doctors in certain situations and in certain ways may be considered an unethical act. Before going into the technicalities of the subject, let us see some of the related case reports.

Warning Issued to Five Doctors

July 9, 2013: The Maharashtra Medical Council (MMC) warned doctors for advertising, which is illegal as per the code of ethics of the Medical Council of India (MCI). A council member told the *Times of India* that these doctors issued advertisements claiming to cure infertility, diabetes, obesity, and other conditions. One of them operated in Mumbai, whereas others traveled here to consult patients. The MMC issued the warning to the doctors and asked them to submit an unconditional apology for violating MCI's code of medical ethics and the Magical Remedies Act and have been warned that their licenses can be suspended if they advertise again.

Mumbai: Doctors Get Notice for Flouting Medical Council of India's Code on Self-advertisement

December 27, 2013; Agency: DNA

The MMC has issued notices to 21 doctors, including four from Mumbai, for violating the MCI code on self-advertisement. The chairman of MMC, said, "*Section 6.1 of the MCI's code of medical ethics says a doctor cannot advertise for himself or herself alone or with other doctors. We found these doctors violating this section.*" The four city doctors who got the notice from the MMC have given an unconditional apology to the MMC.

Sources said one of the doctors was pulled up for an article published in a newspaper on a procedure performed by him more than a decade back and another for writing a column 2 years back that included his photo. According to the MMC, doctors found flouting the rule can invite punishment ranging from a warning letter to cancellation of their registration.

Medical Council of India Derosters Doctors for Advertising

The Hindu-Chennai, April 26, 2013

The MCI has taken action against physicians for reportedly appearing in an advertisement by the hospital where they were working and decided to remove their names from the Medical Register for 15 days for transgressing the medical ethics. The MCI code makes it clear that no doctor should indulge in any advertisement promoting himself or his/her practice. The recent judgment is seen as an "interpretation" of these rules.

Dr KV Babu from Kerala, working on the issues of medical ethics, said, "*This ruling is very interesting.*" He explains "*While we all know that a doctor cannot advertise for himself or herself alone or together with other doctors, as per Section 6.1 of the MCI's Code of Medical Ethics, here, we are being told that it is the duty of individual doctors to inform the hospitals that they would not be a part of any advertisement put out by the hospital.*"

The MCI meeting notes: "After considering all these facts, the Committee is of the opinion that the following doctors whose photos and names appeared in the advertisement have violated provisions of the Indian Medical Council (Professional Conduct, Etiquette and Ethics) Regulations, 2002." It further states: "The Ethics Committee decided to remove the following Names/Registration of the doctors, whose names were mentioned in the advertisement of Saxena Hospital, Sonipat, from the Indian Medical Register/State Medical Register for a period of 15 days."

The MCI says that the code of ethics is clear that in any way the doctors should not participate in advertisements. The code published on the website of MCI mentions that doctors not following the rules would invite censure.

The Indian Medical Association (IMA) President (Dr Jayalal from Tamil Nadu) said that technically action can be taken against the hospital for promoting advertisements, but the MCI has no jurisdiction over hospitals. "Therefore, the MCI can take action only when a complaint is against individual doctors." Dr Ravishankar, former secretary IMA-TN said hospitals can continue to advertise their services, special features, and procedures, but they cannot involve any doctor employees for sure.

Delhi Medical Council Sees Violation in Advertisements and Issues Warning

The Hindu—*"Ad will affect doctor-patient relationship"*

Alarmed over blatant violation of code by several doctors in New Delhi, the *Delhi Medical Council* (DMC) has instructed its committee to have a fresh look at the code so as to reinforce the laws. The council issued warnings to Delhi doctors found to be indulging in deliberate violation of the code rules.

"Allowing doctors and institutions to advertise will result in a few rich and influential ones taking all the publicity. It will, we fear, also adversely affect the dynamics of the doctor-patient relationship, acquiring shades of being a businessman-customer type relationship. Also there is no way to regulate doctors/institutions making false claims. Patients in India have to be taught that when they go by an advertisement they have to be invariably on their guard. It is also important to remember that advertisement money too often comes from the patient's pocket. We welcome the latest move by the DMC and hope that we will be able to clear out the ambiguities in the implementation of the rule," said a member of DMC.

SURROGATE ADVERTISING

The Hindu

The DMC issued a stern warning to the hospitals in the capital for advertising by their doctors and "first-of-its-kind" procedures done.

To ensure patient safety and to put a halt to the aggressive advertisements by some hospitals, DMA will soon put in place a review team to look into the matter and issue warning to the hospitals indulging in marketing of services.

The NMC strictly prohibits doctors and their services being advertised. Similarly, the surrogate advertising is also not allowed. Despite this, establishments in the city are continuing the advertisement on the sly and this is violation of the code.

"The DMC will review all surrogate advertising and if any violation is happening then take appropriate action. The doctors doing 'extraordinary' and 'first-of-its-kind' work should inform and report their respective associations, get peer group review, and then publish in the public domain."

Hospitals claim that there is nothing "wrong" in advertising and providing information to the people. "What else will a medical establishment advertise besides its services and doctors? With so many private hospitals and nursing homes opening in the city it is important that we advertise to make known our presence, tell the people about the services we offer and the fact that patients will be in good hands."

A senior cardiothoracic surgeon from Indraprastha Apollo Hospital said: "*The code of ethics must be followed and doctors should provide information to the general public. When claiming to be doing some procedure for the first time, check the available literature and review with peer group to ensure that correct information is given.*"

NATIONAL MEDICAL COMMISSION ACT

What is unethical in advertising?

- Soliciting patients directly/indirectly by a physician/group of physicians or by hospitals is unethical. Several methods are adopted by doctors or institutions to get referrals. When established hospitals adopt such tactics, it becomes difficult for a newcomer to get a foot hold, therefore they innovate a more aggressive strategy. In such a competition, ultimately, hardly anyone gains but everyone loses. Moreover, this is unethical and illegal.
- A physician shall not make use of his/her name in any form or manner of publicity through any mode, either alone or with others so as to invite attention to his/her professional position, qualification, skill, achievements, associations, appointments, honors, and/or affiliations resulting in his self-aggrandizement.

  In simple words, it means that no doctor should advertise himself by means of his achievements or position; however, this is the clause mostly flouted. News hungry media, especially local newspapers, help such real or surrogate advertising. Any real or projected achievement or attainment of advertiser is printed in the form of news knowing fully well that most of the public accepts it on its face value.

- A physician shall not give to any person, whether for compensation or otherwise:
  - Any approval
  - Any recommendation
  - Any endorsement
  - Any certificate, report, or statement with respect of any drug or medicine
  - Apparatus or appliance or any product or use thereof or any test, or trial thereof, for use in connection with his name, signature, or photograph nor shall he boast of cases, operations, cures, or remedies, or permit the publication of report thereof through any mode.

  All this simply means that no doctor should give his/her endorsement to any pharmaceutical, pathology, or appliance manufacturer or any procedure.
- Printing of self-photograph, or any such material of publicity in the letter head, or on sign board of the consulting room or any such clinical establishment shall be regarded as acts of self-advertisement and unethical conduct on the part of the physician. However, printing of sketches, diagrams, and pictures of human system shall not be treated as unethical.

What is ethical in advertising?

A practitioner is permitted to make various announcements in press regarding:

- Starting of practice
- Changes in type of practice
- Changing the address
- Temporary absence from practice
- Resumption of practice
- Succeeding to another practice
- Declaration of charges to people

Many doctors take advantage of this clause. Whenever going out of station, especially abroad, even for personal visits, advertisement is to show that the doctor will become wiser there by visiting such and such hospital or attending some international conference.

Another loophole used for advertising is the advertisement for appointing staff. Advertisement starts with the beautiful introduction of hospital and services available and ends with two lines about the vacancy in the hospital. No one can challenge this advertisement.

What is happening?

Knowingly or unknowingly, the NMC guidelines are being flouted. Highly educated doctors are expected to know that not knowing the law does not excuse one from punishment. Big signboards of individual practitioners and hospitals can be seen anywhere. Newspaper advertisements are a commonality. Publicizing one's achievements and tall claims through media in the guise of news is a common strategy. Media also encourages such activities by printing special supplements as it gives them revenue.

Is it punishable?

Yes. NMC can punish the erring doctor if a complaint is received. Quantum of punishment is decided by the MCI-NMC after enquiring the matter. It can even amount to cancellation of license to practice.

Why do not we see action being taken?

Action may be initiated if someone complains. As hardly anyone complains, we do not see the punishment being delivered.

Has someone been punished by Medical Council of India/National Medical Commission? There are instances from Maharashtra, Delhi, Haryana, and Madhya Pradesh where MCI/NMC conducted the inquiry, warned the concerned doctors, and taken their apology; however, there is no record of severe punishment to anyone.

ONE MORE CASE STUDY

Local newspapers regularly publish health supplements everywhere. This is their method of getting money from doctors in return of favors done otherwise. In one such supplement, various reputed and senior practitioners of Gwalior gave their advertisements. Two advocates appealed to Gwalior High Court to punish the erring doctors as the MCI does not permit such advertising. They appealed against MCI also for not taking notice of this act.

In response, the MCI issued notice to all these doctors and asked them to appear before MCI at Bhopal. Doctors pleaded ignorance of the law and pressure by the media but finally accepted the mistake done. The MCI strictly warned them and condoned them all after seeking an undertaking from them individually to not to ever indulge in such advertising in future. The court was satisfied with the action taken.

Positive side of this case is that no doctor in Gwalior is now compelled by media to give advertisement, so everyone is saving money.

ADVERTISEMENT THROUGH WEBSITE AND WEBCASTING AND PODCASTING

Many doctors and hospitals maintain their website. Obvious reason is advertising. Webcasting and podcasting have limited reach in our country; therefore, its overall impact may not be much. As this is a new phenomenon, new rules will have to be made. Till then same broad principals about advertising will apply.

No advertising rule; won't work in the digital age:
July 12, 2013
This move of MMC raises a lot of questions whether there is infringement of the rights of the doctors/patients in this digital era. Should not doctors, working long and hard to get where they are, be allowed to market their skills? Or is this completely against the Hippocratic Oath that doctors treat their profession like any other commercial venture?

THE CURRENT SCENARIO: WHAT CONSTITUTES ADVERTISING?

Advertising for self-promotion has not been allowed. But, media and technology are changing the consumer's behavior and health is the second largest searched subject on the net. People take second opinions; look for doctors online, etc. In such a scenario, listing on medical association sites should not be considered an offense. Articles and quotes should also be if they are scientific and do not promote a brand. None of these activities should involve any brand promotion or self-promotion, it should be purely educational.

■ Online Advertising

While making online searches, there are bound to be lists of doctors—most of which is user-generated content and reviews. Just the way people check buying a product, in the same way they check out for doctors and check what other people say. So, it is not totally incorrect to opt for a listing or provide quotes as an influencer. One cannot escape the information age. These days there are two ways of choosing doctors—referrals and online searches. And with increasing superspecialties, it is critical for people to identify and take informed decisions.

Does the NMC need to rethink the no-advertising rule?

Considering the changing dynamics, the NMC should redraft the code to bring more clarity. A lot of doctors have fan following of his patients on social channels where he can educate and keep his patients updated. This relationship building should not be considered unethical when most of the updates are promoting preventive medicine! Many such issues need to be reconsidered.

CONCLUSION

Flip side of all the regulations is that these rules apply on qualified doctors only. Quacks can still advertise on the walls all over city, publish in newspapers and magazines, and even on FM radio stations. They can claim guarantied cure for many incurable diseases. Irony is their license cannot be cancelled as they do no possess any.

In the end, I would like to post a quote:

"Medical Council of India needs to focus on educating ethical practices and provide space to every fellow colleague to be a part of a change and even if many are not willing, effort must not be on reprimanding such doctors because it is never going to serve the purpose. Today anyone who aspires to take up this profession or struggling to establish himself has to go through many personal challenges there is no system in India to provide secure and fulfilling profession for a doctor. He is as novice as anyone who goes through a startup in any venture. I am lucky to be close associates with all types of doctors from GPs to super specialist. Don't just misuse some acquired power under MCI. These are from your community and they are damn good then the older generation and must go through the grind of 22 years of selling career. I have witnessed the whole cycle of an individual entering into college and come out as a qualified Dr and goes to prove himself as successful Dr."

— Dineish S Pardesi

KEY LEARNING POINTS

- Doctor cannot and should not advertise individually by any means and in any form.
- Hospital has certain legal ways to advertise.
- It is difficult to control real and surrogate advertising on online platforms.
- NMC needs to rethink and reframe the "no advertisement rules."

BIBLIOGRAPHY

1. Code Of Medical Ethics Regulations, 2002, Amended Up to 8th October 2016. [Online] Available from https://www.nmc.org.in/rules-regulations/code-of-medical-ethics-regulations-2002/ [Last accessed May, 2024].

59

CHAPTER

Alphabet for Action

Alka Kuthe, Divyangee V Mundhe

INTRODUCTION

Medical profession nowadays is at stake. Cases, both civil and criminal as well as in consumer forum, are often filed complaining of medical negligence against doctors/hospitals/nursing homes. The winds are blowing in favor of the consumers. There has been a continuous increase in the number of legal suits by patients against doctors. To minimize the medicolegal problems, defensive medical practice alone would not prove an adequate solution. It may affect professional confidence and would tax the patients heavily. As per a famous quotation, *"you may not be able to change the winds, but you can definitely adjust the sails"*. Certain safety measures can be adopted to minimize medicolegal problems in addition to improving healthcare delivery system.

A–Z FOR QUICK ACTION

Here is an A, B, C, D,.... Z for taking quick action.

- *A:*
    - Awareness of medicolegal problems; knowing the potential areas of litigation in the medical field is a must. Doctors should have recent updates regarding changes in legislation related to their practice and the happenings in the medicolegal field
    - Accept the changes and challenges in the practice.
    - Alertness of the doctor is of utmost importance.
    - Avoid vague and nonspecific terminologies or short forms.
    - Adjust the doses of the drugs according to weight, especially in patients with renal/hepatic disorders.
    - Avoid prescribing multiple drugs, i.e., shotgun therapy.
    - Attend regularly and personally, whether a patient or a case is going to the Consumer Protection Act (CPA) or not.
- *B*:
    - Be soft and gentle and at the same time be aware of the so-called "social workers" and "ambulance chaser" advocates.
    - Body language of doctors matters.
    - Bodyguards (security) to doctors and nursing homes are preferable.
    - Be careful with the word "P", i.e., Press/police/politician/public prosecutor (lawyer)/paramedical/premedical/pharmacist/pharma company.

- *C*:
    - Cool, calm, and composed attitude is to be inculcated.
    - Communicate and counsel well so as to remove patient's fear and misconception regarding disease. It also helps to build up confidence and faith in doctors.
    - Confirm clinical diagnosis by relevant investigations.
    - Colleague help is to be sought for second and third opinions without hesitation.
    - Consent of the patient may be taken while providing information to the police. Follow the legal procedures or provisions.
    - Commenting loosely on colleagues should never be done.
    - Crisis management committee formation is the need of the hour.
- *D*:
    - Documentation on case paper should be meticulous and elaborate. Updating and maintaining of case sheet should be routine.
    - Do not allow modern diagnostic tests to substitute your clinical acumen.
    - Do not accept substitutes.
    - Degree of the medical practitioner should be recognized by respective councils.
    - Do not disrespect or ignore the courts.
    - Distractions (cell phone, cricket commentary, computer, cinema, and serials) should be kept aloof at the time of examination of the patient.
    - Declaration of death is an art.
- *E*:
    - Expert witness, well conversant with the current trends in that specialty, meticulous and vigilant in patient's care, if called by an alleged doctor then he/she is less likely to be proved careless and negligent.
    - Explain treatment modalities whenever required, especially in complicated cases.
    - Explain the condition of patient and take signature of patient and accompanying person, if possible, at the time of admission and from time to time.
    - Emergencies should be handled carefully. Consult specialists if you feel that there is a possibility of multisystemic involvement.
- *F*:
    - Fees, approximate expenses, and bills should be explained properly, especially in indoor and operative cases.
    - Furnish copies of medical records to police, court, or genuine relatives whenever demanded by procedure.
    - False or bogus certificates should never be issued.
    - Follow the standard protocol of treatment.
    - Failure to diagnose known complications can be taken as negligence.
- *G*:
    - Good personal rapport and compassionate and sensitive communication with the patients and their relatives go a long way in gaining their confidence and maintaining doctor–patient relationship.
    - Give references relevant to case and demand cross-examination in case of litigation.
    - Give guarded prognosis.
- *H*:
    - Honesty toward the profession is always rewarding.
    - History of any drug allergy needs to be recorded, without forgetting.

- *I*:
  - Informed valid consent before performing any operative procedure is important, especially in dealing with minors, before sterilization operation, mentally retarded patients, cases related to marital disturbances, and in complicated cases.
  - Inform police whenever necessary and extend all possible cooperation to them.
  - Involve medical associations, medicolegal cells, voluntary organizations, etc., whenever a legal problem arises.
- *J*:
  - Judgmental error or an error in diagnosis while managing an emergency case may not amount to negligence.
- *K*:
  - Keeping the records meticulously, especially in medicolegal, controversial, or complicated cases can prove the doctor innocent in case any litigation arises in future, but fabrication after any mishap may prove dangerous. Records should be patient-friendly and not just mechanical.
- *L*:
  - Listening patiently, carefully, and attentively to the patient to understand in depth and to gain confidence is an art. One must acquire it.
- *M*:
  - Medical indemnity insurance is one of the possible ways for protection and relief to doctors in case of litigation and claims about malpractice.
  - Multispecialty approach is the right way to combat difficult situations.
  - Mention "diagnosis under review" if the diagnosis is not confirmed.
- N:
  - Negligence is professional misconduct and should always be avoided.
  - Never neglect the treatment while completing the legal formalities, especially in emergency or serious situation.
  - Never behave in a rude, rough, or inhuman manner.
- O:
  - Over-investigations and overprescriptions should be avoided. Clinical diagnosis can be confirmed with relevant investigations (if necessary).
- *P*:
  - Professional auditing would be beneficial to everyone involved in patient's care. Improvement in standards of health services can be done by discussing the work analysis and constructive criticism of errors in acts and omissions.
  - Produce affidavits of colleagues whenever necessary.
  - Prompt recognition and management of the known complication associated with the invasive procedure protects the practitioner from medical negligence.
  - Postmortem examination should be insisted if the cause of death cannot be ascertained.
- *Q*:
  - Quality treatment prevents many problems
  - Qualification and skills decide the ambit of your work.
- *R*:
  - Right investigations at the right time can save a life and lot of litigations in future. Complicated invasive techniques like amniocentesis, chorionic villous biopsy, cardiocentesis, etc., either for diagnostic or for therapeutic purposes need informed written consent.

- *S*:
  - Standard medical service essentially requires adequate and proper infrastructure. There is no substitute for good quality care.
  - Stay calm; avoid surprises, anger, panic, and self-doubt.
- *T*:
  - Timely referral as and when necessary and as per relative's wish to the higher unit is life-saving for the patient and it can avoid legal complications for a doctor as well.
  - Telephonic consultation should be discouraged.
- *U*:
  - Update your core knowledge and clinical acumen by continuous reading, attending continuing medical education (CME), conferences, and clinical meetings regularly, and thereby be a continuing medical educated doctor and not a company's medical representative educated doctor.
  - Update not only your knowledge and skill but also that of the staff. Update facilities and instruments.
- *V*:
  - Vigilance, careful attitude with extra precautionary measures during surgery with proper preoperative and postoperative care and management is important to prevent litigation.
- *W*:
  - Well-organized graded system is recommended while supervising the patients, particularly in a hospital setup. It may prevent a lot of mishappenings.
- *X*:
  - X-ray your thoughts, ideas, and treatment modalities while managing the patient and select the best out of it.
- *Y*:
  - Yearning toward the Almighty and doing a sincere, honest work will definitely help in long run.
- *Z*:
  - Zeal and zest in the practice will help to reach the zenith.

CONCLUSION

Use of alphabets for quick action at the right time can prevent most of the accidents in medical field. Unfortunately, mishaps do happen at times in spite of all the possible care. If doctor–patient relationship is good, the mishap is unlikely to end in litigation. The law is a watchdog and not a bloodhound, and as long as doctors do their duty with reasonable and compassionate care, they will not be held liable even if their treatment is unsuccessful. A kind, courteous, empathetic, and humanity-based attitude and approach toward the patient with medicolegal expert availability in case of need is the ideal strategy to minimize medical litigations and lead a fearless medical practice with minimum stress. Ultimately what remains in the hands of all of us is to pray:

"O God,
Give me the serenity
To change the things that I can,
To accept the things, that I cannot, and
Wisdom to know the difference!"

KEY LEARNING POINTS

- Communicate and counsel properly.
- Documentation should be meticulous.
- Give a guarded prognosis, especially in a critically ill patient.
- Professional indemnity will give protection and relief in case of litigation.
- Crisis management committee is the need of the hour.

BIBLIOGRAPHY

1. Ganguly GM, Chakravorty S. Ways to minimize medical litigation in obstetrics and gynecology in medicolegal aspects. In: Mukharjee GG, Soonawala R, Tank DK (Eds). Obstetrics and Gynecology, 1st edition. New Delhi: Jaypee Brothers Medical Publishers (P) Ltd; 1997. pp. 204-8.
2. Tiwari S. Do's and don'ts for doctors. In: Balwa M, Tiwari S, Tiwari M, Shah N (Eds). Legal Problems in Day-to-Day Pediatric Practice, 2nd edition. Hyderabad: Paras Medical Books Pvt. Ltd; 2010. pp. 199-201.

60

CHAPTER

Consent Forms

(These Forms are to be Printed/Filled in Local/Vernacular Language)

For Indoor Admissions

I/we have been explained and informed (in detail), regarding the disease process, probable outcome and period of hospitalization of the patient. I/we have been explained regarding the provisional diagnosis of the patient --- and the chances/ likelihood of common and major risks, side effects and complications that may occur during the hospital stay or in future.

It is quite possible that during treatment some new findings or complications may arise which may be totally out of control of treating physician. I have been explained that there can be a risk to the life of an otherwise healthy person also. Hence, we have been explained that the doctor will take proper care and doesnot guarantee for cure.

I/we have been informed that there are different modalities of treatment for the illness of the patient and the proper mode will be followed as per the need of the patient from time to time. If there is need for any special investigations, procedures or operations we will be informed accordingly.

For the proper management of the patient there may be need of other specialists, residents, assistants, nursing staff, etc. I give consent for the help of any qualified staff/person in such situation.

We have also been informed regarding the average expenses ---------------------- that may be incurred during the treatment of the patient. All the facilities/modalities of treatment are not available in this hospital. I/we also understand that these expenses may increase if there is need for sophisticated special investigations, treatment or referral. I/we are willing to pay deposit/ advances from time to time.

We understand that it will be our responsibility to bring different medicines, disposables, etc., whenever required and asked for.

I/we have been explained all these in the language known to me/us and I/we are signing this consent form without any pressure/coercion and after satisfying my queries/doubts.

Name of the patient: Age/sex:

Name of the relatives: Witnesses:

Relationship:

Signature: (1)

(2)

Date and time:

For Surgical/Invasive Diagnostic procedures
(These forms are to be printed/filled in local/vernacular language)

Type of Surgery/procedure: --

I/we have been explained and understand about the nature of patient's condition and disease process and the nature of procedure/operation to be performed and the benefits/risks associated with the same. We have also been explained about the failure rate of this procedure/operation.

I/we understand and acknowledge the major risks, complications and side effects (immediate and long-term) associated with the surgery, procedures and the anesthetic drugs used for these procedures.

I/we have been informed that there is always possibility of some unexpected complications or finding after starting the procedure. I hereby consent for the additional surgery/procedure as per the need (if arises). I have been explained that there can be a risk to the life of an otherwise healthy person also.

I/we further state that we have been informed regarding anesthetists (including their procedure/complications), assistants, qualified residents and nursing staff.

We have also been informed that the date and time of surgery or procedure may vary due to circumstances beyond control.

I/we have been explained all these in the language known to me/us and I/we are signing this consent form without any pressure/coercion and after satisfying my queries/doubts.

Name of the patient: Age/sex:

Name of the relatives: Witnesses:

Relationship:

Signature: (1)

(2)

Date and time:

Discharge Against Medical Advise
(These forms are to be printed/filled in local/vernacular language)

My patient was admitted in this hospital since -----------------------
He/she has been suffering from ----------------------------.

The condition of the patient is serious and the treating doctors have informed me not to take discharge. They have also informed me regarding the possible consequences after discharge or during the transfer of the patient. But it is difficult for me to keep the patient in hospital and to continue the treatment. Hence I am taking discharge against medical advice and transferring the patient on our own risk and responsibility. The doctors shall not be responsible for any unexpected complications/consequences.

I/we have been explained all these in the language known to me/us and I/we are signing this form without any pressure/coercion and after satisfying my queries/doubts.

Name of the patient: Age/sex:

Name of the relatives: Witnesses:

Relationship:

Signature: (1)

(2)

Date and time:

Consent for Vaccination
(These forms are to be printed/filled in local/vernacular language)

I/we have been informed about various vaccines available for the immunization of my/our child. We have also been explained about advantages, side effects or complications occurring after the vaccination. I/we have been explained that there can be a risk to the life of an otherwise healthy child also during or after vaccination.

Many new vaccines are now available recently. It has also been explained to us that some of these vaccines are costly and optional. We are willing to immunize our child as per our economic condition, affordability, need, and our knowledge of various vaccines.

I/we have been informed that most of the vaccines may not give 100% protection and there may be possibility of disease even after vaccination.

I/we have been explained all these in the language known to me/us and I/we are signing this form without any pressure/coercion and after satisfying my queries/doubts.

Name of the patient: Age/sex:

Name of the relatives: Witnesses:

Relationship:

Signature: (1)

(2)

Date and time:

CERTIFICATE

This is to certify that Shri/Ms/Master ---
is/was suffering from ---
He/she is/was under my treatment for the same between ---
---.

He/she is/was advised rest during this period.

In continuation of previous Certificate dated ---------------------- he/she is further advised rest for --.

He/she is now fit to resume his/her duties.

Identification marks:
(a)
(b)

Signature of patient:

Date: Signature of doctor:

Seal of hospital/doctor:

POLICE INFORMATION REPORT

To,
The In-Charge
---------------------Police Station.
(Name of Town/City)

Date:
Time:

Name of the patient:
Address:
Date of admission:
Registration no:
Diagnosis:

That this patient had problem, developed complications and deteriorated/has been referred to higher center/discharged/left against medical advice/has been declared dead/was brought dead. The relatives are not willing for postmortem and/are expected to create nuisance.
This is for your information and necessary action.

Name/signature of the receiver:

Buckle no:

Name and signature of informant:

Seal of the hospital/doctor:

REFERRAL LETTER

Name of the patient:
Address:
Date of admission:
Provisional diagnosis:
Final diagnosis (if possible):
Investigations:

Treatment given:

Is being referred to the higher/other center:
Name of the center/hospital:
Reasons for referral:

Please do the needful and if possible inform regarding the plans of future management/prognosis of the patient.

Date: Signature of doctor:

Seal of the hospital/doctor:

(*Note*: All these details can be attached in the form of discharge card)

Index

Page numbers followed by *b* refer to box, *f* refer to figure, and *t* refer to table.

A

B

C

E

I

J

K

L

N

S

T

U

V